Every Decker book is accompanied by a CD-ROM.

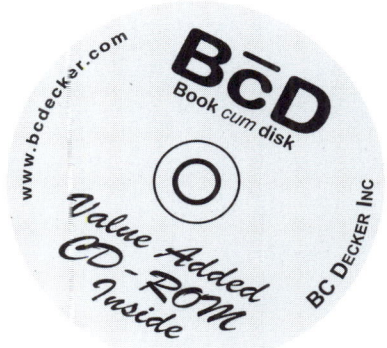

The disk appears in the front of each copy, in its own sealed jacket. Affixed to the front of the book will be a distinctive BcD sticker **"Book *cum* disk"**.

The disk contains the complete text and illustrations of the book, in fully searchable PDF files. The book and disk will be sold *only* as a package; neither will be available independently, and no prices will be available for the items individually.

BC Decker Inc is committed to providing high quality electronic publications that will compliment traditional information and learning methods.

We trust you will find the Book/CD Package invaluable and invite your comments and suggestions.

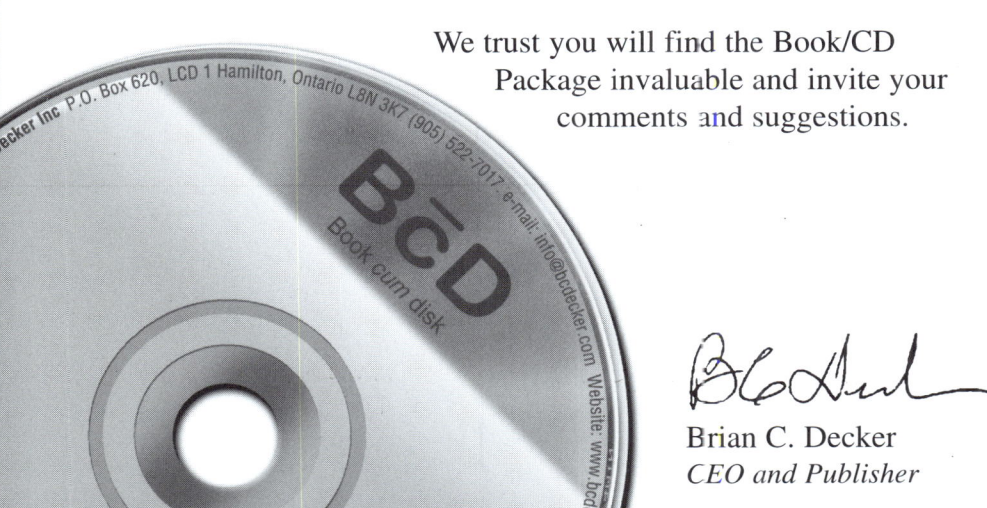

Brian C. Decker
CEO and Publisher

ESTHETICS IN DENTISTRY

SECOND EDITION

VOLUME 2

**ESTHETIC PROBLEMS OF
   INDIVIDUAL TEETH
   MISSING TEETH
   MALOCCLUSION
   SPECIAL POPULATIONS**

Ronald E. Goldstein, DDS
Clinical Professor of Oral Rehabilitation
Medical College of Georgia School of Dentistry
Augusta, Georgia

Adjunct Clinical Professor of Prosthodontics
Boston University Henry M. Goldman School of Dental Medicine
Boston, Massachusetts

Adjunct Professor of Restorative Dentistry
The University of Texas Health Science Center
San Antonio, Texas

Visiting Professor of Oral and Maxillofacial Imaging and Continuing Education
University of Southern California School of Dentistry
Los Angeles, California

Van B. Haywood, DMD, Associate Editor
Professor, Fixed Prosthodontics Section
Department of Oral Rehabilitation
Medical College of Georgia School of Dentistry
Augusta, Georgia

2002
BC Decker Inc
Hamilton • London

BC Decker Inc
20 Hughson Street South
P.O. Box 620, L.C.D. 1
Hamilton, Ontario L8N 3K7
Tel: 905-522-7017; 800-568-7281
Fax: 905-522-7839
e-mail: info@bcdecker.com
website: http://www.bcdecker.com

© 2002 Ronald E. Goldstein

All rights reserved. Without limiting the rights under copyright reserved above, no part of this publication may be reproduced, stored in or introduced into a retrieval system, or transmitted, in any form or by any means (electronic, mechanical, photocopying, recording, or otherwise), without the prior written permission of the publisher.

01 02 03 04 05 / UTP / 9 8 7 6 5 4 3 2 1

ISBN 1-55009-048-8

Printed in Canada

SALES AND DISTRIBUTION

United States
BC Decker Inc
P.O. Box 785
Lewiston, NY 14092-0785
Tel: 905-522-7017; 800-568-7281
Fax: 905-522-7839
E-mail: info@bcdecker.com
Web site: www.bcdecker.com

Canada
BC Decker Inc
20 Hughson Street South
P.O. Box 620, L.C.D. 1
Hamilton, Ontario L8N 3K7
Tel: 905-522-7017; 800-568-7281
Fax: 905-522-7839
E-mail: info@bcdecker.com
Web site: www.bcdecker.com

Foreign Rights
John Scott & Company
International Publishers' Agency
P.O. Box 878
Kimberton, PA 19442
Tel: 610-827-1640
Fax: 610-827-1671
E-mail: jsco@voicenet.com

U.K., Europe, Scandinavia, Middle East
Harcourt Publishers Limited
Customer Service Department
Foots Cray High Street
Sidcup, Kent
DA14 5HP, UK
Tel: 44 (0) 208 308 5760
Fax: 44 (0) 181 308 5702
E-mail: cservice@harcourt_brace.com

Singapore, Malaysia, Thailand, Philippines, Indonesia, Vietnam, Pacific Rim, Korea
Harcourt Asia Pte Limited
583 Orchard Road
#09/01, Forum
Singapore 238884
Tel: 65-737-3593
Fax: 65-753-2145

Australia, New Zealand
Harcourt Australia Pty Limited
Customer Service Department
STM Division, Locked Bag 16
St. Peters, New South Wales, 2044
Australia
Tel: 61 02 9517-8999
Fax: 61 02 9517-2249
E-mail: stmp@harcourt.com.au
Web site: www.harcourt.com.au

Japan
Igaku-Shoin Ltd.
Foreign Publications Department
3-24-17 Hongo
Bunkyo-ku, Tokyo, Japan 113-8719
Tel: 81 3 3817 5680
Fax: 81 3 3815 6776
E-mail: fd@igaku-shoin.co.jp

Notice: The authors and publisher have made every effort to ensure that the patient care recommended herein, including choice of drugs and drug dosages, is in accord with the accepted standard and practice at the time of publication. However, since research and regulation constantly change clinical standards, the reader is urged to check the product information sheet included in the package of each drug, which includes recommended doses, warnings, and contraindications. This is particularly important with new or infrequently used drugs. Any treatment regimen, particularly one involving medication, involves inherent risk that must be weighed on a case-by-case basis against the benefits anticipated. The reader is cautioned that the purpose of this book is to inform and enlighten; the information contained herein is not intended as, and should not be employed as, a substitute for individual diagnosis and treatment.

Contributors

Donald E. Arens, DDS, MSD
Professor, Department of Endodontics
Director, Department of Continuing Education
Indiana University School of Dentistry
Indianapolis, Indiana
Professor of Endodontics
Nova Southern University College of Dental Medicine
Fort Lauderdale, Florida

Gerald Barrack, DDS
Clinical Professor, Restorative Dentistry
Department of Prosthodontics
New York University Dental School
New York, New York

Alberto Caprioglio, DDS, MS
Assistant Professor, Department of Orthodontics
University of Insubria School of Dentistry
Varese, Italy

Claudia Caprioglio, DDS, MS
Visiting Professor, Department of Orthodontics
University of Parma School of Dentistry
Parma, Italy

Damaso Caprioglio, MD, MS
Professor and Chair, Department of Orthodontics
University of Parma School of Dentistry
Parma, Italy

W. Frank Caughman, DMD, MEd
Professor and Chair, Department of Oral Rehabilitation
Medical College of Georgia School of Dentistry
Augusta, Georgia

Daniel C. N. Chan, DMD, MS, DDS
Associate Professor and Section Director of Operative Dentistry
Department of Oral Rehabilitation
Medical College of Georgia School of Dentistry
Augusta, Georgia

Noah Chivian, DDS
Adjunct Associate Professor, Department of Endodontics
University of Pennsylvania School of Dental Medicine
Philadelphia, Pennsylvania
Director Emeritus and Attending in Endodontics
Department of Dentistry
Newark Beth Israel Medical Center
Newark, New Jersey

Roman M. Cibirka, DDS, MS
Associate Professor, Removable Prosthodontics Section
Department of Oral Rehabilitation
Medical College of Georgia School of Dentistry
Augusta, Georgia

James W. Curtis Jr., DMD
Director, Department of Dentistry
Palmetto Richland Memorial Hospital
Columbia, South Carolina

Mark D. Dlugokinski, DDS
Assistant Professor, Operative Dentistry Section
Department of Oral Rehabilitation
Medical College of Georgia School of Dentistry
Augusta, Georgia

Beverley A. Farley, DMD
Private Practice
Irmo, South Carolina

Kevin B. Frazier, DMD
Associate Professor, Operative Dentistry Section
Department of Oral Rehabilitation
Medical College of Georgia School of Dentistry
Augusta, Georgia

F. Michael Gardner, DDS, MA
Associate Professor and Program Director of Postgraduate
    Prosthodontics Program
Department of Oral Rehabilitation
Medical College of Georgia School of Dentistry
Augusta, Georgia

Ronald E. Goldstein, DDS
Private Practice
Atlanta, Georgia
Clinical Professor of Oral Rehabilitation
Medical College of Georgia School of Dentistry
Augusta, Georgia
Adjunct Clinical Professor of Prosthodontics
Boston University Henry M. Goldman School
    of Dental Medicine
Boston, Massachusetts
Adjunct Professor of Restorative Dentistry
The University of Texas Health Science Center
San Antonio, Texas
Visiting Professor of Oral and Maxillofacial Imaging and
    Continuing Education
University of Southern California School of Dentistry
Los Angeles, California

Steven T. Hackman, DDS
Assistant Professor, Operative Dentistry Section
Department of Oral Rehabilitation
Medical College of Georgia School of Dentistry
Augusta, Georgia

Van B. Haywood, DMD
Professor, Fixed Prosthodontics Section
Department of Oral Rehabilitation
Medical College of Georgia School of Dentistry
Augusta, Georgia

John N. Kent, DDS
Boyd Professor and Head, Department of Oral
    and Maxillofacial Surgery
Louisiana State University Health Science Center
New Orleans, Louisiana

Carol A. Lefebvre, DDS, MS
Professor, Removable Prosthodontics Section
Department of Oral Rehabilitation
Medical College of Georgia School of Dentistry
Augusta, Georgia

Michael L. Myers, DMD
Professor and Vice-Chair
Fixed Prosthodontics, Department of Oral Rehabilitation
Medical College of Georgia School of Dentistry
Augusta, Georgia

Steven K. Nelson, DMD
Associate Professor and Assistant Director, Postgraduate
    Prosthodontics Program
Department of Oral Rehabilitation
Medical College of Georgia School of Dentistry
Augusta, Georgia

Linda C. Niessen, DMD, MPH, MPP
Vice-President, Clinical Education
DENTSPLY International
York, PA
Clinical Professor, Department of Public Health Sciences
Baylor College of Dentistry
The Texas A&M Health Science Center
Dallas, Texas

Geoffrey W. Sheen, DDS, MS
Private Practice
Augusta, Georgia
Assistant Clinical Professor, Fixed Prosthodontics Section
Department of Oral Rehabilitation
Medical College of Georgia School of Dentistry
Augusta, Georgia

Asgeir Sigurdsson, cand. odont., MS
Associate Professor and Graduate Program Director
Department of Endodontics
University of North Carolina
School of Dentistry
Chapel Hill, North Carolina

John D. Stover, DDS, MD, PhD
Private Practice
Hilo, Hawaii

Walter F. Turbyfill Jr., DMD
Private Practice
West Columbia, South Carolina

Paul Yurfest, DDS
Private Practice
Atlanta, Georgia

Contributors at Large

Pinhas Adar, MDT, CDT
Oral Design Center, Inc.
Atlanta, Georgia

David A. Garber, DMD
Clinical Professor, Department of Periodontics
Clinical Professor, Department of Oral Rehabilitation
School of Dentistry
Medical College of Georgia
Augusta, Georgia

Cary E. Goldstein, DMD
Clinical Instructor, Department of Oral Rehabilitation
School of Dentistry
Medical College of Georgia
Augusta, Georgia

Cathy Goldstein Schwartz, DDS
Private Practice
Atlanta, Georgia

Angela Gribble Hedlund, DMD
Private Practice
Atlanta, Georgia

Henry Salama, DMD
Assistant Clinical Professor, Department of Periodontics
University of Pennsylvania
Philadelphia, Pennsylvania

Maurice A. Salama, DMD
Assistant Clinical Professor, Department of Periodontics
School of Dentistry
Medical College of Georgia
Augusta, Georgia

Contents

VOLUME 2

Preface vii

Acknowledgments ix

PART 3 Esthetic Problems of Individual Teeth

16. Stains and Discolorations 473
    Van B. Haywood, DMD, W. Frank Caughman, DMD, MEd, Ronald E. Goldstein, DDS

17. Abfraction, Abrasion, Attrition, and Erosion 501
    James W. Curtis Jr., DMD, Beverley A. Farley, DMD, Ronald E. Goldstein, DDS

18. Chipped, Fractured, or Endodontically Treated Teeth 525
    *Daniel C.N. Chan, DMD, MS, DDS, Michael L. Myers, DMD,
    Gerald M. Barrack, DDS, Ronald E. Goldstein, DDS*

19. Endodontics and Esthetic Dentistry 553
    Noah Chivian, DDS, Donald E. Arens, DDS, MSD, Asgeir Sigurdsson, cand. odont., MS

20. Oral Habits 599
    Ronald E. Goldstein, DDS, James W. Curtis Jr., DMD, Beverley A. Farley, DMD

PART 4 Esthetic Problems of Missing Teeth

21. Fixed Replacement of Missing Teeth 635
    Steven K. Nelson, DMD, F. Michael Gardner, DDS, MA, Ronald E. Goldstein, DDS

22. Esthetic Removable Partial Dentures 669
    Roman M. Cibirka, DDS, MS, Carol Lefebvre, DDS, MS, Ronald E. Goldstein, DDS

PART 5 Esthetic Problems of Malocclusion

23. Restorative Treatment of Diastema 703
    Mark D. Dlugokinski, DDS, Kevin B. Frazier, DMD, Ronald E. Goldstein, DDS

24. Restorative Treatment of Crowded Teeth 733
    Geoffrey W. Sheen, DDS, MS, Ronald E. Goldstein, DDS, Steven T. Hackman, DDS

25. Esthetics in Adult Orthodontics 753
    Paul Yurfest, DDS

26. Surgical Orthodontic Correction of Dentofacial Deformity 775
    John N. Kent, DDS, John D. Stover, DDS, MD, PhD

PART 6 Esthetic Problems of Special Populations

27. Esthetics in Pediatric Dentistry 805
    Claudia Caprioglio, DDS, MS, Alberto Caprioglio, DDS, MS, Damaso Caprioglio, MD, MS

28. Esthetics: the Complete Denture 831
    Walter F. Turbyfill Jr., DMD

29. Geresthetics: Esthetic Dentistry for Older Adults 853
    Linda C. Niessen, DMD, MPH, MPP, Ronald E. Goldstein, DDS

Appendix E: Manufacturer Index 875

Appendix F: Product Index 877

Index 878

VOLUME 1

PART 1 Principles of Esthetics
1. Concepts of Dental Esthetics
2. Esthetic Treatment Planning
3. Marketing
4. Legal Considerations
5. Photography
6. Biology of Esthetics
7. Pincus Principles
8. Creating Esthetic Restorations through Special Effects
9. Divine Proportion
10. Understanding Color

PART 2 Esthetic Treatments
11. Cosmetic Contouring
12. Bleaching Discolored Teeth
13. Composite Resin Bonding
14. Etched Porcelain Restorations: Veneers and Inlays/Onlays
15. Crown Restoration

VOLUME 3

PART 7 Problems of Facial Appearance
30. Facial Considerations in Esthetic Restorations
31. Esthetic Plastic Surgery in Relation to Esthetic Dentistry
32. Cosmetic Adjuncts to Dental Esthetics
33. Esthetic Considerations in the Performing Arts

PART 8 Esthetic Problems of Supporting Structures
34. Periodontic Considerations in Esthetic Dentistry
35. Esthetic Considerations in Implant Dentistry

PART 9 Problems of the Esthetic Emergency
36. Esthetic Emergencies
37. Esthetic Repairs

PART 10 The Esthetic Failure
38. How to Prevent and Correct Esthetic Failures

PART 11 Chairside Procedures for Esthetic Dentistry
39. Tooth Preparation in Esthetic Dentistry
40. Impressions for Esthetic Dentistry
41. Esthetic Temporization
42. The Esthetic Try-In
43. Cementation of Restorations

PART 12 Maximizing Restorative Materials for Esthetic Dentistry
44. Restorative Materials in Esthetic Dentistry
45. Esthetic Principles in Constructing Ceramic Restorations
46. Maintenance of Esthetic Restorations

Preface

In Volume 1 of *Esthetics in Dentistry*, I dealt with two basic areas of esthetic dentistry: principles and treatments. This second volume covers four specific areas of dental esthetics: the problems of individual teeth, missing teeth, malocclusion, and the special populations of children and the elderly.

Although esthetic dentistry continues to grow as a major part of overall dentistry, our initial emphasis must always concentrate on basic oral health principles. Only when these fundamentals are considered can and should we move on to the more complicated and complex interdisciplinary problems that we see in an increasing number of patients.

Although planning a patient's treatment should consist of seeing the entire face rather than an individual tooth, the concept of how that individual tooth is managed must be integrated into the overall goals of both patient and practitioner. Thus, we begin with treatments for individual teeth, such as stains and discolorations, erosion, abfraction, attrition, abrasion and erosion, chipped, fractured and endodontically treated teeth, and especially oral habits. Then we graduate into the more complex problems of missing teeth. Whereas the patient may enter our practice desiring a new crown or several restorations, our approach must consider the question, "Does the patient want an improved smile?" Or is he or she content with the tooth color, shape, and arrangement of the current smile? Every patient should routinely be given the option of improving the overall smile before deciding on the treatment for a single tooth or teeth.

The individual tooth defect often presents a most difficult esthetic problem. Solutions to the problems of discolorations and stains, caries, fractures, erosion, and other rather common—and not so common—related maladies are discussed in detail. An orderly transition is made from simple treatment of individual teeth through to the more complex treatment. The degree of success by which the dentist treats individual tooth problems is a measure of what he or she can achieve in more complex cases.

Treatment planning and restoring teeth with endodontic problems are two of the most perplexing problems every dentist periodically faces. Thus, this volume includes two chapters that deal with endodontic considerations when planning esthetic restorations. We have assembled some of the world's outstanding authorities on this subject to write these chapters.

In an effort to help our patients protect their naturally beautiful smiles, as well as to assist them in achieving longer life with their esthetic restorations, there is an important new chapter on personal habits and how we can control them. We can and must spend more time communicating with our patients about how important their oral care is, as well as minimizing or helping them to eliminate any destructive habits.

The problem of missing teeth is one that plagues countless humans, and yet the esthetic replacement of a missing tooth or teeth is really one of the toughest assignments we all face. However, the ability to restore the natural dentition successfully is possible not only through the use of new materials and techniques but most of all because of the desire to spend the time necessary to accomplish an esthetic result.

Fixed and removable replacement bridges have been divided into two chapters. The preferred method of replacement, the fixed partial denture, is presented in the first chapter. Methods or replacement from the simple cantilevered bridge to highly complex procedures of telescoping and cross-linkage are all discussed from an esthetic viewpoint. The second chapter deals with removable techniques of restoring the missing tooth. Again, emphasis is on an esthetic approach from the simple, yet popular, clasp designs and how to make them more attractive to the more sophisticated means of precision attachment replacement. The discussion of tooth replacement through implantology will be found in Volume 3.

Until the publishing of the first edition of *Esthetics in Dentistry* in 1976, almost all dental texts and articles dealing with the subject of dental esthetics were approached from the standpoint of full denture esthetics. Practically all of the early work in research was in this area. The approach used in this volume is concise yet effective. Ultimately, if all else fails and there is no hope to save the teeth or no desire for implant prosthesis, esthetic dentistry's answer is the full denture. Although it is realized that numerous young people have or are in need of full dentures, it is primarily a geriatric problem. So we have included an outstanding chapter on full-denture prosthesis.

There is no greater human suffering than that of the facially deformed individual who cannot hide his or her defect. There is no greater feeling of accomplishment than to successfully treat and aid one who has this disorder. This deformity can range from a malocclusion such as diastema or crowded teeth to a severe Class III or other facial deformity. The five chapters in this section deal with this problem. The major problems of diastema and crowded teeth have separate chapters covered from a restorative standpoint. An alternative method of treatment of crowded teeth and other occlusal deformities is covered in a separate chapter on cosmetic contouring. There are two chapters contributed by colleagues: one covers the entire field of esthetics in orthodontics. The last chapter of this section encompasses surgical treatment of malocclusion. New techniques now offer positive solutions to heretofore virtually hopeless esthetic problems.

Thus, the dentist has at his or her disposal many ways to approach the deformities of malocclusion. Correction of these problems usually involves three choices: repositioning, restoration, or removal. Somewhere in the "three R's" lies an esthetic compromise or solution to almost any problem. The right decision is not simple; it is hoped that after study of this section it will be easier to make.

Esthetics begins with the child, so a new chapter written by three leading practitioners from Italy provides an interesting look at how to achieve the best smiles in one's youth.

The esthetic problems of children are basically the same as those of adults and deserve the same attention. In fact, many times the child may suffer more than the adult from the same esthetic problem. Because the formative years of children are extremely important, children should be treated as proactively as possible where dental esthetics is concerned. Based on this premise, most of Chapter 22 is handled in atlas form, showing types of esthetic problems and treatment for children. Cross-references are provided to avoid duplication of specific techniques shown elsewhere in the text since the method of treatment is almost identical.

It can also be anticipated, as the public has become more informed about prevention, that more people will be helping their teeth for much longer periods of time. In fact, the final chapter in this volume deals with the ever-increasing market for geriatric dentistry or "geresthetics," as I termed it many years ago. With baby boomers being more able and willing to invest in their oral care than other age groups, as well as being the first generation to have benefited from community water fluoridation and preventive dentistry programs, this group represents promising prospects for esthetic dentistry as its constituents reach age 65 with virtually intact natural dentition. At age 65, American adults can expect to live another 17 years, with these adults making more of this part of their lives than any previous generation.

Practicing dentistry is not easy. Practicing esthetic dentistry steps up to the more complex technologies and psychological understanding of the needs, wants, desires, and expectations of our patients, as well as some of the frustrations and limitations of what we can provide. With the publication of this volume, we are two-thirds of the way home.

Ronald E. Goldstein

> This book is lovingly dedicated to the future of our family:
> Katie, Jennie, Brett, Max, Landon, Gracie, Matthew, and William.

Acknowledgments

I spend 3 days per week (36 hours) working on patients, and the other 4 days I devote mostly to my lectures, articles, and, finally, to producing this text. That is why I am so appreciative of all of the people who have helped me produce this second of a 3-volume set.

First and foremost, I am indebted to the patient persistence and hard work of Susan Hodgson, who has dedicated so much time and effort to making sure that the text is easy to understand and that all of the details have been taken care of. Even when I was content, Susan wasn't, and I am appreciative of her devotion to making this a better volume.

A special thanks to Van Haywood, who was a valuable organizer early on, particularly during the task to get on board some of the very best contributing authors, especially those at the Medical College of Georgia, who helped bring this volume up to date. I want to thank all of the contributors whom Van and I were able to motivate to join us for this second volume. In every case, the individual was overly committed to his or her teaching tasks, as well as other projects, so it took all of us longer; however, perseverance paid off, and almost everyone came through! The demands on dental school faculty are so heavy today that it is difficult for them to take time away from their day-to-day activities, lectures, and student supervision for outside writing projects, so I am appreciative of the special efforts of our contributors from the Medical College of Georgia: Frank Caughman, Roman Cibirka, Kevin Frazier, Geoff Sheen, Dan Chan, Michael Gardner, Steve Hackman, Carol Lefebvre, Steve Nelson, Michael Myers, Mark Dlugokinski, James Curtis, and Beverly Farley.

Always a source of advice and assistance whenever needed, Stephen Moss helped me secure the contribution of three wonderful Italian practitioners, Claudia Caprioglio, Alberto Caprioglio, and their father, Damaso Caprioglio, who produced an excellent chapter on pediatric dentistry, in record time!

A big thanks to Linda Niessen, who just doesn't know how to say no and says "yes" with such enthusiasm that it always amazes me. She not only agreed to co-author the chapter on gerestherics with me, she also packed up her laptop and took a flight to Atlanta to sit with me for a day working out the details. I always appreciate her beyond-the-call-of-duty effort.

My appreciation also goes to Gerald Barrack, who lent us his expertise in restoring endodontically treated teeth. There are no busier endodontists than Noah Chivian, Don Arens, and Asgeir Sigurdsson and no more qualified individuals to produce the excellent chapter on endodontic contributions to esthetic dentistry. Jack Turbyfill had finished his chapter some time ago on the complete denture, but in his effort to be the best, he rewrote it, and the result was well worth his effort.

Jack Kent wrote an excellent chapter in the first edition of *Esthetics in Dentistry*. I am glad to have he and John Stover update their chapter since they helped to establish the standards in their specialty. I am also indebted to Paul Yurfest, who took considerable time out from his schedule to update the chapter that he cowrote with my late uncle, Marvin Goldstein, and their partner, Mike Burns.

Personally, I can't thank enough my valuable executive assistant, Candace Paetzhold, who is always willing to help with whatever the demands of the day call for. Our other assistants, Elaine Canning and Ruth McCormick, pitch in when needed to help us, as do my excellent dental assistants Angie Pitts and Claudia Madrigal, who offer me such great help at all times. I am thankful for my long-time dental assistant, Charlene Bennett, who keeps us technologically up to date and is especially valuable in our educational projects. I am also appreciative of my personal assistant, Mona Frastaci, who always reminds me of the details that I seem to forget from time to time.

Brian Decker and Susan Cooper at BC Decker have been tolerant of our time limitations but were committed to making sure that this volume is the best it could be. As in the first volume, Andy Rideout continues to create outstanding illustrations.

I want to reiterate my thanks to my partners—David Garber, Maurice and Henry Salama, Angela Gribble Hedlund, and Brian Beaudreau—for their clinical material and advice.

As in the last volume, I again thank my family for their continued support in all of my endeavors. I especially want to thank my precious wife Judy for proofing chapters and offering valuable constructive criticism at every level. My three dentist children, Cary (his wife Jody and children Max, Landon, and Gracie), Cathy (her husband Steve and children Katie, Jennie, and Brett), and Ken, who continue to be a source of pride for me, as does my physician son, Rick (his wife Amy and children Matthew and William), who helps to keep me alive!

PART 3

ESTHETIC PROBLEMS OF INDIVIDUAL TEETH

Chapter 16

Stains and Discolorations

Van B. Haywood, DMD, W. Frank Caughman, DMD, MEd, Ronald E. Goldstein, DDS

Each year, millions of individuals change toothpaste, purchase ineffective preparations, and even change their dentists in their quest for "whiter teeth." Many an attractive smile is marred by some discoloration or stain, either on an individual tooth or on all teeth (Figures 16–1A and B). There are many causes and corresponding treatments for these stains and discolorations. The dentist needs to be able to both diagnose and treat the various discolorations. Some treatments must be performed in the dental office, some can be performed at home by the patient, and some are a combination of office and home treatments.

Some of the clinical appearances of discolorations have been described in Volume 1, Second Edition. Generally, stains can be divided into extrinsic (located on the outside of the tooth) and intrinsic (located within the tooth). Moreover, extrinsic stains can become intrinsic over time. Hence, stains can originate from the outside in or from the inside out. The clinical appearance can be in a variety of colors. Table 16–1 provides a summary of tooth discolorations and associated conditions.

Some examples of these different discolorations can be seen in Figures 16–2 to 16–13. Additionally, the discoloration can either be of a generalized nature or specific to one tooth or one location on a tooth (Table 16–2).

A number of treatment options should be considered, in order of increasing aggressiveness (Table 16–3).

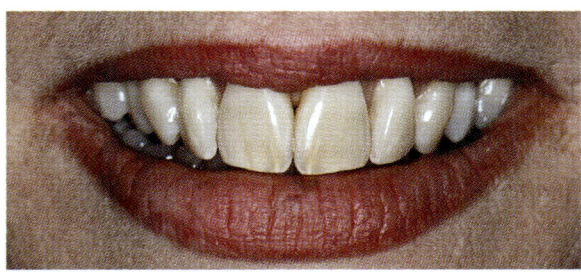

Figure 16–1A: An otherwise attractive smile is marred by discolored teeth.

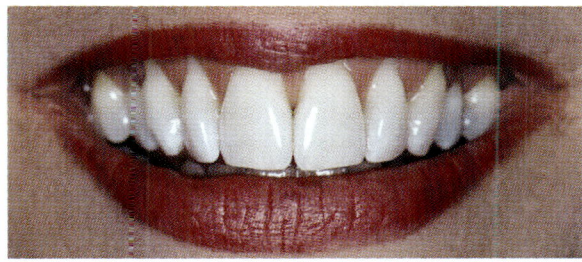

Figure 16–1B: After tooth lightening, the smile is much more pleasing.

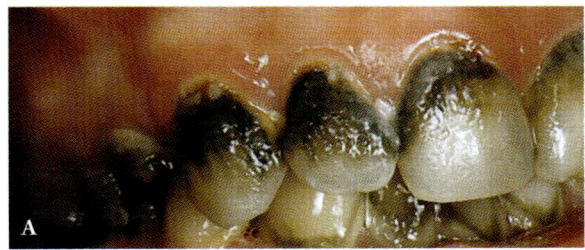

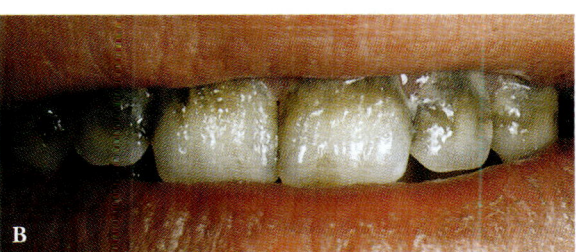

Figure 16–2A and B: Total neglect resulted in severe staining of this patient's teeth.

474 Esthetics in Dentistry

TABLE 16–1. Common Discolorations and Associated Causes

TOOTH DISCOLORATION	ASSOCIATED CONDITION
Yellow	Aging Calcific metamorphosis Loss of vitality Tetracycline ingestion Amoxicillin syrup[81] Stannous fluoride Imipenem for cystic fibrosis[98] Amelogenesis imperfecta[43]
Opaque	Fluorosis Sickle cell anemia[87] Osteogenesis imperfecta[72]
White	Fluorosis Chronic kidney failure[10] Hypomineralization
Brown	Fluorosis[26] Smoking[84] Coffee[29] Soy sauce[16] Cola Tea[30] Calcific metamorphosis Loss of vitality Chlorhexidine ingestion[1,34,70] Iron[74] Tetracycline ingestion Antitartar toothpaste[28] Osteogenesis imperfecta[72] Chlorhexidine glucamate (Hibitane) disinfectant[11] Tannic acid[85] Ochronosis[43] Dental materials[106]
Black	Occupational: glass blowers[99] Betel nut chewers[91] Pipe/cigar smokers[92] Dental materials (pins) Caries
Blue	Tetracycline ingestion Osteogenesis imperfecta[72]
Green	Hyperbilirubinemia[95] Congenital biliary atresia[83,110] Occupational: brass factory[27] Marijuana smoking Nasmyth's membrane
Orange	Poor oral hygiene Chromic acid fumes
Red	Internal resorption Congenital erythropoietic porphyria[31] Periapical granuloma in lepromatous leprosy[93]
Gray	Death[9,68] Tetracycline ingestion for cystic fibrosis[7,67,90] Minocycline for acne in adults[6,12,24,88,89,94,97,109] Dentinogenesis imperfecta[21] Amalgam restorations Cyclosporine[38]

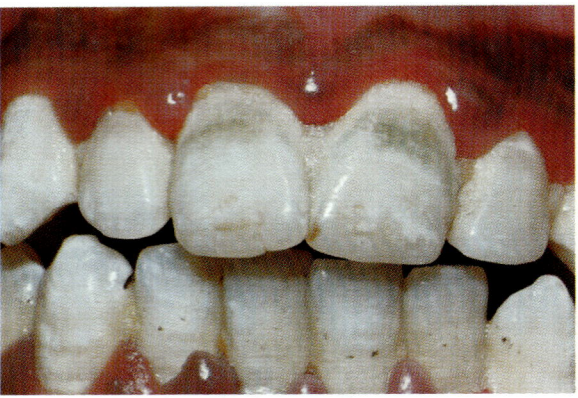

Figure 16–3: Green stain associated with poor oral hygiene and gingival inflammation.

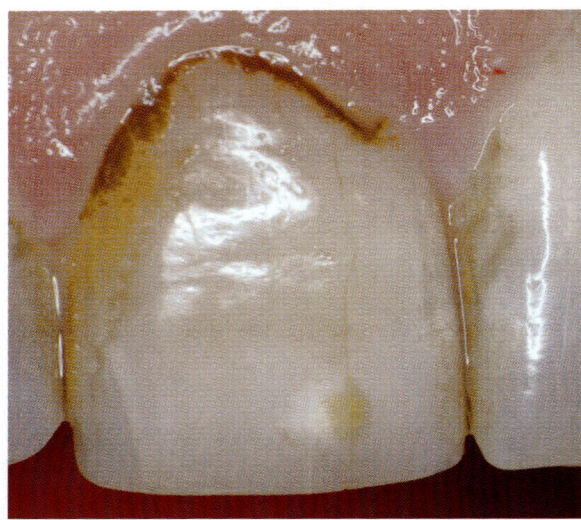

Figure 16–4: Orange stain appears as a thick brick-red, orange, or yellow line on the cervical third of the involved teeth, usually the incisors, and is associated with poor oral hygiene.

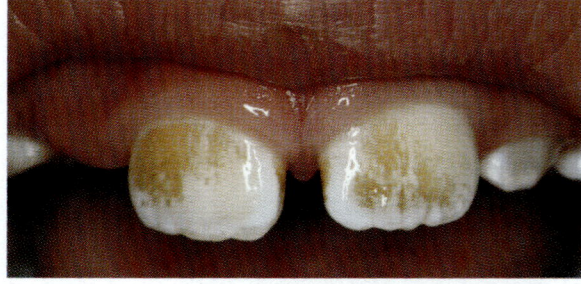

Figure 16–5: Orange-brown stain may cover more of the facial area from poor oral hygiene and ingestion of chromagenic foodstuffs.

Stains and Discolorations 475

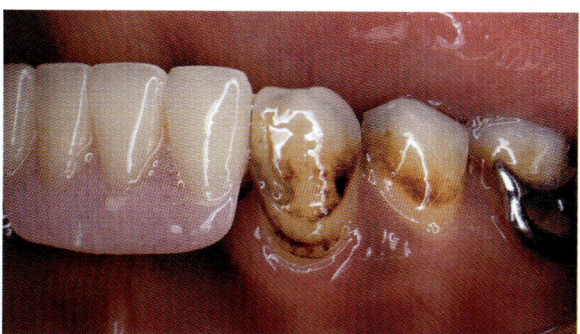

Figure 16–6: Black tobacco stain from dipping snuff for 15 years.

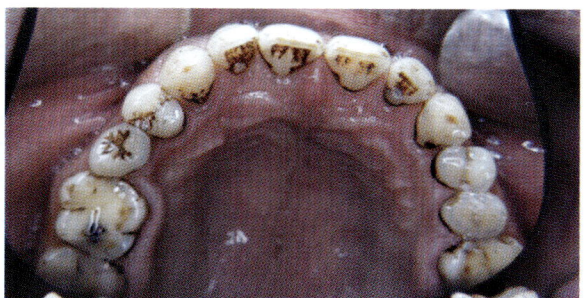

Figure 16–7: Black stain from chewing betel nuts.

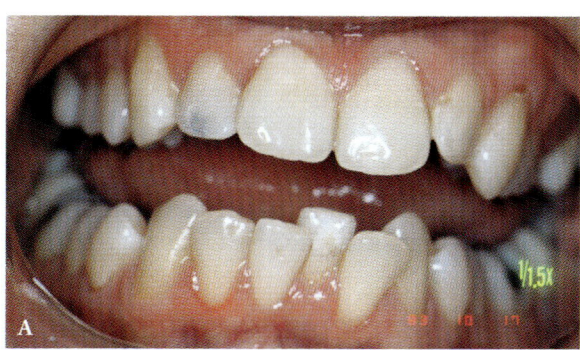

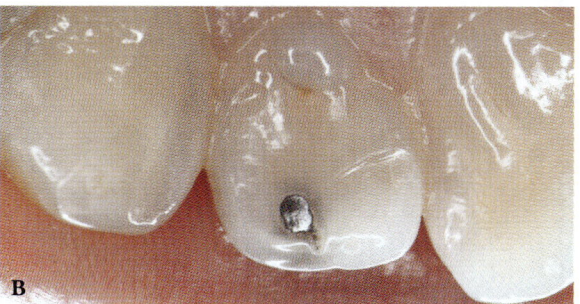

Figure 16–8A and B: Gray stain on lateral incisor (A) is a result of an amalgam restoration on the lingual surface of the tooth (B).

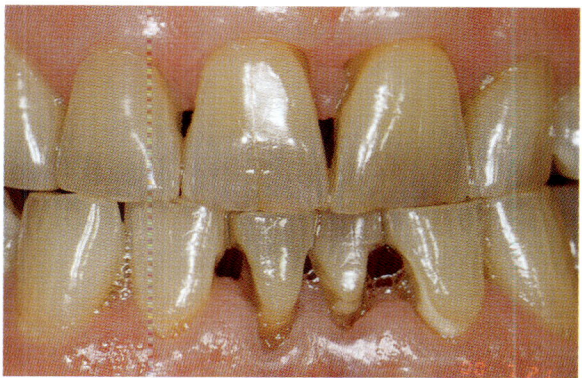

Figure 16–9: Brown stain and overall discoloration of teeth from 20 years of pipe smoking.

EXTRINSIC STAINS

Prior to final diagnosis of the stain or discoloration, a complete prophylaxis should be performed to remove minor surface staining. Occasionally, an air polisher will be used on the posterior occlusal surfaces to help diagnose whether the grooves are stained or carious. The diagnosis of occlusal decay is better done by visual means rather than by tactile sensation with an explorer. Proponents of the visual method explain that some grooves will not "stick" but will have decay, whereas others will stick mechanically due to their surface topography but will contain no decay.

Diagnosis for decay is difficult in deep groves. If there is a possibility, first use an air-abrasive or some other method to remove the organic pellicle and any caries present and then either fill or seal

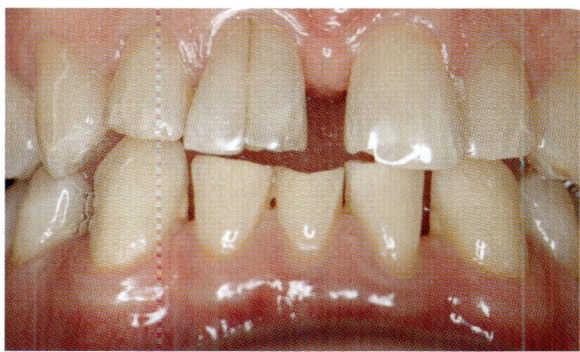

Figure 16–10: Staining can occur in tooth defects such as the vertical crack line on the central incisor.

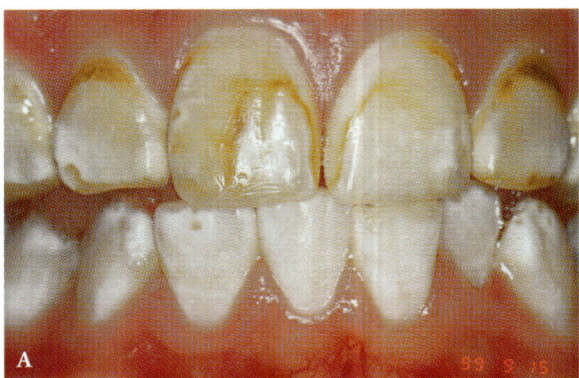 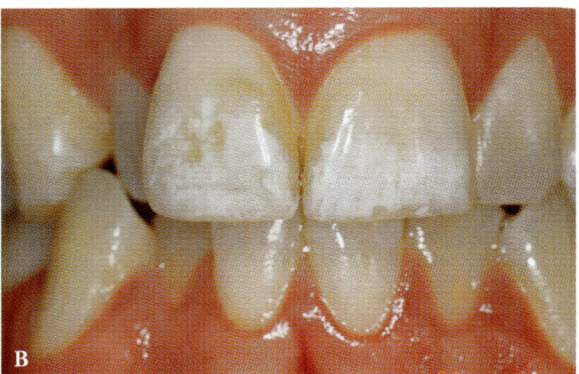

Figure 16–11A and B: Enamel fluorosis can be seen as either mostly brown *(A)* or mostly white *(B)* discolorations.

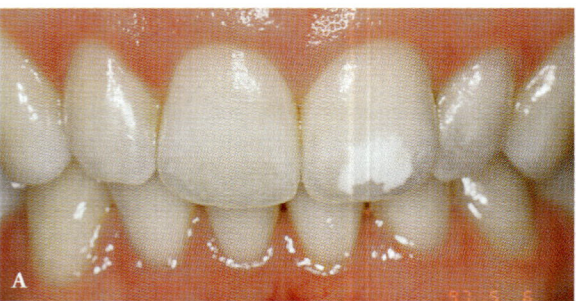 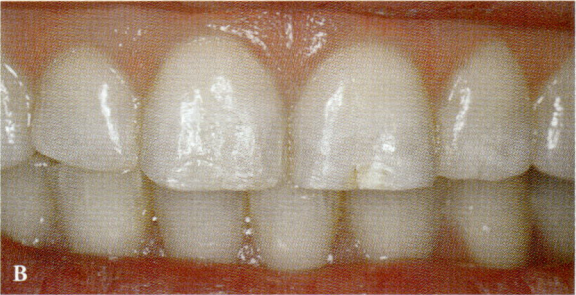

Figure 16–12A and B: Trauma to primary teeth can result in a large white-spot discoloration *(A)* or a less noticeable white and brown defect *(B)*.

the tooth rather than merely watch the area.[80] Patients who complain about discolored grooves will be better served with a highly filled tinted or opaque sealant rather than a clear sealant through which the groove can be seen. Additionally, clear sealants that were chemically cured may exhibit an amber or yellow discoloration over time and require replacement (Figure 16–14). Prior to the placement of a sealant, the grooves should be cleaned of organic matter.[107] The cleaning of grooves can be mechanically accomplished by use of a ¼ round bur in a high-speed handpiece or air abrasion. Placing 3% hydrogen peroxide in the grooves is a chemical option to débride the grooves.[17] If peroxide is used, the cessation of bubbling will indicate that the grooves are clean. A caries detection agent (Seek Caries Indicator, Ultradent Products, South Jordan, UT) can also be used to help determine if caries are present. A sealant can then be placed to prevent further staining. Some sealants have acetone water chasers to improve the bond to the enamel (UltraSeal, Ultradent Products).

Another extrinsic stain is one caused by the use of a mouthrinse containing chlorhexidine. This product is often prescribed to promote gingival

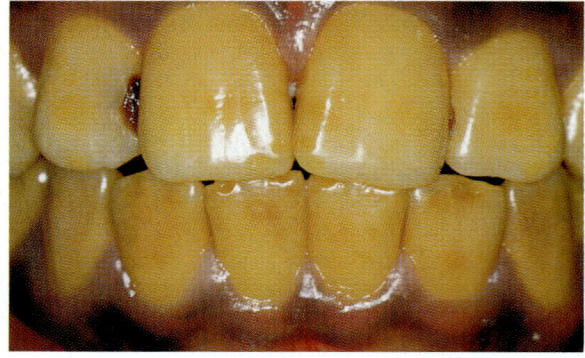

Figure 16–13: Yellow teeth caused by ingestion of iron over a long period of time.

TABLE 16–2. Clinical Appearance and Causes of Discoloration

CLINICAL PRESENTATION	CONSIDERATIONS
Single dark tooth (radiograph needed for diagnosis of pathology)	Vital: bloodborne pigments from trauma, calcific metamorphosis, internal resorption Nonvital: blood stains during endodontic therapy, remaining pulp material in chamber, restoration type (amalgam) or leaking, internal resorption
Generalized discoloration of all of the teeth	From smoking (extrinsic or intrinsic), chromagenic foods, drugs (tetracycline), diseases, or aging, or genetically inherited
Localized discoloration to one tooth	White spots: surface or subsurface fluorosis, white surface demineralization Brown spots: fluorosis, formation defects
Localized discoloration to one area on all of the teeth	Chromagenic foods, chlorhexidine, smoking (extrinsic), often associated with plaque and poor oral hygiene
Discoloration associated with a restoration	Amalgam: show-through because of thin enamel, stained dentin Composite: staining of margins, staining beyond margins, complete discoloration of restoration
Discoloration associated with caries	Aproximal and occlusal stained additionally by food or saliva
Tooth defects: pitted, poorly formed	Facial, lingual, or incisal defects from fever or trauma during development, genetics (peg laterals or deep grooves)
Translucency: dark incisal	Finger test on lingual to determine translucency; may appear darker with bleaching due to loss of further color

TABLE 16–3. Treatment Options for Stained Teeth

TREATMENT OPTIONS	INTRINSIC	EXTRINSIC
Prophlylaxis		X
Air polisher		X
Bleaching external with 10% or more CP	X	X
Bleaching external with 35% HP	X	
Bleaching internal with 10% CP	X	
Bleaching internal with 35% HP	X	
Sealant or preventive resin	X	
Macroabrasion: handpiece, burs, disks		X
Microabrasion: rubber dam and acid		X
Resurface and seal restoration		X
Replace restoration	X	X
Replace portion of restoration (composite to mask over amalgam)	X	X
Veneer (partial or complete, composite or ceramic)	X	
Crown (PFM, porcelain butt, all ceramic)	X	

CP = carbamide peroxide; HP = hydrogen peroxide; PFM = porcelain fused to metal.

health. The dark stain resulting from the product's use is a major disadvantage to an otherwise very beneficial product. Some patients are able to overcome this disadvantage by employing 10% carbamide peroxide in a bleaching tray periodically (Figures 16–15A and B). This approach is possible only if the patient is a reasonable candidate for bleaching or if his or her teeth are already as light as they can become. Otherwise, more frequent prophylaxis is required for esthetics.

TOOTHPASTES

Once the dental office has removed the extrinsic stains, the patient can use a toothpaste to maintain the whiteness of his or her teeth.

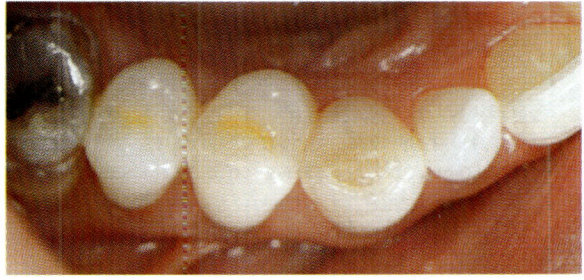

Figure 16–14: Clear sealants that were chemically cured tend to yellow over time, becoming unesthetic.

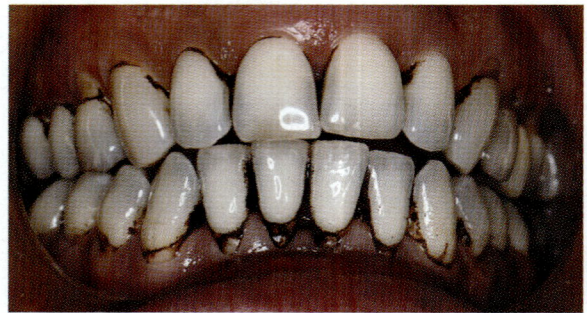

Figure 16–15A: Patient on regular use of chlorhexidine rinse for gingival treatment shows marked staining of teeth.

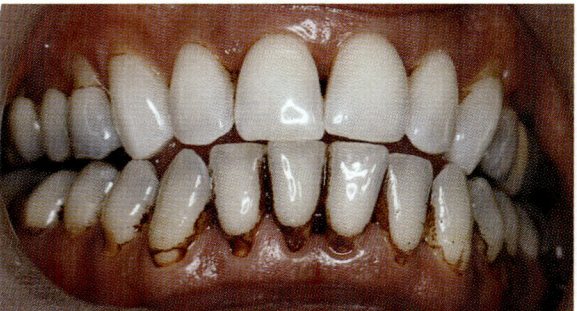

Figure 16–15B: Stains were removed, and the patient continued with chlorhexidine use while simultaneously bleaching the maxillary arch. After 3 months of treatment, there is markedly less staining on the maxillary teeth.

There are a number of toothpastes on the market advertised for whitening, and patients are always seeking something that they can use at home to obtain whiter teeth. The U.S. Food and Drug Administration allows any toothpaste that removes stains to make claims as a whitening toothpaste. However, the mechanism of action of the different toothpastes is generally divided into three categories[36,48]:

- *Abrasive toothpastes.* The original whitening toothpastes, commonly referred to as the "smoker's toothpaste," remove extrinsic stains by mechanical abrasion, which can make the tooth appear whiter. However, overuse of these toothpastes will eventually reduce enamel, causing the teeth to appear more yellow due to the show-through of the dentin. These toothpastes are not recommended, especially in persons who are aggressive with their toothbrushing technique or use a hard toothbrush.

- *Chemical toothpastes.* Some toothpastes attempt to remove stains by changing the surface chemistry of the tooth so that plaque and tarter will not adhere. These types of "tarter control" toothpaste act much like teflon on a frying pan, and if there is no plaque or tarter on the tooth, there is less substrate to be stained. One of the problems with this approach is that, in some patients, these types of toothpastes cause marked sensitivity. Another class of chemical toothpastes that have become popular since the advent of bleaching are those that contain peroxide. Many of these products also contain baking soda. Baking soda is a mild abrasive, but the peroxide acts by chemical means. The problem with the use of a peroxide dentifrice for whiter teeth is that the contact time on the tooth is too short to produce any noticeable whitening. However, a peroxide-containing toothpaste may be useful in color maintenance after the dentist has whitened the teeth.

- *Cosmetic toothpastes.* Most of the whitening toothpastes should be classified as a cosmetic, in that they apply something to the surface of the tooth. Most whitening toothpastes contain titanium dioxide, which is essentially a "sticky white paint." This "paint" then adheres to the cracks and crevices on the tooth and to the embrasures, giving the illusion of whiter teeth. However, cosmetic toothpastes are only temporary and do not change the inherit tooth color.

The color of make-up, lipstick, or clothes can also impact the perceived color of a patient's teeth. Just as certain colors of clothing make the complexion look either whiter or more tanned, so do certain redder colors of lipstick make the teeth appear whiter. In the same manner, a whiter complexion (or white make-up, as used by a circus clown) makes the teeth appear more yellow. Some patients may wish to consult with a color or make-up specialist to improve other aspects of their appearance than their teeth.[65] Improvements in areas of the face and head will, in turn, have an impact on the color of the teeth. Generally the color of the teeth should closely match the color of the sclera (white part) of the eye for a natural appearance.[8,49,53]

INTRINSIC STAINS

Much of the etiology of internal stains has been discussed in the first volume of this textbook. Typically, bleaching with 10% carbamide peroxide in a custom-fitted tray easily treats discolorations due to aging, smoking, or chromogenic foods, and beverages (Figures 16–16A and B and 16–17A and B). Although these types of stains generally require only 2 to 6 weeks of bleaching treatment, some are more stubborn. Nicotine staining of long-term duration may require as long as 3 months of nightly treatment (Figures 16–18A and B).[48] Tetracycline staining may take anywhere from 2 to 12 months

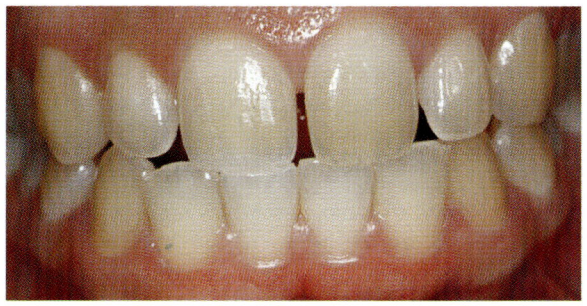

Figure 16–16A: Some teeth darken over time from chromagenic foods. Some patients' teeth are just naturally yellow.

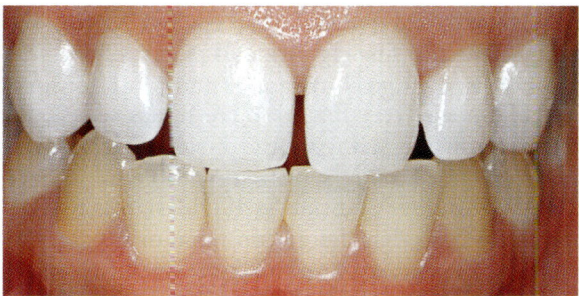

Figure 16–16B: Whitening of the maxillary teeth using 10% carbamide peroxide in a custom tray results in a more pleasing smile. This patient is now interested in closing the spaces.

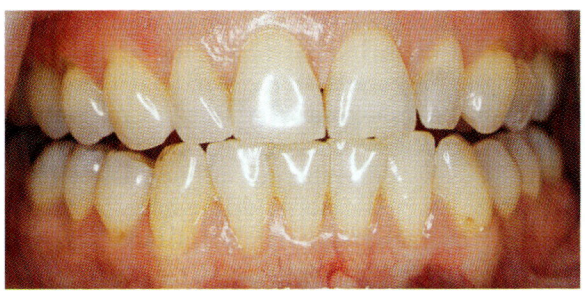

Figure 16–17A: Some teeth darken through natural aging.

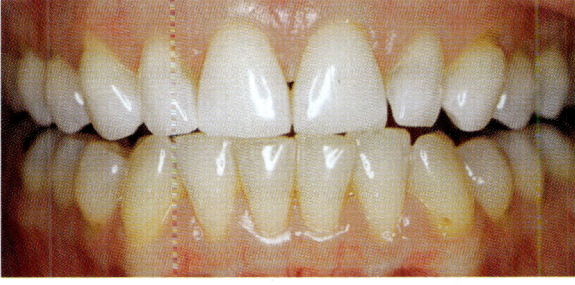

Figure 16–17B: Whitening of the maxillary teeth using 10% carbamide peroxide in a custom tray produces a normal progression of color from gingival to incisal edge but offers a more pleasing, younger look to the patient.

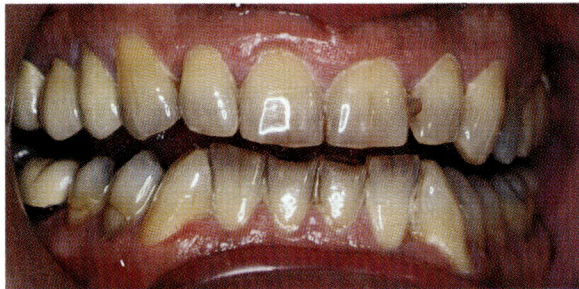

Figure 16–18A: Years of pipe smoking have caused the extrinsic nicotine stain to become intrinsic.

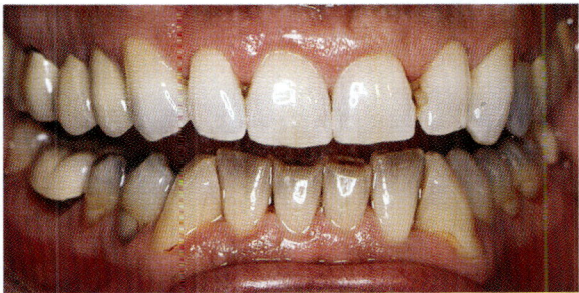

Figure 16–18B: Whitening, using at-home treatment of 10% carbamide peroxide in a custom-fitted tray, was necessary to remove the stubborn nicotine stains.

of nightly treatment.[49] Patients must be counseled regarding realistic expectations for the outcomes of bleaching. Long-term treatment is best presented as one that is worthwhile but may not produce the desired results.[8]

TRAY DESIGN OPTIONS FOR AT-HOME BLEACHING

The original tray design for bleaching was a thin, somewhat rigid material that extended onto the gingival tissue. The rigidity and extent of the tray often caused gingival irritations and tooth sensitivity. The newer tray materials are much softer and have eliminated many of the mechanical gingival irritation and tooth sensitivity problems (Figure 16–19). Another addition to tray design is to scallop the tray so that there is minimal or no gingival contact. This design minimizes the chemical gingival irritation experienced by some patients. However, the scalloped design requires the use of a viscous, sticky, somewhat insoluble material that adheres to the tooth and tray, or there is the potential for saliva to wash the material from the tray. The final addition to tray design is the use of reservoirs or spacers to avoid the tightness of the tray on the tooth and to allow better seating of the tray when loaded with a thick viscous material. This design may also supply additional material for bleaching but, conversely, may waste additional material or lessen the comfort of the tray if not properly fabricated.[53]

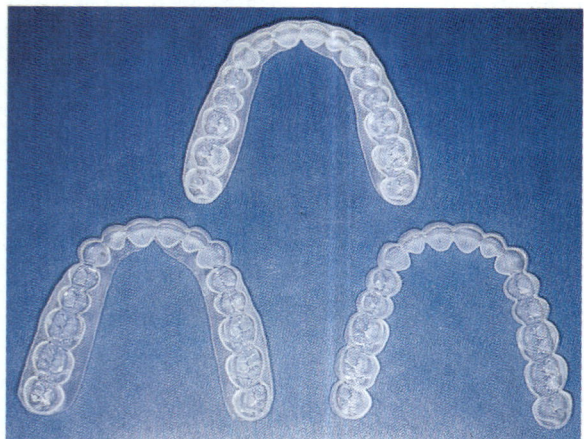

Figure 16–19: Tray design can be scalloped or nonscalloped, with or without reservoirs. The choice depends on the bleaching material used and patient and clinical issues.

The choice of the type of tray design used must include consideration of the type of bleaching material used, the gingival characteristics of the patient, the concerns of the patient, and the arch to be treated.[55] Some runny, low-viscosity bleaching materials are best applied with a nonscalloped no-reservoir tray, which is the easiest to fabricate and the most comfortable to wear. However, if the patient has thin facial gingival tissue, the facial side of the tray may be scalloped to avoid gingival irritation. If the patient does not like the taste, the lingual may be left unscalloped since rarely does gingival irritation occur on the palate. Concern for contact of peroxide with any soft tissue would warrant a tray scalloped on the facial and lingual surfaces.[52]

In the same manner, reservoirs are not required for successful bleaching with any material,[61] but reduce the tightness of the tray to aid in the seating of the tray with the thick viscous materials.[33] However, on the mandibular arch, the shape of the teeth and the facial occlusal contacts make the placement of reservoirs impractical or provide very little benefit. Since most mandibular teeth are slightly malaligned, a no-reservoir tray can be used with any material on the mandible. Scalloping is also more irritating to the patient on the mandibular arch due to the small narrow teeth. Both the tongue and lips may be irritated by the edges, so often a nonscalloped design is preferable for all materials on the mandible. The nonscalloped design helps overcome the influence of gravity, salivary glands, and the tongue for retention of the material in the tray. Only highly viscous materials can be retained in the scalloped, reservoired mandibular tray design.

With the nonscalloped tray design, the dental office still has the option of scalloping the tray if the patient experiences gingival irritation. Chemical irritation may be related more to the base vehicle of the bleaching material than the carbamide peroxide. Current bleaching materials vary greatly in base vehicles, flavoring, stabilizers, thickeners, and ingredients other than carbamide peroxide. If the material is more water soluble, it is less likely to cause gingival irritation. Also, less viscous materials require better tray adaptation, which can be better accomplished with a nonscalloped tray.

Another variation in tray design concerns the patient with temporomandibular dysfunction. For patients in this category, any alteration of the occlusal surfaces of the arch could precipitate some discomfort or pain. One solution is to make a scalloped reservoired tray that does not extend beyond the facial cusp tips.[69] This approach avoids changes in the occlusion. This design must be used in conjunction with a thick sticky material because that can help retain the tray in the mouth.

SINGLE DARK TEETH

A single tooth may become dark either from trauma, after completion of endodontic therapy, or from internal resorption. The first step in the treatment of this tooth is to take a radiograph to determine if there is any periapical pathology and to pulp test the tooth for vitality.[57]

If the single dark tooth tests vital, there are two options for treatment. One option is when the patient wishes to lighten the other teeth as well. The other option is when the patient only wants to bleach the single tooth. If the patient wants to lighten all teeth, a conventional bleaching tray is fabricated, and carbamide peroxide is placed on all of the teeth. When the unaffected teeth cease to lighten, treatment is continued by placing the material only on the darkened tooth until it matches the color of the other teeth (Figures 16–20A and B).

There are several techniques for those patients who only wish to lighten the single tooth. The fabrication of a single-tooth bleaching tray has been previously described.[46] The single-tooth bleaching technique involves the use of a nonscalloped tray, with or without reservoirs. In this tray design, the tooth-imprint areas on either side of the darkened tooth are removed to allow the bleach to contact only one tooth. Other techniques for single dark teeth involve a scalloped tray with adjacent teeth molds removed[23] or use of a polycarbonate crown former to carry the material.[108] The more conventional treatment of a single dark tooth would be the use of an in-office power bleaching technique as described in Chapter 12, *Esthetics in Dentistry*, Volume 1, 2nd Edition. This procedure uses 35% hydrogen peroxide on the single tooth isolated with a rubber dam. However, it is not possible to predict the number of visits required, thus making the total cost unknown. The patient must be informed that treatment may take two to six visits to achieve a successful lightening, with a fee necessary for each visit that may be comparable to the total at-home whitening fee.[8] Also, the dangers to both the dentist and the patient of burns from handling the high concentration of peroxide are a concern. In-office bleaching does offer some shortening of time but not necessarily a better outcome due to the tendency to terminate treatment prematurely because of cost concerns. Another popular approach is to initiate treatment with in-office bleaching, followed by at-home bleaching until the process is completed.[39]

If a single dark tooth does not test vital, the radiograph is negative for periapical pathology, and the patient has had no symptoms, the treatment can be the same as a single dark vital tooth without initia-

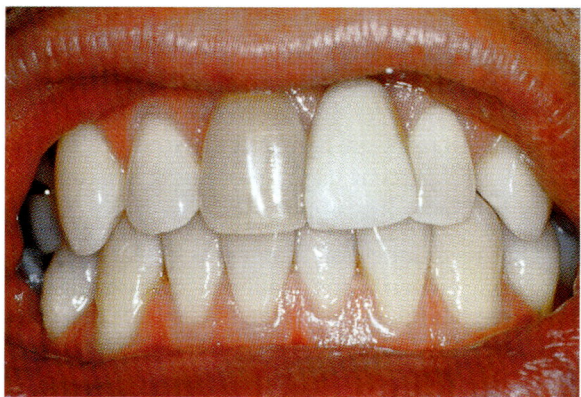

Figure 16–20A: Because of trauma, one central incisor was lost and was replaced by an acrylic removable partial denture. The other single right central incisor is discolored. Photograph courtesy of Dr. Kevin Frazier.

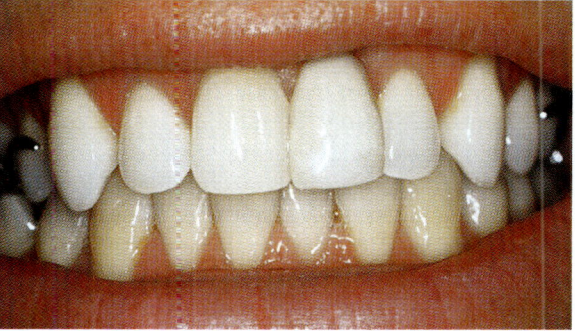

Figure 16–20B: The patient may start with the dark tooth followed by lightening of all of the teeth or continue placing bleaching material in the single dark tooth mold after the remaining teeth have lightened. The artificial tooth is also polished to match the texture of the natural teeth. Photograph courtesy of Dr. Kevin Frazier.

tion of endodontic therapy. However, the patient should be informed that there is a chance that the tooth may need a root canal should symptoms eventually occur. There has been only one report in the literature of a nonvital tooth requiring endodontic therapy after bleaching, but that situation used 35% hydrogen peroxide for in-office bleaching, not 10% carbamide peroxide for home bleaching.[40] Other options listed in the first volume of this textbook include intentional endodontic therapy and the walking bleach technique or in-office power bleaching. Additionally, when successful endodontic therapy cannot be accomplished due to a calcified canal, some reports describe the creation of an artificial pulp chamber for the subsequent walking bleach technique.[2]

Other situations for dark teeth occur after the tooth has received endodontic therapy. If the tooth has not been restored, or if the treating dentist is not certain that all of the remaining pulp material has been removed from the tooth, then some form of inside bleaching should be performed. This would involve removal of the restoration and débridement of the pulp chamber. The traditional walking bleach technique has been described previously,[86] as well as the thermocatalytic technique.[32] Both techniques were popular until reports were published of external root resorption.[42,69,75] There are many hypotheses for this resorption. A review of the literature on root resorption since 1979 indicates several common themes between the case reports[37]: no sealer over the gutta-percha, heat, and trauma.[45] Other speculations include a lack of cement–enamel junction (CEJ) in 10% of teeth where a dentin gap between cementum and enamel is present and alteration of the pH of the surrounding bone from peroxide exit or cellular damage from overheating. In addition to the concern for potential external resorption, general concerns exist with both bleaching techniques. Common concerns include the possibilities of chemical burns from handling 35% hydrogen peroxide clinically, the need for fresh solutions to be effective, the unknown number of office visits required, and the possibility of overlightening the tooth. The walking bleach technique also presents the difficulty of maintaining the provisional seal between appointments. The difficulty with the thermocatalytic technique is determining and controlling the proper heating temperature.

Some suggestions have been offered to avoid these concerns.[104] These include the use of sodium perborate alone for walking bleach,[64] the use of calcium hydroxide powder postbleaching to neutralize the pH,[4] and a catalase after internal bleaching to inactivate the peroxide.[96] All options stress the importance of placing a sealer over the gutta-percha and avoidance of the use of heat. If heat is used, the temperature should not exceed that which would cause discomfort on a vital tooth. Probably the safest treatment options are the use of sodium perborate alone and the use of 10% carbamide peroxide sealed in the pulp chamber in the walking bleach fashion.[105]

INSIDE-OUTSIDE BLEACHING TECHNIQUE

In 1996, a technique was described (company product catalogue, Ultradent Products) using 10% carbamide peroxide applied in a tray to a tooth prepared for conventional walking bleaching but not sealed.[77] In this situation, the outside and the inside of the nonvital tooth are lightened using a fresh solution applied daily. For this approach to be indicated, the vital teeth and the open nonvital teeth must require lightening or the adjacent vital teeth must exhibit a light shade already. Other recent articles have described or researched the technique.[13,14,73,101] The advantage of leaving the tooth open for multiple applications is that the patient does not have to return to the office to apply fresh solution if one treatment is insufficient. This ease of continual treatment at home avoids the uncertainty of cost to the patient and the number of office visits. In difficult discolorations, this technique can afford both a reduction in time and fee and avoid the safety concerns to the tooth from the higher concentrations of peroxide. Ten percent carbamide is approximately equal to 3% hydrogen peroxide.

The technique for use with a thick, sticky whitening material and scalloped tray design is as follows: a radiograph is taken to ensure the adequacy of the endodontic therapy and the level of the CEJ. Written consent is obtained, and photographs are taken. Alginate impressions are made, and stone casts are generated. Bleaching trays are fabricated of the scalloped, reservoired design, according to the manufacturer's instructions, from a thermoplastic tray material.[52] The bleaching tray is fitted, observing carefully that the gingivae will not be irritated by contact with the tray.

In the nonvital tooth, access is made through the lingual endodontic opening and the pulp chamber contents are removed. Gutta-percha is removed 2 to 3 mm apical to the CEJ. The remaining gutta-percha is sealed using glass ionomer (or composite or resin-ionomer) 2 to 3 mm in thickness (Figure 16–21). After the glass ionomer has set, the chamber is cleaned by etching with 35% phosphoric acid for 2 minutes and then rinsing with water. No other restorative material is placed above the glass ionomer base so the access orifice is not sealed. Bleaching material will be placed both in the tooth orifice and in the bleaching tray to apply the material from the inside and the outside simultaneously in the following manner.

Patients are instructed in the technique for inserting a cotton ball into the opening in the tooth during the day when the bleaching tray is not being used. This is done to prevent accidental packing of food into the orifice. The cotton ball is removed after each meal by means of twisting a toothpick inserted into the cotton. The coronal orifice is irrigated with a water syringe to ensure the removal of debris, and a fresh ball of cotton is inserted. At bedtime, the cotton is removed again, and the tooth is irrigated as before. The 10% carbamide peroxide is loaded into the bleaching tray and injected into the tooth orifice. The tray is seated, and excess material is removed with a finger or toothbrush. The patient then wears the loaded tray during the night. On removal of the tray in the morning, the internal chamber of the tooth is irrigated again with water using a syringe, and a cotton ball is inserted into the chamber by the patient. Patients bleach their teeth until the vital teeth no longer change color and the nonvital tooth matches the color of the vital teeth. Patients are cautioned not to bite with the front teeth during the duration of the treatment. The disadvantage of this technique is that it requires excellent patient compliance and skills for treatment and a responsible patient who will return to the office in a timely manner to have the orifice closed with a restoration on completion of treatment. There is no concern for caries during the active treatment phase since carbamide peroxide is anticariogenic and the pH is elevated beyond the level of carious activity.[71] However, once treatment is complete, the orifice must be restored.

CLOSURE OF INTERNAL BLEACHING

On return to the office after completion of the inside-outside or conventional walking bleaching technique, the orifice to the nonvital tooth is débrided and temporarily sealed for 2 weeks with a noneugenol-containing temporary cement. A noneugenol-containing material is used to avoid future contamination of the acid-etched composite restoration, which will be used to close the orifice to the canal and make any final minor color adjustments by varying the composite color internally. Placement of the final restoration is delayed for 2 weeks to allow the oxygen generated during bleaching to dissipate from the tooth and the shade to stabilize. The presence of residual oxygen in the tooth results in a reduction of bond strengths[79] and an artificially light shade. Two weeks after termination of bleaching, the bond strength potential will have returned to normal,[82] and the shade will have stabilized.[5] This shade stabilization (a slight darkening) is thought to occur from the change in optical qualities of the tooth after the residual oxygen generated during the oxidation process of bleaching has diminished. Two weeks after completion of bleaching, the temporary stopping is removed, and the orifice is occluded using an acid-etched composite.

If the tooth needs any further lightening, a slight modification of the shade can be accomplished by the selection of a lighter composite to restore the internal root and coronal portions of the tooth. For

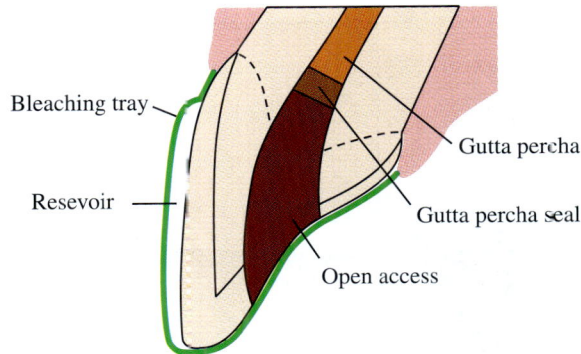

Figure 16–21: Schematic drawing of preparing the nonvital tooth for inside-outside bleaching using 10% carbamide peroxide when more rapid results are desirable.

years, the lightest shade of composite available was a B1 on the Vita shade guide (Vident, Brea, CA). Now, with the advent of teeth bleached lighter than B1, companies have introduced shades of composite lighter than B1 (COSMEDENT, Chicago, IL; Ultradent Products). These may be used for final color corrections and diastema closure or restorations to the bleached tooth (Figure 16–22). Should the tooth subsequently discolor, it is preferable not to remove composite but rather to rebleach the tooth from the outside using the conventional nightguard vital bleaching technique (Figure 16–23).

WHY IS BLEACHING OF ANTERIOR ENDODONTICALLY TREATED TEETH BECOMING MORE PREVALENT?

There has been an increase in the opportunities to bleach endodontically treated anterior teeth due to research on the longevity of other treatment options.[102] At one time in dentistry, all teeth that had received endodontic therapy subsequently received a post and core followed by a full crown. However, it has been found that the use of the post and core did not strengthen the tooth as originally thought, but often the preparation of the post space weakened the tooth. The best method to obtain strength for an endodontically treated tooth is to maximize the amount of remaining dentin and have a 2-mm ferrule of tooth structure internally above the margins. The current opinion is that an anterior endodontically treated tooth does not automatically require crowning but should be restored with an acid-etched composite if possible. A crown should be used only if indicated on a vital tooth in the same condition. A post and core is used only if there is a need to generate a core form to retain the crown. Hence, there are more teeth that are sound structurally, but discolored, and for which bleaching is the treatment of choice. Posterior teeth receiving endodontic therapy continue to require full-coverage restorations in almost all situations to avoid vertical tooth fracture.

TOOTH SENSITIVITY DURING VITAL BLEACHING

Tooth sensitivity during bleaching is the most prevalent side effect to treatment, and the dental office should be prepared to offer different treatment options. Tooth sensitivity experienced during bleaching can be treated actively or passively by the dentist (Table 16–4). Passive treatment consists of reducing either the duration of each treatment (fewer hours) or the frequency of treatment (skip days).[44] Originally, the only active treatment cited was the use of a neutral fluoride gel placed in the tray at the onset of sensitivity. One early report of a laboratory bleaching experiment on the use of stannous fluoride during bleaching had suggested that fluoride was contraindicated.[41] However, this recommendation may have been a result of the staining nature of the stannous fluoride used in the study. Some current bleaching products now incorporate a neutral fluoride with no apparent compromise of the bleaching process (15% Opalescence with Fluoride, Ultradent Products). One report has also indicated a reduction in sensitivity by having the patient apply the neutral fluoride for 3 weeks nightly prior to initiation of

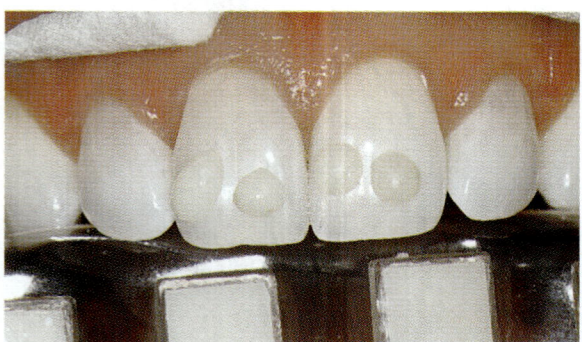

Figure 16–22: The darkest sample of composite in this photograph is a B1 shade. Shades lighter than B1 are necessary for some bleached teeth.

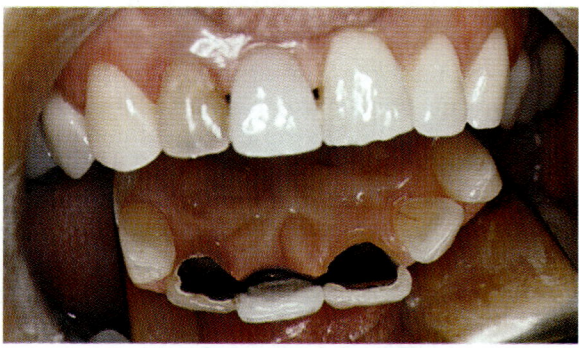

Figure 16–23: Some nonvital teeth are inaccessible to retreatment by internal bleaching due to subsequent restorative treatment but can be lightened again from the outside.

TABLE 16–4. Treatment Approaches for Tooth Sensitivity during Bleaching

PASSIVE	ACTIVE
Reduce treatment time (night to day wear)	Apply neutral fluoride in the tray
Reduce treatment frequency (skip a night)	Apply 3–5% potassium nitrate in the tray
Alter carbamide peroxide concentrations or brands	Pretreat with either fluoride or potassium nitrate

the bleaching process.[100] The mechanism of action of fluoride is as a tubular blocker.

Another active approach to treating sensitivity involves the use of 5% or less concentrations of potassium nitrate applied in the bleaching tray.[50,56] Potassium nitrate is generally found in desensitizing toothpastes,[103] which are applied via brushing. This application technique generally takes 2 weeks to see results. However, a recent report has shown that the application of the material for longer periods of time (1–8 hours) via a tray is effective in relieving tooth/root sensitivity.[66] Because the application of toothpaste in a bleaching style tray can cause gingival irritations in some patients, dental companies have now introduced products of potassium nitrate with and without fluoride in a base carrier (Desentize, DEN-MAT, Santa Monica, CA; UltraEZ, Ultradent Products; Relief, Discus Dental, Culver City, CA). The mechanism of action of potassium nitrate is different from that of fluoride. Potassium nitrate is thought to act in one of two ways: to chemically depolarize the nerve to inhibit refiring[63,76] or to release the nitric oxide radical, which reduces sensations to the nerve.[78] Whatever the mechanism, it is a good adjunct for any type of chronic sensitivity, as well as bleaching sensitivity.

LOCALIZED BROWN DISCOLORATION

Typically, brown discoloration is associated with high fluoride ingestion.[22] The discoloration is generally localized to sporadic areas on the tooth. Usually, microabrasion is considered the primary treatment.[3] Microabrasion is the application of acid and pumice to selectively remove the enamel surface discolorations.[20] However, nightguard vital bleaching has been shown to successfully remove brown discolorations.[58,72,88] It is estimated that 80% of these brown discolorations are amenable to bleaching with 10% carbamide peroxide.[54] Recent articles have shown removal of brown discoloration after 4 to 6 weeks of bleaching, with no return or need for additional treatment at 7 years recall (Figures 16–24A to C).[59] Certainly, attempting bleaching first avoids the removal of the fluoride-rich enamel layer, and microabrasion[19] or macroabrasion[62] can be attempted (Figures 16–25A and B) should bleaching not be successful.[18,47] When time is of the utmost importance to the patient, a combination approach can be most effective.

LOCALIZED WHITE DISCOLORATION

As with brown discolorations, white discolorations are often associated with high fluoride ingestion, high fever, or other disturbances during enamel formation. Bleaching does not remove white spots and may occasionally make them lighter during treatment, but it does lighten the surrounding tooth so as to make the white spot less noticeable (Figures 16–26A and B).[44] During bleaching, the white spot may get whiter, but on termination of the bleaching it generally returns to its original color. It is thought that these white spots are differently formed portions of enamel that respond differently to the bleaching material. Teeth with white spots undergoing bleaching often develop a "splotchy look" during the first week or two of bleaching. However, patients should be encouraged to continue through this stage so that the darker portions of the teeth can "catch up." Often, malformed parts of enamel below the surface of the tooth contribute to this splotchy appearance. On termination of bleaching, the white spots return to their original color. Bleaching with 10% carbamide peroxide is still the first treatment of choice because it can lighten the other portions of the tooth so that the white spot is no longer as noticeable.

CHOOSING MICROABRASION OR BLEACHING

Historically, micro- or macroabrasion has been recommended for removal of white spots. These treatments should be considered as the second level of treatment only if bleaching is unsuccessful. The only time microabrasion is considered as the first

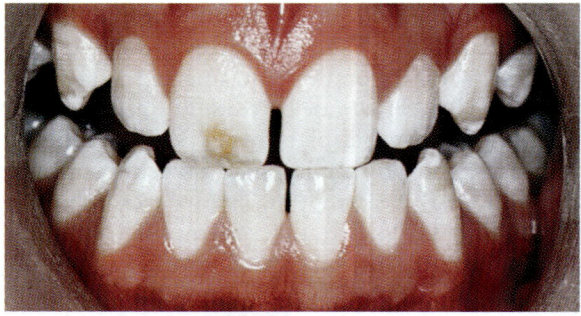

Figure 16–24A: A single dark brown spot, possibly from trauma to the primary tooth, is present in this 13-year-old male. The remaining teeth are already very white.

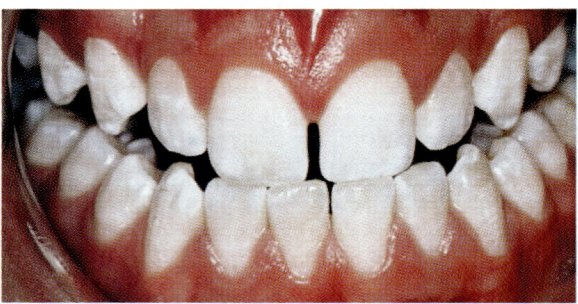

Figure 16–24B: The teeth are treated for 5 weeks nightly with 10% carbamide peroxide, resulting in the removal of the brown area without changing the surface characteristics or removing the fluoride-rich layer of enamel.

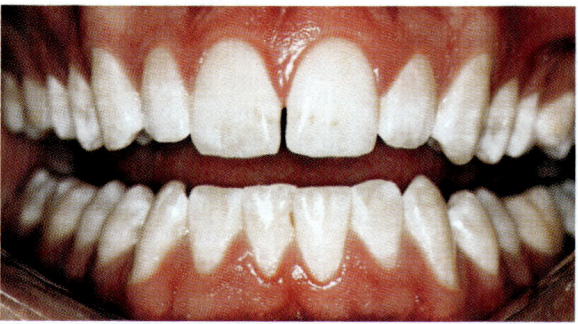

Figure 16–24C: With no further whitening treatment, the brown spot has not returned for 7 years.

treatment is when the teeth have a soft, chalky appearance rather than hard, shiny enamel, or the discoloration is obviously unnatural and known not to respond to bleaching, such as stark white discolorations. If microabrasion is attempted first on a single white spot, the white spot can become whiter as the operator progresses subsurface, requiring removal of more tooth structure and replacement of loss tooth structure with a composite (Figures 16–27A to C). If bleaching has not pre-

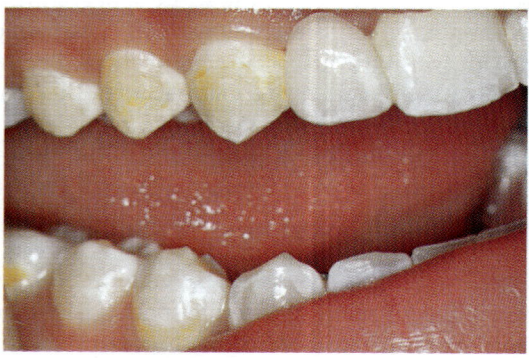

Figure 16–25A: Yellow-brown stain that appears rough adjacent to a resin-bonded fixed partial denture.

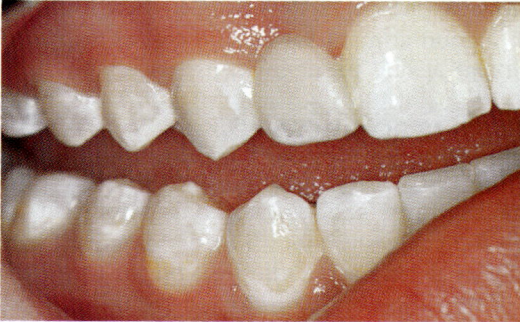

Figure 16–25B: Microabrasion is used to remove the stain and smooth and polish the surface of the tooth without altering the shade of the adjacent teeth.

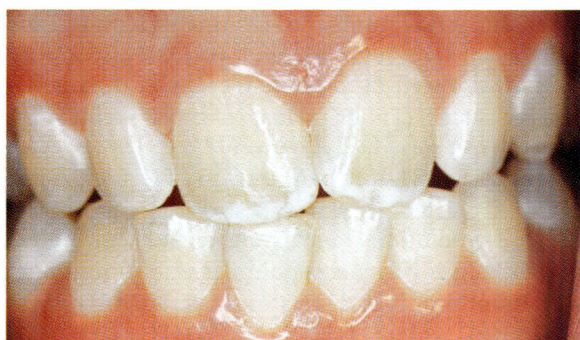

Figure 16–26A: White spots on the incisal edges are accentuated by the yellow of the teeth.

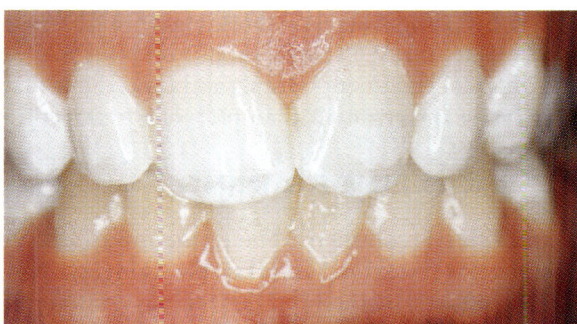

Figure 16–26B: After 5 weeks of nightly treatment with 10% carbamide peroxide, the white is less noticeable because the yellow has been removed.

viously been performed, the shade of the composite will have to match the current shade of the teeth, which may be undesirable. Also, if generalized whitish areas on the teeth are removed, the teeth often appear more yellow, requiring bleaching afterward. Again, it is more efficient to leave the fluoride-rich layer of enamel intact and attempt bleaching first, and then try microabrasion fol-

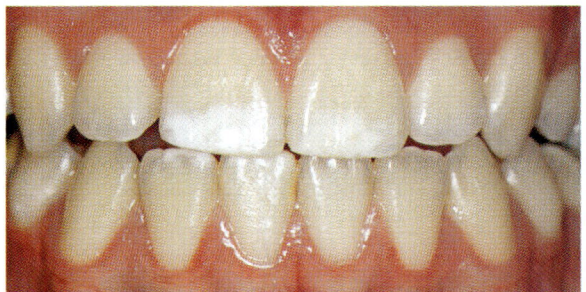

Figure 16–27A: White spots may be considered for microabrasion, but the depth of the discoloration is unknown. Bleaching is generally the first treatment of choice.

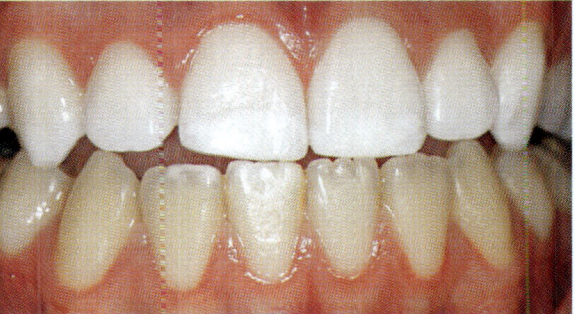

Figure 16–27B: After bleaching for 6 weeks with 10% carbamide peroxide, the white is less noticeable but still a distraction.

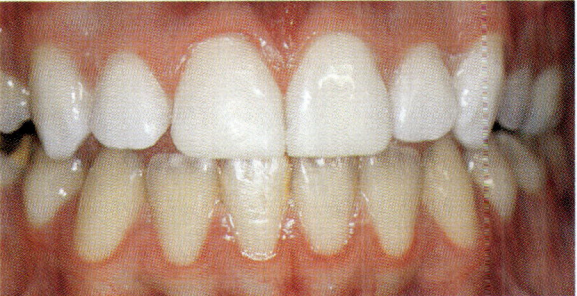

Figure 16–27C: On initiating removal of the white areas, they became whiter and extended deeper into the tooth, requiring removal and composite bonding. The composite bonding is completed using the shade of the bleached teeth to restore a natural coloration.

lowed by composite resin bonding with the new shade if necessary. Patients should be informed of the different treatment options and procedures that may be necessary rather than only one treatment.

TETRACYCLINE STAINING

Tetracycline is considered one of the most difficult tooth stains to remove. In-office bleaching is a possible treatment method but generally is contraindicated due to the number of treatments required and the concurrent high fee and patient discomfort. With the advent of at-home bleaching, these tetracycline stains can be managed more easily.[49,51,60] Treatment times may vary from 2 months to 1 year (Figures 16–28A to C, 16–29A and B, 16–30A and B, 16–31A and B). Patients are seen monthly to replenish solutions and evaluate for continuing color change. Patients should agree to a minimum of 2 months of nightly treatment before deciding to

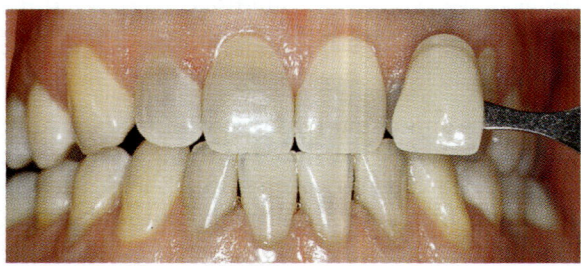

Figure 16–28A: Patient with moderately tetracycline-stained teeth is considering bleaching or veneers. Bleaching is initiated to either resolve the issue or provide a lighter base onto which the veneers can be placed.

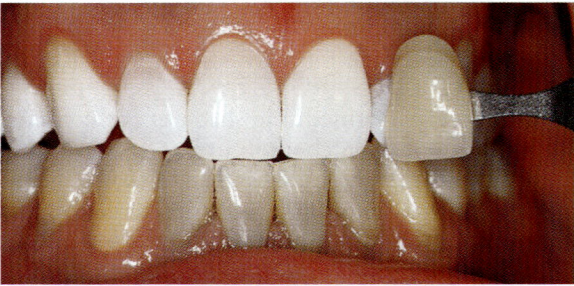

Figure 16–28B: Four months of bleaching of the maxillary arch using 10% carbamide peroxide produces a remarkable shade change.

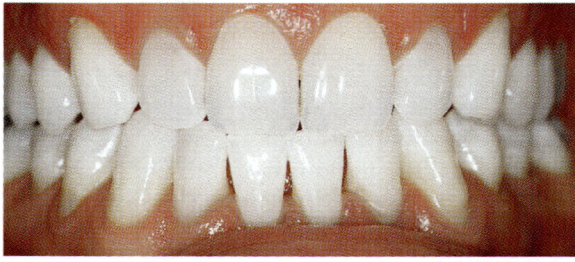

Figure 16–28C: The mandibular arch is subsequently lightened.

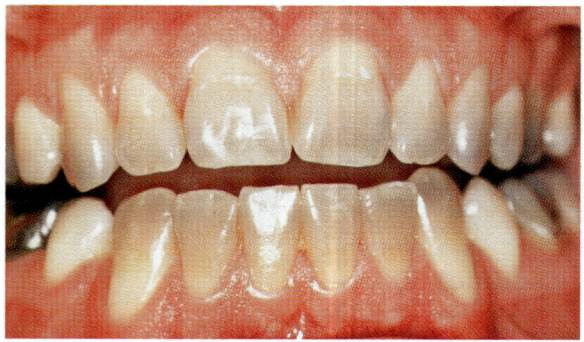

Figure 16–29A: Moderately tetracycline-stained teeth.

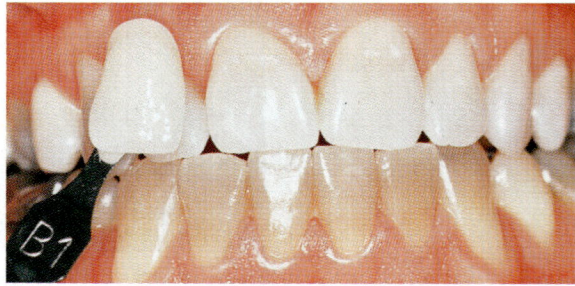

Figure 16–29B: In a research study, these teeth were bleached for 6 months nightly with a 10% carbamide peroxide. Not all results will be this good, especially if the discoloration is blue/gray or at the gingival third.

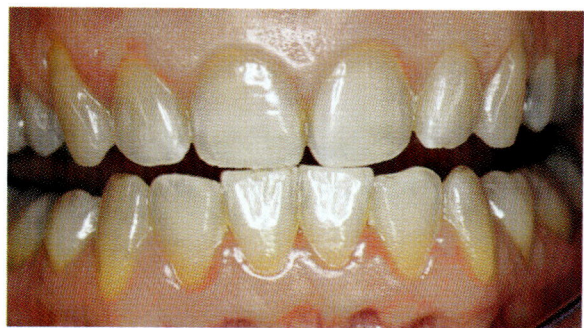

Figure 16–30A: Moderately tetracycline-stained teeth.

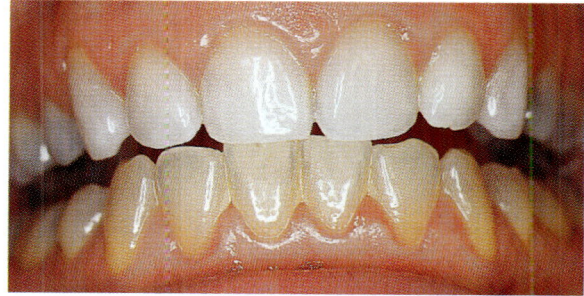

Figure 16–30B: After only 2 months of treatment, the results are satisfactory. Patients with tetracycline-stained teeth should commit to at least 2 months of treatment.

proceed to more aggressive treatment. Fees are generally the cost of a monthly office recall visit and additional material. Once lightening is observed, patients should continue treatment until a month has passed with no obvious color change. Dark tetracycline stains located in the gingival third of the tooth or dark blue or gray stains have the least favorable prognosis. However, even in these situations, there can be some improvement. This improvement may be sufficient for the patient's esthetic demands. However, compliance by the patient is necessary for success. Patients with tetracycline staining often view the at-home bleaching regime similar to a weight loss or an exercise program. Application of the bleaching material at night becomes a regular part of their routine. There is no increase in side effects with this long-term bleaching since most side effects occur in the initial weeks of treatment.

BLEACHING AND PORCELAIN VENEERS

Bleaching may not produce an acceptable result on all tetracycline-stained teeth, but it can provide the patient with a better idea of how his or her smile will appear with whiter teeth. Often, bleaching is the stepping stone to veneers. Once the patient has seen what a little color change will do for his or her appearance, he or she is often more excited about completing the restorative process. Even when veneers are the ultimate goal, bleaching lightens the underlying tooth, decreasing the masking needs of the veneers, which results in a more vital final restoration. If the tooth shade regresses after the placement of the veneers, the teeth can be rebleached through the lingual surfaces (Figures 16–32A to D).

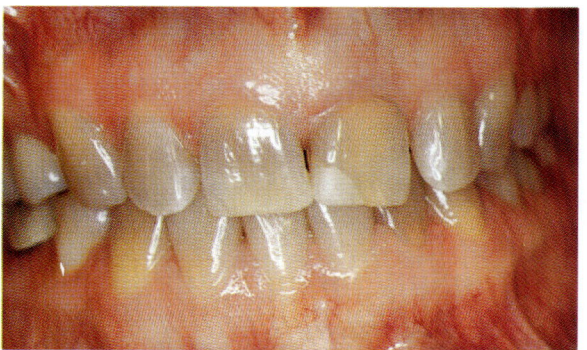

Figure 16–31A: Moderately tetracycline-stained teeth, with one nonvital central incisor with a Class IV composite needing replacement.

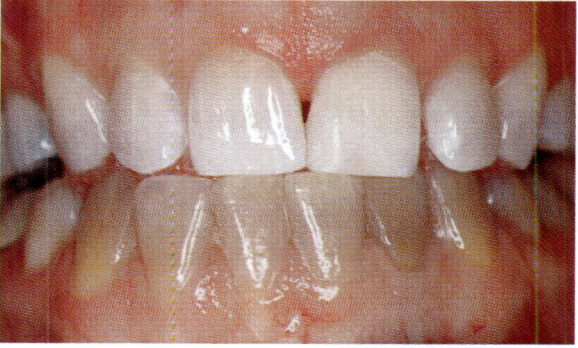

Figure 16–31B: Teeth are bleached with 10% carbamide peroxide in a tray for 12 months nightly. The Class IV composite is removed, and the pulp chamber is cleaned. A lighter than B1 composite is used to restore the root portion, followed by a tooth matching the Class IV composite.

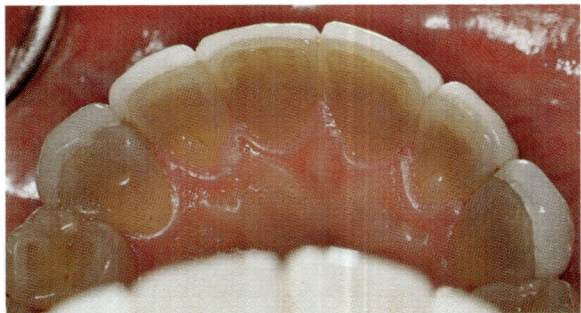

Figure 16–32A: Extent of the discoloration is evident from the lingual view of the maxillary teeth and the unrestored mandibular teeth.

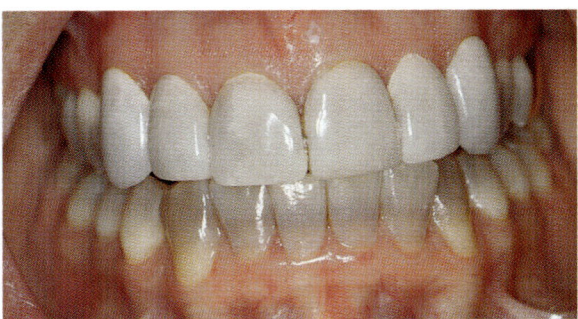

Figure 16–32B: Porcelain veneers were placed over tetracycline-stained teeth, but the appearance of the teeth is still gray due to show-through of the tooth discolorations.

Bleaching and Other Restorations

Bleaching does not change the color of other restorations. In fact, existing restorations tend to appear darker as the adjacent teeth lighten. Patients should be informed of the possible need for replacement of restorations in the esthetic area should there be a color mismatch post-treatment (Figures 16–33A and B). However, the color stability of restorations can also be a benefit to the clinician. Usually, crowns that match adjacent natural teeth are placed. Over time, the teeth may have darkened to the point where they no longer match the crowns. Rather than replace the otherwise acceptable crown with a darker shade crown, bleaching is the treatment of choice. In these instances, the patient can carefully bleach the teeth until the natural teeth return to the shade they were when the crowns were fabricated (Figures 16–34A and B). To avoid overbleaching the teeth, patients are instructed to apply the whitening solution for only 1 to 2 hours a day until they see how responsive the natural teeth will be to the process. This avoids a color mismatch, where the teeth become lighter than the crowns from bleaching, which would require replacing the crowns with a lighter shade to be esthetic.

COMPOSITE RESIN RESTORATIONS

Discoloration of Composites

Stains to composite resin restorations can occur in the body of the composite, on the surface of the composite, or at the restoration margins. Bulk discoloration of chemically cured composites was common before the advent of light-curing. Benzoyl peroxide, which is the chemical initiator in all chemically cured composites, is not color stable and will cause the restoration to darken over time. This phenomenon may necessitate the replacement of many otherwise serviceable restorations. Darkening of light-cured composites is a result of

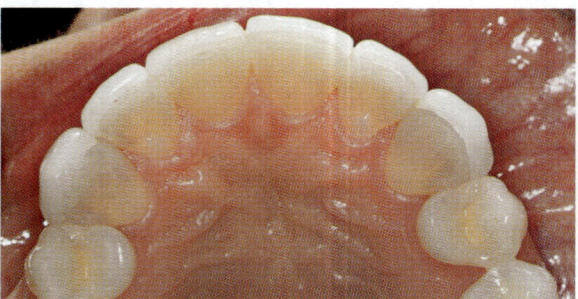

Figure 16–32C: After bleaching the tetracycline-stained teeth for 9 months, the lingual view demonstrates the extent of tooth color change.

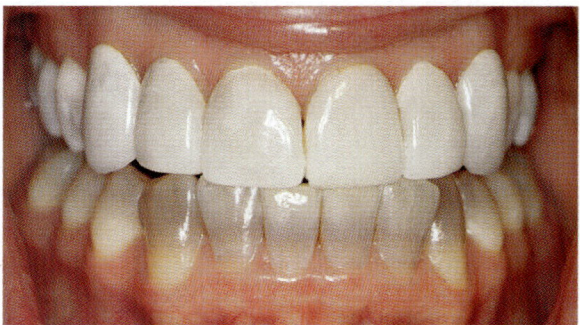

Figure 16–32D: A facial view of the veneers shows that they appear lighter because the underlying tooth is lighter.

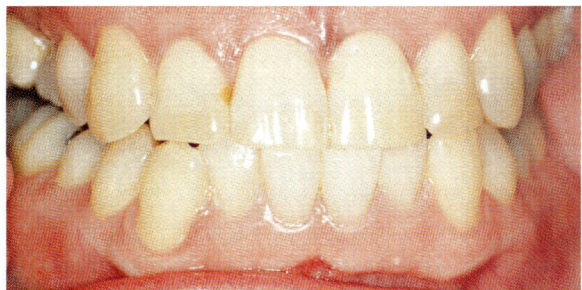

Figure 16–33A: The composite on the mesial of the lateral incisor is somewhat discolored but not markedly noticeable.

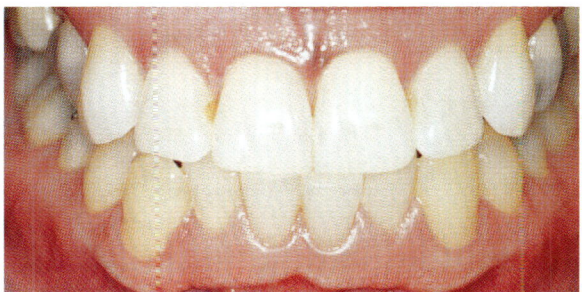

Figure 16–33B: After bleaching, the composite restoration is much more noticeable.

extrinsic stains from food, drink, or oral habits. Orange stain can be the result of chromagenic bacteria. If these stains recur after thorough prophylaxis, refer the patient to an oral pathologist for culture, which will help determine a specific antibiotic to help prevent the recurrence of the bacteria (Figures 16–35A and B). These stains can often be removed by merely repolishing the restoration. Care must be taken not to use certain aggressive cleaning devices during prophylaxis (ie, Prophy-jet air polisher, DENTSPLY Professional, York, PA) because these technologies can roughen the surface finish of composite restorations.[35]

It is not uncommon for staining to occur at the margins of composite restorations as the restorations age. If the staining is superficial, it can often be removed by bleaching, air abrasion, or the use of diamond or finishing burs. After stain removal, the composite's margins should be etched for 15 seconds with 32 to 37% phosphoric acid, rinsed, and resealed with a bonding agent or surface sealant. When a marginal stain is not easily removed by conservative finishing techniques, the affected area should be mechanically removed because of the possible presence of recurrent decay. If on penetration and exploration the stain is found to be superficial, the restoration's margins can be repaired with fresh composite. If the stain is extensive, the entire restoration should be replaced. The postfinish application of a surface sealant (Fortify, Bisco, Schaumburg, IL; Optiguard, KerrDental, Romulus, MI) has been shown to improve the composite's marginal integrity over time and can provide a more esthetic restoration by sealing surface irregularities.[25]

USING COMPOSITE TO MASK EXISTING AMALGAMS

Occasionally, a patient may present with an otherwise satisfactory amalgam restoration and either a fractured cusp in an esthetic area or discoloration of the tooth from the amalgam. Complete removal of the amalgam may jeopardize the status of the tooth, but esthetics remains a consideration. In these cases, composite may be used to mask the dis-

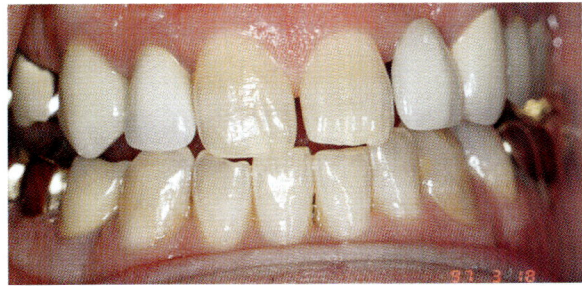

Figure 16–34A: All of the maxillary teeth except the central incisors had porcelain-fused-to-metal restorations placed 17 years previously. The natural teeth no longer match the restorations.

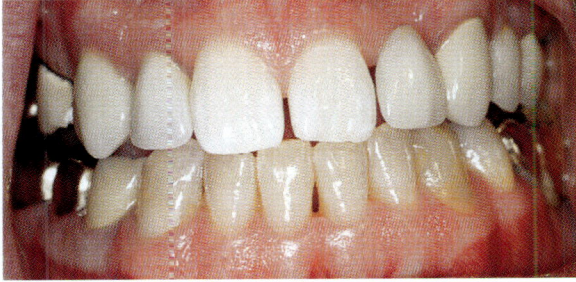

Figure 16–34B: The teeth are lightened until the natural teeth return to the shade that originally matched the porcelain, providing an esthetic smile again with minimal expense.

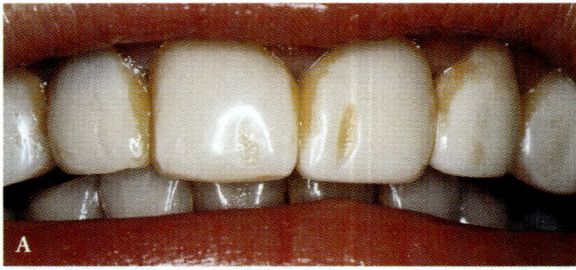
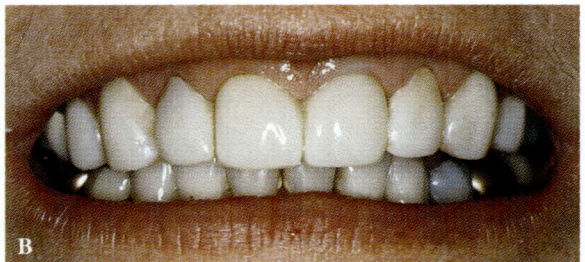

Figure 16–35A and B: This orange stain on the surface of these composite resin veneers was caused by chromagenic bacteria.

coloration of the existing amalgam or replace the missing tooth structure (Figures 16–36A to C). These procedures can provide a conservative alternative to crowns or at least an intermediate treatment option until the crowns can be initiated.

Show-through of the discoloration is often seen on the mesiofacial surface of a maxillary first premolar or molar. In this situation, the operator would remove the amalgam to the proximal contact, providing for 1- to 2-mm bulk of composite.

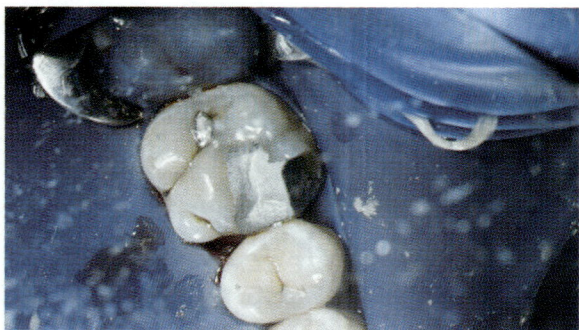

Figure 16–36A: Fractured tooth structure in an esthetic area reveals an unacceptable display of amalgam. From the occlusal view, the amalgam is acceptable and would require extensive removal for replacement.

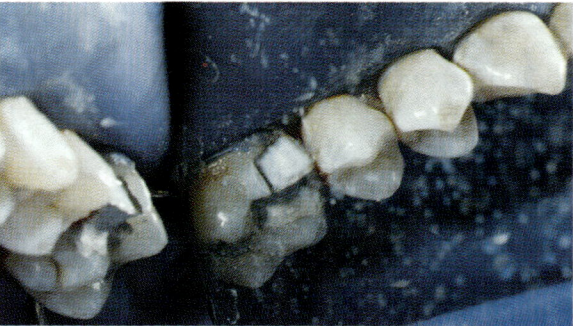

Figure 16–36B: The amalgam is masked using opaque composite and adhesive technology.

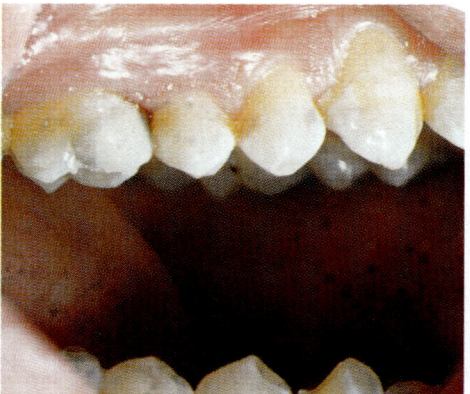

Figure 16–36C: The facial view exhibits the minimal need for composite to retain the success of the amalgam restoration.

Mechanical retention can be placed in the amalgam, or a chemical approach for bonding can be adopted. The surface of the amalgam is cleaned and roughened using an air abrasive with 50- to 60-micron aluminum oxide particles. Next, any adjoining tooth structure is etched with 32 to 35% phosphoric acid. The prepared surface of the amalgam and etched tooth is covered with a universal bonding system or a thin layer of Panavia cement (J. Morita USA, Irvine, CA).[15] An appropriate opaque shade of composite resin is applied, shaped, and cured before final contouring and polishing.

Still another question that routinely arises is the patient who desires his or her posterior good amalgam restorations replaced with tooth-colored restorations. Some dentists have advocated leaving part of the old but serviceable amalgam in and resurfacing the restorations with composite resin. The major problem with this technique is the initial or eventual show-through of the old amalgam, making it virtually impossible to diagnose future potential caries.

DISCOLORATIONS AROUND PORCELAIN VENEERS

Marginal staining of porcelain veneers may necessitate the replacement of otherwise acceptable restorations. Marginal staining can result from any of three clinical situations, as follows:

1. The cement line may become obvious after several years if a dual-cured or chemically cured composite luting agent was used instead of a more color-stable light-cured resin cement. Also, unsightly margins may develop when extensive stains accumulate on improperly polished margins. However, the eventual esthetic failure of laminates may be due to advance marginal staining. The final potential cause of unsightly margins is marginal leakage. This occurs when the tooth-composite bond becomes compromised. Whereas the first two margin discolorations present only an esthetic concern, staining as a result of leakage may signal a problem with decay under the restoration. As stated earlier, nightguard bleaching with 10% carbamide peroxide may be helpful as both a therapeutic and a diagnostic procedure. If the stain around the veneer is removed by the at-home bleaching, the margin can be refinished[58] and/or resealed and the veneer salvaged.

2. Discoloration can be microleakage due to failure of the adhesive cement or an inadequate bond at virtually any part of the laminate. Because of the physiologic problems associated with maintaining an adequate bond in the cervical area, this leakage is most often seen associated with the cervical portion of the laminate. Treatment of this problem generally consists of replacement of the laminate. However, it is sometimes possible to repair the gingival aspect with composite resin (Figures 16–37A to E). If this treatment option is selected, it is advisable to use an abrasive technology device to avoid any unnecessary trauma or injury to the remaining porcelain. Often, jet-black stain caused by chromogenic bacteria is found underneath the defective part of the laminate.

3. Both vital and endodontically treated teeth under veneers may darken over time. Bleaching may be a conservative treatment for this condition. In this instance, the bleaching material is applied to the surface of the tray that contacts the lingual surface of the tooth. The bleaching of the underlying tooth may return the veneered tooth to an acceptable shade.

ESTHETIC CONSIDERATIONS FOR FACIAL COMPOSITE RESTORATIONS

There are several factors that should be kept in mind when esthetically restoring the Class V restoration:

1. *Color match.* For most patients, the objective will be to correctly match the present tooth shade. If using composite resin, a microparticle restorative material is preferred rather than a hybrid composite since there will usually be no occlusal force with which to deal and the polishability of a microfilled composite will be of benefit to the patient. Generally, a slightly darker shade should be applied first at the cervical-most portion of the restoration, followed by either a blending body tone or translucent shade to help create a natural look to the tooth. If the patient is bleaching his or her teeth first, wait 2 to 3

weeks following termination of bleaching before appointing the patient for the restorative procedures.

2. *Gingival seal.* Perhaps the most difficult procedure to accomplish is obtaining an effective gingival seal when bonding the Class V restoration. However, failure to obtain proper gingival adhesion will eventually result in either the restoration becoming debonded or the subsequent microleakage can result in a gray-black stain that can, in time, be detected. Use of a rubber dam is the best way to avoid contamination. If a rubber dam is not used, then the placement of a gingival retraction cord 10 to 15 minutes prior to restoring the tooth may help prevent crevicular contamination.

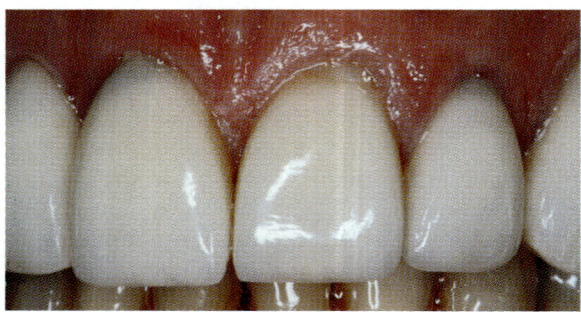

Figure 16–37A: These porcelain laminate veneers have been in this patient's mouth for over 10 years and are now showing signs of gingival leakage.

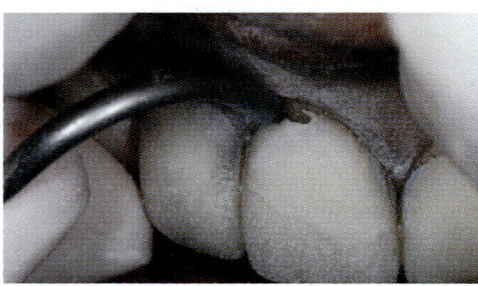

Figure 16–37B: Air abrasion is used instead of a bur to remove the portion of the porcelain over the leakage to avoid potential damage to the remaining portions of the well-bonded laminate veneer.

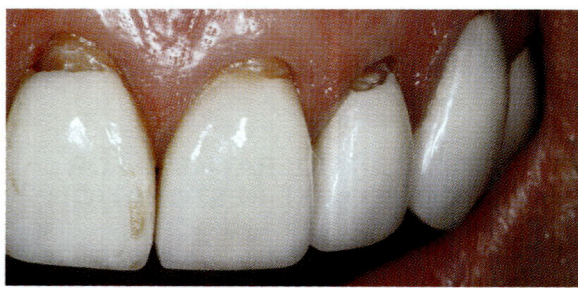

Figure 16–37C: The preparations have now been completed on the three incisor teeth, and they are ready for repair using composite resin bonding.

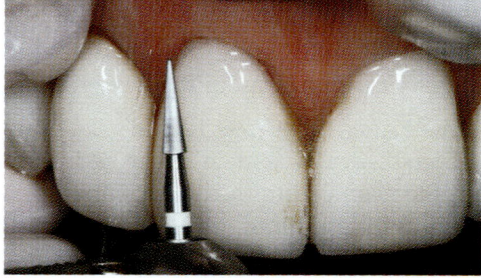

Figure 16–37D. A 30-bladed carbide bur (ET6UF, Brasseler, Savannah, GA) is used to refine the margins.

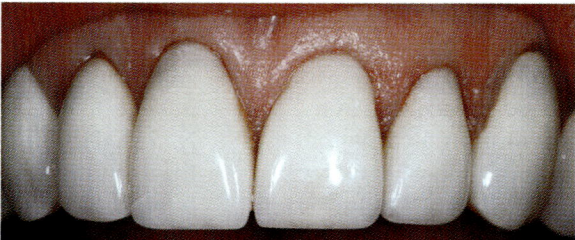

Figure 16–37E: The completed repairs show a close color match of composite to the porcelain.

3. *Shape.* After color, the shape of the restoration becomes the most important element of an esthetic restoration. Using the overlay technique (see Chapter 13, *Esthetics in Dentistry,* Volume 1, 2nd Edition), be sure to slightly overbuild the restoration so that sufficient material remains to finish and polish the restoration. Both building up and contouring of the restoration should be accomplished by viewing the tooth not only from the facial aspect but also occlusally and laterally to best obtain the correct silhouette form.

Although the patient may tend to focus on specific discolorations or stains, it is important for the dentist to remain objective and view the stains in the context of the entire smile and face. In other words, will removal of the stain truly satisfy the patient's quest to look better, or will a more comprehensive approach not only improve the tooth color but also provide a smile that would better improve his or her self-image? The answer to this question may be found in esthetic computer imaging. Actually showing your patient the difference in just removing the stains and changing the smile provides the truest form of informed consent.

SUMMARY

The staining or discoloration of teeth can be indicative of a variety of clinical situations, ranging from severe systemic conditions that may be life threatening to the mere build-up of extensive stains as a result of oral habits. Therefore, the first step in the treatment of a patient whose chief complaint is stains or discolorations is the diagnosis of the cause of the discoloration. The diagnosis will dictate the appropriate treatment options from which to choose. It is incumbent on the dentist to select the most conservative treatment option for the specific stain, while preparing the patient for subsequent treatments should the selected one not be effective.

References

1. Addy M, Moran J. Extrinsic tooth discoloration by metals and chlorhexidine. II. Clinical staining produced by chlorhexidine, iron and tea. Br Dent J 1985;159:331–4.

2. Albers HF. Home bleaching. ADEPT Rep 1991;2(1):9–17.

3. Ames JW. Removing stains from mottled enamel. J Am Dent Assoc 1937;24:1674–7.

4. Baratieri LN, Ritter AV, Monteiro S Jr, et al. Nonvital tooth bleaching: guidelines for the clinician. Quintessence Int 1995;26:597–608.

5. Ben-Amar A, Liberman R, Gorfil C, Bernstein Y. Effect of mouthguard bleaching on enamel surface. Am J Dent 1995;8(1):29–32.

6. Berger RS, Mandel EF, Hayes TJ, Grimwood RR. Minocycline staining of the oral cavity. J Am Acad Dermatol 1989;21:1300–1.

7. Blacharsh C. Dental aspects of patients with cystic fibrosis: a preliminary clinical study. J Am Dent Assoc 1977;95:106–10.

8. Blankenau R, Goldstein RE, Haywood VB. The current status of vital toothwhitening techniques. Compendium 1999;20:781–94.

9. Borrman H, Du Chesne A, Brinkmann B. Medico-legal aspects of postmortem pink teeth. [Review] Int J Legal Med 1994;106:225–31.

10. Bublitz A, Machat E, Scharer K, et al. Changes in dental development in paediatric patients with chronic kidney disease. Proc Eur Dialys Transpl Assoc 1981;18:517–23.

11. Budtz-Jorgensen E. Hibitane in the treatment of oral candidiasis. J Clin Periodontol 1977;4:117–28.

12. Caro I. Discoloration of the teeth related to minocycline therapy for acne. [Letter] J Am Acad Dermatol 1980;3:317–18.

13. Carrilo A, Trevino MVA, Haywood VB. Simultaneous bleaching of vital teeth and an open-chamber nonvital tooth with 10% carbamide peroxide. Quintessence Int 1998;29:643–8.

14. Caughman WF, Frazier KB, Haywood VB. Carbamide peroxide whitening of nonvital single discolored teeth: case reports. Quintessence Int 1999;30:155–61.

15. Caughman WF, Kovarick RE, Rueggeburg FA, Snipes WB. The bond strength of Panavia EX to air-abraded amalgam. Int J Prosthodont 1991;4:276–81.

16. Chan KC, Hormati AA, Kerber PE. Staining calcified dental tissues with food. J Prosthet Dent 1981;46:175–8.

17. Christensen GJ. Fluoride made it: why haven't sealants? J Am Dent Assoc 1992;123:89–90.

18. Coll JA, Jackson P, Strassler HE. Comparison of enamel microabrasion techniques: Prema Compound versus a 12-fluted finishing bur. J Esthet Dent 1991; 3:180–6.

19. Croll TP. Enamel micro abrasion: the technique. Quintessence Int 1989;20:395–400.

20. Croll TP, Cavanaugh RR. Enamel color modification by controlled hydrochloric acid-pumice abrasion. I. Technique and examples. Quintessence Int 1986;17: 81–7.

21. Croll TP, Sasa IS. Carbamide peroxide bleaching of teeth with dentinogenesis imperfecta discoloration: report of a case. Quintessence Int 1995;26:683–6.

22. Dean HT. Chronic endemic dental fluorosis. JAMA 1936;107:1269–73.

23. Denehy GE, Swift EJ Jr. Single-tooth home bleaching. Quintessence Int 1992;23:595–8.

24. Di Benedetto DC. Tetracycline staining in an adult. J Mass Dent Soc 1985;34:183–217.

25. Dickinson GL, Leinfelder KF. Assessing the long-term effect of a surface penetrating sealant. J Am Dent Assoc 1993;124:68–72.

26. Donoghue AM, Ferguson MM. Superficial copper staining of the teeth in a brass foundry worker. Occup Med 1996;46:233–4.

27. Ellingsen JE, Eriksen HM, Rolla G. Extrinsic dental stain caused by stannous fluoride. Scand J Dent Res 1982;90(1):9–13.

28. Eriksen HM, Jemtland B, Finckenhagen HJ, Gjermo P. Evaluation of extrinsic tooth discoloration. Acta Odontol Scand 1979;37:371–5.

29. Eriksen HM, Nordbo H. Extrinsic discoloration of teeth. [Review] J Clin Periodontol 1978;5:229–36.

30. Eriksen HM, Nordbo H, Kantanen H, Ellingsen JE. Chemical plaque control and extrinsic tooth discoloration. A review of possible mechanisms. J Clin Periodontol 1985;12:345–50.

31. Fayle SA, Pollard MA. Congenital erythropoietic porphyria—oral manifestations and dental treatment in childhood: a case report. Quintessence Int 1994;25: 551–4.

32. Feinman RA, Goldstein RE, Garber DA. Bleaching teeth. Chicago: Quintessence, 1987.

33. Fisher DE. Dental bleaching compositions and methods for bleaching teeth surfaces. US Patent #5,376,006, Dec 27, 1994.

34. Formicola AJ, Deasy MJ, Johnson DH, Howe EE. Tooth staining effects of an alexidine mouthwash. J Periodontol 1979;50:207–11.

35. Frazier KB. Aesthetic dentistry. Stuttgart: Georg Thieme, 1998.

36. Frazier KB. An overview of tooth whitening procedures. J Pract Hygiene 1998;7:32–33.

37. Friedman S. Internal bleaching: long-term outcomes and complications. J Am Dent Assoc 1997;128: 51S–5S.

38. Funakoshi Y, Ohshita C, Moritani Y, Hieda T. Dental findings of patients who underwent liver transplantation. J Clin Pediatr Dent 1992;16:259–62.

39. Garber DA, Goldstein CE, Goldstein RE, Schwartz CG. Dentist monitored bleaching: a combined approach. Pract Periodont Aesthetic Dent 1991;3:22–6.

40. Glickman GN, Frysh H, Baker FL. Adverse response to vital bleaching. J Endod 1992;18:351–4.

41. Golub J. Home bleaching may lure new patients. DENTIST Mag 1989;1, 35, 43.

42. Harrington GW, Natkin E. External resorption associated with bleaching of pulpless teeth. J Endod 1979;5:344–8.

43. Hayes PA, Full C, Pinkham J. The etiology and treatment of intrinsic discolorations. J Can Dent Assoc 1986;52:217–20.

44. Haywood VB. Nightguard vital bleaching: current information and research. Esthet Dent Update 1990; 1(2):7–12.

45. Haywood VB. Bleaching of vital and nonvital teeth. Curr Opin Dent 1992;2:142–9.

46. Haywood VB. History, safety, and effectiveness of current bleaching techniques and applications of the nightguard vital bleaching technique. Quintessence Int 1992;23:471–88.

47. Haywood VB. Bleaching and microabrasion options. Esthet Dent Update 1995;6:99–100.

48. Haywood VB. Achieving, maintaining, and recovering successful tooth bleaching. J Esthet Dent 1996;8(1):31–8.

49. Haywood VB. Bleaching tetracycline-stained teeth. Esthet Dent Update 1996;7(1):25–26.

50. Haywood VB. Bleaching of vital teeth. Current concepts. Quintessence Int 1997;28:424–5.

51. Haywood VB. Extended bleaching of tetracycline-stained teeth: a case report. Contemp Esthet Restor Pract 1997;1(1):14–21.

52. Haywood VB. Nightguard vital bleaching: construction of NGVB prosthetic. Dent Today 1997;16:86–91.

53. Haywood VB. Nightguard vital bleaching: current concepts and research. J Am Dent Assoc 1997;128:19S–25S.

54. Haywood VB. Whitening teeth by nightguard vital bleaching. Pract Rev Pediatr Dent 1998;8(6):1.

55. Haywood VB. Current status and recommendations for dentist-prescribed, at-home tooth whitening. Contemp Esthet Restor Pract Suppl 1999;3(1):2–10.

56. Haywood VB, Caughman WF, Frazier KB, Myers ML. Tray delivery of potassium nitrate-fluoride to reduce bleaching sensitivity. Quintessence Int 2001;32:1005–9.

57. Haywood VB, Heymann HO. Response of normal and tetracycline-stained teeth with pulp-size variation to nightguard vital bleaching. J Esthet Dent 1994;6:109–14.

58. Haywood VB, Heymann HO, Kusy RP, et al. Polishing porcelain veneers: an SEM and spectral reflectance analysis. Dent Mater 1988;4:116–21.

59. Haywood VB, Leonard RH. Nightguard vital bleaching removes brown discoloration for 7 years: a case report. Quintessence Int 1998;29:450–1.

60. Haywood VB, Leonard RH, Dickinson GL. Efficacy of six-months nightguard vital bleaching of tetracycline-stained teeth. J Esthet Dent 1997;9(1):13–19.

61. Haywood VB, Leonard RH, Nelson CF. Efficacy of foam liner in 10% carbamide peroxide bleaching technique. Quintessence Int 1993;24:663–6.

62. Heymann HO, Sockwell CL, Haywood VB. Additional conservative esthetic procedures. In: CM Sturdevant, ed. The art and science of operative dentistry. 3rd edn. St. Louis: CV Mosby, 1995:643–7.

63. Hodosh M. A superior desensitizer—potassium nitrate. J Am Dent Assoc 1974;88:831–2.

64. Holmstrup G, Palm AM, Lambjerg-Hansen H. Bleaching of discolored root-filled teeth. Endod Dent Traumatol 1988;4:197–201.

65. Jackson C Color me beautiful. New York: Ballantine, 1985.

66. Jerome CE. Acute care for unusual cases of dentinal hypersensitivity. Quintessence Int 1995;26:715–6.

67. Jordan RE, Boksman L. Conservative vital bleaching treatment of discolored dentition. Compend Cont Educ Dent 1984;5:803–5.

68. Kirkham WR, Andrews EE, Snow CC, et al. Postmortem pink teeth. J Forensic Sci 1977;22:119–31.

69. Lado EA. Bleaching of endodontically treated teeth: an update on cervical resorption. Gen Dent 1988;36:500–1.

70. Leard A, Addy M. The propensity of different brands of tea and coffee to cause staining associated with chlorhexidine. J Clin Periodontol 1997;24:115–8.

71. Leonard RH, Austin SM, Haywood VB, Bentley CD. Change in pH of plaque and 10% carbamide peroxide solution during nightguard vital bleaching treatment. Quintessence Int 1994;25:819–23.

72. Levin LS. The dentition in the osteogenesis imperfecta syndromes. Clin Orthop 1981;159:64–74.

73. Liebenberg WH. Intracoronal lightening of discolored pulpless teeth: a modified walking bleach technique. Quintessence Int 1997;28:771–7.

74. Lokken P, Birkeland JM. Dental discolorations and side effects with iron and placebo tablets. Scand J Dent Res 1979;87:275–8.

75. Madison S, Walton R. Cervical root resorption following bleaching of endodontically treated teeth. J Endod 1990;16:570–4.

76. Markowitz K. Tooth sensitivity: mechanism and management. Compend Dent Educ 1992;14:1032–46.

77. Materials and procedures manual. South Jordan, UT: Ultradent Products Inc., 1996.

78. McCormack K, Davies R. The enigma of potassium ion in the management of dentine hypersensitivity: is nitric oxide the elusive second messenger? Pain 1996;68:5–11.

79. McGuckin RS, Thurmond BA, Osovitz S. In vitro enamel shear bond strengths following vital bleaching. J Dent Res 1991;70:377.

80. Mertz-Fairhurst EJ, Smith CD, Williams JE, et al. Cariostatic and ultraconservative sealed restorations: six-year results. Quintessence Int 1992;23:827–38.

81. Meyboom RH, Verduijn MM, Steenvoorden MG, et al. Reversible tooth discolorations during oral use of antibiotics. Ned Tijdschr Geneeskd 1996;140:207–9.

82. Miles PG, Pontier JP, Bahiraei D, Close J. The effect of carbamide peroxide bleach on the tensile bond strength of ceramic brackets: an in vitro study. Am J Orthod Dentofac Orthop 1994;106:371–5.

83. Morisaki I, Abe K, Tong LS, et al. Dental findings of children with biliary atresia: report of seven cases. ASDC J Dent Child 1990;57:220–3.

84. Ness L, Rosekrans D deL, Welford JF. An epidemiologic study of factors affecting extrinsic staining of teeth in an English population. Community Dent Oral Epidemiol 1977;5:55–60.

85. Nordbo H. Discoloration of dental pellicle by tannic acid. Acta Odontol Scand 1977;35:305–10.

86. Nutting EB, Poe GS. A new combination for bleaching teeth. J South Calif Dent Assoc 1963;31:289.

87. Okafor LA, Nonnoo DC, Ojehanon PI, Aikhionbare O. Oral and dental complications of sickle cell disease in Nigerians. Angiology 1986;37:672–5.

88. Parkins FM, Furnish G, Bernstein M. Minocycline use discolors teeth. J Am Dent Assoc 1992;123:87–9.

89. Poliak SC, DiGiovanna JJ, Gross EG, et al. Minocycline-associated tooth discoloration in young adults. JAMA 1985;254:2930–2.

90. Primosche RE. Tetracycline discoloration, enamel defects, and dental caries in patient with cystic fibrosis. Oral Surg Oral Med Oral Pathol 1980;50:301–8.

91. Reichart PA, Lenz H, Konig H, et al. The black layer on the teeth of betel chewers: a light microscopic, microradiographic and electronmicroscopic study. J Oral Pathol 1985;14:466–75.

92. Reid JS, Beeley JA, MacDonald DG. Investigations into black extrinsic tooth stain. J Dent Res 1977;56:895–9.

93. Rendall JR, McDougall AC. Reddening of the upper central incisors associated with periapical granuloma in lepromatous leprosy. Br Oral Surg 1976;13:271–7.

94. Rosen T, Hoffmann TJ. Minocycline-induced discoloration of the permanent teeth. J Am Acad Dermatol 1989;21:569.

95. Rosenthal P, Ramos A, Mungo R. Management of children with hyperbilirubinemia and green teeth. J Pediatr 1986;108:103–5.

96. Rotstein I. Role of catalase in the elimination of residual hydrogen peroxide following tooth bleaching. J Endod 1993;19:567–9.

97. Salman RA, Salman DG, Gilckman RS, et al. Minocycline induced pigmentation of the oral cavity. J Oral Med 1985;40:154–7.

98. Scanlon N, Wilsher M, Kolbe J. Imipenem induced dental staining. [Letter] Aust N Z J Med 1997;27:190.

99. Schiodt M, Larsen V, Bessermann M. Oral findings in glassblowers. Community Dent Oral Epidemiol 1980;8:195–200.

100. Schwartz AG, Dunkel CE. The use of neutral sodium fluoride as a pre-bleaching treatment regime and its effect on dentinal sensitivity. [Abstract] National Dental Hygiene Association Meeting, New Orleans, 1998.

101. Settembrini L, Gultz J, Kaim J, Scherer W. A technique for bleaching nonvital teeth: inside/outside bleaching. J Am Dent Assoc 1997;128:1283–4.

102. Shillingburg HT, Hobo S, Whitsett LD, et al. Fundamentals of fixed prosthodontics. 3rd edn. Chicago: Quintessence, 1997.

103. Silverman G, Berman E, Hanna CB, et al. Assessing the efficacy of three dentifrices in the treatment of dentinal hypersensitivity. J Am Dent Assoc 1996;127:191–201.

104. Trope M. Cervical root resorption. J Am Dent Assoc 1997;128:56S–9S.

105. Vachon C, Vanek P, Friedman S. Internal bleaching with 10% carbamide peroxide in vitro. Pract Periodont Aesthet Dent 2000;10:1145–54.

106. Van der Burgt TP, Plasschaert AJ. Tooth discoloration induced by dental materials. Oral Surg Oral Med Oral Pathol 1985;60:666–9.

107. Waggoner WF, Siegal M. Pit and fissure sealant application: updating the technique. J Am Dent Assoc 1996;127:351–61.

108. Wahl MJ. At-home bleaching of a single tooth. J Prosthet Dent 1992;67:281–2.

109. Wolfe ID, Reichmister J. Minocycline hyperpigmentation: skin, tooth, nail, and bone involvement. Cutis 1985;33:457–8.

110. Zaia AA, Graner E, de Almeida OP, Scully C. Oral changes associated with biliary atresia and liver transplantation. J Pediatr Dent 1993;18:38–42.

Additional Resources

Goldstein RE. Esthetics in dentistry. Philadelphia: JB Lippincott, 1976:162–74.

Goldstein RE. Diagnostic dilemma: to bond, laminate or crown. Int J Periodont Restor Dent 1987;87:9–30.

Goldstein RE. Solving tooth color problems in esthetic dentistry. Presented at Hinman Dental Meeting, Clinical Topics in Dentistry, University of Nebraska Medical Center, #81, 1992.

Goldstein RE. Change your smile. 3rd edn. Carol Stream, IL: Quintessence, 1997.

Goldstein RE, Feinman RA, Garber DA. Esthetic considerations in the selection and use of restorative materials. Dent Clin North Am 1983;27:723–31.

Goldstein RE, Adar P. Special effects and internal characterization. J Dent Technol 1989;17:11.

Goldstein RE, Garber DA. Complete dental bleaching. Chicago: Quintessence, 1995.

Goldstein RE, Garber DA, Goldstein CE, et al. The changing esthetic dental practice. J Am Dent Assoc 1994;125:1447–57.

Goldstein RE, Goldstein CE. Is your case really finished? J Clin Orthod 1988;22:702–13.

Haywood VB. Current status of nightguard vital bleaching. Compendium 2000;21(Suppl 28):S10–7.

Haywood VB. Supervised at-home bleaching is safest, most effective. Dent Prod Rep 2000;May:82–91.

Haywood VB. Tooth whitening in your practice: treatment time and fee schedules. Contemp Esthet Restor Pract 2000;4(11):12–5.

Haywood VB, Heymann HO. Nightguard vital bleaching. Quintessence Int 1989;20:173–6.

Robinson FG, Haywood VB. Bleaching and temporomandibular disorder using a half tray design: a clinical report. J Prosthet Dent 2000;83:501–3.

Wolfe YL. Turn the white on: your healthy smile. Prevention 1997;May:49.

Chapter 17

Abfraction, Abrasion, Attrition, and Erosion

James W. Curtis Jr., DMD, Beverley A. Farley, DMD, Ronald E. Goldstein, DDS

Modern dental practices frequently encounter patients who exhibit various forms of wear to the dentition. The wear may present as abfraction, abrasion, attrition, and/or erosion. During their lifetime, many people will experience the effects of one or more of these conditions. The stresses of today's fast-paced lifestyle may lead to various habits that can directly cause or contribute to these problems. The etiologies of abfraction, abrasion, attrition, and erosion may be interrelated. Therefore, multiple conditions may be seen in a single patient (Figures 17–1A to C).

A review of the literature frequently reveals confusion, controversy, and contradiction concerning the terminology and etiology related to the loss of tooth structure due to noncarious processes. For example, erosion, as used in the dental literature, indicates the loss of tooth structure due to chemical dissolution. However, corrosion is the better term to denote the physical deterioration of a material (including teeth) by a chemical or electrochemical process. Erosion is actually the abrasive destruction of a material that occurs as a result of movement of liquid or gas, with or without solid

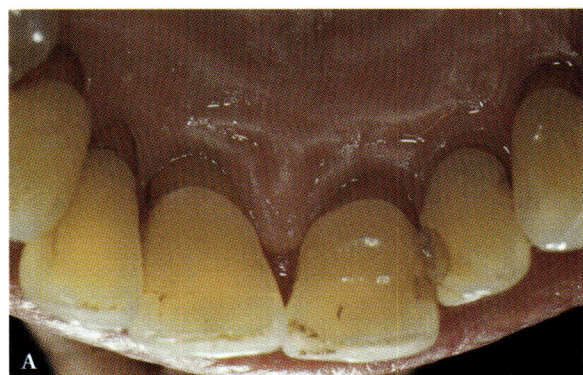

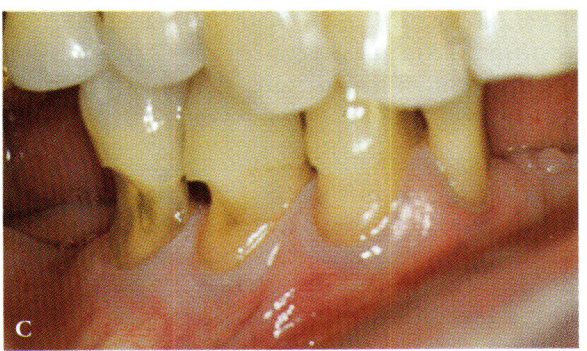

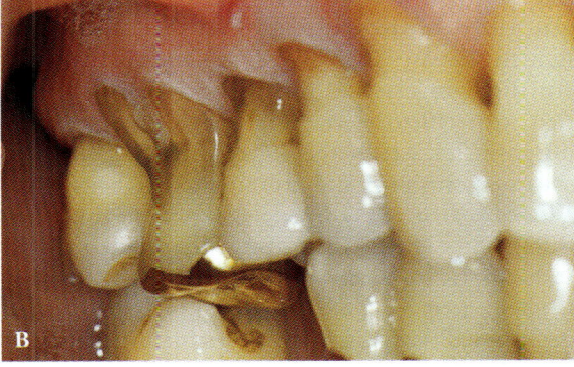

Figure 17–1A to C: These photographs illustrate the complex dental condition of a 71-year-old male: (A) The palatal cervical regions of the maxillary anterior teeth exhibit sharp, wedge-like lesions that are characteristic of abfraction. These areas would be difficult, if not impossible, to have resulted from toothbrush abrasion. (B) The buccal aspects of the maxillary posterior teeth show smooth, concave configurations that are consistent with toothbrush abrasion and/or erosion. (C) The buccal surfaces of the mandibular teeth have lesions that possess components of both abfraction (sharp margins in the occlusal regions) and abrasion (concave geometry and gingival recession in the cervical regions).

particles, over the surface of the material. In this chapter, each term will be defined in an effort to eliminate any confusion.

Often, the lines between the chemical and physical forces that cause noncarious tooth structure loss are blurred. When the etiologic factors of more than one of these conditions are simultaneously present, the resultant loss of tooth structure will be accelerated or magnified. As an example, bulimics who brush their teeth immediately after regurgitation may increase the rate of enamel loss. This is due to the greater effect of abrasion on acid-etched enamel. In assessing these various conditions, the possibility of multifactorial etiology should always be kept in mind.[93]

In the new millennium, it is important to recognize that wear of the dentition has been present since the origin of humankind. Young provides an extremely interesting summary of the literature relating to dental wear in the aboriginal populations of Australia and New Zealand.[113] The anthropologic studies of the University of Adelaide Dental School show the gamut of "development, progressive modification, and adaptability of the human occlusion to the demands of the environment before Western culture shock."[113] Through these studies, it was shown that human dentition was better able to withstand wear than the plaque-induced diseases that are primarily related to modern diets. In essence, these data support the fact that wear enhances the efficiency of teeth for the purposes for which they were intended: incising, shearing, crushing, and grinding foods. Begg wrote a series of articles on his analysis of prehistoric dentitions.[14–17] These articles provide insight into the orthodontic implications of dental wear as it relates to the preservation of dental arch integrity. Barrett determined that Australian aborigines with abrasive diets did not have significant malocclusion from a functional perspective.[6]

In 1958, Barrett noted that teeth in modern populations rarely exhibit the patterns of wear seen occurring in a natural fashion in aboriginal civilizations.[5] Herein lies part of the dilemma faced by the profession today. Radical changes in our environment and diet over the past few centuries have altered the extent and type of wear present in teeth.[64] These same dietary alterations have increased the prevalence of plaque-related dental diseases and the subsequent effects of such diseases.[61] Further compounding the picture are cultural shifts that have led to heightened awareness and the demand for esthetic dentistry.[109] Ultimately, as a profession, it is important that we recognize the anthropologic evidence related to tooth wear and the consequences of basic stomatognathic function on the longevity of teeth and restorations.

ABFRACTION

Abfraction is a wedge-shaped cervical lesion that results from repeated tooth flexure caused by occlusal loading. Other terms have also been suggested for this phenomenon, including noncarious cervical lesions and stress corrosion. Although these lesions have been recognized for years, their etiology has been debated. Numerous hypotheses were put forward over time to explain the cause of these lesions. The most common theory was that of toothbrush abrasion occurring independently or in conjunction with acid erosion.[88] However, the sharp angles and frequent subgingival location of these cervical lesions cannot be adequately explained by any of the previous hypotheses. It was not until the early to mid-1980s that the concept of tensile stress as the etiology of these lesions came to the forefront.[66,75,76] Sufficient experimental and clinical evidence has now been garnered to establish the primary etiology of these lesions as tensile stress of occlusal origin.[4,19,26,34,42,44,46,47,65,68,87,98] However, even in light of strong scientific evidence, this topic remains highly controversial.

As lateral occlusal forces are generated during mastication and parafunction, flexure of the tooth occurs at the cervical fulcrum (Figure 17–2). This flexure concentrates tensile stresses that disrupt the chemical bonds of the crystalline structure of enamel and dentin. Small molecules then enter the microfractures and prevent the reformation of the chemical bonds. Loss of tooth structure ultimately occurs in the regions of concentrated stresses. After the initiation of these lesions, they may be accelerated by acid erosion and/or abrasion.

When abfractions are restored, there tend to be relatively high failure rates if the occlusal problems that initiated the lesions are not corrected. This is true for both nonbonded and bonded restorations.[23,36,45,50,51,73,77,82,85,87] Although not reported in the literature, some clinicians suspect that the

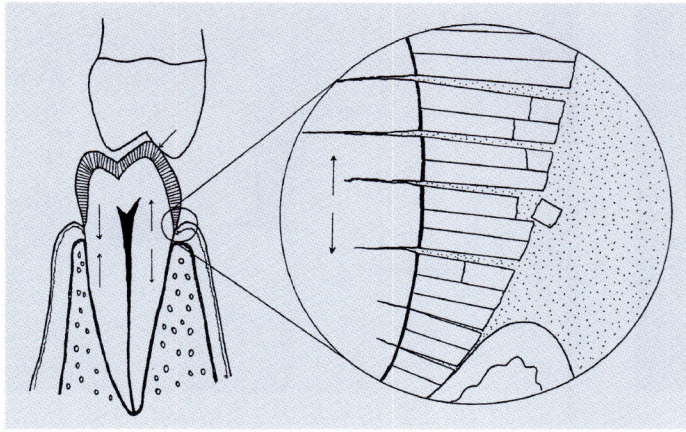

Figure 17–2: Model of tensile stress etiology of abfraction. Lateral forces create tension and compression in the cervical region, as indicated by arrows. Magnified section shows disruption of hydroxyapatite crystals of enamel and microfractures of dentin. When small molecules enter microcracks, re-establishment of chemical bonds is prevented. These areas are more susceptible to destruction from factors such as abrasion and chemical dissolution. (Reproduced with permission from Lee WC, Eakle S. Stress-induced cervical lesions: review of advances in the past 10 years. J Prosthet Dent 1996;75:488.[67])

occasional case of facial porcelain debonding in ceramic-metal crowns used to restore teeth with abfractions is caused by the same stresses that caused the original lesions. This apparently occurs when the facial crown margin has been placed at the same level as the apical aspect of the abfraction and the occlusal disharmony has not been corrected. Again, the key to restorative success for abfraction is control of the destructive occlusal forces that initially caused the lesions.

Case Studies

A 34-year-old female presented for routine examination. She expressed no complaints related to tooth sensitivity or occlusal dysfunction. Sharp angles of the cervical lesions on the mandibular left first premolar and first molar (mesial root) can be seen in Figure 17–3A. Although the lesions are darkly stained, the dentin and cementum are not cariously involved. There is no associated gingival recession on these teeth. Further clinical examination revealed other abfractions. Occlusal analysis demonstrated centric relation prematurities and a 2.5-mm left anterolateral shift from centric relation to maximum intercuspation. During left lateral movement, the patient exhibited group function, with the heaviest contacts occurring on the teeth with the abfractions (Figure 17–3B). The patient was questioned in detail after the clinical examination and eventually disclosed occasional muscle symptoms that helped support the diagnosis of nocturnal bruxism.

The case is a 42-year-old male with a complaint related to the space between the maxillary left central and lateral incisors. He reported that the space

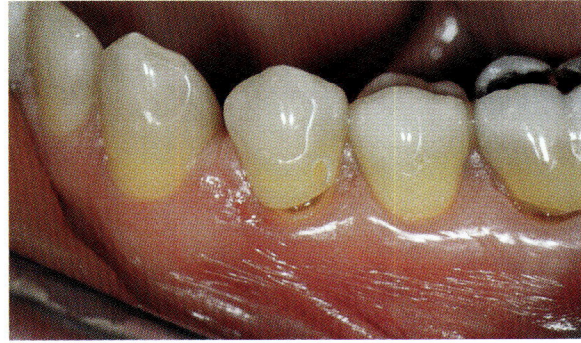

Figure 17–3A: This 34-year-old woman does not show caries or gingival recession associated with the cervical lesions of the first premolar and mesial root of the first molar.

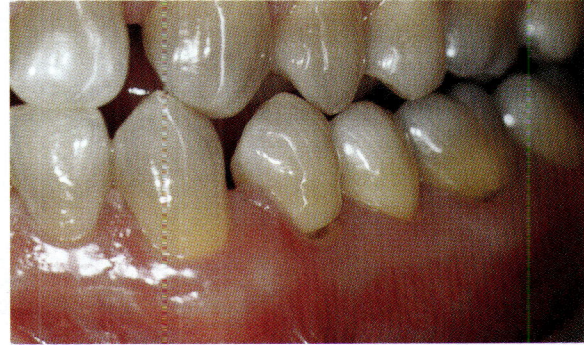

Figure 17–3B: During left lateral movement, the patient exhibited group function, with the heaviest contacts occurring on the teeth with the abfractions.

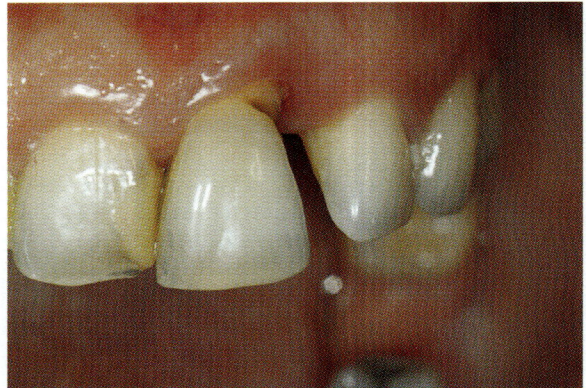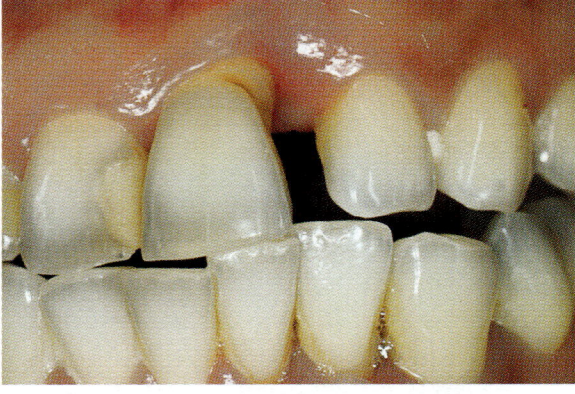

Figure 17–4A: This 42-year-old male has a space between the left lateral and central incisors.

Figure 17–4B: It is easy to see that traumatic occlusion could have played a role in the development of the cervical lesion on the distolabial area.

had been present as long as he could remember, but that it had increased over time. Although he was aware of the notching defect on the central incisor, he could not recall how long it had been present (Figure 17–4A). The abfraction extended from the midfacial to the distolingual line angle. The discrepancy in the sizes of the maxillary central incisors can be seen in the figure. There was significant gingival recession, particularly on the distal aspect of the left central incisor, that was accompanied by gingival inflammation and a probing defect of 4 to 5 mm. Further, there was a marked right shift of the dental midline and the solid contact between the maxillary and mandibular left central incisors in protrusion (Figure 17–4B).

This 28-year-old man has an asymptomatic abfraction with gingival recession on the maxillary right first premolar. The angle of the lesion is extremely acute and extends approximately 2 mm into the facial surface of the tooth at its greatest depth (Figure 17–5). Examination reveals malpositioning of the mandibular canine and a hint of abfractions on the mandibular premolars and shows a major mesiofacial wear facet on the affected maxillary premolar.

A 60-year-old woman presented with posterior bite collapse and poor health of the dentition despite having received extensive dental care over

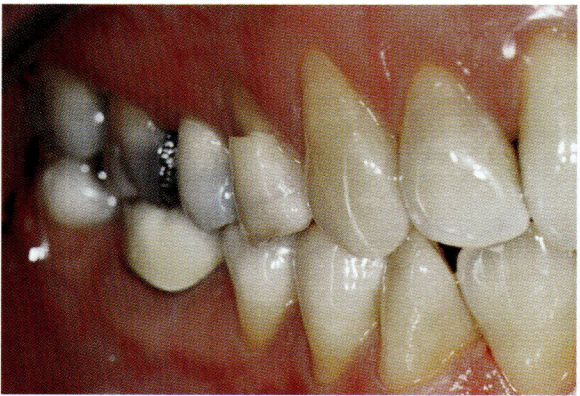

Figure 17–5: This 28-year-old man has asymptomatic abfraction and gingival recession as well as malpositioning of the mandibular canine and a major wear facet on the affected maxillary premolar.

Abfraction, Abrasion, Attrition, and Erosion

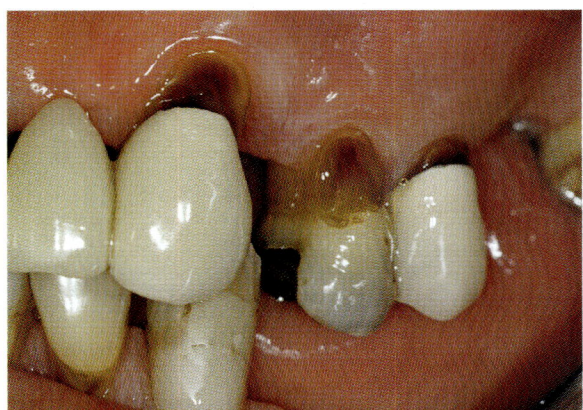

Figure 17–6: This 60-year-old woman exhibited stained abfractions on the maxillary cuspid and premolars that are noncarious but require restoration.

the years. Stained abfractions on the maxillary premolars and canine can be seen in Figure 17–6. Although the dentin was markedly stained, it was hard and noncarious. The mandibular left lateral incisor also exhibited an abfraction. Her mandibular partial denture (not shown) had been fabricated approximately 12 years previously and accommodated the gross occlusal plane discrepancy.

A 70-year-old male presented with an extreme loss of tooth structure owing to abfraction. Figure 17–7 shows the severe nature of the abfractions on the palatal surfaces of all posterior teeth on the right side. Both molars had exposures of the pulp chambers due to the abfractions. The pulp tissue in the second molar was clearly visible and vital, but the first molar was necrotic. Neither tooth was symptomatic. The maxillary left region was similarly involved. The mandibular arch also had generalized abfractions, but they were not as severe as those in the maxilla.

ABRASION

The loss of tooth structure due to repeated mechanical contact with objects other than teeth is termed abrasion. This process is considered to be pathologic. Any object placed against the teeth can cause abrasion. Evidence exists of various forms of abrasion in prehistoric populations.[2,24,39,40,110] A number of dental specimens recovered from the Sima de los Huesos Middle Pleistocene cave site in Spain exhibited a particular type of interproximal grooves between the posterior teeth. The grooves were found only in adults and were apparently caused by the habitual probing of the interdental spaces with rigid objects (ie, prehistoric toothpicks). Particles in the diet likely enhanced this abrasive phenomenon.[18] This same condition is seen in present-day societies. Other articles present information on various forms of tooth sharpening.[80,108]

Numerous oral habits cause abrasion; these are further discussed in Chapter 20. Examples of these habits include the localized occlusal defects seen in some pipe smokers who clench the pipe stem or individuals who chew on pens and pencils. Incisal notching is fairly common among seamstresses who hold pins or needles between the anterior teeth. Unusual cases of abrasion are reported in the dental literature and are discussed in Chapter 20.

Case Studies

The most conservative restoration of Class V defects is composite resin bonding. It generally requires little or no tooth reduction, thereby retaining as much tooth structure as possible to an already compromised tooth. A typical procedure can be seen in Figures 17–8A to I, which show a 45-year-old man with evidence of gingival and incisal abrasion, erosion, and abfraction. It is important to convey to patients that by treating these types of defects as early as possible, less tooth structure is lost and more enamel is present to enable a stronger bonded restoration.

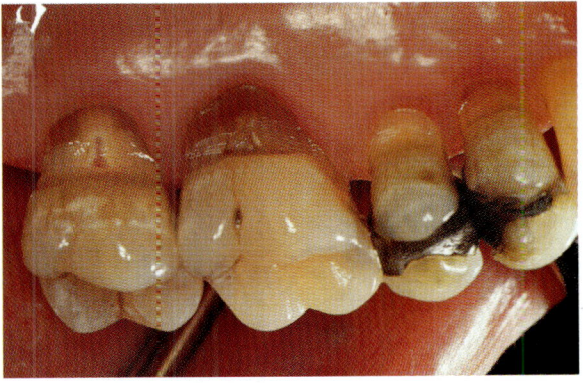

Figure 17–7: This is an excellent example of how extreme loss of tooth structure due to abfraction can exist and invade the pulp chamber without causing any symptoms.

506   Esthetics in Dentistry

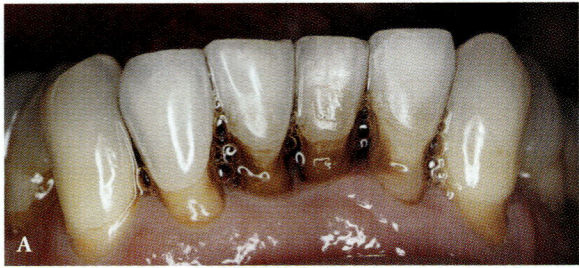 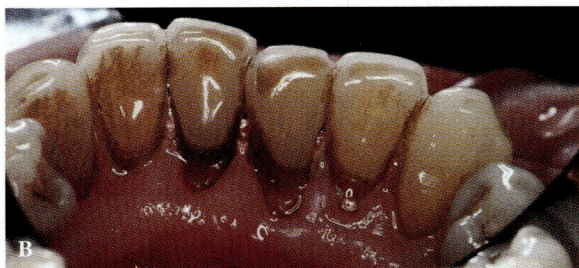

Figure 17–8A and B: This 45-year-old man shows extreme tooth loss due to combination lesions both gingivally and incisally of abrasion, erosion, and abfraction.

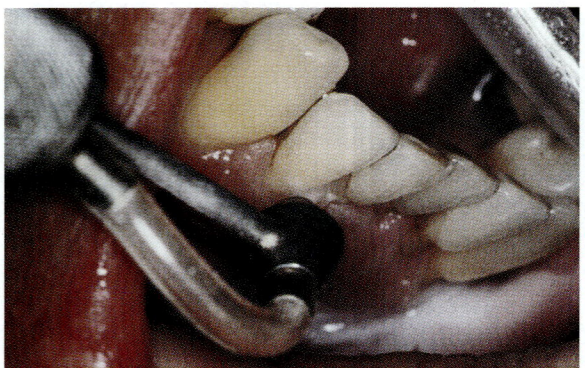

Figure 17–8C: An air polisher is used to remove stain.

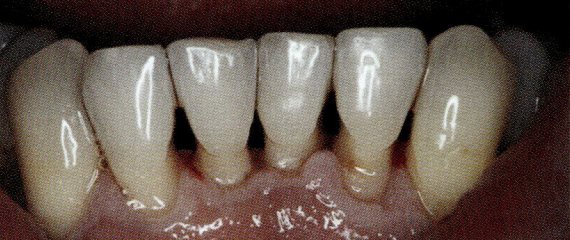

Figure 17–8D: Note how clean the teeth appear after a thorough prophylaxis with an air polisher.

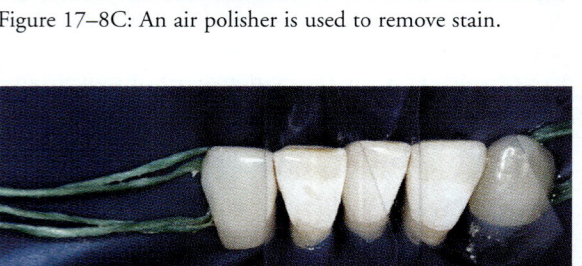

Figure 17–8E: A rubber dam is placed, mylar strips are applied, and the teeth to be restored are etched.

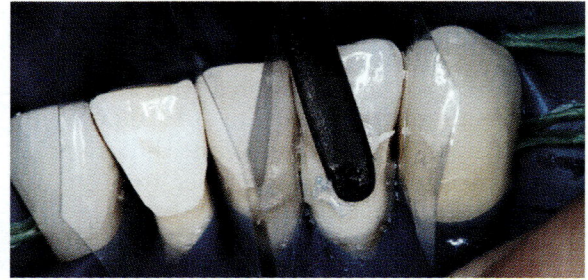

Figure 17–8F: A dentin/enamel bonding agent is applied, then a dentin/enamel resin, and finally an appropriate tooth-colored microfilled composite resin is placed using a Goldstein #3 composite instrument (Hu-Friedy, Chicago, IL).

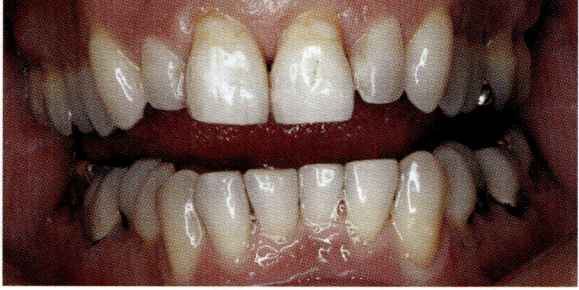

Figure 17–8G: Careful shade selection and attention to detail should produce an invisible margin.

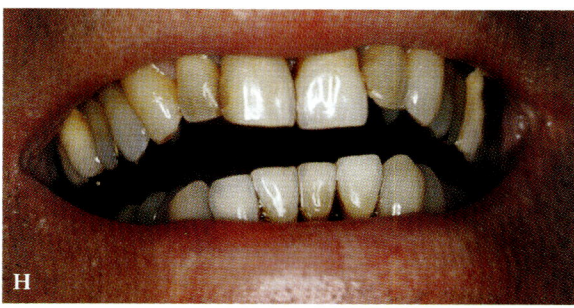
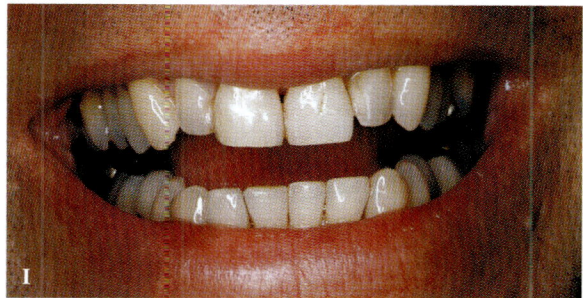

Figure 17–8H and I: Although early intervention is the best approach, restoring the defects at any point is both functionally and esthetically beneficial. Bonding is especially effective in preventing further damage to the tooth surface it covers.

Figure 17–9A shows a 29-year-old female who has abrasion and gingival recession confined to the anterior left segment, involving the canine and two incisors on that side. Closer examination revealed the smooth, rounded nature of the abraded areas (Figure 17–9B). Although she could not recall her specific age at the time, she reported that she was told by a hygienist that her brushing technique was improper when she was a teenager. She stated that she was instructed in brushing and flossing by this hygienist and had noted no progression of the recession since that time. For the past 8 years, she has been a patient in the same dental practice, and the clinical charting indicates that there has been no worsening of the problem. She has been informed about gingival surgery to correct the defects but has declined since she does not show her teeth when smiling.

ATTRITION

Attrition is the loss of tooth structure from tooth-to-tooth contact. According to the classic definition, attrition was considered to be a physiologic process occurring primarily from tooth contact during mastication. The wear from attrition may be seen on the occlusal surfaces of posterior teeth, the incisal edges of anterior teeth, the palatal surfaces of maxillary anterior teeth, and the labial surfaces of mandibular anterior teeth. The affected surfaces are usually hard, smooth, and shiny. However, the teeth may be sharp and jagged in certain cases. The areas of attrition may exhibit a yellowish-brown discoloration if the wear has penetrated the enamel. Wear may also occur interproximally, causing mesial drifting and broadening of proximal contacts.

Young mouths typically do not exhibit severe attrition. However wear may be seen in the primary and mixed dentitions (Figure 17–10). Numerous articles have reported on wear in children and adolescents.[1,8,53,78,79,84,95,96] As expected, increasing wear is seen with increasing age. This, as well as the fact that men exhibit more wear as they age, was demonstrated in a study of 586 subjects aged 45 and older.[35]

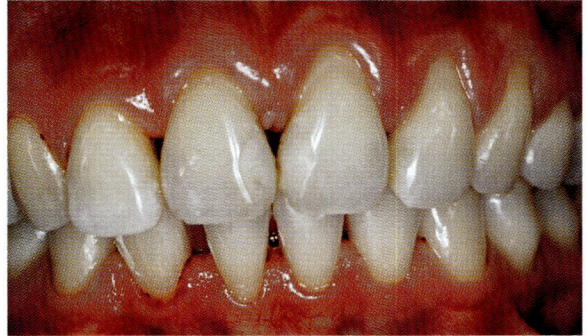

Figure 17–9A: A 29-year-old female with abrasion confined to the maxillary left canine and lateral and central incisors.

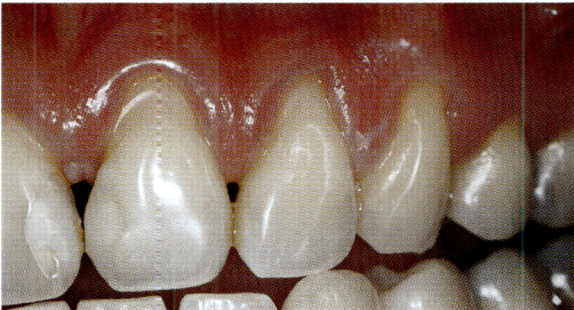

Figure 17–9B: Close examination reveals smooth, rounded, abraded areas that are suspected to be the result of improper brushing.

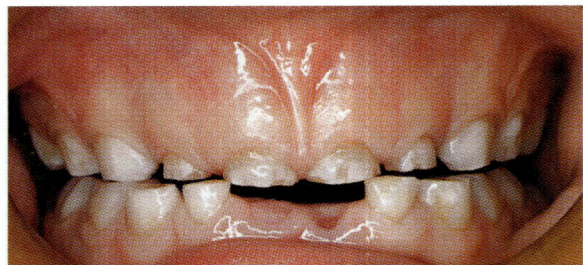

Figure 17–10: This young girl demonstrated severe wear and attrition in her mixed dentition.

There is growing evidence that attrition is more likely the result of pathologic conditions and environmental factors. Thus, the classic definition of attrition as an entirely physiologic process is being challenged. It is well established that teeth rarely contact during mastication, and there are many other factors that more likely contribute to this type of wear. These factors include bruxism, clenching, diet, malocclusion, and abrasive particles in the environment.[12,22,32,52,55,56,60,72,74,89,90,94,97] Dust in the tree top canopy has been shown to contribute to wear in primates.[107] Chronic exposure to dust and dirt can also cause increased wear in humans. This can occur in agricultural settings[49] or be associated with various industrial settings, such as cement factories.[102]

Bruxism

Bruxism can lead to extreme loss of occlusal and incisal tooth structure (Figures 17–11A to J). For example, a young woman was treated for her defective restorations in 1968 (see Figures 17–11D and E). Although she continued with routine maintenance appointments for a few years, she never accepted the advice to have a bite appliance constructed to treat her bruxism habit. Thirty-one years later, she returned with an extremely worn dentition as seen in Figures 17–11F, G, and H. Crown lengthening and full crowns were necessary to restore this patient's smile.

Bruxism may also produce abfractions in the cervical regions.[62] Patients with bruxism may experience symptoms of myofascial pain dysfunction syndrome or related disorders.[65,106] It is imperative to look closely at wear patterns in patients suspected of bruxism and evaluate for other signs and symptoms of occlusal dysfunction.

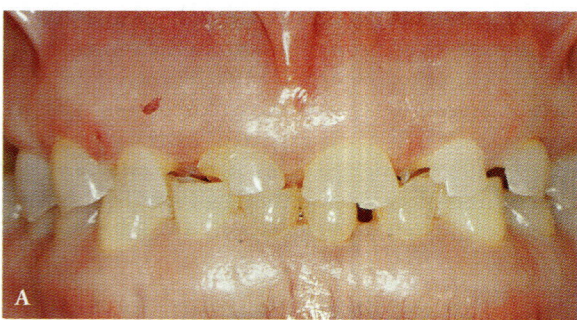
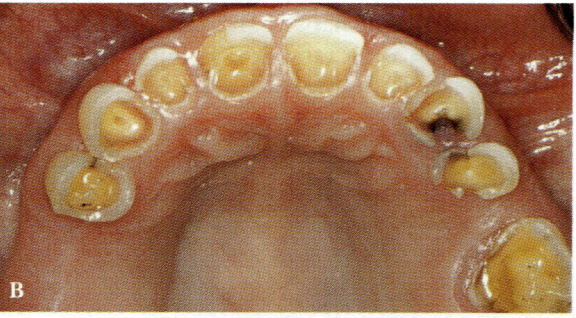
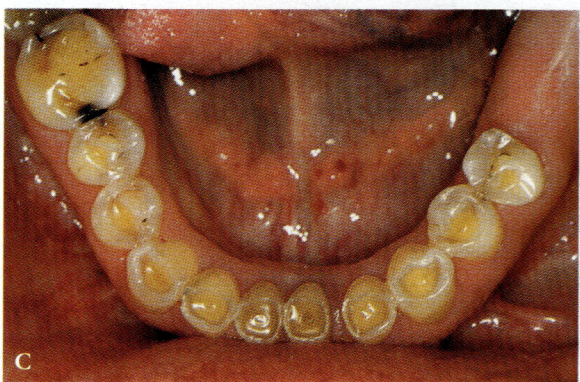

Figure 17–11A to C: This case illustrates the severe damage that can be caused by bruxism. The patient is a 56-year-old male who reports that his wife tells him he grinds his teeth while she is trying to sleep. He is also a farmer and is exposed to dust for extended periods of time for much of the year. The combined bruxism and environmental factors have likely contributed to the extreme wear present. As is most commonly seen with cases in which the wear progresses slowly, there has been no discernible loss of vertical dimension, as evidenced by lip position and speech patterns. Note the traumatic occlusal relationship when the patient is in complete intercuspation (A). Views of the severe wear of the maxillary and mandibular arches. Note the calcified, exposed pulp chambers and caries (B and C).

Abfraction, Abrasion, Attrition, and Erosion

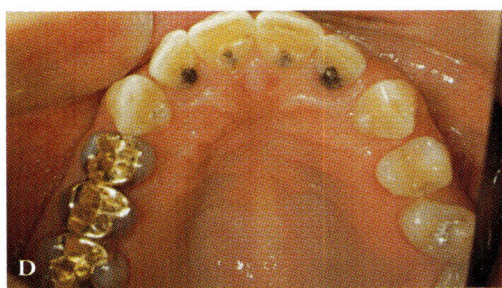 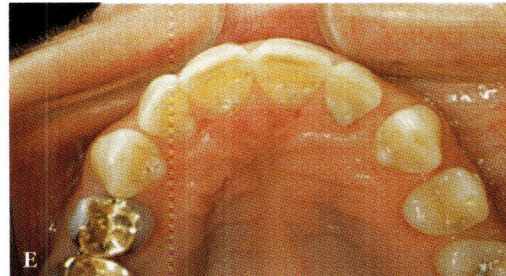

Figure 17–11D and E: This young woman's defective amalgam restorations were replaced in 1968 with tooth-colored restorations. At that time, and during the ensuing few years of maintenance recalls, she was advised to have a bite appliance constructed for her severe bruxism habit.

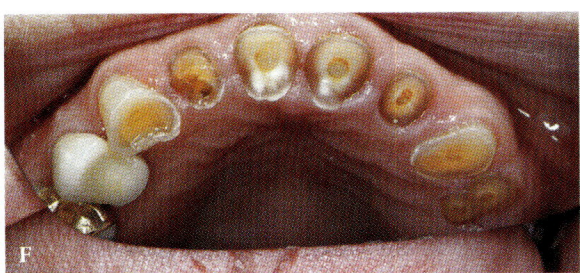 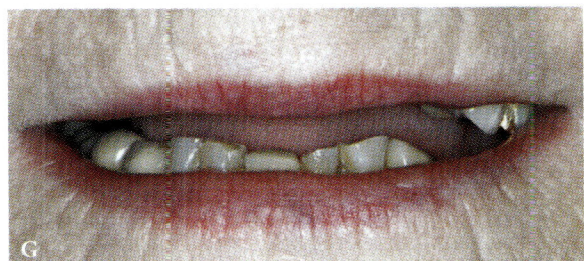

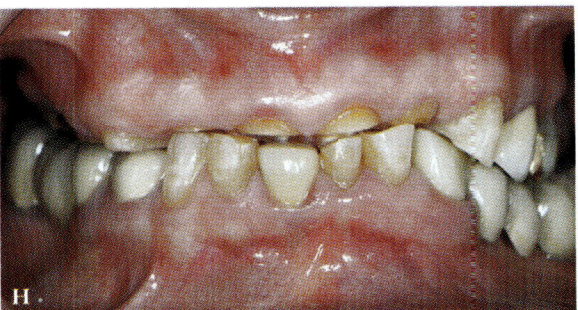

Figure 17–11F to H: She returned 31 years after her first appointment with an extremely worn dentition.

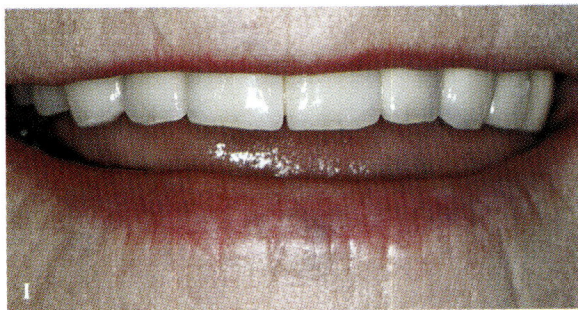 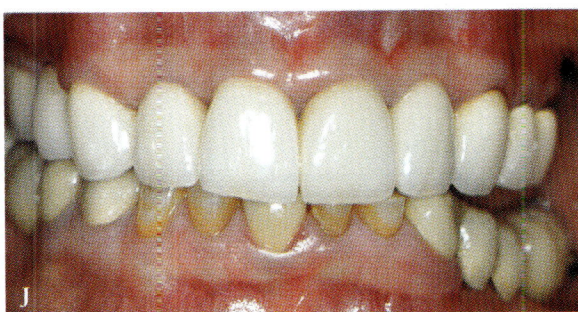

Figure 17–11I and J: Treatment consisted of crown lengthening and full crowns, which restored the patient's smile and her self-confidence.

Due to the gradual loss of tooth structure that most commonly occurs with bruxism, there is rarely loss of the vertical dimension of occlusion. Attempting to increase the vertical dimension is often the first thought of many dentists when planning the restoration of the severely worn dentition. This approach, however, may be ill advised. Instead, the use of various occlusal appliances may prevent or slow the loss of tooth structure and is highly recommended (if not mandatory) following occlusal rehabilitation of a patient with bruxism. Periodontal surgery to increase the clinical length of worn crowns prior to restoration is often a useful adjunct.[13] Nel and colleagues described a variety of techniques that can be used in restoring wear from bruxism.[81]

When the patient's main esthetic complaint is not showing enough tooth structure when speaking or smiling, several treatment alternatives should be considered. These include the following:

1. *Orthodontics.*[36,63] Repositioning the teeth should be the first treatment option when both functional and esthetic improvements can be achieved. Although patient motivation may not be easily obtained, the slow eruption of anterior teeth combined with functional orthodontic intervention can many times result in the ideal solution to this problem. Therefore, it is wise to seek an orthodontic consultation before providing the patient with alternative treatment plans.

2. *Prosthodontics.*[10,20,21,33,59,99] Depending on the patient's intraoral condition, it may be possible to formulate a restorative plan consisting of either reshaping mandibular anterior teeth to permit lengthening of the maxillary anteriors or slightly opening the vertical dimension. The best scenario is the patient who has worn the anterior teeth but has maintained vertical dimension with the posterior teeth. If this patient is treated with either direct composite resin bonding, porcelain laminates, or full crowns, it will be essential to make and insist that the patient wear a protective nightguard or bruxing appliance after the restorations are placed.

In most instances, it will not be easy to determine if the patient has actually lost vertical dimension. If esthetics is the primary motivating factor and the patient insists on a restorative solution, the best option is to determine if it is possible to slightly open (or restore) the vertical dimension. This can best be accomplished by slightly increasing the vertical dimension on a properly articulated, mounted set of diagnostic casts. A wax-up or mock-up using composite resin of the new occlusal scheme, at the increased vertical dimension, can be completed. An acrylic or composite resin appliance is then fabricated and cemented over the unprepared teeth. The patient should wear these temporary restorations for approximately 3 months to ensure that the new occlusal relationship is comfortable. If there is temporomandibular joint or muscle discomfort, the occlusion can be adjusted until the patient is comfortable. However, if it is necessary to adjust the occlusion to the previous vertical dimension, it will be impossible to continue with this plan of action. Instead, another option should be attempted: either orthodontics or rearranging the incisal guidance of the anteriors if function permits (Figures 17–12A to J). This usually requires shortening or beveling the mandibular incisors and lengthening the maxillary incisors.

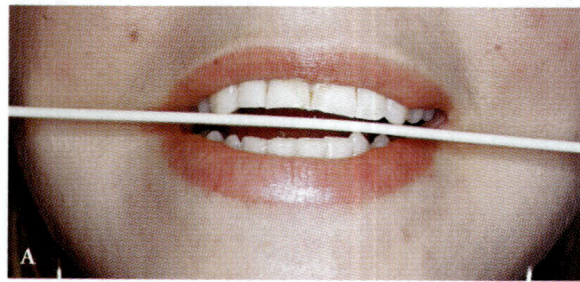 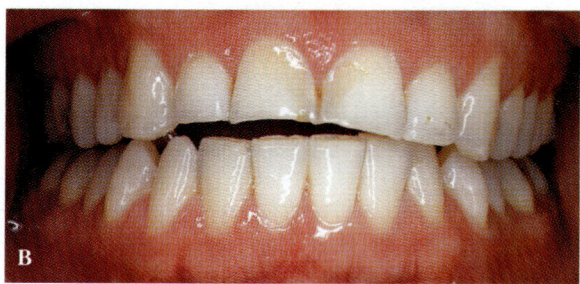

Figure 17–12A and B: This 23-year-old female presented with advanced anterior incisal wear.

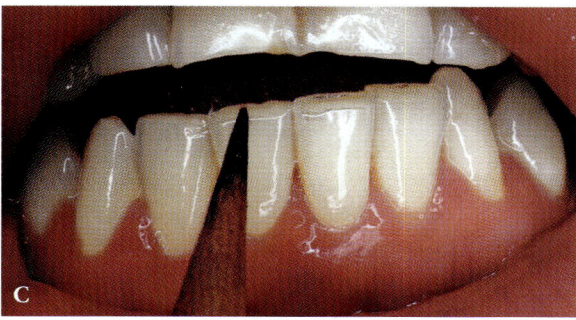
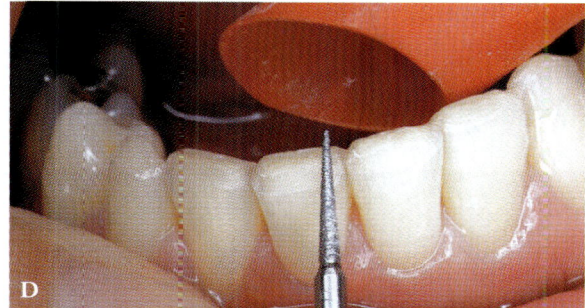

Figure 17–12C and D: The lower incisors were shortened and slightly beveled with a diamond stone.

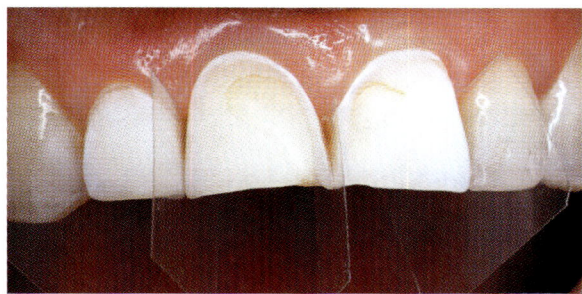
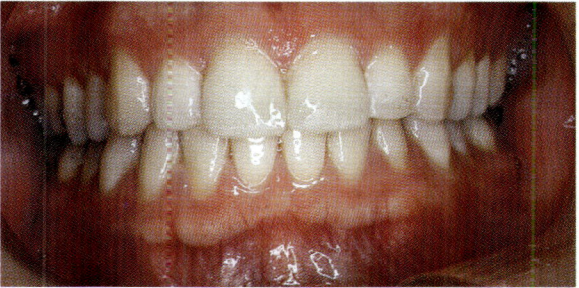

Figure 17–12E: The maxillary right lateral and central incisors were etched and veneered with composite resin to add length.

Figure 17–12F: The final result shows a younger-appearing incisal plane.

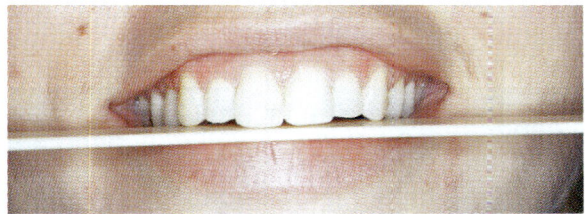

Figure 17–12G: Note the improvement of the smile line by comparing this figure with Figure 17–12A.

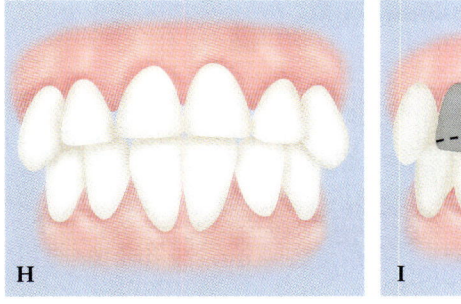
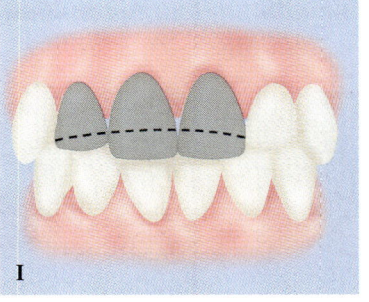
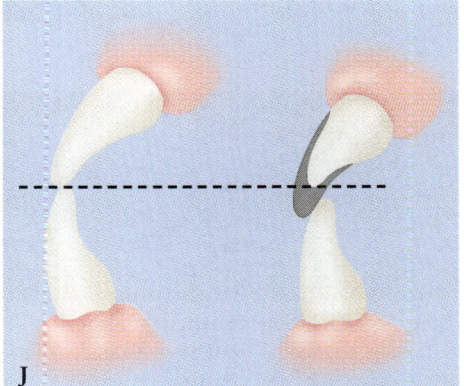

Figure 17–12H to J: These diagrams show how this procedure was accomplished. A balance was achieved by shortening and beveling the mandibular anteriors (J) to compensate for the lengthening of the maxillary incisal edges.

3. *Overlay denture.* In elderly patients, it may be possible to create the desired esthetics and functionally restore the lost occlusion with an overlay denture. This serves as an economic alternative and an interim solution (Figures 17–13A to H), especially when there is loss of vertical dimension.

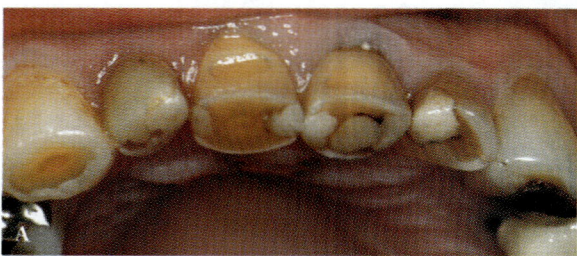
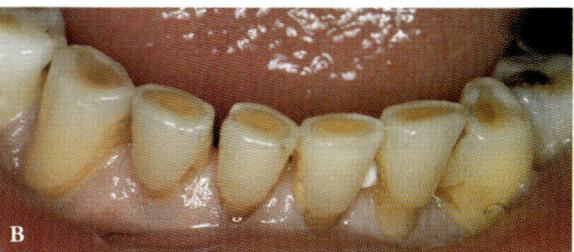

Figure 17–13A and B: This 70-year-old man showed advanced incisal and occlusal wear on both the maxillary and mandibular teeth.

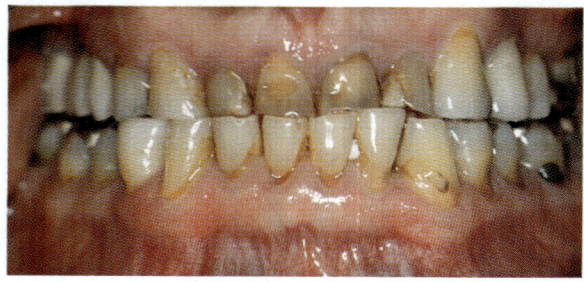

Figure 17–13C: The anterior view shows, in addition to advanced wear, that the maxillary anterior teeth are in crossbite.

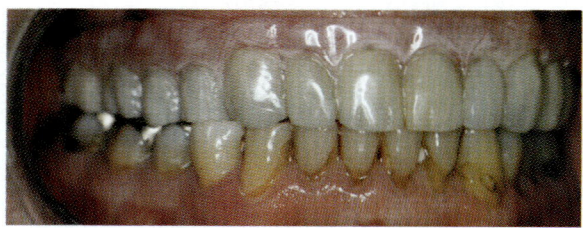

Figure 17–13D: A removable all-acrylic overdenture that was made to fit over the patient's natural dentition was constructed to correct the crossbite, improve esthetics, and restore the vertical dimension.

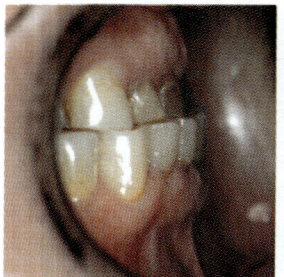

Figure 17–13E: The extent of the patient's crossbite can easily be seen in this lateral view.

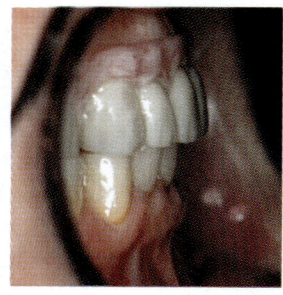

Figure 17–13F: The corrected crossbite seen in this lateral view also provided the patient with additional lip support.

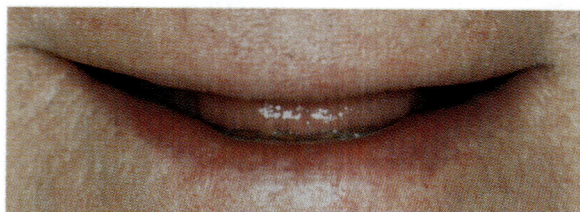

Figure 17–13G: The patient complained of looking older because he showed no teeth when he smiled. This was partially due to tooth wear and collapsed lip support.

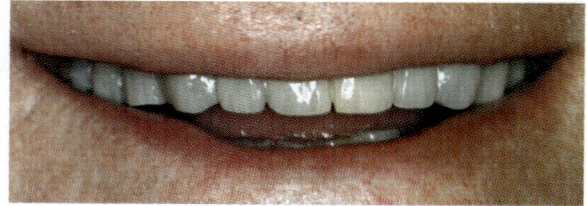

Figure 17–13H: Note the pleasing esthetics achieved with the removable overdenture, which provided increased support, correction of the crossbite, and additional tooth length.

Case Studies

This is a 24-year-old male who is a heavy bruxer. In addition to severe wear of the dentition, he had buttressing bone (tori) throughout the mouth, as shown in Figure 17–14. In the mandibular right second molar region, a piece of this dense cortical bone had become necrotic and was sequestrating.

The 29-year-old female shown in Figures 17–15A to D is an admitted bruxer. The total loss of the buccal cusp of the mandibular second premolar can be seen in Figure 17–15A and the wear of the lingual cusp of the opposing maxillary second premolar in Figure 17–15B. The static occlusal relationship is shown in Figure 17–15C. The working

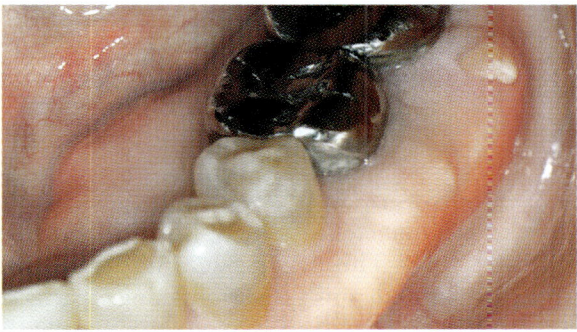

Figure 17–14: This 24-year-old male produced severe wear due to his heavy bruxing habit. Note the sequestrating bone in the molar region that had become necrotic.

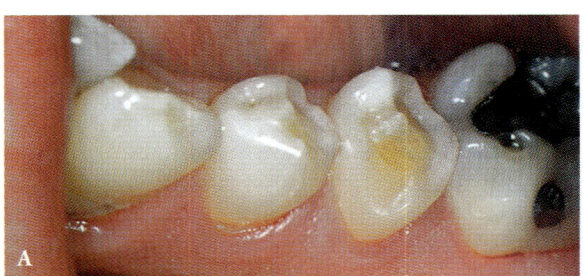
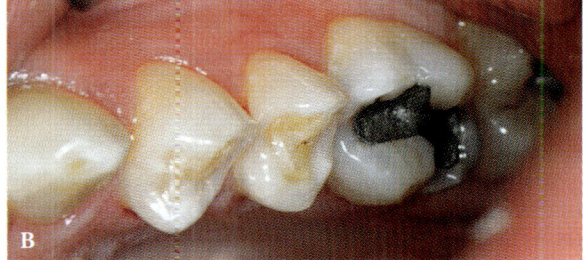

Figure 17–15A and B: Note the total loss of the buccal cusp of the mandibular second premolar *(A)* and the wear of the lingual cusp of the opposing maxillary second premolar *(B)* caused by bruxism.

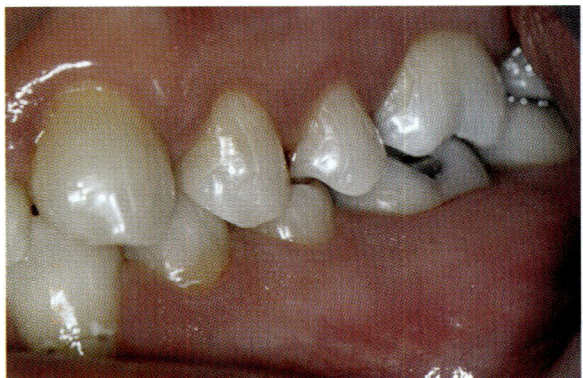
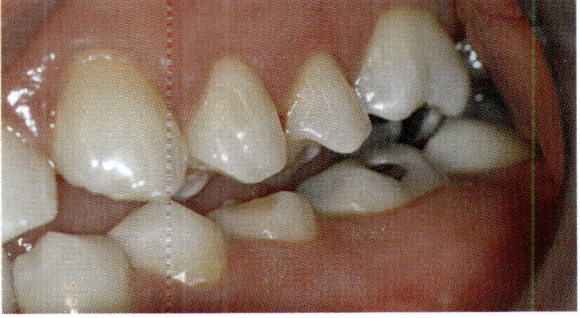

Figure 17–15C: This shows the occlusal relationship.

Figure 17–15D: The grinding may have been precipitated by the working prematurities between the maxillary first molar and the mandibular first and second molars.

prematurities between the maxillary first molar and mandibular first and second molars, shown in Figure 17–15D, may have precipitated the grinding.

EROSION

Dental erosion is a perplexing and frustrating problem. It is defined as the noncarious loss of tooth structure due to chemical dissolution not related to acids produced by dental plaque. It can present as a solitary lesion or involve a significant number of teeth. In certain medical conditions, such as gastroesophageal reflux disease (GERD) and bulimia, the erosive lesions have a characteristic pattern.[9,11,25,27,37,83,86,91,92,112]

There have been a number of theories regarding the etiology of erosion, and there are numerous extrinsic causes of erosion.[7,43,54,57,71,100] These include environmental, dietary, medication, and lifestyle factors. Chronic contact with acidic fumes in factories that produce or use acids has been cited as a notable cause of erosion.[29,30,101,103,104] Another environmental cause of erosion is prolonged swimming in pools with a low pH. Dietary factors receive widespread attention and likely affect the greatest number of people.[76] Wine has been shown to lead to erosion in wine makers,[38] wine tasters,[111] and wine merchants.[28] Carbonated soft drinks and other acidic beverages play a major role in the development of erosive lesions and dental caries.[3,41,48,58,69,105] Whether the causes are acidic foods or beverages, the frequency and time of consumption are major lifestyle factors that contribute to erosion. Certain medications[70] and oral hygiene products have also been implicated in the development of dental erosion. It is well known that a drop in oral pH below 5.5 initiates demineralization. Salivary flow rates and the buffering capacity of saliva also affect demineralization. Additionally, it has been postulated that extreme alkaline conditions promote chelation of calcium out of teeth. Treatment of these types of lesions should only be done when the causative problem is under control. Otherwise, restorations will have too short a lifespan, ending in esthetic failure. It is acceptable, however, to use provisional restorations during the corrective phase.

Case Studies

A 28-year-old woman had a severe bulimic condition over the course of many years (Figures 17–16A to C). However, she underwent successful treatment and desired to restore her smile. Since so much tooth structure had been eroded, it was necessary to place provisional restorations followed by crown lengthening (Figure 17–16D) and eventual replacement with the final ceramic-metal restorations (Figures 17–16E to G).

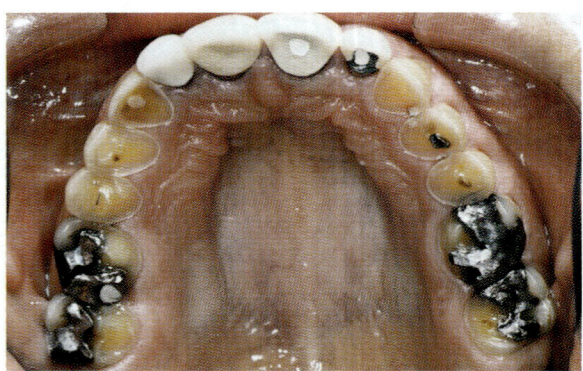

Figure 17–16A: This 28-year-old woman had a history of bulimia. After several years of therapy, she wanted to correct the damage caused by the bulimic condition. Note the severe occlusal erosion.

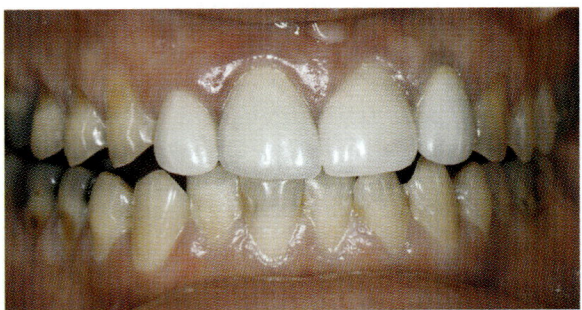

Figure 17–16B: The labial erosion seen here also contributed to the discoloration that bothered the patient.

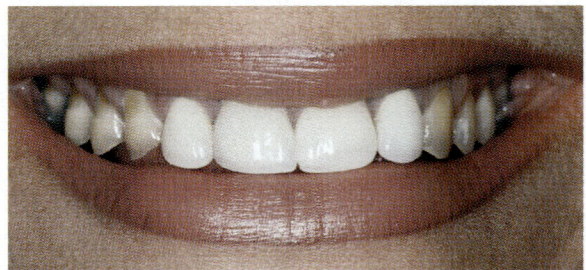

Figure 17–16C: This before picture shows the severe labial erosion present on the posterior teeth.

Abfraction, Abrasion, Attrition, and Erosion

This is a 62-year-old man with angina pectoris. He developed the habit of holding his nitroglycerine tablets between his teeth on the right side of the mouth. As a result of this unusual behavior, erosive lesions affected the right first molars. Figure 17–17 illustrates the defects on the mandibular right first molar.

DIFFERENTIAL DIAGNOSIS

Proper diagnosis is required to achieve successful treatment outcomes. As noted at the beginning of this chapter, patients may simultaneously have more than one of the conditions described. Thus, when occlusal or incisal changes are noted, the cervical

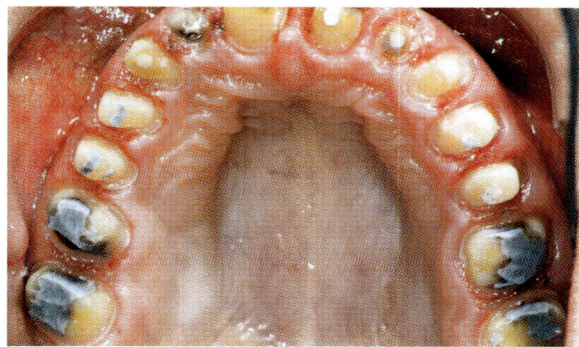

Figure 17–16D: Crown lengthening and build-ups with composite resin were necessary before making the impressions for the final restorations.

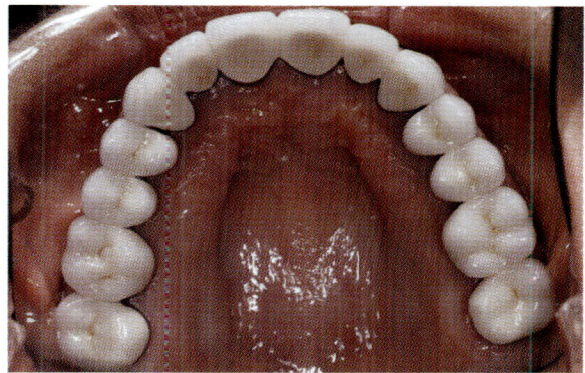

Figure 17–16E: The final splinted restorations were constructed using ceramic-metal.

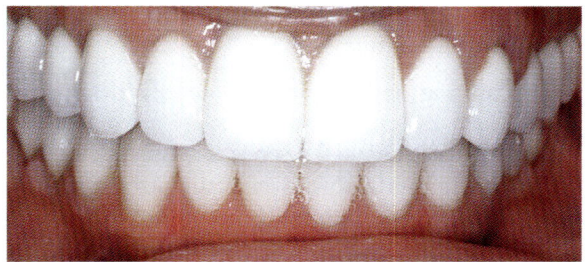

Figure 17–16F: The five splinted crowns restored this attractive lady's smile. Note how light a shade the patient selected.

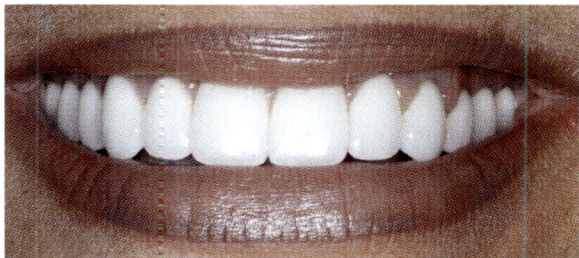

Figure 17–16G: The new, improved shapes and shade helped to accomplish the smile desired by the patient.

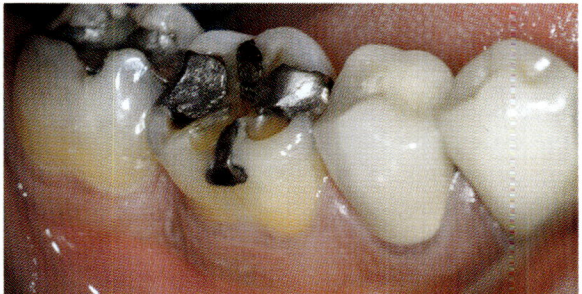

Figure 17–17: The habit of retaining nitroglycerine tablets between the teeth on the right side of the mouth resulted in erosive lesions as seen here on the mandibular right first molar.

regions of the teeth should also be closely examined. Likewise, the occlusal scheme should be fully evaluated if cervical notches or defects are found.

When evaluating a patient who has any of these lesions, it is necessary to correctly diagnose the condition and address the etiologic factors. Many patients with these conditions may be asymptomatic and/or unaware of them. In addition, they may have received "routine" dental care in the past and be surprised when these conditions are brought to their attention. In the case of bruxism, some patients are so surprised that they actually deny the problem. If this is the case, the best way to demonstrate to them that they have a bruxing problem is through visual images. A variety of means are available to illustrate the problem, including intraoral photographs, surgical microscopes, intraoral or extraoral video images, and diagnostic casts. With the aid of even simple visual references, the patient can be shown the extent of the damage that has been done and how he or she is causing it.[31] Once the patient is convinced of the problem, the next step is attempting to determine when it is occurring. If it occurs primarily during waking hours, the patient may be able to control or correct the problem. If it occurs during sleep, an appliance will be necessary to control the bruxing and/or prevent further damage to the dentition.

A key criterion when examining a suspected abfraction is the presence of lateral occlusal stresses during mastication or parafunctional movements. Thus, signs of attrition in the form of notable wear facets and/or loss of anterior guidance are highly probable when abfraction is present. The orientation of the long axis of the tooth in relation to occlusal loading should also be evaluated. The physical characteristics of abfraction are that of a sharp, angular defect, and these lesions may be located completely beneath the marginal gingiva. Abrasion in the cervical region can usually be distinguished from abfraction by the smooth, rounded nature of the lesion. Minimal to extreme gingival recession, with or without mucogingival defects, will likely accompany abrasion. Gingival recession may also be seen with abfraction but is not a hallmark of these defects.

Certain forms of abrasion are related to specific oral habits. The abraded areas may be localized, such as with pen or pencil chewing or with pipe stem clenching. Chapter 20 addresses these and the deleterious effects of numerous other oral habits.

Dental practitioners should have a high level of suspicion when they see generalized lingual erosion of the maxillary anterior teeth. Bulimia or GERD will be the likely cause. It is important to carefully obtain a history that will allow proper diagnosis. Individuals with GERD will more readily provide information that will assist in the diagnosis. Patients who suffer from bulimia may be reluctant to reveal their condition and are sometimes outwardly defensive when questioned concerning the issues related to their eating disorder. Often, however, a dentist may be the first medical professional to recognize signs of bulimia and can be instrumental in initiating an appropriate referral to address the overall condition.

Dentists must be diligent when they examine patients. They must look beyond the routine of caries, periodontal diseases, and missing teeth and closely evaluate patients for the loss of tooth structure due to noncarious processes. When these conditions are found, dentists must take the time to assess potentially interrelated etiologic factors by obtaining a proper history and performing a thorough clinical examination.

Discovering and helping to identify destructive habits, such as bruxism, needs to be a team effort. Frequently, the dental hygienist or assistant can be the observant individual who calls attention to a potential problem before it becomes an esthetic deformity. Team educational meetings are useful in teaching staff exactly what signs to observe. Knowing the correct anatomy of anterior and posterior teeth is of considerable value in being able to recognize even minor cusp or incisal edge changes that are a result of bruxism. Thus, the esthetics of the patient's smile not only depends on good oral hygiene but also becomes a shared team responsibility to keep it looking as good as possible throughout life.

References

1. Abreu Tabarini HS. Dental attrition of Mayan Tzutujil children—a study based on longitudinal materials. Bull Tokyo Med Dent Univ 1995;42:31–50.

2. Alexandersen V, Noren JG, Hoyer I, et al. Aspects of teeth from archeological sites in Sweden and Denmark. Acta Odontol Scand 1998;56:14–9.

3. al-Hiyasat AS, Saunders WP, Sharkey SW, Smith GM. The effect of a carbonated beverage on the wear of human enamel and dental ceramics. J Prosthodont 1998;7:2–12.

4. Bader JD, McClure F, Scurria MS, et al. Case-control study of non-carious cervical lesions. Community Dent Oral Epidemiol 1996;24:286–91.

5. Barrett MJ. Dental observations on Australian aborigines. Continuously changing functional occlusion. Aust Dent J 1958;58:39–52.

6. Barrett MJ. Functioning occlusion. Ann Aust Coll Dent Surg 1969;2:68–80.

7. Bartlett DW. The causes of dental erosion. Oral Dis 1997;3:209–11.

8. Bartlett DW, Coward PY, Nikkah C, Wilson RF. The prevalence of tooth wear in a cluster sample of adolescent schoolchildren and its relationship with potential explanatory factors. Br Dent J 1998;184:125–9.

9. Bartlett DW, Evans DF, Smith BG. The relationship between gastro-oesophageal reflux disease and dental erosion. J Oral Rehabil 1996;23:289–97.

10. Bartlett DW, Ricketts DN, Fisher NL. Management of the short clinical crown by indirect restorations. Dent Update 1997;24:431–6.

11. Bartlett DW, Smith BG. The dental impact of eating disorders. Dent Update 1994;21:404–7.

12. Bauer W, van den Hoven F, Diedrich P. Wear in the upper and lower incisors in relation to incisal and condylar guidance. J Orofac Orthop 1997;58:306–19.

13. Becker W, Ochsenbein C, Becker BE. Crown lengthening: the periodontal-restorative connection. Compend Cont Educ Dent 1998;19:239–40, 242, 244–6.

14. Begg PR. Stone age man's dentition. Am J Orthod 1954;40:298–312.

15. Begg PR. Stone age man's dentition. Am J Orthod 1954;40:373–83.

16. Begg PR. Stone age man's dentition. Am J Orthod 1954;40:462–75.

17. Begg PR. Stone age man's dentition. Am J Orthod 1954;40:517–31.

18. Bermudez de Castro JM, Arsuaga JL, Perez PJ. Interproximal grooving in the Atapuerca-SH hominid dentitions. Am J Phys Anthropol 1997;102:369–76.

19. Bevenius J, L'Estrange P, Karlsson S, Carlsson GE. Idiopathic cervical lesions: in vivo investigation by oral microendoscopy and scanning electron microscopy. A pilot study. J Oral Rehabil 1993;20:1–9.

20. Bishop K, Bell M, Briggs P, Kelleher M. Restoration of a worn dentition using a double-veneer technique. Br Dent J 1996;180:26–9.

21. Bishop K, Kelleher M, Briggs P, Joshi R. Wear now? An update on the etiology of tooth wear. Quintessence Int 1997;28:305–13.

22. Bishop KA, Briggs PF, Kelleher MG. Modern restorative management of advanced tooth-surface loss. Prim Dent Care 1994;1:20–3.

23. Boghosian A. Clinical evaluation of a filled adhesive system in Class 5 restorations. Compend Cont Educ Dent 1996;17:750–7.

24. Borrman H, Engstrom EU, Alexandersen V, et al. Dental conditions and temporomandibular joints in an early Mesolithic bog man. Swed Dent J 1996;20:1–14.

25. Bouquot JE, Seime RJ. Bulimia nervosa: dental perspectives. Pract Periodont Aesthet Dent 1997;9:655–63.

26. Braem M, Lambrechts P, Vanherle G. Stress-induced cervical lesions. J Prosthet Dent 1992;67:718–22.

27. Brown S, Bonifazi DZ. An overview of anorexia and bulimia nervosa, and the impact of eating disorders on the oral cavity. Compend Cont Educ Dent 1993;14: 1594, 1596–1602, 1604–8.

28. Chaudhry SI, Harris JL, Challacombe SJ. Dental erosion in a wine merchant: an occupational hazard? Br Dent J 1997;182:226–8.

29. Chikte UM, Josie-Perez AM, Cohen TL. Industrial dental erosion—a case report. J Dent Assoc S Afr 1996; 51:647–50.

30. Chikte UM, Josie-Perez AM, Cohen TL. A rapid epidemiological assessment of dental erosion to assist in settling an industrial dispute. J Dent Assoc S Afr 1998; 53:7–12.

31. Cook DA. Using crayons to educate patients about front-tooth wear patterns. J Am Dent Assoc 1998;129: 1149–50.

32. da Silva AM, Oakley DA, Hemmings KW, et al. Psychosocial factors and tooth wear with a significant component of attrition. Eur J Prosthodont Restor Dent 1997;5:51–5.

33. Darbar UR, Hemmings KW. Treatment of localized anterior toothwear with composite restorations at an increased occlusal vertical dimension. Dent Update 1997;24:72–5 [published erratum appears in Dent Update 1997;24:157].

34. Dawid E, Meyer G, Schwartz P. The etiology of wedge-shaped defects: a morphological and function-oriented investigation. J Gnathol 1991;10:49–56.

35. Donachie MA, Walls AW. The tooth wear index: a flawed epidemiological tool in an aging population group. Community Dent Oral Epidemiol 1996;24:152–8.

36. Douglas WH. Form, function and strength in the restored dentition. Ann R Austra Coll Dent Surg 1996;13:35–46.

37. Evans RD, Briggs PF. Tooth-surface loss related to pregnancy-induced vomiting. Prim Dent Care 1994;1:24–6.

38. Ferguson MM, Dunbar RJ, Smith JA, Wall JG. Enamel erosion related to winemaking. Occup Med 1996;46:159–62.

39. Formicola V. Interproximal grooving: different appearances, different etiologies. Am J Phys Anthropol 1991;86:85–7.

40. Frayer DW. On the etiology of interproximal grooves. Am J Phys Anthropol 1991;85:299–304.

41. Gedalia I, Dakuar A, Shapira L, et al. Enamel softening with Coca-Cola and rehardening with milk or saliva. Am J Dent 1991;4:120–2.

42. Goel VK, Khera SC, Ralston JL, Chang KH. Stresses at the dentinoenamel junction of human teeth—a finite element investigation. J Prosthet Dent 1991;66:451–9.

43. Grenby TH. Methods of assessing erosion and erosive potential. Eur J Oral Sci 1996;104:207–14.

44. Grippo JO. Abfractions: a new classification of hard tissue lesions of teeth. J Esthet Dent 1991;3:14–9.

45. Grippo JO. Noncarious cervical lesions: the decision to ignore or restore. J Esthet Dent 1992;4(Suppl):55–64.

46. Grippo JO. Bioengineering seeds of contemplation: a private practitioner's perspective. Dent Mater 1996;12:198–202.

47. Grippo JO, Simring M. Dental "erosion" revisited. J Am Dent Assoc 1991;122:41–7.

48. Harrison JL, Roeder LB. Dental erosion caused by cola beverages. Gen Dent 1991;39:23–4.

49. Healy WB. Soils and dental research. N Z Dent J 1998;94:114.

50. Heymann HO, Sturdevant JR, Bayne S, et al. Examining tooth flexure effects on cervical restorations: a two year clinical study. J Am Dent Assoc 1991;122:41–7.

51. Horsted-Bindslev P, Knudsen J, Baelum V. 3-year clinical evaluation of modified Gluma adhesive systems in cervical abrasion/erosion lesions. Am J Dent 1996;9:22–6.

52. Hudson JD, Goldstein GR, Georgescu M. Enamel wear caused by three different restorative materials. J Prosthet Dent 1995;74:647–54.

53. Hugoson A, Ekfeldt A, Koch G, Hallonsten AL. Incisal and occlusal tooth wear in children and adolescents in a Swedish population. Acta Odontol Scand 1996;54:263–70.

54. Imfeld T. Dental erosion. Definition, classification and links. Eur J Oral Sci 1996;104:151–4.

55. Jagger DC, Harrison A. An in vitro investigation into the wear effects of selected restorative materials on enamel. J Oral Rehabil 1995;22:275–81.

56. Jagger DC, Harrison A. An in vitro investigation into the wear effects of selected restorative materials on dentine. J Oral Rehabil 1995;22:349–54.

57. Jarvinen VK, Rytomaa II, Heinonen OP. Risk factors in dental erosion. J Dent Res 1991;70:942–7.

58. Johansson AK, Johansson A, Birkhead D, et al. Dental erosion associated with soft-drink consumption in young Saudi men. Acta Odontol Scand 1997;55:390–7.

59. Josephson CA. Restoration of mandibular incisors with advanced wear. J Dent Assoc S Afr 1992;47:419–20.

60. Kelleher M, Bishop K. The aetiology and clinical appearance of tooth wear. Eur J Prosthodont Restor Dent 1997;5:157–60.

61. Kerr NW. Dental pain and suffering prior to the advent of modern dentistry. Br Dent J 1998;184:388.

62. Khan F, Young WG, Daley TJ. Dental erosion and bruxism. A tooth wear analysis from south east Queensland. Aust Dent J 1998;43:117–27.

63. Kokich VG. Esthetics and vertical tooth position: orthodontic possibilities. Compend Cont Educ Dent 1997;18:1225–31.

64. Langsjoen OM. Dental effects of diet and coca-leaf chewing on two prehistoric cultures of northern Chile. Am J Phys Anthropol 1996;101:475–89.

65. Lavigne GJ, Rompre PH, Montplaisir JY. Sleep bruxism: validity of clinical research diagnostic criteria in a controlled polysomnographic study. J Dent Res 1996;75:546–52.

66. Lee WC, Eakle WS. Possible role of tensile stress in the etiology of cervical erosive lesions of teeth. J Prosthet Dent 1984;52:374–80.

67. Lee WC, Eakle WS. Stress-induced cervical lesions: review of advances in the past 10 years. J Prosthet Dent 1996;75:487–94.

68. Levitch LC, Bader JD, Shugars DA, Heymann HO. Non-carious cervical lesions. J Dent 1994;22:195–207.

69. Lussi A, Jaeggi T, Jaeggi-Scharer S. Prediction of the erosive potential of some beverages. Caries Res 1995;29:349–54.

70. Lussi A, Portmann P, Burhop B. Erosion on abraded dental hard tissues by acid lozenges: an in situ study. Clin Oral Investig 1997;1:191–4.

71. Lussi A, Schaffner M, Hotz P, Suter P. Dental erosion in a population of Swiss adults. Community Dent Oral Epidemiol 1991;19:286–90.

72. Mair LH, Stolarski TA, Vowles RW, Lloyd CH. Wear: mechanisms, manifestations and measurement. Report of a workshop. J Dent 1996;24:141–8.

73. Matis BA, Cochran M, Carlson T. Longevity of glass-ionomer restorative materials: results of a 10-year evaluation. Quintessence Int 1996;27:373–82.

74. Mayhall JT, Kageyama I. A new, three-dimensional method for determining tooth wear. Am J Phys Anthropol 1997;103:463–9.

75. McCoy G. The etiology of gingival erosion. J Oral Implantol 1982;10:361–2.

76. McCoy G. On the longevity of teeth. J Oral Implantol 1983;11:248–67.

77. Miller MB. Restoring class V lesions. Part 2: abfraction lesions. Pract Periodont Aesthet Dent 1997;9:505–6.

78. Millward A, Shaw L, Smith AJ, et al. The distribution and severity of tooth wear and the relationship between erosion and dietary constituents in a group of children. Int J Paediatr Dent 1994;4:151–7.

79. Milosevic A, Lennon MA, Fear SC. Risk factors associated with tooth wear in teenagers: a case control study. Community Dent Health 1997;14:143–7.

80. Murray CG, Sanson GD. Thegosis—a critical review. Aust Dent J 1998;43:192–8.

81. Nel JC, Marais JT, van Vuuren PA. Various methods of achieving restoration of tooth structure loss due to bruxism. J Esthet Dent 1996;8:183–8.

82. Neo J, Chew CL. Direct tooth-colored materials for noncarious lesions: a 3-year clinical report. Quintessence Int 1995;27:183–8.

83. Nunn JH. Prevalence of dental erosion and the implications for oral health. Eur J Oral Sci 1996;104:156–61.

84. Nystrom M, Kononen M, Alaluusua S, et al. Development of horizontal tooth wear in maxillary anterior teeth from five to 18 years of age. J Dent Res 1990;69:1765–70.

85. Osborne-Smith KL, Burke FJ, Farlane TM, Wilson NH. Effect of restored and unrestored non-carious cervical lesions on the fracture resistance of previously restored maxillary premolar teeth. J Dent 1998;26:427–33.

86. O'Sullivan EA, Curzon ME, Roberts GJ, et al. Gastroesophageal reflux in children and its relationship to erosion of primary and permanent teeth. Eur J Oral Sci 1998;106:765–9.

87. Powell LV, Johnson GH, Gordon GE. Factors associated with clinical success of cervical abrasion/erosion restorations. Oper Dent 1995;20:7–13.

88. Radentz WH, Barnes GP, Cutright DE. A survey of factors possibly associated with cervical abrasion of tooth surfaces. J Periodontol 1976;47:148–54.

89. Richards LC, Miller SL. Relationships between age and dental attrition in Australian aboriginals. Am J Phys Anthropol 1991;84:159–64.

90. Ritchard A, Welsh AH, Donnelly C. The association between occlusion and attrition. Aust Orthod J 1992;12:138–42.

91. Ruffs JC, Koch MO, Perkins S. Bulimia: dentomedical complications. Gen Dent 1992;40:22–5.

92. Rytomaa I, Jarvinen V, Kanerva R, Heinonen OP. Bulimia and tooth erosion. Acta Odontol Scand 1998;56:36–40.

93. Seow WK. Clinical diagnosis of enamel defects: pitfalls and practical guidelines. Int Dent J 1997;47:173–82.

94. Shaw L. The epidemiology of tooth wear. Eur J Prosthodont Restor Dent 1997;5:153–6.

95. Silness J, Berge M, Johannessen G. Longitudinal study of incisal tooth wear in children and adolescents. Eur J Oral Sci 1995;103:90–4.

96. Silness J, Berge M, Johannessen G. Re-examination of incisal tooth wear in children and adolescents. J Oral Rehabil 1997;24:405–9.

97. Smith BG, Robb ND. The prevalence of toothwear in 1007 dental patients. J Oral Rehabil 1996;23:232–9.

98. Spranger H. Investigation into the genesis of angular lesions at the cervical region of teeth. Quintessence Int 1995;26:183–8.

99. Stewart B. Restoration of the severely worn dentition using a systematized approach for a predictable prognosis. Int J Periodont Rest Dent 1998;18:46–57.

100. ten Cate JM, Imfeld T. Dental erosion, summary. Eur J Oral Sci 1996;104:241–4.

101. Touminen M, Touminen R. Dental erosion and associated factors among factory workers exposed to inorganic acid fumes. Proc Finn Dent Soc 1991;87:359–64.

102. Touminen M, Touminen R. Tooth surface loss among people exposed to cement and stone dust in the work environment in Tanzania. Community Dent Health 1991;8:233–8.

103. Touminen M, Touminen R. Tooth surface loss and associated factors among factory workers in Finland and Tanzania. Community Dent Health 1992;9:143–50.

104. Touminen ML, Touminen RJ, Fubusa F, Mgalula N. Tooth surface loss and exposure to organic and inorganic acid fumes in workplace air. Community Dent Oral Epidemiol 1991;19:217–20.

105. Touyz LZ. The acidity (pH) and buffering capacity of Canadian fruit juice and dental implications. J Can Dent Assoc 1994;60:454–48.

106. Tsolka P, Walter JD, Wilson RF, Preiskel HW. Occlusal variable, bruxism and temporomandibular disorders: a clinical and kinesiographic assessment. J Oral Rehabil 1995;22:849–56.

107. Ungar PS, Teaford MF, Glander KE, Pastor RF. Dust accumulation in the canopy: a potential cause of dental microwear in primates. Am J Phys Anthropol 1995;97:93–9.

108. Ungar PS, Fennell KJ, Gordon K, Trinkaus E. Neanderthal incisor beveling. J Hum Evol 1997;32:407–21.

109. Vallitu PK, Vallitu AS, Lassila VP. Dental aesthetics—a survey of attitudes in different groups of patients. J Dent 1996;24:335–8.

110. Villa G, Giacobini G. Subvertical grooves of interproximal facets in Neanderthal posterior teeth. Am J Phys Anthropol 1995;96:51–62.

111. Wiktorsson AM, Zimmerman M, Angmar-Mansson B. Erosive tooth wear: prevalence and severity in Swedish winetasters. Eur J Oral Sci 1997;105:544–50.

112. Yettram AL, Wright KWJ, Rickard HM. Finite element stress analysis of the crowns of normal and restored teeth. J Dent Res 1976;55:1004–11.

113. Young WG. Anthropology, tooth wear, and occlusion ab origine. J Dent Res 1998;77:1860–3.

Additional Resources

Abdullah A, Sherfudhin H, Omar R, Johansson A. Prevalence of occlusal tooth wear and its relationship to lateral and protrusive contact schemes in a young adult Indian population. Acta Odontol Scand 1994;52:191–7.

al-Hiyasat AS, Saunders WP, Sharkey SW, et al. Investigation of human enamel wear against four dental ceramics and gold. J Dent 1998;26:487–95.

al-Hiyasat AS, Saunders WP, Sharkey SW, et al. The abrasive effect of glazed, unglazed, and polished porcelain on the wear of human enamel, and the influence of carbonated soft drinks on the rate of wear. Int J Prosthodont 1997;10:269–82.

Altshuler BD. Eating disorder patients. Recognition and intervention. J Dent Hyg 1990;64:119–25.

Attin T, Koidl U, Buchalla W, et al. Correlations of microhardness and wear in differently eroded bovine dental enamel. Arch Oral Biol 1997;42:243–50.

Attin T, Zirkel C, Hellwig E. Brushing abrasion of eroded dentin after application of sodium fluoride solutions. Caries Res 1998;32:344–50.

Beckett H. Dental abrasion caused by a cobalt-chromium denture base. Eur J Prosthodont Restor Dent 1995;3:209–10.

Berge M, Johannessen G, Silness J. Relationship between alignment conditions of teeth in anterior segments and incisal wear. J Oral Rehabil 1996;23:717–21.

Blair FM, Thomason JM, Smith DG. The traumatic anterior overbite. Dent Update 1997;24:144–52.

Bohmer CJ, Klinkenberg-Knol EC, Niezen-de Boer MC, et al. Dental erosions and gastro-oesophageal reflux disease in institutionalized intellectually disabled individuals. Oral Dis 1997;3:272–5.

Bowles WH, Wilkinson MR, Wagner MJ, Woody RD. Abrasive particles in tobacco products: a possible factor in dental attrition. J Am Dent Assoc 1995;126:327–31.

Brady JM, Woody RD. Scanning microscopy of cervical erosion. J Am Dent Assoc 1977;94:726–9.

Briggs P, Bishop K. Fixed prostheses in the treatment of tooth wear. Eur J Prosthodont Restor Dent 1997;5:175–80.

Briggs PF, Bishop K, Djemal S. The clinical evolution of the 'Dahl Principle.' Br Dent J 1997;183:171–6.

Burke FJ, Whitehead SA, McCaughey AD. Contemporary concepts in the pathogenesis of the Class V non-carious lesion. Dent Update 1995;22:28–32.

Carlson-Mann LD. Recognition and management of occlusal disease from a hygienist's perspective. Probe 1996;30:196–7.

Donachie MA, Walls AW. Assessment of tooth wear in an ageing population. J Dent 1995;23:157–64.

Douglas WH. Considerations for modeling. Dent Mater 1996;12:203–7.

Evans RD. Orthodontics and the creation of localised inter-occlusal space in cases of anterior tooth wear. Eur J Prosthodont Restor Dent 1997;5:69–73.

Goldstein RE. Esthetics in dentistry. Philadelphia: JB Lippincott, 1976:162–74

Goldstein RE. Current concepts in esthetic treatment. Proceedings of the Second International Prosthodontic Congress; 1979; Los Angeles, CA, Chicago: Quintessence, 1979:310–2.

Goldstein RE. Esthetics in dentistry. J Am Dent Assoc 1982;104:301–2.

Goldstein RE. Diagnostic dilemma: to bond, laminate, or crown? Int J Periodont Restor Dent 1987;87(5):9–30.

Goldstein RE. Finishing of composites and laminates. Dent Clin North Am 1989;33:305–18.

Goldstein RE, Feinman RA, Garber DA. Esthetic considerations in the selection and use of restorative materials. Dent Clin North Am 1983;27:723–31.

Goldstein RE, Garber DA, Schwartz CG, Goldstein CE. Patient maintenance of esthetic restorations. J Am Dent Assoc 1992;123:61–6.

Goldstein RE, Garber DA, Goldstein CE, et al. The changing esthetic dental practice. J Am Dent Assoc 1994;125:1447–57.

Gregory-Head B, Curtis DA. Erosion caused by gastroesophageal reflux: diagnostic considerations. J Prosthodont 1997;6:278–85.

Hacker CH, Wagner WC, Razzoog ME. An in vitro investigation of the wear of enamel on porcelain and gold in saliva. J Prosthet Dent 1996;75:14–7.

Haines DJ, Berry DC, Poole DFG. Behavior of tooth enamel under load. J Dent Res 1963;42:885–8.

Hazelton LR, Faine MP. Diagnosis and dental management of eating disorder patients. Int J Prosthodont 1996;9:65–73.

Imfeld T. Prevention of progression of dental erosion by professional and individual prophylactic measures. Eur J Oral Sci 1996;104:215–20.

Irish JD, Turner CG 2nd. Brief communication: first evidence of LSAMAT in non-native Americans: historic Senegalese from West Africa. Am J Phys Anthropol 1997;102:141–6.

Isacsson G, Bodin L, Selden A, Barregard L. Variability in the quantification of abrasion on the Bruxcore device. J Orofac Pain 1996;10:362–8.

Johansson A. A cross-cultural study of occlusal tooth wear. Swed Dent J Suppl 1992;86:1–59.

Kaidonis JA, Richards LC, Townsend GC, Tansley GD. Wear of human enamel: a quantitative in vitro assessment. J Dent Res 1998;77:1983–90.

Kiliaridis S, Johansson A, Haraldson T, et al. Craniofacial morphology, occlusal traits, and bite force in persons with advanced occlusal tooth wear. Am J Orthodont Dentofac Orthop 1995;107:286–92.

Knight DJ, Leroux BG, Zhu C, et al. A longitudinal study of tooth wear in orthodontically treated patients. Am J Orthod Dentofac Orthop 1997;112:194–202.

Lambrechts P, van Meerbeek B, Perdigao J, et al. Restorative therapy for erosive lesions. Eur J Oral Sci 1996;104:229–40.

Leinfelder KF, Yarnell G. Occlusion and restorative materials. Dent Clin North Am 1995;39:355–61.

Lussi A. Dental erosion clinical diagnosis and case history taking. Eur J Oral Sci 1996;104:191–8.

Lyttle HA, Sidhu N, Smyth B. A study of the classification and treatment of noncarious cervical lesions by general practitioners. J Prosthet Dent 1998;79:342–6.

Magnusson T. Is snuff a potential risk factor in occlusal wear? Swed Dent J 1991;15:125–32.

McIntyre JM. Erosion. Aust Prosthodont J 1992;6:17–25.

Meurman JH, ten Cate JM. Pathogenesis and modifying factors of dental erosion. Eur J Oral Sci 1996;104:199–206.

Millward A, Shaw L, Smith AJ. Dental erosion in four-year-old children from differing socioeconomic backgrounds. ASDC J Dent Child 1994;61:263–6.

Milosevic A. Tooth wear: an aetiological and diagnostic problem. Eur J Prosthodont Restor Dent 1993;1:173–8.

Milosevic A. Toothwear: aetiology and presentation. Dent Update 1998;25:6–11.

Milosevic A, Brodie DA, Slade PD. Dental erosion, oral hygiene, and nutrition in eating disorders. Int J Eat Disord 1997;21:195–9.

Milosevic A, Lo MS. Tooth wear in three ethnic groups in Sabah (northern Borneo). Int Dent J 1996;46:572–8.

Mixson JM, Spencer P, Moore DL, et al. Surface morphology and chemical characterization of abrasion/erosion lesions. Am J Dent 1995;8:5–9.

Morley J. The esthetics of anterior tooth aging. Curr Opin Cosmet Dent 1997;4:35–9.

Nemcovsky CE, Artzi Z. Erosion-abrasion lesions revisited. Compend Cont Educ Dent 1996;17:416–8.

Neo J, Chew CL, Yap A, Sidhu S. Clinical evaluation of tooth-colored materials in cervical lesions. Am J Dent 1996;9:15–18.

Nunn J, Shaw L, Smith A. Tooth wear—dental erosion. Br Dent J 1996;180:349–52.

Owens BM, Gallien GS. Noncarious dental "abfraction" lesions in an aging population. Compend Cont Educ Dent 1995;16:552–62.

Pintado MR, Anderson GC, DeLong R, Douglas WH. Variation in tooth wear in young adults over a two-year period. J Prosthet Dent 1997;77:313–20.

Plavcam JM, Kelley J. Evaluating the "dual selection" hypothesis of canine reduction. Am J Phys Anthropol 1996;99:379–87.

Ramp MH, Suzuki S, Cox CF, et al. Evaluation of wear: enamel opposing three ceramic materials and a gold alloy. J Prosthet Dent 1997;77:523–30.

Robb ND, Cruwys E, Smith BG. Regurgitation erosion as a possible cause of tooth wear in ancient British populations. Arch Oral Biol 1991;36:595–602.

Robertson PB, DeRouen TA, Ernster V, et al. Smokeless tobacco use: how it affects the performance of major league baseball players. J Am Dent Assoc 1995;126:1115–21.

Sakaguchi RL, Brust EW, Cross M, et al. Independent movement of cusps during occlusal loading. Dent Mater 1991;7:186–90.

Schmidt U, Treasure J. Eating disorders and the dental practitioner. Eur J Prosthodont Restor Dent 1997;5:161–7.

Seligman DA, Pullinger AG. The degree to which dental attrition in modern society is a function of age and of canine contact. J Orofac Pain 1995;9:266–75.

Seligman DA, Pullinger AG. A multiple stepwise logistic regression analysis of trauma history and 16 other history and dental cofactors in females with temporomandibular disorders. J Orofac Pain 1996;10:351–61.

Silness J, Berge M, Johannessen G. A 2-year follow-up study of incisal tooth wear in dental students. Acta Odontol Scand 1995;53:331–3.

Smith BG, Bartlett DW, Robb ND. The prevalence, etiology and management of tooth wear in the United Kingdom. J Prosthet Dent 1997;78:367–72.

Sognnaes RF, Wolcott RB, Xhonga FA. Dental erosion I. Erosion-like patterns occurring in association with other dental conditions. J Am Dent Assoc 1972;84:571–6.

Suzuki S, Cox CF, Leinfelder KF, et al. A new copolymerized composite resin system: a multiphased evaluation. Int J Periodont Restor Dent 1995;15:482–95.

Suzuki S, Suzuki SH, Cox CF. Evaluating the antagonistic wear of restorative materials when placed against human enamel. J Am Dent Assoc 1996;127:74–80.

Tay FR, Gwinnett AJ, Pang KM, Wei SH. Structural evidence of a sealed tissue interface with a total-etch wet-bonding technique in vivo. J Dent Res 1994;73:629–36.

Teo C, Young WG, Daley TJ, Sauer H. Prior fluoridation in childhood affects dental caries and tooth wear in a south east Queensland population. Aust Dent J 1997;42:92–102.

Tyas MJ. The Class V lesion—aetilogy and restoration. Aust Dent J 1995;40:167–70.

Ungar PS, Teaford MF. Preliminary examination of non-occlusal dental microwear in anthropoids: implications for the study of fossil primates. Am J Phys Anthropol 1996;100:101–13.

van Foreest A, Roeters J. Restorative dental treatment of abraded canine teeth in a Sumatran tiger (*Panthera tigris sumatrae*). J Vet Dent 1997;14:131–6.

Vandewalle KS, Vigil G. Guidelines for the restoration of Class V lesions. Gen Dent 1997;45:254–60.

Villa G, Giacobini G. Dental microwear. Morphological, functional and phylogenetic correlations. Ital J Anat Embryol 1998;103:53–84.

West NX, Maxwell A, Hughes JA, et al. A method to measure clinical erosion: the effect of orange juice consumption on erosion of enamel. J Dent 1998;26:329–35.

Yaacob HB, Park AW. Dental abrasion pattern in a selected group of Malaysians. J Nihon Univ Sch Dent 1990;32:175–80.

Yap AU, Neo JC. Non-carious cervical tooth loss: part 1. Dent Update 1995;22:315–8.

Yap AU, Neo JC. Non-carious cervical tooth loss. Part 2: management. Dent Update 1995;22:364–8.

Zero DT. Etiology of dental erosion—extrinsic factors. Eur J Oral Sci 1996;104:162.

CHAPTER 18

CHIPPED, FRACTURED, OR ENDODONTICALLY TREATED TEETH

Daniel C.N. Chan, DMD, MS, DDS, Michael L. Myers, DMD,
Gerald M. Barrack, DDS, Ronald E. Goldstein, DDS

New caries prevention and health measures and improved oral care will help more patients keep more of their teeth disease free for a lifetime. However, one thing in "dental life" is almost a certainty: teeth will continue to fracture. Although sports injuries can be greatly reduced with proper protective gear, our daily lives are conducive to all sorts of accidents causing patients to fracture their teeth. The frequency of permanent incisor fractures in children is reported to range from 5 to 20%.[2,17] The loss of tooth substance in these situations is likely to be more horizontal than vertical.

Most tooth fractures are minor and seldom involve pulp. This chapter discusses such simple fractures, as well as treatment of teeth with pulpal and endodontic intervention (Table 18–1). One example of a more serious fracture involving the pulp is also presented with an explanation of techniques for handling this problem. Difficult fracture cases are usually emergencies. With our population living longer and retaining most of their teeth, the incidence of cracks in teeth also seems to be increasing. A tabulated review of cracked tooth syndrome, treatment options, and other considerations is included for easy reference (Table 18–2).

Conservative restorative dentistry is always the goal in treating esthetic problems, and the fractured tooth is no exception. The most conservative treatment would obviously be cosmetic contouring, or the reshaping of the natural teeth, provided that it does not negatively alter the esthetics of the smile (Figures 18–1A and B). Decades ago, the

TABLE 18–1. Coronal Chips or Fractures

DIAGNOSIS	SITUATION	TREATMENT OPTIONS	CONSIDERATIONS
No pulpal involvement	Small chip (enamel involvement only)	Recontour Composite repair	Occlusion
	Medium chip (dentin exposure)	Rebond fractured piece Composite repair	Shine-through effect; esthetics; occlusion
	Large chip (dentin exposure)	Rebond Repair Veneers (composite or porcelain)	Auxiliary retention; occlusion
Pulpal involvement	Direct pulp cap Endodontic treatment required: (i) conventional access with adequate tooth structure (ii) extensive tooth loss; post and core required	Restore as for large chip Composite restoration Cast post and core Prefabricated post and core	Pulpotomy or partial pulpotomy Material choice: conventional glass ionomers, resin modified glass ionomer, composite resin, amalgam, and cast metal. Post materials: nickel-containing stainless steel, non–nickel-containing stainless steel, commercially pure titanium, titanium alloy, zirconia polycrystals, and carbon fibers.

TABLE 18–2. Cracked Tooth Syndrome

DIAGNOSIS	SITUATION	TREATMENT OPTIONS	CONSIDERATIONS
Intracoronal fractures	Affect enamel only Craze lines affecting enamel, dentin, and possibly the pulp	No treatment indicated	Long vertical craze line on anterior teeth
	Fractured cusp		
	Supragingival	Remove the affected cusp; full-crown/ onlay coverage	Good prognosis
	Subgingival	Periosurgery, crown lengthening, orthodontic extrusion, full crown/onlay	Prognosis guarded
	Cracked tooth	Endodontics, full crown	Questionable prognosis
	Split tooth	Extraction; removal of mobile segment	Easily disclosed crack, movable segment; poor prognosis
	Vertical root fracture	Extraction or removal of fractured root	Difficult to diagnosis; poor prognosis
Extracoronal fractures	Subgingival	Periosurgery, crown lengthening, orthodontic extrusion	Prognosis guarded
	Vertical root fracture	Extraction or removal of cracked root	Difficult to diagnose; poor prognosis

full crown restoration was the treatment of choice. Today, in addition to cosmetic contouring, the conservative solution is a choice between direct bonding with composite resin and laminating with porcelain.[11,12,14] These choices are based on several factors:

- *Amount of tooth destruction present.* Generally, small chips or fractures are easily restored with direct bonded composite resin (Figures 18–2A and B). The esthetic result is excellent and provides the patient with an economic, one-appointment solution without any anesthesia.[9,10] However, if the patient continues to chip or fracture the bonding, then porcelain would be a better alternative (Figures 18–3A to F). In the event that the enamel is severely compromised, requiring a more extensive restoration, the patient may ultimately be better off with a porcelain laminate. The fractured area is then replaced with the stronger and more durable porcelain. However, it may be a wise choice to select composite resin bonding as an interim restoration. This minimizes any further trauma to the tooth by additional preparation and allows observation time for any pulpal problem; moreover, the bonded solution can last for an indefinite period of time (Figures 18–4A to F).[12]

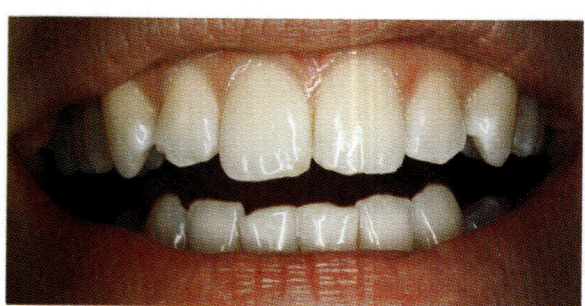

Figure 18–1A: This 21-year-old girl had chipped her anterior incisors when she was a teenager.

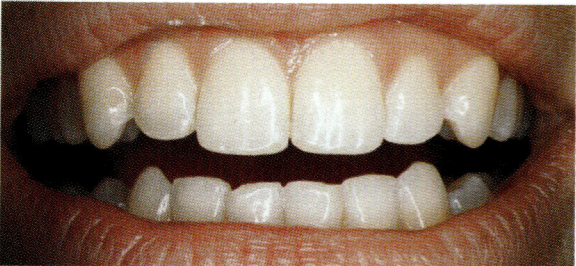

Figure 18–1B: Cosmetic contouring was the most conservative treatment available and was performed in a less than 1-hour appointment.

Chipped, Fractured, or Endodontically Treated Teeth 527

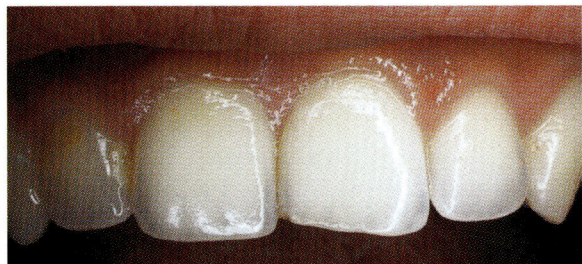

Figure 18–2A: This teenager chipped her maxillary front teeth.

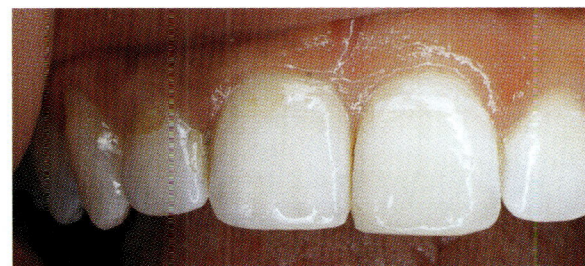

Figure 18–2B: The left central incisor was bonded with composite resin.

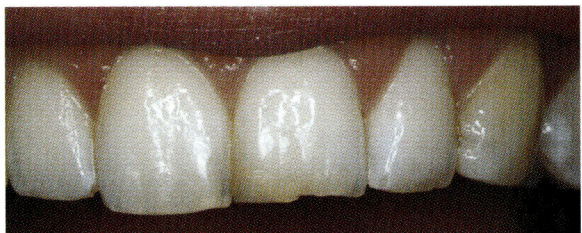

Figure 18–3A: This young lady fractured her maxillary anterior incisors. Despite numerous bonding repairs, she continued to refracture the teeth. Because she also objected to the incisal translucency, she was treatment planned for three porcelain laminates.

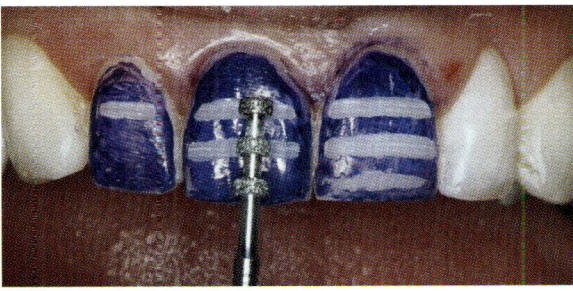

Figure 18–3B: The initial preparations for the three porcelain laminates were done with a 0.5-mm depth cutter (Brasseler LVS System, Brasseler, Savannah, GA).

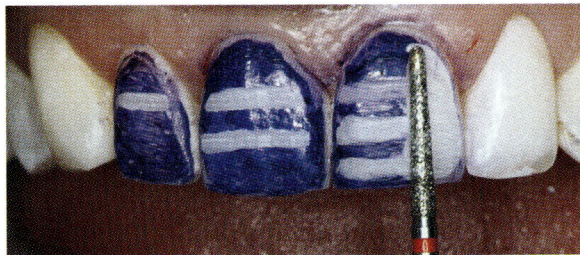

Figure 18–3C: The two-grit diamond is used to reduce the enamel to the predetermined depth cut.

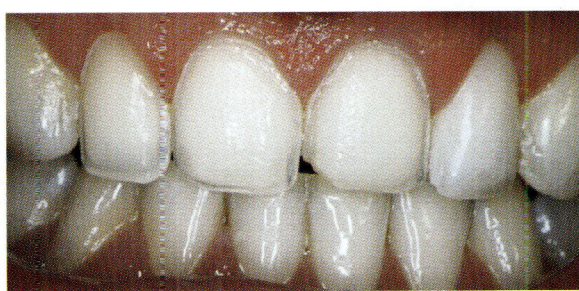

Figure 18–3D: The final preparations.

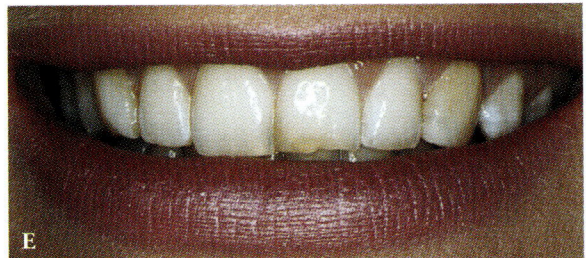

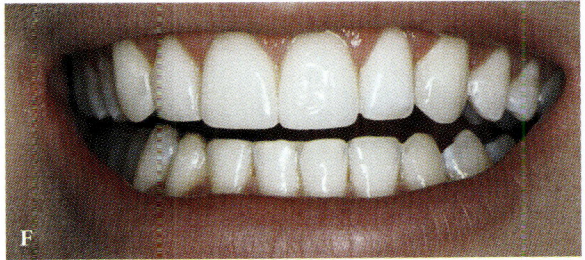

Figure 18–3E and F: Three porcelain laminates were placed on the central incisors and right lateral. The new laminates also achieved the objective to eliminate the incisal translucency.

528 Esthetics in Dentistry

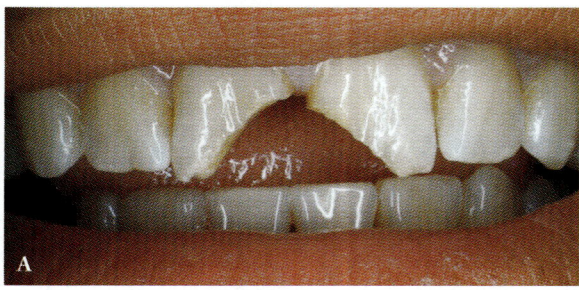
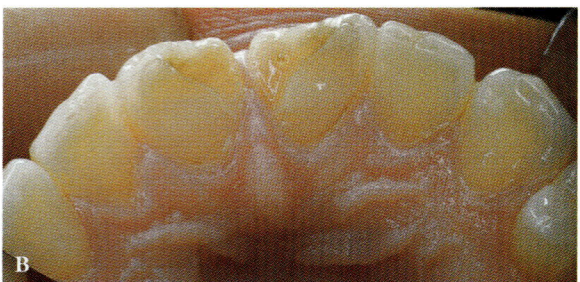

Figure 18–4A and B: This 17-year-old student fractured her central incisors on the edge of a swimming pool.

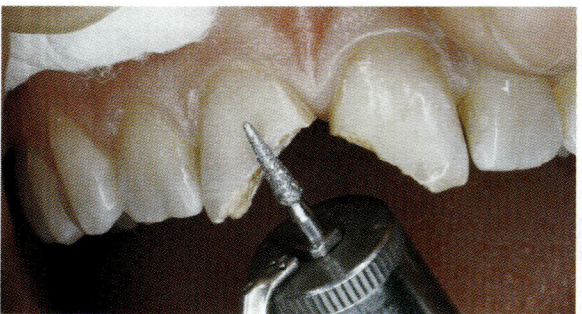

Figure 18–4C: A long bevel is placed using an extra coarse diamond.

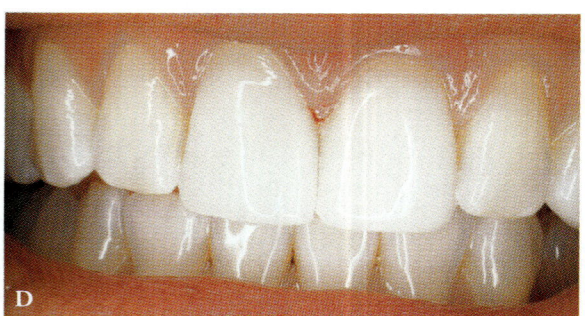
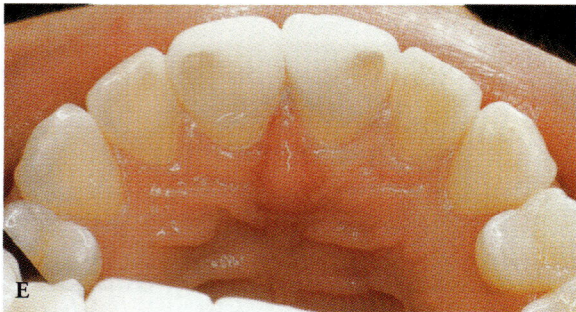

Figure 18–4D and E: The central incisors are bonded with composite resin.

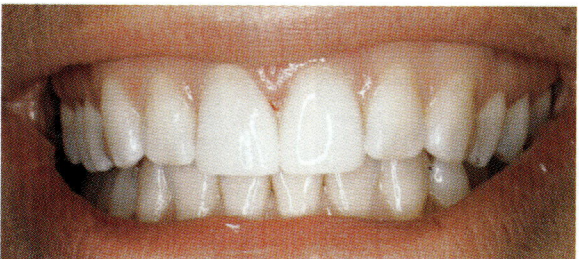

Figure 18–4F: Five years later, the patient has continued to be maintained with composite resin restorations.

- *Longevity required.* If the patient does not mind the added cost, increased longevity can be achieved with the porcelain laminate. However, the patient needs to be informed about the limited life expectancy of each restorative option. Patients must also be made aware of the periodic maintenance required, proper home care, and any dietary restrictions necessary to obtain the longest life possible.[14]

- *Economic considerations.* Although the cost savings of direct bonding might not be realized if numerous repairs are considered, it still may be easier for the patient to pay lesser amounts over the many years during which the direct bonded restoration can stay in place.

- *Occlusal factor.* If an end-to-end occlusal relationship or increased occlusal requirement exists, porcelain may again provide more durability, depending on the design of the laminate. It is essential to protect the incisal edge with sufficient porcelain to resist fracture. An example of this condition is seen in a patient who fractured a tooth (Figure 18–5A). During the clinical examination, this patient expressed his desire for a younger and brighter smile. The teeth were then prepared, and an impression was made for six porcelain laminate veneers. To help protect the occlusion, porcelain was wrapped incisally to the lingual surface (Figure 18–5B). What began as an emergency visit to repair a fractured tooth resulted in enhancing this patient's entire smile (Figure 18–5C).

It is essential to use these opportunities to present each patient with alternatives that not only correct the immediate problem but also improve the entire smile.

In the final analysis, although direct bonding will generally be the method most often selected, there are definite situations for which porcelain laminate will be the technique of choice. The advantages and disadvantages of direct bonding, laminating, and crowns are outlined in Tables 18–3 to 18–5 for comparison.[12]

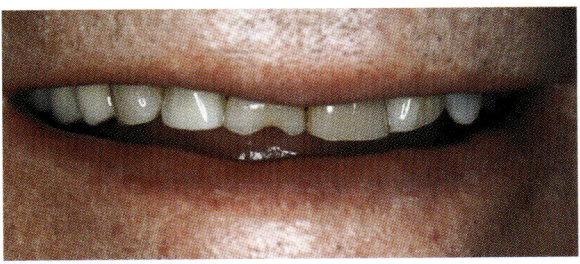

Figure 18–5A: This 65-year-old man had fractured his right central incisor. Because he desired a younger and brighter looking smile, six porcelain laminates were treatment planned.

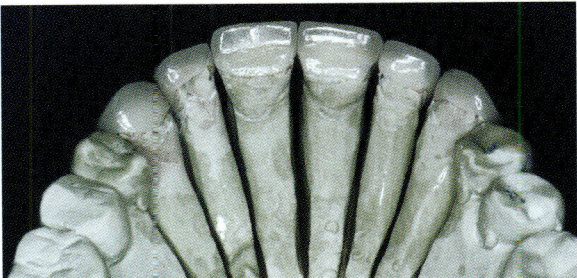

Figure 18–5B: This patient had an end-to-end bite, which required additional incisal edge reinforcement.

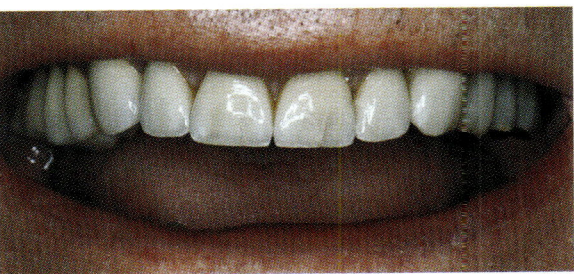

Figure 18–5C: Note the improvement in this man's smile with a lighter shade and teeth that are more proportionate to each other.

TABLE 18–3. Advantages and Disadvantages of Bonding

Advantages
- Conserves tooth structure
- Easier to match or blend in tooth shade
- Less expensive than crowning
- Immediate repair
- Reduces possible trauma of a crown preparation for badly damaged teeth
- No anesthesia required
- Painless repair
- Can improve shape and shade if necessary

Disadvantages
- Can stain more easily than porcelain laminate or a crown
- Needs periodic refinishing
- Some maintenance required
- Must have sufficient enamel left to be able to bond it
- Must be repaired or replaced in approximately 5 to 8 years
- Not appropriate for use in posterior teeth

TABLE 18–4. Advantages and Disadvantages of Porcelain Laminates

Advantages
- Excellent esthetics
- Improved edge strength
- Better retention of surface finish
- Fewer repairs required
- Does not stain
- Conserves tooth structure

Disadvantages
- May require anesthesia
- More costly than bonding
- Usually requires two appointments
- Some tooth preparation indicated
- Cannot alter color once cemented

CHIPS OR FRACTURES WITHOUT PULPAL INVOLVEMENT

Conservative Bonding Techniques for Long-Term Results

PROBLEM: A 27-year-old male presented with fractured maxillary central incisors involving the incisal edges (Figure 18–6A). Because the patient preferred not to reduce the tooth structure, a bonded composite resin was the material of choice to restore the fractured edges.

TREATMENT: Since the left central incisor overlapped the right one, the mesial surface of the left central was reshaped slightly to reduce the amount of overlapping in an attempt to create an illusion of straightness (Figure 18–6B). These fractures were old and not sensitive, so no protective base was required. In a new fracture or pulp exposure, the fracture site would have been protected first with glass ionomer liner. A large particle composite restoration was used for strength and to help blend in translucency. The restorations were finished with conventional composite resin finishing techniques (see Chapter 13, *Esthetics in Dentistry*, Volume 1, 2nd Edition).

Fourteen years later, the patient came in with a small fracture in the bonding material of the central incisor (Figure 18–6C). The teeth were reveneered with hybrid composite resin to improve his smile once more (Figure 18–6D). Although this patient may well be the exception to the rule of an average life expectancy of 5 to 8 years, his case does point out the fact that many patients would have preferred the restoration replaced long before the slight discoloration took place. However, careful maintenance, including good oral hygiene and prudent dietary habits, helped account for the extended life of these restorations. The tooth can always be laminated or crowned if bonding does not work, but once the enamel is reduced for a full crown, it can never be bonded or laminated. In the future, better bonding and laminating materials will, no doubt, become available.

TABLE 18–5. Advantages and Disadvantages of Crowning

Advantages
- Can ideally change color and shape of teeth
- Longest lasting esthetic restoration
- Lasts approximately 5 to 15 years
- Less likely to require repairs

Disadvantages
- Must reduce the enamel and dentin
- Most expensive form of replacement
- Possibility of pulp irritation
- More chance for periodontal problems if margin is subgingival
- Requires anesthesia
- Difficult to repair

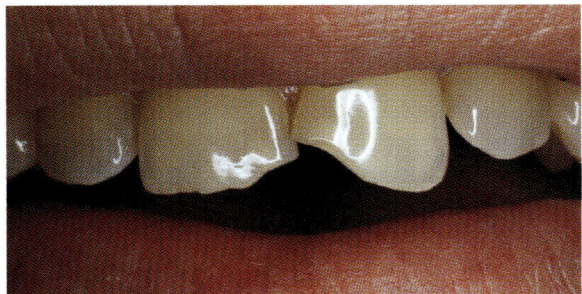

Figure 18–6A: This 27-year-old man fractured his maxillary central incisors.

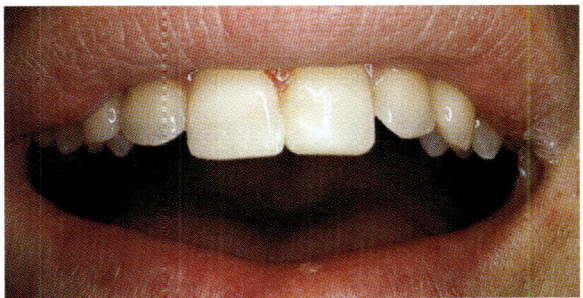

Figure 18–6B: After light cosmetic contouring to the left central incisor, both central incisors were bonded with a large particle composite resin.

Bonding Original Tooth Fragment

Simonsen first suggested that fractured original tooth segments could be bonded back together.[26] If the patient has a "clean" break and brings in the fractured piece of enamel, it is entirely possible and many times advisable to attempt reattachment by acid etching both the tooth itself and the fragment. Light polymerized tooth-colored resin cement is applied to both pieces and the fracture piece is carefully fit and polymerized 1 minute labially and 1 minute lingually.

Additional modifications have taken place, and there are newer techniques that are variations on the original philosophy.[27] For instance, Croll advocated attaching the two segments together, first with a glass ionomer light polymerized liner (Vitrebond, 3M ESPE, St. Paul, MN) and then reinforcing labially and lingually with composite resin.[6] Many variations of such bonding are reported in the literature.[2,18,31,32,33]

Bonding the original tooth fragment is not limited to the anterior region. Posterior teeth fractures, especially in the case of premolars, can be successfully bonded together. The long-term survival of such repairs is reported to be in the 5-year range.[2,24] However, in these cases, the bonded teeth are best viewed as a temporary restoration awaiting partial or full crown coverage. Liebenberg reported using resin-bonded partial-coverage ceramic restorations to treat incomplete fractures.[22,23]

CHIPS OR FRACTURES WITH PULPAL INVOLVEMENT

In the event that the pulp is exposed, two choices exist:

- *Pulpotomy.* If the root apex is open, this is the preferred treatment according to several sources.[4,5] Ehrmann described the procedure beginning with coronal pulp removal, which will allow root maturation to proceed only with closure of the apex then taking place.[8]

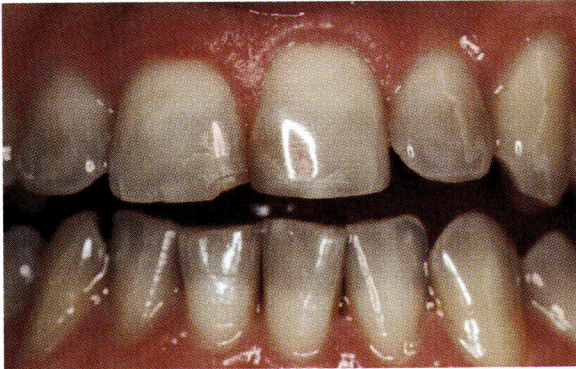

Figure 18–6C: Fourteen years later, this patient fractured the bonding on the right central incisor.

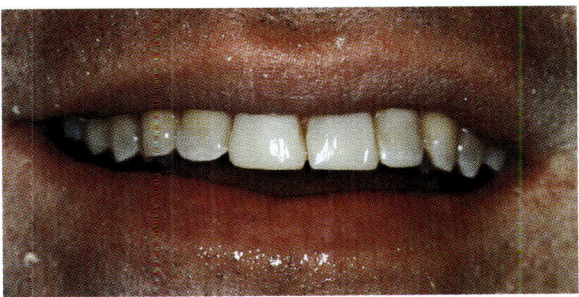

Figure 18–6D: The central incisors were reveneered and the left lateral was also bonded to achieve an even more attractive smile.

Following closure, a radicular pulpectomy is done and is usually followed by endodontic therapy plus construction of a post and core.

- *Partial pulpotomy.* Another view has been expressed by Cvek, who suggested a partial pulpotomy in permanent incisors with complex root fractures, regardless of whether the apex was open.[7] Basically, the technique consists of a 2-mm-depth removal of the coronal pulp with sterile saline being used to control bleeding. Next, a calcium hydroxide pulp liner (Dycal Caulk, DENTSPLY/Caulk, Milford, DE) is used and is covered with a composite resin. Ehrmann concluded that this latter technique seems to be the method of choice, citing fewer traumas and preserving most of the pulp as two advantages.[8] He reported that of 35 cases, 33 were successful and retained their vitality, with the longest follow-up being 8 years.

The consideration for a chipped or fractured tooth is whether the pulp is damaged. If it has been exposed, the tooth should be protected with a pulp-capping material (calcium hydroxide) and covered with a tooth-colored restorative material for at least 6 weeks. A recommended technique after pulp capping is bonding with a composite resin. Kanca reported the success of a case with a 5-year follow-up.[20]

The responsibility of the dentist is to preserve the natural dentition. In some circumstances, this is impossible, but it is an ideal for which to aim. To achieve this goal, it may be necessary to call on colleagues for assistance. Who is credited with the result is unimportant. What is important is for the patient to receive the best possible treatment and advice.

This point is well illustrated by the actual treatment of a patient with fractures of the maxillary central incisors that extended lingually beneath the crest of the bone and exposed the pulps. The patient's dentist consulted an oral surgeon who recommended endodontic treatment. Before final restorative therapy was chosen, consultations were held with an oral surgeon, a pediatric dentist, and two general practitioners. The case that follows involved consultation with other dental specialists and shows an esthetic result that was worth the effort.[15]

Preservation of Fractured Maxillary Central Incisors through Interdisciplinary Therapy

PROBLEM: A general practitioner saw a 12-year-old girl who had been in an accident. He referred her to an oral surgeon for removal of both maxillary permanent central incisors, which had been fractured horizontally and vertically, exposing the pulps. The oral surgeon thought that the teeth might be saved and referred the patient to an endodontist. After endodontic therapy on both teeth (Figures 18–7A and B), the patient returned to the general practitioner, who consulted the pediatric dentist. The two agreed that someone skilled in cosmetic restorative procedures should be called on for the reconstruction.

TREATMENT: Because saving teeth was a step-by-step procedure involving endodontic treatment, periodontal surgery, and reconstructive techniques, the treatment plan could be changed if one of the suggested treatments failed. Endodontic therapy had already been completed on both central incisors. These surgical procedures were performed

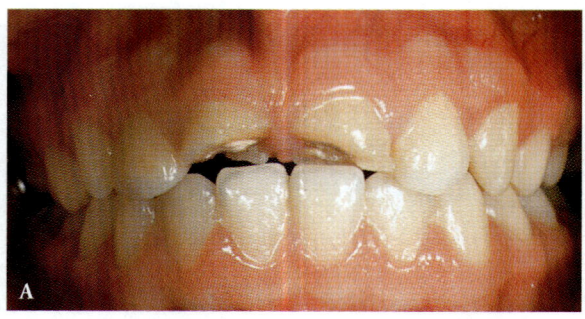
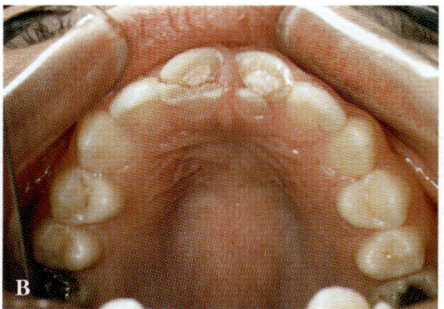

Figure 18–7A and B: Although this 12-year-old girl was referred to an oral surgeon for a postaccident extraction of both fractured central incisors, he wisely referred the patient to an endodontist in an attempt to save the teeth.

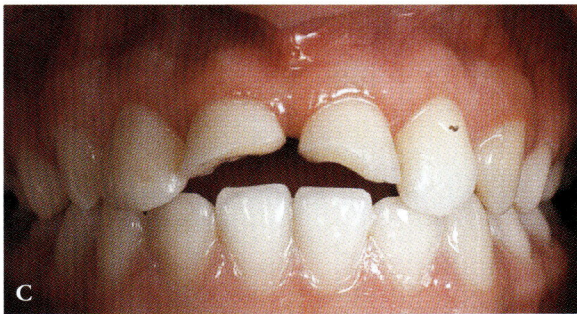
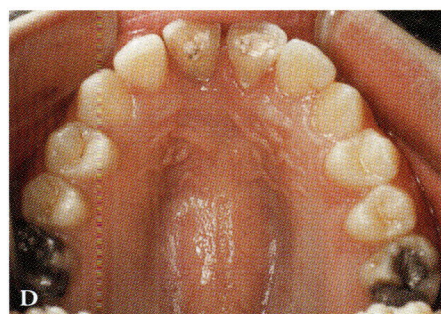

Figure 18–7C and D: Following endodontic therapy and removal of the fractured tooth fragments, periodontal surgery to lengthen the exposed crowns was performed.

next: removal of the tooth fragments that were fractured vertically, labial and lingual gingivectomy and gingivoplasty, palatal ostectomy, and labial frenectomy (Figure 18–7C). Approximately 5 mm of palatal plate was removed to expose new margins on the fractured teeth (Figure 18–7D). After the tissue healed, gold posts were constructed and cemented on the two maxillary incisors (Figures 18–7E to H). Final preparations were made, and impressions for aluminous porcelain crowns were made. The two crowns were seated (Figures 18–7I and J). Figure 18–7K is a radiograph of the teeth at the end of treatment.

The parents have been told that these crowns will probably have to be replaced when the patient is older because the margins may be exposed. However, they might last longer because of the higher marginal attachment. Because of the age of the child, the anticipated cost of the treatment, and the presumed lack of dental knowledge of the parents, the pediatric dentist and the general practitioner

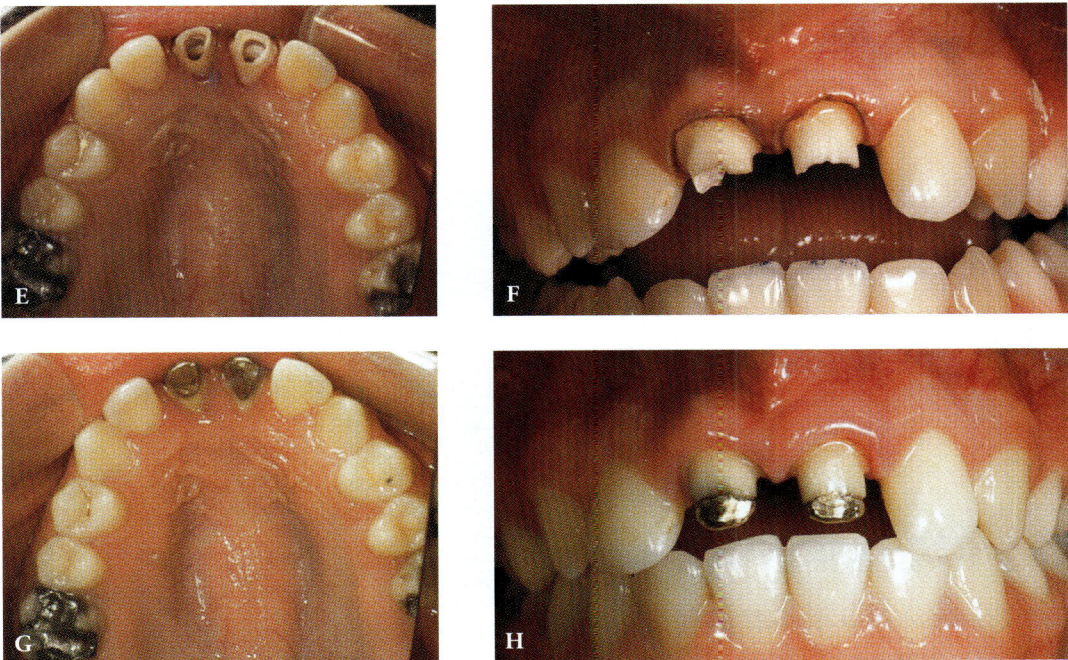

Figure 18–7E to H: Next, two posts and cores were constructed for the endodontically treated teeth.

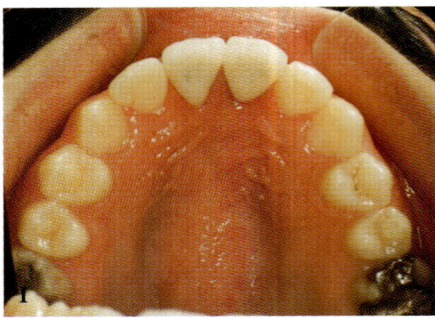 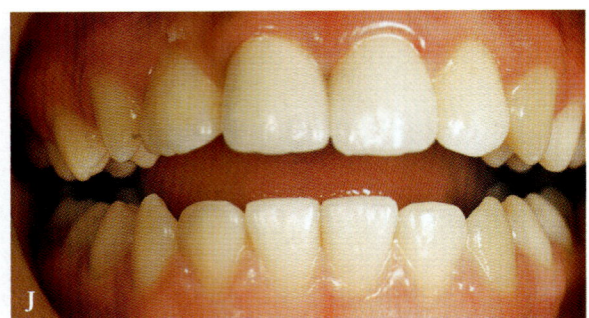

Figure 18–7I and J: Two aluminous porcelain crowns were constructed and inserted on the central incisors.

who were to do the treatment explained the reconstruction procedures at length. Although the endodontic therapy had been completed, the father informed the two dentists that he had decided to have "both teeth pulled and a plate put in." A subsequent conference convinced the parents that this would not be the wisest course to follow if restorative procedures could be performed. Their expression of thanks at the end of the treatment justified the time spent persuading the family to accept the outlined treatment plan.

RESULT: Dentists sometimes assume, incorrectly, that because a tooth is fractured beneath the periodontal ligament and into the bone, it cannot be saved. Proper surgical and reconstructive techniques can save these roots for many years, sometimes indefinitely.

Dentists may also assume, again incorrectly, that because of the expense or difficulty of treatment, a patient or his or her family would prefer to sacrifice a tooth. Not knowing what value the patient places on a tooth, the dentist should give the patient the opportunity to decide. It is almost always better to save a tooth. The patient can clean it more easily with floss, and the root support helps share occlusal load.

The purpose of this case is not to show the skill of the operator but to call attention to the fact that, even though extraordinary measures are needed, it may be possible to preserve the natural dentition. To do so may involve multiple referrals and consul-

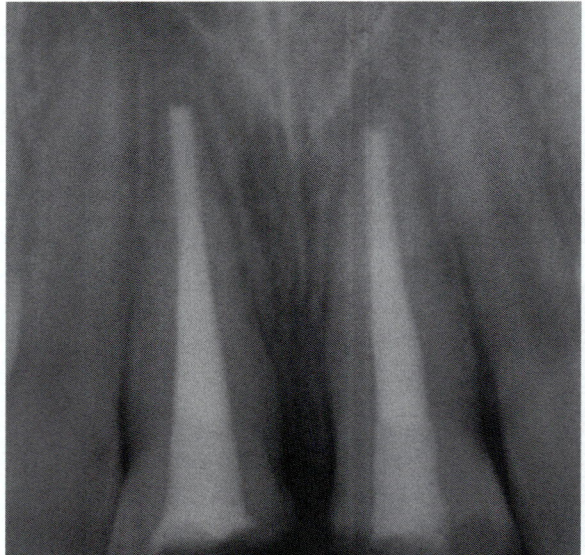

Figure 18–7K: Post-treatment radiograph of the two fractured and restored central incisors.

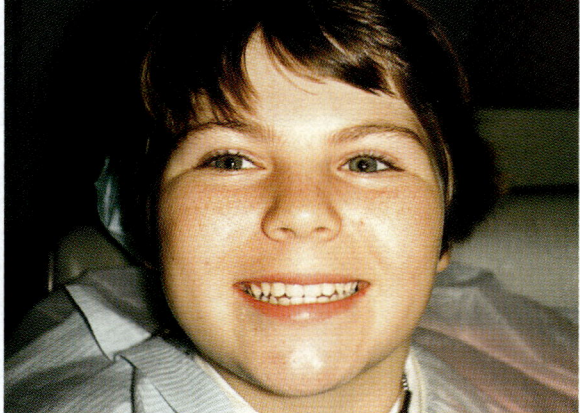

Figure 18–7L: A total team approach was necessary to save this young lady's maxillary incisors. Both she and her parents appreciated the benefits of interdisciplinary care.

Chipped, Fractured, or Endodontically Treated Teeth

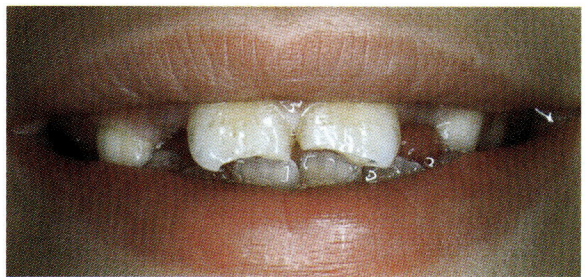

Figure 18–8A: This 6-year-old girl fractured her maxillary central incisors in an accident.

tations, but the good result (Figure 18–7L) and the knowledge that possibilities exist should be considered before a patient is allowed to lose a tooth. The function of dentistry is to maintain the integrity of the dental arch and to preserve the dentition. For this patient, at least, this goal was achieved.

LIFE EXPECTANCY WITH COMPOSITE RESINS

Although the average life expectancy is 3 to 8 years, the fact is that some patients may experience a much longer and more useful restoration life (see Figures 18–6A to D).[14] These restorations are, for the most part, noninvasive, and the bonded restoration offers a good measure of protection to the tooth while odontoblastic activity is taking place at the damage site. They can also continue to be reveneered rather than replaced for an indefinite period of time (Figures 18–8A to E). When replacement is necessary, if full crown coverage is the treatment of choice, it can be done with less chance of pulp involvement.

POSTERIOR RESTORATIONS

In these areas, it is even more important to place a protective base and use the etching technique on enamel walls and dentin. Marginal leaks can be minimized by this technique. In addition, patients

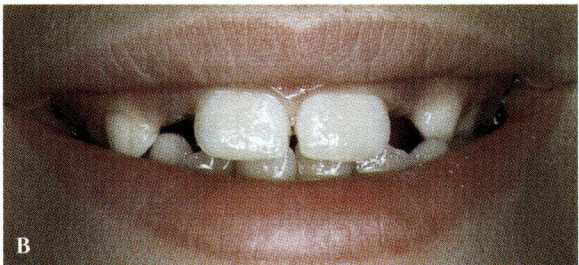

Figure 18–8B and C: The two central incisors were beveled and bonded with composite resin.

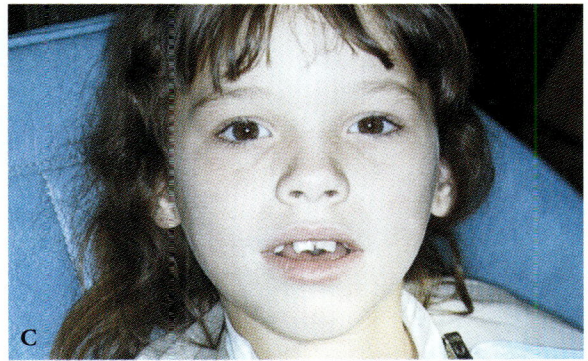

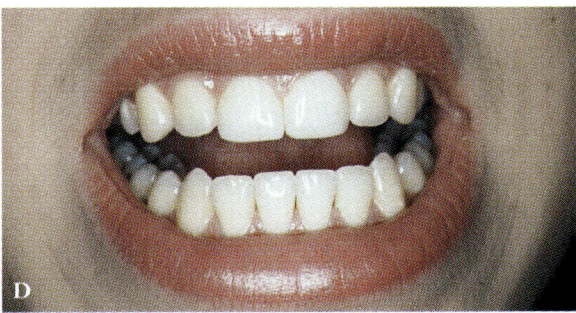

Figure 18–8D and E: Ten years later, the patient still retains her original bonding, although reveneering has been done to maintain appearance.

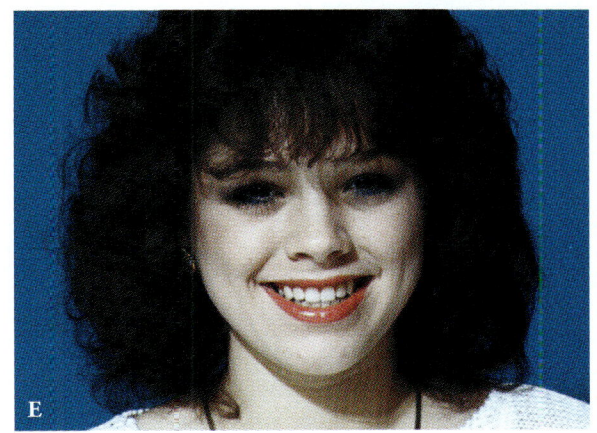

must be advised of the possibility of replacing the restorations every 3 to 8 years.

Several methods of restoring the simple fracture have been shown in this chapter, although all seem to arrive at the same conclusion: the final measure of success is how these bonds respond to oral fluids. With further investigation, stronger materials and stronger bonds will be developed that may warrant reinserting restorations as improved materials become available. Thus, in certain cases, it may be to the patient's advantage not to destroy tooth structure for full-coverage procedures at present. However, when small pieces break off of posterior teeth, bonding can be used either as an interim or the final restoration if it is not in an occluding area where it may be under too much stress. If it is, then porcelain may be the best choice (Figures 18–9A to C).

In the final analysis, the full crown remains a viable option, especially if esthetic changes are to be made that may not be possible with a more conservative treatment. Also, some patients prefer the long-lasting benefit that the full crown provides.[13]

RESTORATION OF ENDODONTICALLY TREATED FRACTURED TEETH

Principles

The philosophy for the restoration of endodontically treated teeth has changed significantly in recent years. Traditional concepts were that nonvital teeth were so weakened by root canal therapy that they

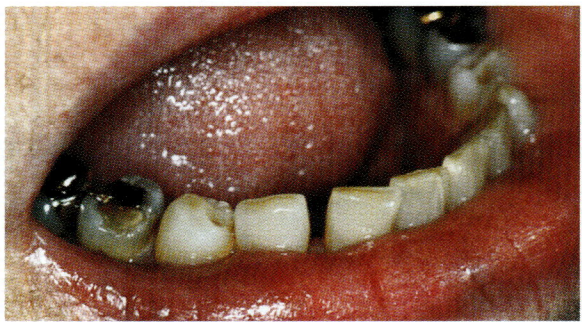

Figure 18–9A: This 60-year-old woman fractured the bucco-occlusal surface of her mandibular right second bicuspid. Because the fracture was in an occluding area and was previously repaired with composite resin bonding, the patient opted for the longer lasting protection of a full crown.

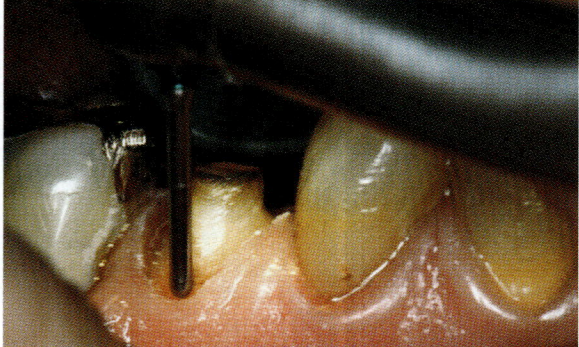

Figure 18–9B: Full shoulder margins are prepared with a TPE diamond (Shofu, Menlo Park, CA) or TGE diamond (Premier, King of Prussia, PA).

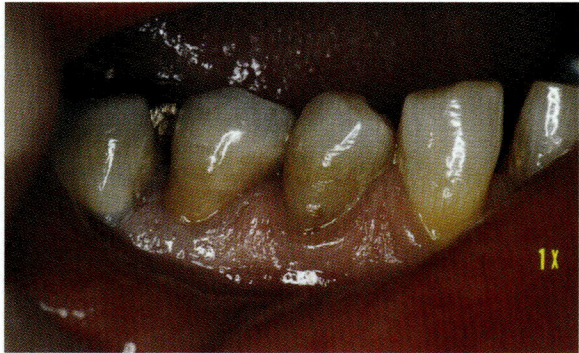

Figure 18–9C: The final crown shows how well ceramics can mimic the natural tooth and esthetically blend with the existing dentition.

required a post to reinforce the root in the same manner that concrete is reinforced with steel rods. Further, it was believed that these teeth also needed to be crowned to protect the tooth from fracture.

Clinical experience and research studies have, in some cases, produced a dramatic shift in the way endodontically treated teeth are restored.[1,2,19,21,25] Endodontically treated teeth have certain characteristics that are well known by clinical dentists. First, the loss of vitality results in a change in color over time. This can result in an unacceptable esthetic result. These teeth are structurally compromised due to the access opening required to accomplish root canal therapy. Additionally, these teeth often have extensive restorations or caries, further compromising their strength and structural integrity. Endodontically treated teeth also seem to be brittle because of the loss of vitality. Clinical experience has shown that these teeth seem to have an increased risk of fracture.

There is no large body of in vivo scientific literature to determine how to best restore endodontically treated teeth. However, there are several good retrospective studies that provide some guidance. From these studies, it is clear that anterior teeth have different characteristics and require a different clinical approach than posterior teeth. Another conclusion that can be made is that endodontically treated anterior teeth do not automatically require restoration with a crown. In fact, most endodontically treated anterior teeth will have the same longevity whether or not they have been crowned.

So, the clinical options for restoration of an anterior tooth are dictated by the condition and the functional and esthetic requirements of the tooth. If the tooth is relatively intact, it should simply be restored with a composite resin restoration. If it has changed color, then bleaching of the tooth would also be indicated. If the existing restorations or caries are moderate in size or include the incisal edge, then a porcelain veneer could be the appropriate choice for treatment. In many instances, bleaching of the endodontically treated tooth prior to restoration with composite resin or a porcelain veneer will provide a better esthetic result.

Three major reasons for using crowns are (1) if the tooth is badly broken down, (2) a significant change in tooth contour is desired, or (3) if the tooth is to be used as an abutment for a fixed or removable partial denture. Most anterior teeth in this condition have little sound remaining tooth structure and will require a post and core restoration to support and retain the crown. This concept is supported by most studies. Such a patient can be seen in Figures 18–10A to H. Post restorations used in anterior teeth fall into two broad types: (1) the prefabricated post with a core material to replace the missing coronal tooth structure and (2) the cast metal post and core that is custom made for the tooth (Figure 18–10I).

As previously mentioned, posterior teeth require a different treatment approach than is indicated for anterior teeth. Posterior teeth usually have a greater bulk of remaining tooth structure

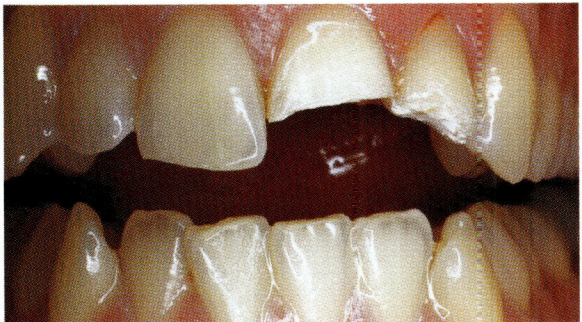

Figure 18–10A: This young lady fractured her left central and lateral incisors in an accident. Because the original teeth had protruded before fracturing, the patient requested that the restoration be accomplished with an improved appearance in the most permanent treatment available.

than anterior teeth. Also, the occlusal forces on posterior teeth are significantly greater than anterior teeth. Retrospective studies of posterior teeth that have had root canal therapy indicate that these teeth are much more likely to fracture if they are not crowned. Therefore, conclusions from research indicate that posterior teeth that have had root canal therapy should always be restored with

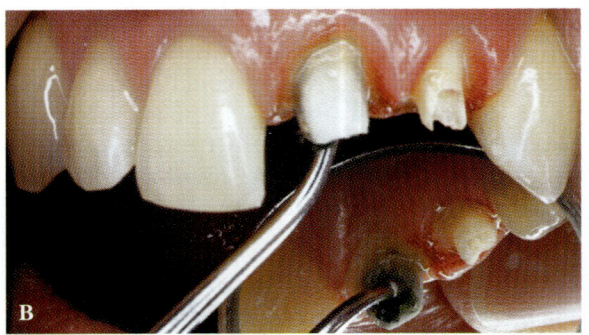

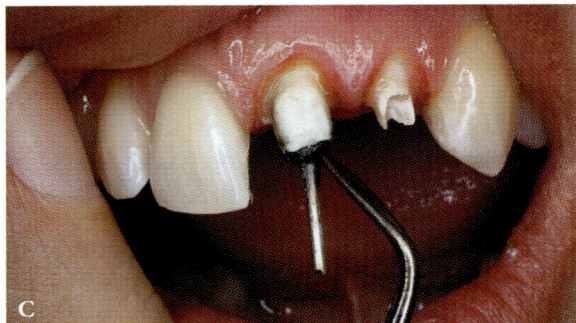

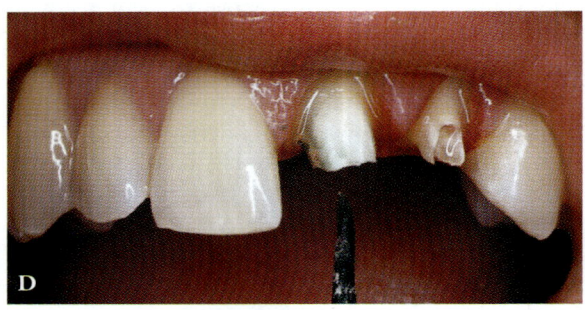

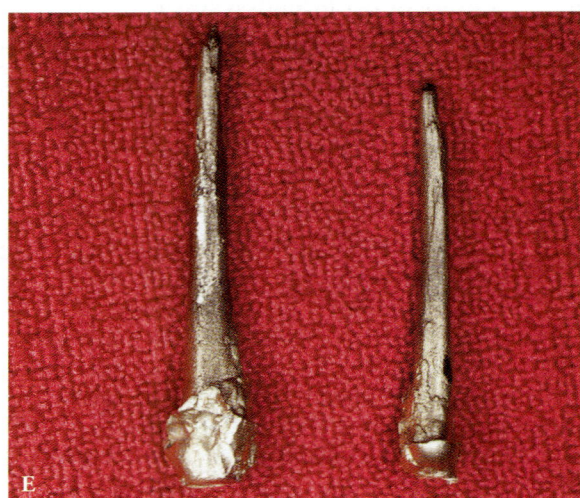

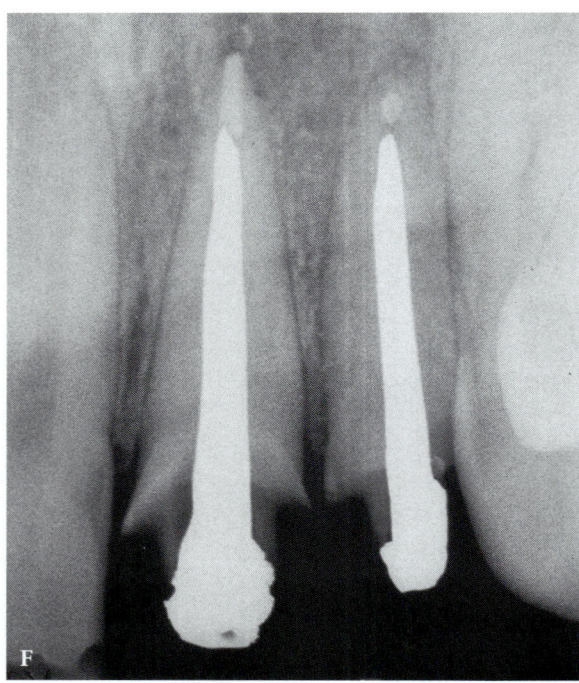

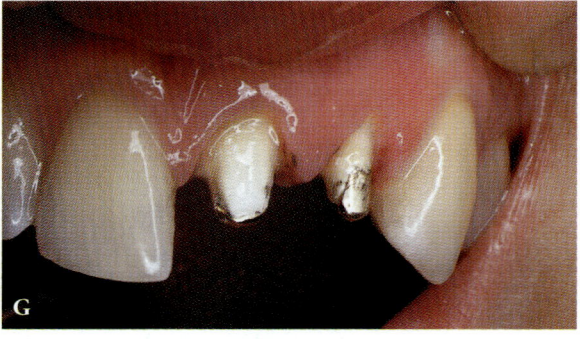

Figure 18–10B to G: Following endodontic therapy, two cast posts were constructed and cemented to place in the prepared incisors.

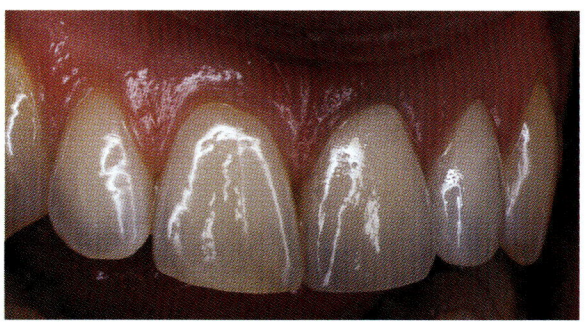

Figure 18–10H: The final all-ceramic crowns were bonded to place. Note the natural result of both the shade and texture of the crowned teeth.

a restoration that provides coronal coverage. The basic principle for posterior teeth is that the restoration should provide for cuspal coverage or protection. This can be accomplished with a crown (either full or partial coverage) or even an onlay. The only exception to this rule might be for a premolar that has a minimal endodontic access and at least one intact marginal ridge. In this instance, if the occlusion is favorable (ie, canine disclusion), a small two-surface bonded composite could be considered.

Unlike anterior teeth, which almost always require a post to retain the core, posterior teeth seldom need a post. The retention for the core or foundation can usually be obtained by taking advantage of the undercuts present in the pulp chamber, especially in molars. So if amalgam is used for the core, it is simply condensed into the pulp chamber. If a composite resin core material is used, it can be retained both by dentin bonding and the pulp chamber. If the tooth has hardly any coronal tooth structure (ie, level with the gingival margin), a cemented, prefabricated post can be used to provide the required retention for the core restoration. Small premolars are more likely to need a post restoration because there may not be sufficient retention for the core.

In summary, endodontically treated anterior teeth do not always need to be crowned; when they are to be crowned, a post may or may not be required. Posterior teeth always need a crown (ie, cuspal coverage) but rarely require a post. The purpose of a post is to retain the core; it does not reinforce the root.[29,30]

Post Design

Several principles must be considered in post selection and design. These principles apply for either prefabricated or cast posts. Design characteristics include length, diameter, shape, surface configuration or texture, method of attachment, and material. Many of these characteristics have been studied extensively by in vitro studies. In addition, several retrospective studies give guidance concerning optimum factors for post selection and design.

Retention of a post increases with increasing length. The post should at least be equal in length to the clinical crown or two-thirds of the root length, whichever is greater (Figure 8–10J). At least 4 mm of gutta-percha should be left in the apex of the root to maintain the apical seal. In contrast to post length, post diameter has little influence on retention. In fact, increasing post diameter requires removal of additional tooth structure and simply weakens the tooth, increasing the risk of a vertical root fracture. Therefore, the post should not be any larger in diameter than is absolutely necessary. The general guidelines are that the post should not be greater than one-third of the diameter of the root at the cement–enamel junction and that at least 1 mm of dentin thickness should be maintained at all levels of the root. Generally, it is best not to enlarge the post space any greater than the space created

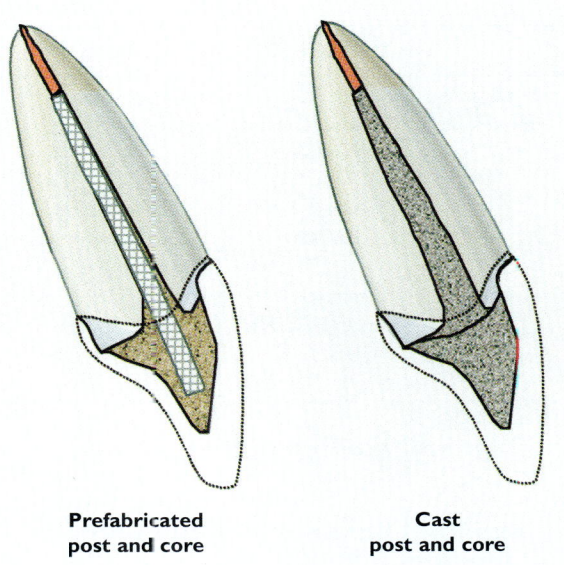

Figure 18–10I: Options for post and core restorations.

540 Esthetics in Dentistry

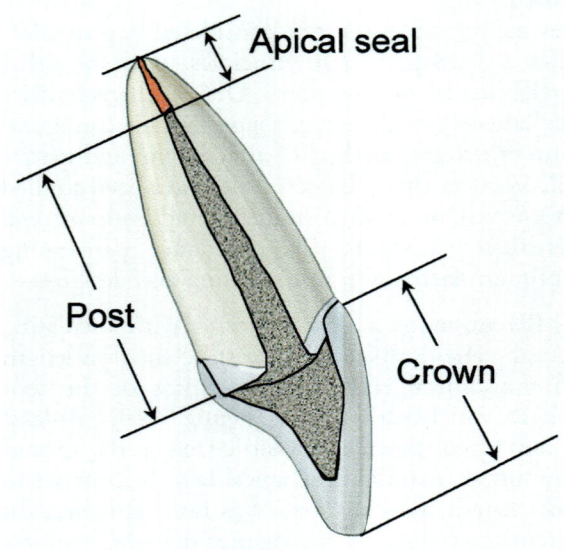

Figure 18–10J: Optimum post length.

during root canal therapy. Too aggressive flaring of the canal during root canal therapy or enlargement of the canal space for a post will surely compromise the tooth. In the same vein, the shape of the post should be parallel rather than tapered. A tapered post design creates a wedging force within the root of the tooth. Conversely, parallel posts produce less stress and fewer vertical root fractures.

The surface configuration or texture has a significant influence on post retention. A smooth-surface or polished post is less retentive than a textured (eg, sandblasted) post. Post designs that are serrated or crosshatched or have some other retentive design exhibit the best resistance to dislodgment.

One other design parameter is the mode of attachment. A post can have a passive fit in the tooth root and be retained by cement, or it can be actively retained (threaded like a screw) and retention gained by virtue of the threads (with or without the aid of cement). However, threaded posts create the potential for a significant wedging force within the tooth root and should be avoided. Parallel posts with proper length and a retentive surface design can obtain more than adequate retention. In situations when it is not possible to obtain the optimum length or shape, the required retention is much better and gained more safely by using a stronger cement (ie, resin) than by using a threaded post.

There are several different materials that can be used for posts, including stainless steel, titanium, zirconium (tooth colored), ceramic, and polymers (Table 18–6). The material used for the post is

TABLE 18–6. Materials for Prefabricated Posts

	MATERIAL	INDICATIONS	ADVANTAGES	DISADVANTAGES
Metallic				
Stainless steel	Nickel-containing (ASM 300)		Superior physical properties, radiopaque, excellent corrosion resistance	Nickel content (possible allergic response), metallic color
	No nickel (ASM 400)	General use; particularly suited for situations requiring high strength	Superior physical properties, radiopaque	Poor corrosion resistance, metallic color
Titanium	Commercially pure titanium (99%)		Moderate strength, biocompatibility	
	Alloy Ti-Al-V		Superior physical properties, biocompatibility	Metallic color, not as radiopaque as stainless steel, difficult to cut
Nonmetallic				
Ceramic	Zirconia polycrystals	Situations requiring high esthetic demand; all-ceramic crowns	Tooth color, light transmission, high strength	Lack of long-term clinical results
Fiber-polymer composite	Carbon fibers		High strength, modulus of elasticity equal to dentin	No long-term clinical results, dark color, fiber–polymer matrix interface may degrade

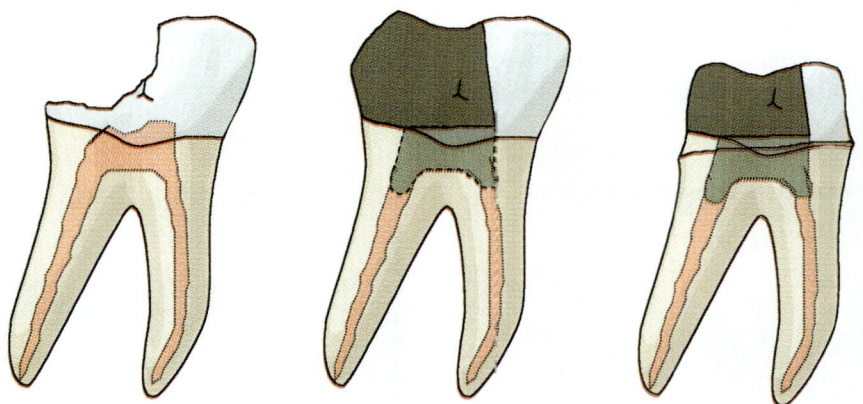

Figure 18–11: Amalgam or composite resin core.

much less important than the design and size of the post (ie, preservation of tooth structure) unless esthetics becomes a consideration. If so, a tooth-colored post should be considered.

Sequence of Treatment for Posterior Teeth (Molars and Large Premolars)
The core build-up for a posterior tooth should be placed prior to crown preparation. A sufficient amount of time should have elapsed since completion of the root canal therapy to be confident that it has been successful. The tooth should be asymptomatic and not sensitive to percussion. Following root canal therapy, the typical molar will have a large existing restoration. All restorative materials and caries should be removed. The gutta-percha should be removed from the pulp chamber. The gutta-percha can be removed 1 to 2 mm into the canal orifices to increase retention (Figure 18–11). If there is at least one cusp remaining and the pulp chamber has walls of 2 to 3 mm in depth, a post is not required for retention of the core. The core may be either amalgam or composite resin (Table 18–7).

The advantage of composite resin is that it may be prepared immediately. Composite resin also offers the advantage of dentin bonding and a relatively simple technique for core placement. The main disadvantage of composite resin is that it is subject to water absorption and microleakage. It should only be used in posterior applications when it is possible to place the crown margins at least 2 mm beyond (ie, apical to) the resin–tooth interface. A composite resin core material of contrasting color should be used to minimize the risk of inadvertently preparing the preparation margin on composite resin. For an amalgam core, a metal matrix band or copper band can be used as a retainer. If the crown preparation needs to be completed the same day the core is placed, a fast-setting amal-

TABLE 18–7. Core Materials

	INDICATIONS	ADVANTAGES	DISADVANTAGES
Conventional glass ionomers	Only for blockout of undercuts	Fluoride release	Low fracture toughness and strength, solubility
Resin-modified glass ionomer	Partial core build-up with adequate tooth structure present	Fluoride release, moderate strength, tooth color	
Composite resin	Core with prefabricated posts in anterior teeth	Tooth color, dentin bonding	Plastic deformation, absorbs moisture, dimensionally unstable
Amalgam	Cores for posterior teeth	Strength	Low early strength, metallic color
Cast metal	Cast post and core	Strength, core joined to post, biocompatibility	Cost, metallic color

gam can be used. After 15 minutes, the core is hard enough to begin the crown preparation. The crown margin should be extended 1 mm apical to the amalgam–tooth interface (Figures 18–12A to F).

For molars, if there is little remaining tooth structure or the pulp chamber is shallow, then a post should be used to provide retention for the core (Figure 18–13A). Usually, only one post is

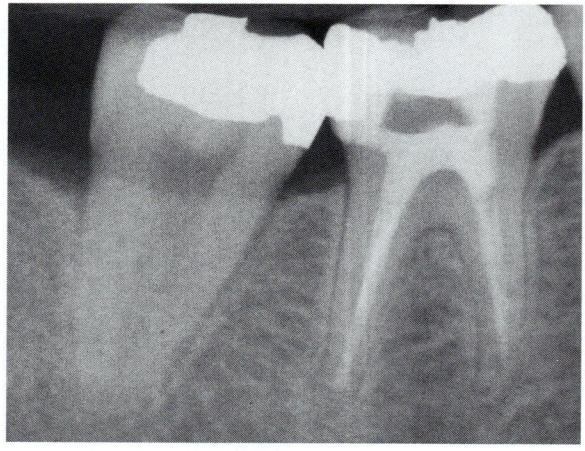

Figure 18–12A: Periapical radiograph showing tooth #30 after successful root canal treatment.

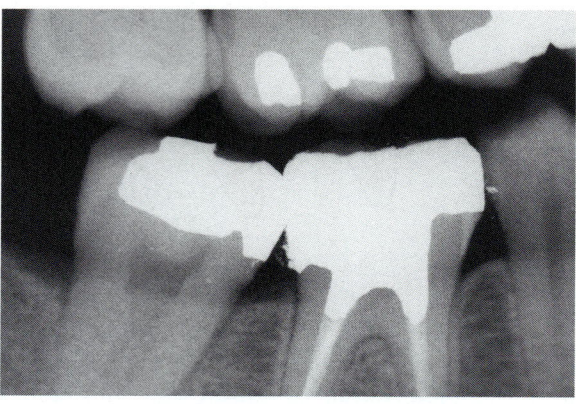

Figure 18–12B: Bitewing radiograph showing tooth #30 with amalgam core build-up completed. Note that the core material extends approximately 2 mm into the canal orifices for increased retention.

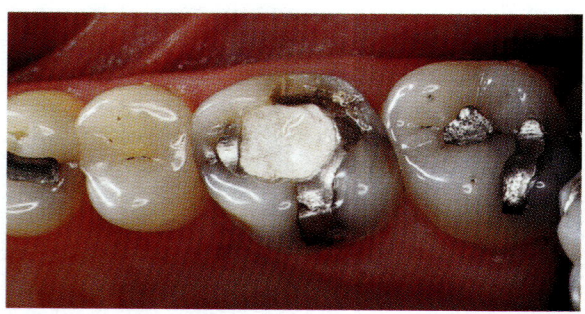

Figure 18–12C: Tooth #14 after successful root canal treatment.

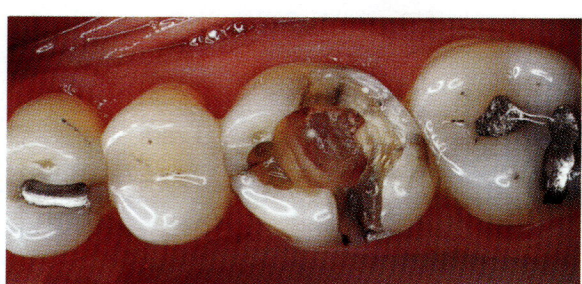

Figure 18–12D: Removal of temporary restorative material and remaining amalgam. Gutta-percha from the pulp chamber was removed for core retention.

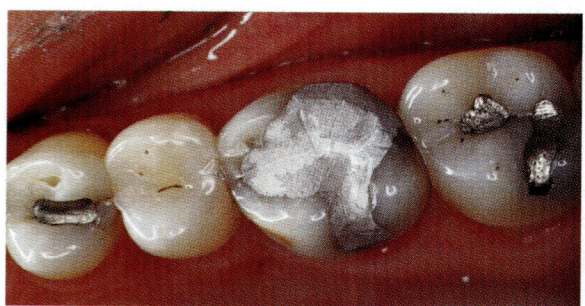

Figure 18–12E: Completed core build-up on tooth #14.

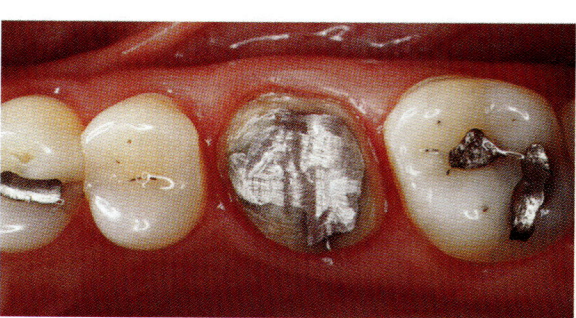

Figure 18–12F: Completed crown preparation on tooth #14.

Chipped, Fractured, or Endodontically Treated Teeth 543

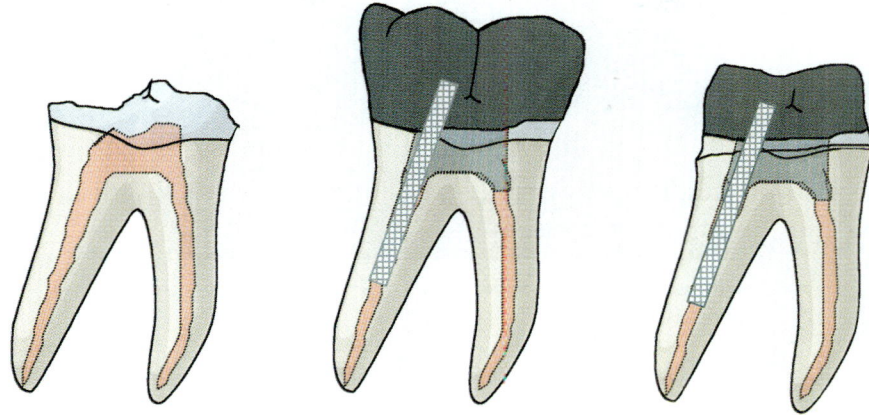

Figure 18–13A: Prefabricated post with core.

needed. A prefabricated post should be cemented into the largest canal. In mandibular molars, this will typically be the distal canal. No attempt should be made to place a post in the mesial canal of a mandibular molar as the distal wall of the mesial root is thin and easily perforated. For maxillary molars, a single post in the lingual canal is adequate. Because the direction of the post is divergent from the pulp chamber, it creates excellent retention for the core (Figures 18–13B to F).

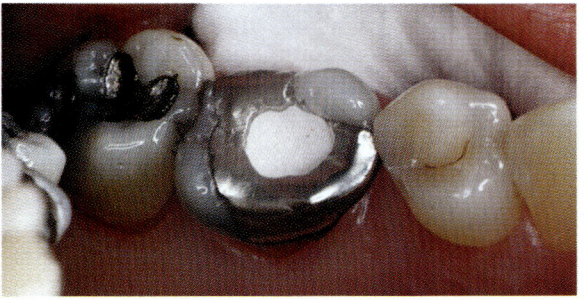

Figure 18–13B: Tooth #3 after successful root canal treatment.

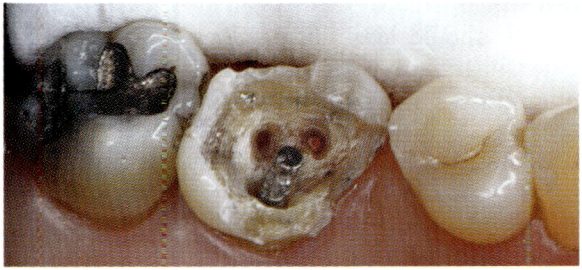

Figure 18–13C: Inadequate pulp chamber wall height and lack of remaining tooth structure evident after removal of previous restorative materials. Additional retention with prefabricated post is indicated.

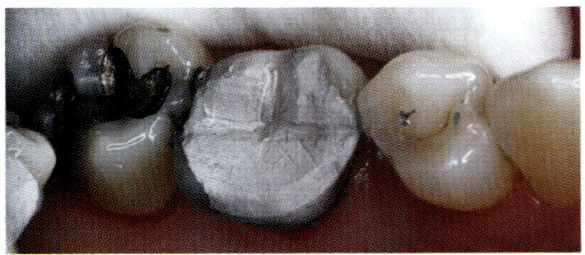

Figure 18–13D: Completed core build-up on tooth #3.

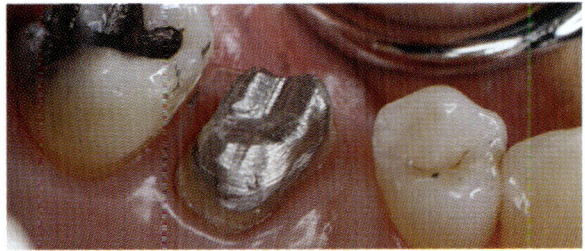

Figure 18–13E: Completed crown preparation on tooth #3. Note that the preparation margin extends apical to the core–tooth interface.

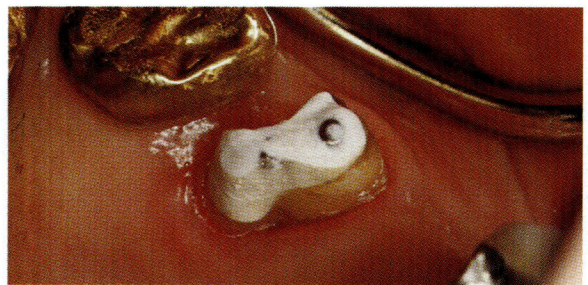

Figure 18–13F: Composite resin may also be used as core material.

Sequence for Anterior Teeth

For anterior teeth, the decision to use a prefabricated post versus a cast post and core is best made after the crown preparation is completed (Table 18–8). The appropriate amount of incisal and axial reduction should be created. Then the amount of remaining sound tooth structure can be evaluated to make the decision about the post type. The prefabricated post and core is indicated when there is a moderate amount of remaining tooth structure or there are significant undercuts in the canal or pulp chamber that would require excessive removal of tooth structure. It should also allow the preparation of the crown margin at least 2 mm beyond the core to minimize the risk of water absorption. The advantage of this technique is that it conserves tooth structure, decreases the risk of root fracture, and is less expensive and time consuming. There are several disadvantages with the prefabricated post technique. The core of a prefabricated post and core is not as strong as a cast post and core. There is a risk of mechanical failure of the core since the composite resin core materials do not bond to the cemented posts, and, as previously mentioned, the resin core is susceptible to water absorption. It is also not indicated when the long axis of the root is significantly different from the long axis of the core.

The cast post and core is indicated when there is a minimal amount of remaining tooth structure or the core will be very close to the crown margin (less than 1 mm). It may also be needed when the core does not align with the root or there is a deep vertical overlap resulting in minimal occlusal clearance. The advantage of the cast post and core is that it is strong and will fit irregular or flared canals. The major disadvantages are that it is expensive, time consuming, and less conservative (requires more tooth reduction to eliminate undercuts or for canal enlargement).

Post Preparation

After the decision has been made for either a cast post and core or a prefabricated post and core, the canal preparation should be initiated. The gutta-percha may be removed with either a hot instrument (plugger) or with a rotary instrument. The rotary instrument is more convenient, and there is no risk of burning the patient. A noncutting drill

TABLE 18–8. Post and Core Options for Anterior Teeth

	INDICATIONS	ADVANTAGES	DISADVANTAGES
Prefabricated post and core	Moderate amount of remaining tooth structure Undercuts in canal or chamber Crown margin can be prepared ≥ 2 mm past core	Conserves tooth structure, decreased risk of root fracture, less expensive, simple technique, less time consuming	Not as strong as cast post and core, failure may occur at post–core interface
Cast post and core	Minimal amount of remaining tooth structure Core close to preparation margin Core does not align with root	Strong, fits irregular canals	Expensive, time consuming, less conservative

(Gates Glidden, Miltex, York, PA, or Peeso reamer, Miltex) is the proper instrument for this step. The noncutting drill should be smaller in diameter than the existing canal space so that it only removes gutta-percha. A high-speed bur or an end-cutting drill from a prefabricated post kit should never be used to remove the gutta-percha because the risk of perforation is too great. The tooth is measured on a radiograph, a reference point is established on the tooth, and the gutta-percha is carefully removed to the desired depth, leaving a minimum of 4 mm for the apical seal. Ideally, a minimum of 10 mm of length should be obtained. The canal preparation should be the same at this point regardless of the type of post that is planned. No attempt should be made at this time to enlarge the canal; the goal of this step is to establish the proper post length.

The post space length and preservation of gutta-percha in the apical portion of the root can be verified with a radiograph at this time. Digital radiographs are a distinct advantage as they save considerable time and require much less radiation, thus allowing the operator to take multiple views during the entire procedure. Combined with digital radiography, the use of an intraoral camera or surgical microscope can provide an excellent view of the canal and an inherent safety factor in preventing perforation. Next, the canal should be shaped with the drills provided with the post system. Enlargement of the canal should be kept to a minimum, remembering that the tooth becomes weaker as more tooth structure is removed. The canal should not be enlarged any greater than is necessary to accommodate the post (Figure 18–14). The typical maxillary lateral incisor should not be enlarged to more than 0.040 inches in diameter. Maxillary central incisors may be enlarged to a diameter of 0.050 inches. If the coronal portion of the canal is flared, the canal should not be enlarged to achieve parallel walls as this will unnecessarily weaken the root. In this case, it would be better to use a tapered, prefabricated post design or a cast post and core in combination with a resin cement.

The choice of material type is probably less significant than adhering to accepted design principles (ie, adequate length, parallel shape). The most commonly used prefabricated post types are stainless steel, titanium, or titanium alloy. The prefabricated post can be cemented with any acceptable cement, including glass ionomer or zinc phosphate cement. If the post is shorter than desired or the canal is tapered, a resin cement should be considered. For the core, composite resin has the necessary strength, provides dentin bonding, and is the material of choice to use with prefabricated posts in anterior teeth. Figures 18–15A to G show two examples of the use of post and composite resin build-up.

If a cast post and core is indicated, the pattern can be made either by a direct or indirect technique (Figure 18–16). For the direct technique, undercuts in the canal or pulp chamber must be blocked out. Then a direct pattern can be made using the appropriate-size plastic post from the post system and making the core with autopolymerizing acrylic resin. With the indirect technique, an impression of the tooth is obtained using a plastic post to record the post space. The post can be cast in either a noble or non-noble metal (Figure 18–17). For smaller-diameter posts, a type III gold alloy is inad-

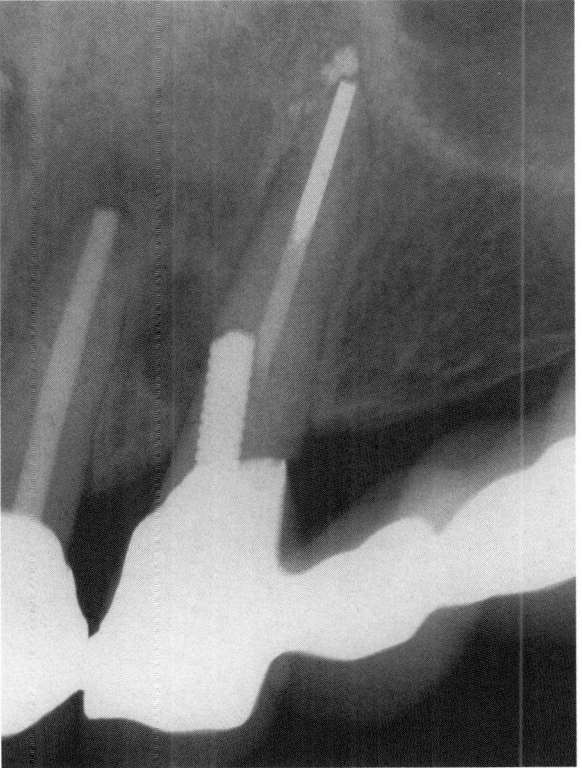

Figure 18–14: Improper post and core technique leading to clinical failure.

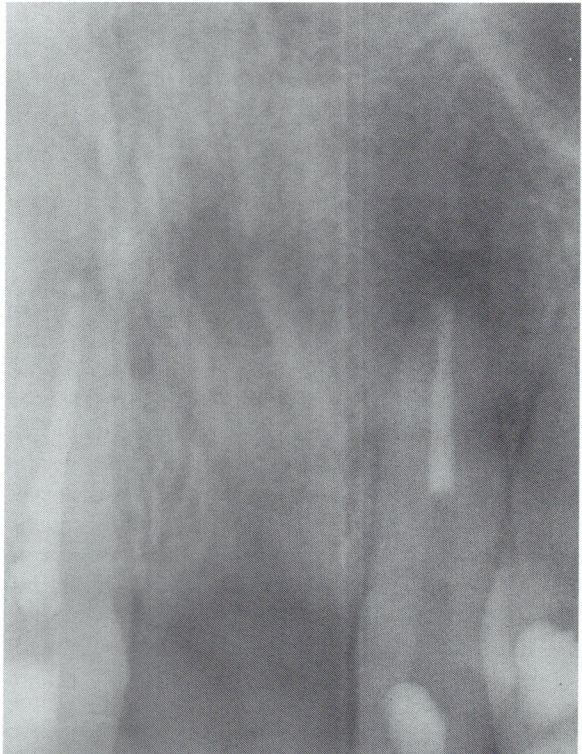

Figure 18–15A: Periapical radiograph showing tooth #7 after post space preparation.

visable as it does not provide adequate strength. The use of a non-noble alloy (Ni-Cr-Be) provides the potential for resin bonding of the post to the dentin surface of the canal. This may be desirable for short posts or for tapered canals.

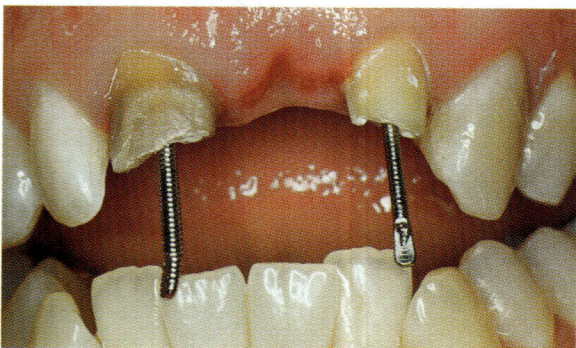

Figure 18–15B: Try-in of prefabricated posts. The post should be at least equal in length to the clinical crown or two-thirds of the root length.

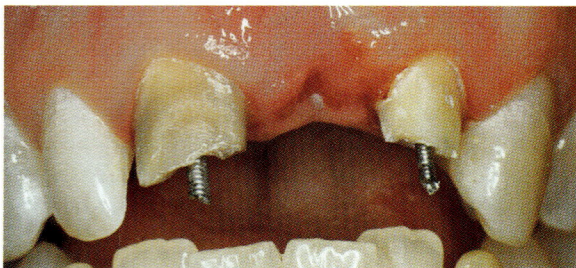

Figure 18–15C: Prefabricated post cut to length and cemented.

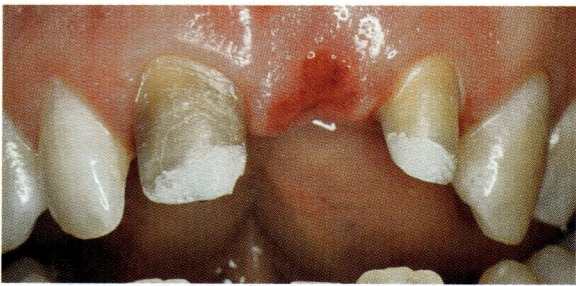

Figure 18–15D: Teeth #8 and #10 restored with composite core build-up material and prepared to receive porcelain-fused-to-metal crowns.

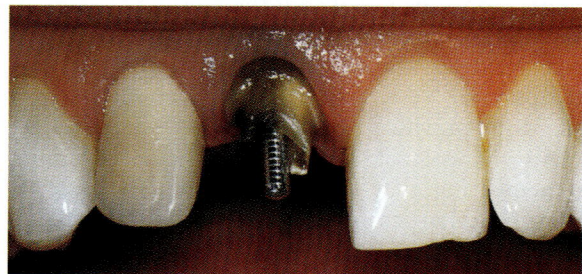

Figure 18–15E: In another patient, tooth #8 with a prefabricated post cut to length and cemented.

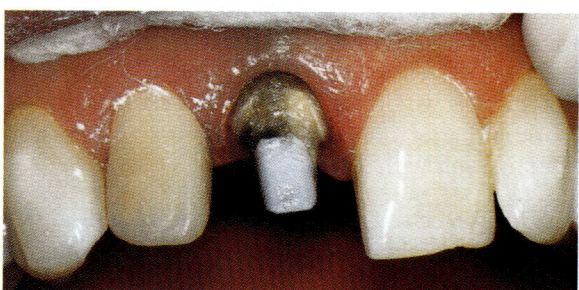

Figure 18–15F: Tooth #8 restored with composite core build-up material.

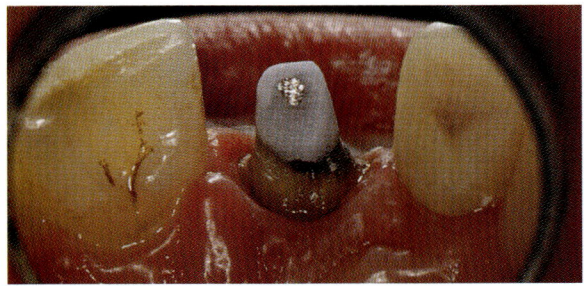

Figure 18–15G: Mirror view of the lingual surface of tooth #8. Note the ferrule design with 1 to 2 mm of vertical tooth structure beyond the restorative margin.

For cementation of the post, a groove or vent should be created along the length of the post to allow for excess cement. If using zinc phosphate or glass ionomer cements, a Lentulo spiral drill (DENTSPLY/Caulk) should be used to place the cement into the canal. This will result in the maximum retention for the post. After the cement has set, the excess is removed, and the core material is placed (prefabricated post) or the impression procedures are initiated (cast post and core).

For resin cement, the instructions for the bonding and cementation procedures for the cement should be followed. This may include placing cement on the post rather than into the canal to prevent overly rapid set of the cement. One advantage of using resin cement is that the core material can be placed immediately after the post is seated. Then the cement and core resin can set simultaneously and bond together. This technique works especially well when retrofitting a post to an existing crown (reverse post crown repair).

Sequence for Premolars

The type of foundation restoration for a premolar is determined by the amount of available tooth structure. This requires making an estimation of the amount of tooth structure that will remain after the crown preparation. If there is a moderate amount of tooth structure, the tooth can be restored like a molar using amalgam or composite as the core material. Similar to a molar, the retention for the core would be gained by either mechanical retention and/or dentin bonding. If there is minimal tooth structure, it is best to use the same treatment sequence as described for an anterior tooth. First, the tooth is prepared for the indicated crown. Then the

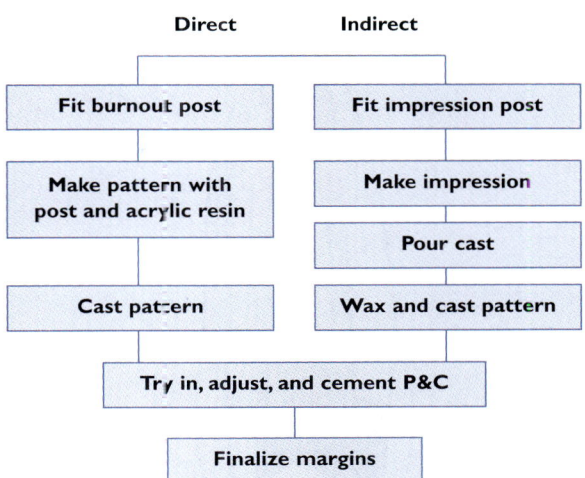

Figure 18–16: Cast post and core.

amount of remaining tooth structure is evaluated. If the premolar has two roots, prefabricated posts can be cemented in the two canals (Figures 18–18A and B). It is usually not possible or even necessary to make these posts very long because of canal curvature. However, because the canals are usually not parallel, following placement of the core, the posts and core are virtually impossible to dislodge. For a small premolar, composite resin is a better core material than amalgam because the prefabricated posts weaken the amalgam. If there is minimal or no coronal tooth structure, a cast post should be considered, especially for a single rooted premolar.

Principles for Crown Preparation

The proper preparation of the tooth after completion of the post and core restoration is very impor-

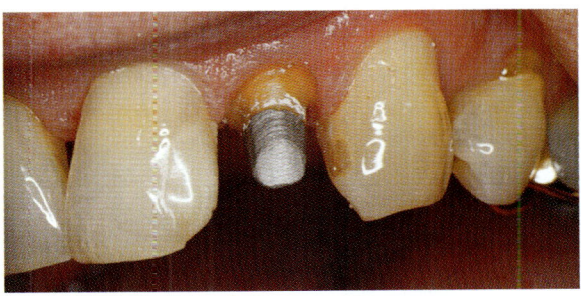

Figure 18–17: Similar case restored with cast post and core. The decision between restoring a tooth with a prefabricated post or cast post and core depends on how much intact tooth structure is remaining.

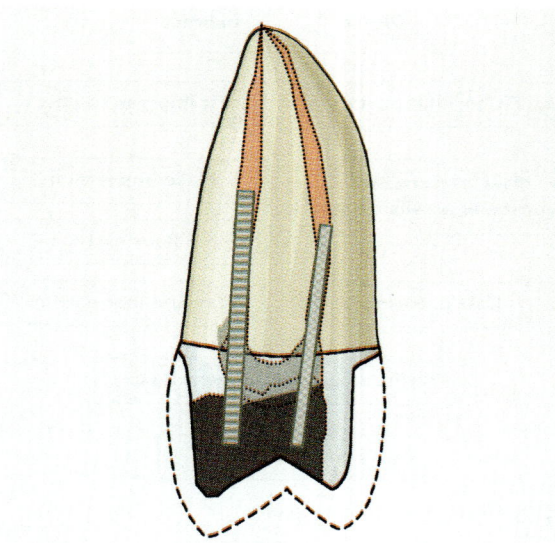

Figure 18–18A: Prefabricated post for additional core retention.

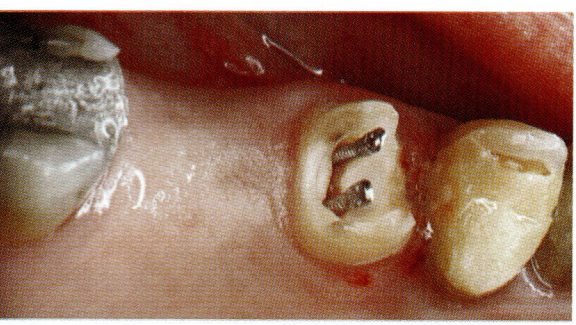

Figure 18–18B: Prefabricated posts in the two canals of a premolar prior to core placement. It is usually not possible to make these posts very long because of canal curvature. Because canals are usually not parallel to each other, the core is well retained by posts.

tant. Even with the ideal canal preparation and post restoration, the post has a tremendous potential to act as a wedge in the tooth root. This can result in initiation of a vertical root fracture and subsequent loss of the tooth. The best way to protect the tooth (ie, the root) against this wedging force is by the creation of a ferrule design in the crown preparation on the tooth.[3,16,18,21,28] The ferrule design is the encirclement of 1 to 2 mm of vertical tooth structure by the crown. This encirclement, like metal bands on a barrel, helps protect the tooth from fracture. It resists the wedging forces that would be transmitted to the post from the occlusion. To create an adequate ferrule, the margin usually must be prepared further apical. Often, this requires a crown-lengthening procedure to gain sufficient tooth length to prepare the ferrule (Figure 18–19). This principle of creating a ferrule around the tooth is probably the single most important principle in the restoration of endodontically treated teeth (Figures 18–20A to C). If an adequate ferrule is obtained, the type, material, and design of the post and core become much less important. Conversely, if a ferrule is not obtained, then the tooth is at risk of fracturing no matter what type of post and core is used. This is especial-

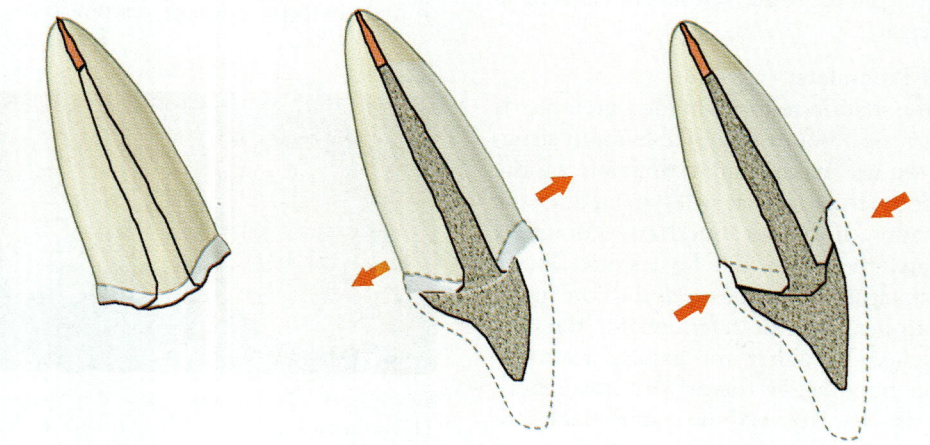

Figure 18–19: Ferrule design resists wedging force of post.

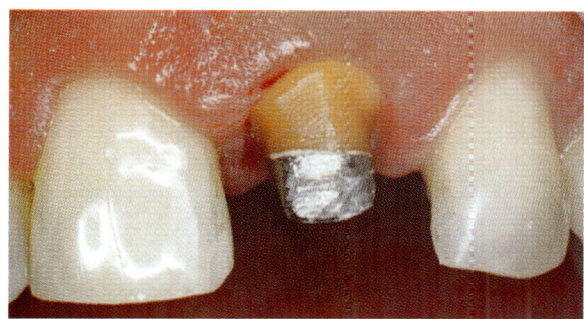

Figure 18–20A: Proper ferrule design on preparation for porcelain-fused-to-metal crown.

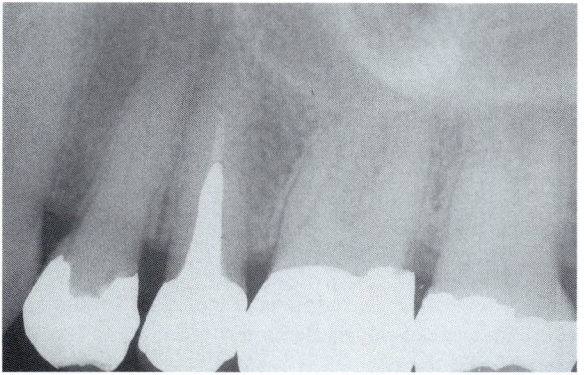

Figure 18–20B: Radiograph showing cast post and core after cementation. Note that the post is more than one-third of the diameter of the root at the cement–enamel junction and is tapered. Tooth preparation did not exhibit ferrule design.

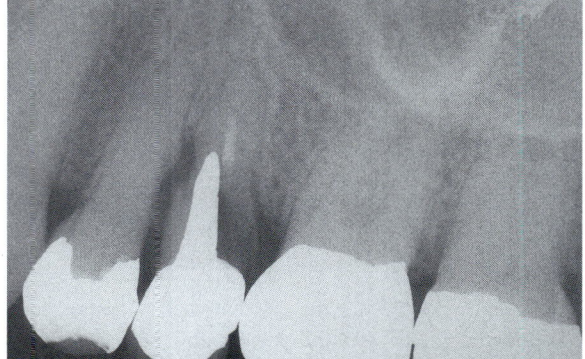

Figure 18–20C: Same clinical case as in Figure 18–20B after 8 years. Note the oblique root fracture. Such a fracture could be prevented by a more conservative post in combination with proper ferrule design in the crown preparation.

ly true for teeth that are expected to carry a heavy load such as a removable partial denture or fixed partial denture abutment or in patients who exhibit excessive wear or bruxism.

References

1. Andreasen JO, Andreasen FM. Essentials of traumatic injuries to the teeth. Copenhagen: Munksgaard, 1990.

2. Andreasen FM, Noren JG, Andreasen JO, et al. Long-term survival of fragment bonding in the treatment of fractured crowns: a multicenter clinical study. Quintessence Int 1995;26:669–81.

3. Assif D, Bitenski A, Pilo R, Oren E. Effects of post design on resistance to fracture of endodontically treated teeth with complete crowns. J Prosthet Dent 1993; 69:36–40.

4. Bader JD, Shugars DA, Robertson TM. Using crowns to prevent tooth fracture. Community Dent Oral Epidemiol 1996;24:47–51.

5. Cavalleri G, Zerman N. Traumatic crown fractures in permanent incisors with immature roots: a follow-up study. Endodont Dent Traumatol 1995;11:294–6.

6. Croll TP. Rapid reattachment of fractured crown segment: an update. J Esthet Dent 1990;2:1–5.

7. Cvek MA. A clinical report on partial pulpotomy and capping with calcium hydroxide in permanent incisors with complicated crown fracture. J Endod 1978;4:232–7.

8. Ehrmann EH. Restoration of a fractured incisor with exposed pulp using original tooth fragment: report of a case. J Am Dent Assoc 1989;118:183–5.

9. Fahl N Jr. Predictable aesthetic reconstruction of fractured anterior teeth with composite resins: a case report. Pract Periodont Aesthet Dent 1996;8(1):17–31.

10. Fahl N Jr. Optimizing the esthetics of Class IV restorations with composite resins. J Can Dent Assoc 1997;63:108–11, 114–5.

11. Goldstein RE. Chipped or fractured teeth. In: Esthetics in dentistry. Philadelphia: JB Lippincott, 1976:54–64.

12. Goldstein RE. Diagnostic dilemma: to bond, laminate, or crown. Int J Periodont Restor Dent 1987;7:5, 8–29.

13. Goldstein RE. Esthetic principles for ceramo-metal restorations. Dent Clin North Am 1988;21:803–22.

14. Goldstein RE. Repairing fractured teeth. In: Change your smile. 3rd edn. Carol Stream, IL: Quintessence, 1997:89–106.

15. Goldstein RE, Levitas TC. Preservation of fractured maxillary central incisors in an adolescent: report of a case. J Am Dent Assoc 1972;84:381.

16. Hemmings KW, King PA, Setchell DJ. Resistance to torsional forces of various post and core designs. J Prosthet Dent 1991;66:325–9.

17. Hunter ML, Hunter B, Kingdon A, et al. Traumatic injuries to maxillary incisor teeth in a group of South Wales school children. Endod Dent Traumatol 1990;6:260–4.

18. Hyde TP. A reattachment technique for fractured incisor tooth fragments: a case history and discussion of alternative techniques. Primary Dent Care 1995;2(1):18, 20–2.

19. Isidor F, Brondum K, Ravnholt G. The influence of post length and crown ferrule length on the resistance to cyclic loading of bovine teeth with prefabricated titanium posts. Int J Prosthodont 1999;12:78–82.

20. Kanca J 3rd. Replacement of a fractured incisor fragment over pulpal exposure: a long-term case report. Quintessence Int 1996;27:829–32.

21. Libman WJ, Nicholls JI. Load fatigue of teeth restored with cast posts and cores and complete crowns. Int J Prosthodont 1995;8:155–61.

22. Liebenberg WH. Esthetics in the cracked tooth syndrome: steps to success using resin-bonded ceramic restorations. J Esthet Dent 1995;7:155–66.

23. Liebenberg WH. Use of resin-bonded partial coverage ceramic restorations to treat incomplete fractures in posterior teeth: a clinical report. Quintessence Int 1996;27:739–47.

24. Munskgarrd ZC, Hojtred L, Jorgensen EAW, et al. Enamel-dentin crown fractures bonded with various bonding agents. Endod Dent Traumatol 1991;7:73–77.

25. Saupe WA, Gluskin AH, Radke RA Jr. A comparative study of fracture resistance between morphologic dowel and cores and a resin-reinforced dowel system in the intraradicular restoration of structurally compromised roots. Quintessence Int 1996;27:483–91.

26. Simonsen RJ. Restoration of a fractured central incisor using original tooth fragment. J Am Dent Assoc 1982;105:646–8.

27. Simonsen RJ. Traumatic fracture restoration: an alternative use of the acid-etch technique. Quintessence Int 1979;10:15–22.

28. Sorensen JA, Engelman MJ. Ferrule design and fracture resistance of endodontically treated teeth. J Prosthet Dent 1990;63:529–36.

29. Sorensen JA, Martinoff JT. Intracoronal reinforcement and coronal coverage: a study of endodontically treated teeth. J Prosthet Dent 1984;51:780–4.

30. Sorensen JA, Martinoff JT. Clinical significant factors in dowel design. J Prosthet Dent 1984;52:28–35.

31. Strassler HE. Aesthetic management of traumatized anterior teeth. Dent Clin North Am 1995;39:181–202.

32. Vissichelli VP. Restoration of a fractured maxillary central incisor by using the original tooth fragment. Gen Dent 1996;44:238–40.

33. Walker M. Fractured-tooth fragment reattachment. Gen Dent 1996;44:434–6.

Additional Resources

Bakland LK, Milledge T, Nation W. Treatment of crown fractures. J Calif Dent Assoc 1996;24(2):45–50.

Goldstein RE. Current concepts in esthetic treatment. Proceedings of the Second International Prosthodontic Congress; 1979; Los Angeles, CA, Chicago: Quintessence, 1979:310–2.

Goldstein RE. Esthetics in dentistry. J Am Dent Assoc 1982;104:301–2.

Goldstein RE. Finishing of composites and laminates. Dent Clin North Am 1989;33:305–18.

Goldstein RE. Change your smile. 3rd edn. Carol Stream, IL: Quintessence, 1997.

Goldstein RE, Feinman RA, Garber DA. Esthetic considerations in the selection and use of restorative materials. Dent Clin North Am 1983;27:723–31.

Goldstein RE, Garber DA, Schwartz CG, Goldstein CE. Patient maintenance of esthetic restorations. J Am Dent Assoc 1992;123:61–6.

Goldstein RE, Garber DA, Goldstein CE, et al. The changing esthetic dental practice. J Am Dent Assoc 1994;125:1447–57.

Patel DK, Burke FJ. Fractures of posterior teeth: a review and analysis of associated factors. Dent Clin North Am 1995;39:181–202.

Rauschenberger CR, Hovland EJ. Clinical management of crown fractures. Dent Clin North Am 1995;39:25–51.

Takatsu T, Sano H, Burrow MF. Treatment and prognosis of a vertically fractured maxillary molar with widely separated segments: a case report. Quintessence Int 1995;26:479–84.

CHAPTER 19

ENDODONTICS AND ESTHETIC DENTISTRY

Noah Chivian, DDS, Donald E. Arens, DDS, MSD, Asgeir Sigurdsson, cand. odont., MS

Part of the success of esthetic dentistry depends on the dentist's ability to use teeth that have pulps compromised by trauma or injury. The role of the endodontist or general dentist performing endodontic procedures is to clearly intercept or eliminate the potential for problems. An equally important role is to respond to pulpal disease after esthetic restorations have been completed.

Endodontics has clearly established its role in providing the foundation needed to rebuild the dentition to form, function, health, and esthetics. As long as there is sufficient tooth structure to restore and a healthy periodontal complex for support, root canal therapy is the treatment of choice when a pulp is diseased or compromised by restorative demands. Although regional differences in techniques and materials exist, there is general agreement within the endodontic community on principles, that is, strict adherence to the endodontic triad of microbial disinfection and control, débridement, and the sealing of the canal system. With proven and predictable success rates, dentists can include endodontically treated teeth in their esthetic restorative treatment plans with the utmost degree of confidence.

TREATMENT PLANNING

Endodontics should be incorporated into the multidisciplined treatment process when the ultimate esthetic design is being determined. Treatment sequencing can be established and painful episodes and disruption of the restorative schedule avoided if the pulpal health and any previously root canal–treated teeth are evaluated early in the planning stages. The patient should be informed that the overall treatment plan is dynamic and may change as conditions arise. It is equally important to evaluate the patient's radiographs, and if deep existing amalgam or other restorations will be redone as part of the treatment plan, the patient should be advised of future problems owing to the depth of those restorations. If, at a later time, there are complications such as an inflamed pulp or pain following final cementation, the patient has at least been forewarned. This problem is sometimes complicated by difficulty in seeing the depth of certain tooth-colored restorations.

The removal of existing restorations, excavation of decay, and paralleling of multiple abutments may require periodic reassessment and endodontic reconsideration. Sensitive teeth that do not respond to palliative measures within a reasonable period of time may require pulpectomy. There is nothing more disheartening to a patient who has completed 18 months of combined orthodontic, periodontic, and restorative treatment than to experience a "toothache" shortly after final cementation. Although pulpal problems cannot always be predicted, a great majority can be avoided with insight, careful evaluation, and good judgment.

CLINICAL EVALUATION

The success of any reconstructive treatment plan depends on the health of the pulp, the periradicular area, and/or the quality of the existing root canal therapy of the teeth to be restored. In an effort to determine this condition, a standardized evaluating procedure should include the following:

- Communication that includes listening and recording
- Visual examination
- Periodontal probing
- Thermal tests
- Electric tests
- Cavity tests

- Periapical tests
  - Percussion
  - Palpation
- Bite tests
- Radiographic evaluation

History

Besides knowing the medical condition of the patient, the diagnostician should ask the patient about past dental experiences. Their desires and objectives should be clearly defined. If neglect is evident, the reasons for the neglect should be determined and discussed. If phobia and anxieties exist, the extensiveness of the case should be explained and relaxation techniques should be offered to ensure a comfortable and pain-free treatment experience. In addition, when a professional air of confidence, concern, and care is exhibited by the doctor, the patient's faith and interest can be gained. Once this rapport is established, the patient becomes far more receptive to accepting and entering a treatment program regardless of its difficulty and their apprehensions. The quality of treatment is inversely proportional to the level of stress experienced by the patient and the doctor during the procedure. Again, warning your patient about the potential for existing restorations to require future endodontic treatment is vital for continued patient trust.

Communication

Listen, Learn, and Record. Dentists are the professionals who must perform the tests, interpret the results, and design a treatment based on the information gathered. When the diagnosis is not evident, the dentist must turn to the patient for that one pinpointing clue. Sir William Osler, the famous English physician, once said, "Listen, listen, listen —for the patient is giving you the diagnosis." This statement is profound. The diagnostician must not only ask sufficient and leading questions to obtain as much information as possible but must also listen carefully to interpret the verbal response and its expressed meaning. Patients should be quoted verbatim in the chart, and their answers must become a permanent record for review.

Visual Examination

Direct examination of each tooth with some method of magnification (loupes or a microscope) is essential to locate fracture lines, decay, or defective restorations.

Transillumination via a fiber-optic light may be of great assistance in detecting color shifts in a crown (Figures 19–1A and B). A tooth with a pink or reddish hue would more than likely indicate internal hemorrhage from a recent injury (Figure 19–2), a dental procedure (Figure 19–3), or gingival tissue hyperplasia that has invaded a coronal cavity produced by caries or resorption (Figures 19–4A to D).

A gray, blue, or black color might indicate blood infiltrate hemostasis within the dentinal tubules

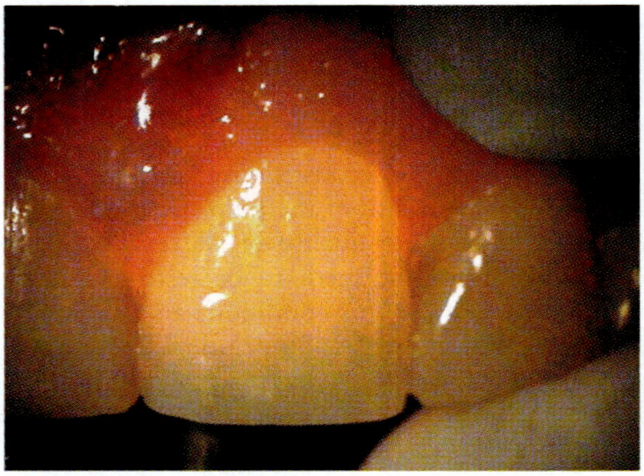

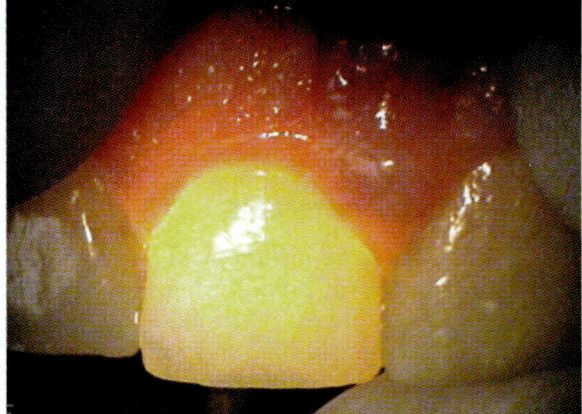

Figure 19–1A: Transillumination of a maxillary left central incisor with a necrotic pulp.

Figure 19–1B: Transillumination of the adjacent tooth with a vital pulp. Because there is active blood flow through the live pulp tissue, the tooth appears brighter to the fiber-optic light than the adjacent tooth with a necrotic pulp.

and chamber, long-term necrotic tissue (Figure 19–5), or silver precipitants from certain root canal sealers and filling materials (Figures 19–6A to C). A yellow or brown (Figures 19–7A and B) unrestored crown often represents a physiologically calcified nonpathologic obliteration of the root chamber/canal. Pharmacologically affected (ie, tetracycline-stained) teeth may vary in color from yellow to black (Figures 19–8A to C), and their drug fluorescence and etiology may be verified by using an ultraviolet or Woods black light.

The reader is referred to the chapter on bleaching as many of these discolorations can be reduced or eliminated by oxidizing techniques and agents without requiring endodontic intervention.

Teeth with vertical fractures have a diagnostic constant. The transilluminated light does not pass through the fracture line, but the crown beyond the fracture (Figures 19–9A and B) or the opposite cusp(s) (Figure 19–10) appears darker. Periodontal probing, cold testing, and a bite test will possibly assist in confirming the diagnosis of cracked tooth syndrome.

Periodontal Probing

The depth of the sulcus and individual pockets are of concern to the treating dentist or endodontist. There are two main reasons for that concern. One is that if there is a combined periodontal endodontic problem associated with a tooth, the true cause of the problem is not only difficult to diagnose but could also be even more difficult to manage during treatment. The second issue is that if there is an isolated, narrow, but deep periodontal pocket somewhere around the tooth, a vertical root fracture has to be ruled out prior to any further restorative treatment. The pocket could be just a draining sinus tract from a necrotic and infected pulp. Endodontic therapy would then be indicated, and the pocket should heal without any periodontal therapy within days after the initial endodontic visit. The pocket could also be associated with a vertical root fracture, and if that is the case, the prognosis of the tooth is hopeless. Endodontic therapy would not clear up the pocket, nor would periodontal therapy. Extraction of the tooth or removal of the root would be the only treatment option.

Thermal Pulp Tests

In an effort to determine the vitality of a pulp, the cold test is probably the most commonly advocated. In the past, an "ice pencil" (water frozen in sterilized anesthetic cartridge and removed) (Figure 19–11) or an ice cube was the only consistent way to chill a tooth. But there are several problems with using frozen water: it is not very cold, so the stimulus may not be intense enough to penetrate through a porcelain crown, and cold water from the pencil could leak on adjacent teeth or gingival tissue, giving a false impression of pulpal vitality in the tooth that is being tested. However, in a tooth with an acute pulpitis, an ice pencil is an effective diagnostic tool. Recently, 1,1,1,2-tetrafluoroethane has become available in spray form (Endo-Ice, Hygenic, Akron, OH) (Figure 19–12). This gas is relatively cold (–26°C), enough to penetrate through most crowns, and more importantly, the

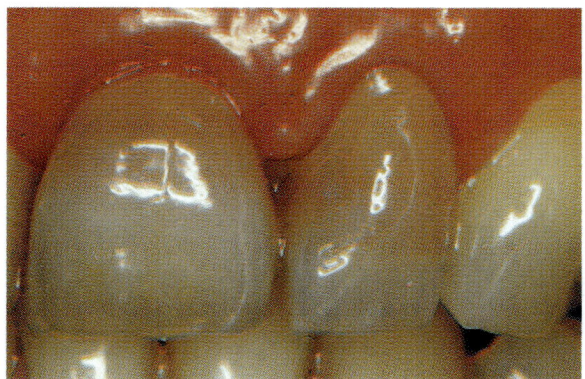

Figure 19–2: The maxillary central and lateral incisor teeth experienced a concussion injury and there was subsequent extravasation of blood causing the reddish hue.

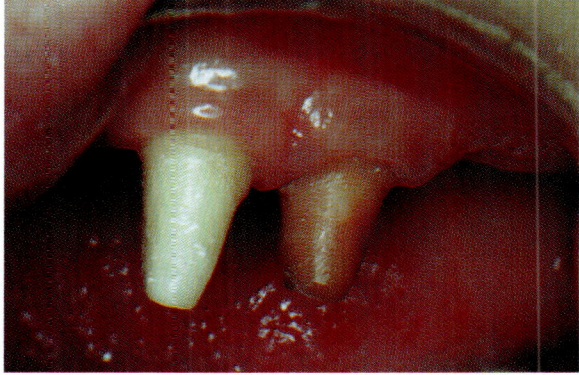

Figure 19–3: One week following crown preparation, the tooth structure was red, signifying extravasation of blood and the need for pulp extirpation.

556 Esthetics in Dentistry

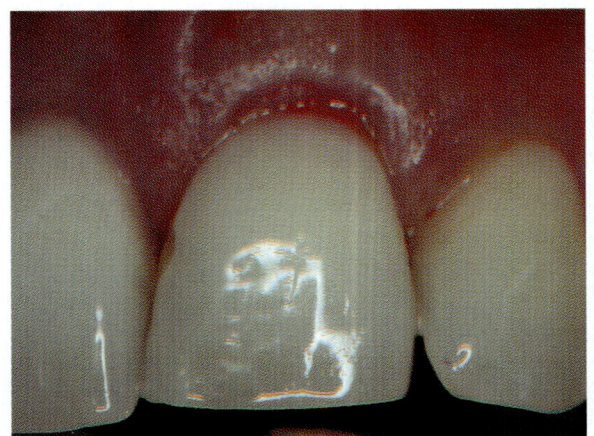

Figure 19–4A: Pink spot as a result of external resorption.

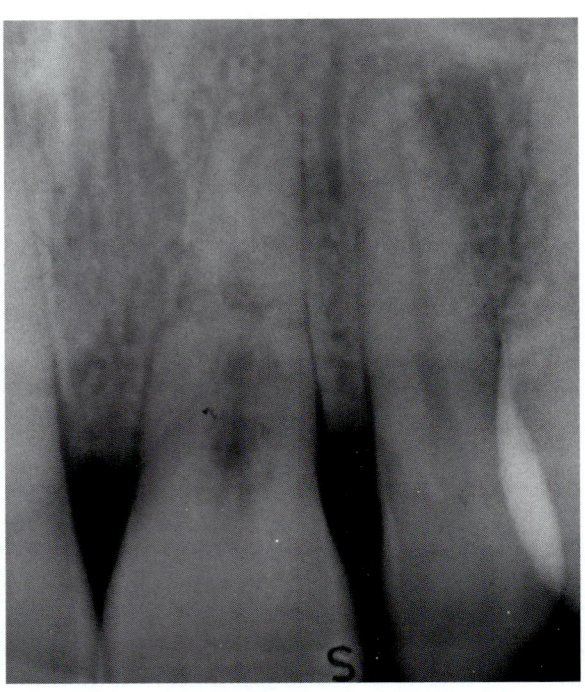

Figure 19–4B: Radiograph of the same tooth showing external resorption.

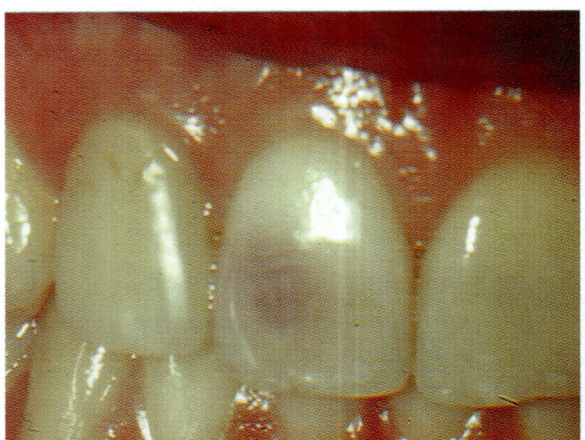

Figure 19–4C: Pink spot as a result of internal resorption.

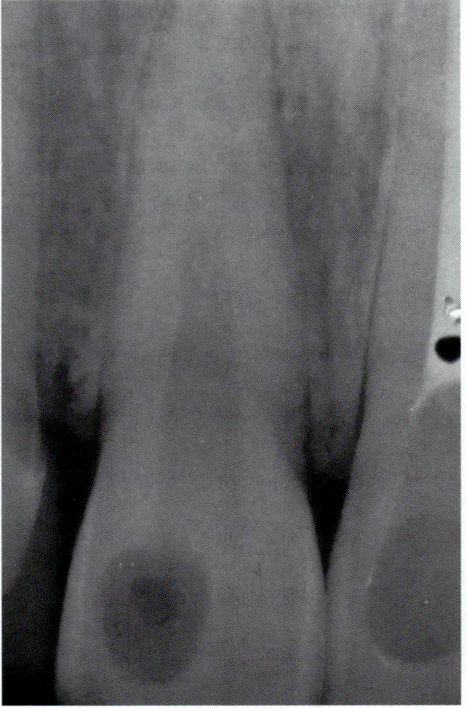

Figure 19–4D: Radiograph of the same tooth showing internal resorption.

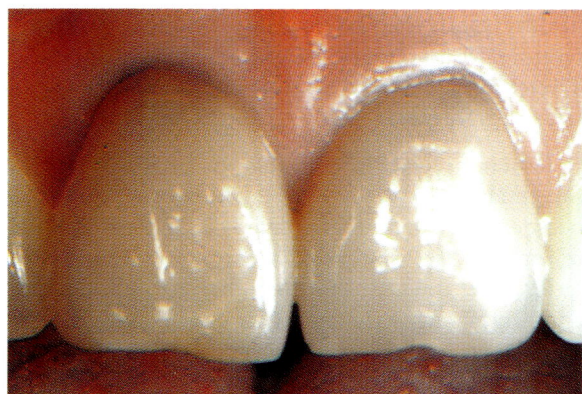

Figure 19-5: Discolored maxillary central incisors with necrotic pulps.

ice crystals will not turn into liquid prior to evaporating; rather, they will rapidly turn into gas on the tooth's surface. The use of this system is simple and inexpensive, the gas is sprayed on a cotton applicator, and then the chilled cotton is placed on the tooth that is to be tested.

Dry ice cylinders (Odontotest Thermal Pulp Tester, Miltex, York, PA) are also a very good way to investigate pulpal response to cold. Carbon dioxide is very cold (−70°C), so it will penetrate most if not all restorations, and like tetrafluoroethane, it will evaporate without turning into liquid on the tooth. There was some concern initially that the extreme cold would be dangerous to pulp, dentin, and/or the enamel, but in a series of studies by Peters et al.[23] and Ingram et al.,[13] they demonstrated that it did not do any damage to any structures investigated.[13]

The response of a normal, healthy, vital pulp is sharp and quickly dissipates once the stimulus is removed. If the response is quicker, more intense, and prolonged, it usually indicates an irreversible pulpitis. When calcified pulp chambers or constricted canals exist, the response from an otherwise

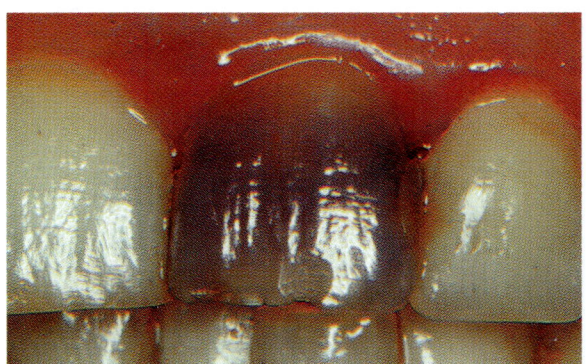

Figure 19-6A: Discoloration from silver-containing root canal cement.

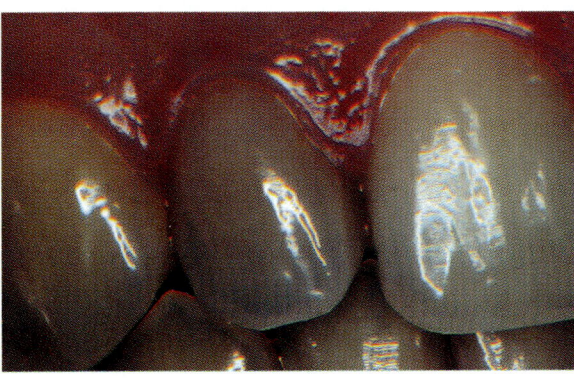

Figure 19-6B: Gray color of crown from a post.

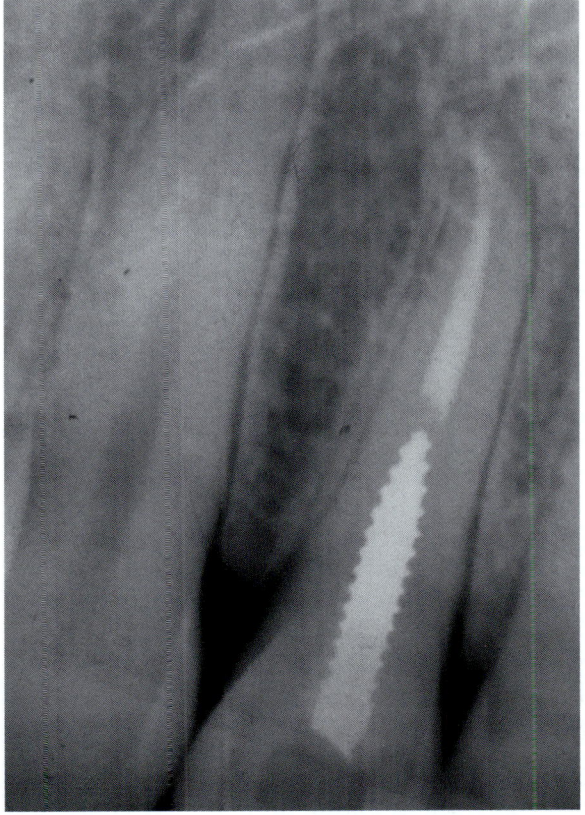

Figure 19-6C: Same radiograph as 19-6B. An unnecessary post that caused the discoloration.

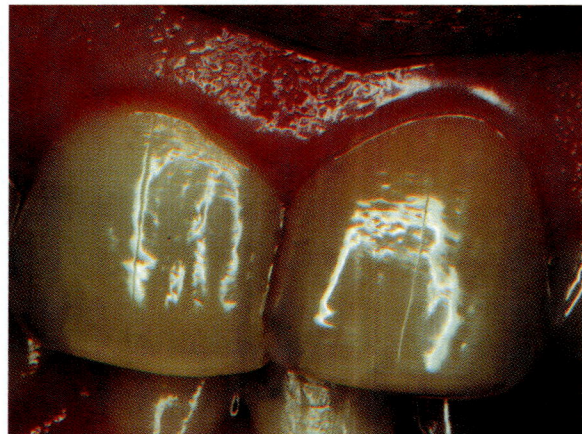

Figure 19–7A: The crown of this maxillary central incisor discolored gradually over a 3-year period following a concussion injury. The complete fill-in of the pulp chamber with dentin is the cause of the yellowish brown hue. In the absence of periapical radiographic changes and clinical symptoms, endodontic therapy is not indicated.

healthy tooth may be delayed or nonexistent. The reduced conductivity can mislead the operator. Therefore, other tests must be used to confirm negative responses.

When faced with teeth that are heavily restored, the final tests can be delayed until the tooth has been excavated, and the patient is in a provisional restoration. By wisely testing prior to final cementation, the true status of the pulp may be validated, and any changes that may have arisen during the fabrication interval can be appraised.

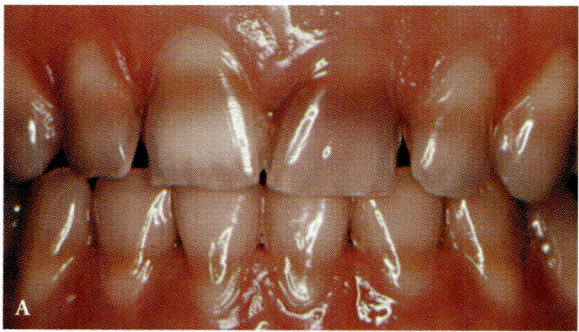
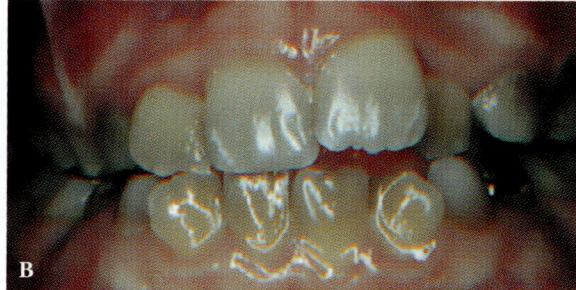
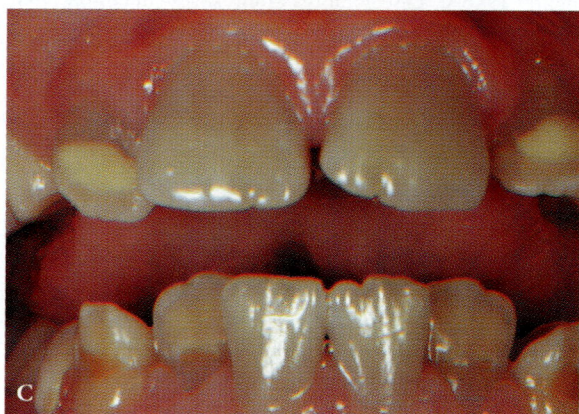

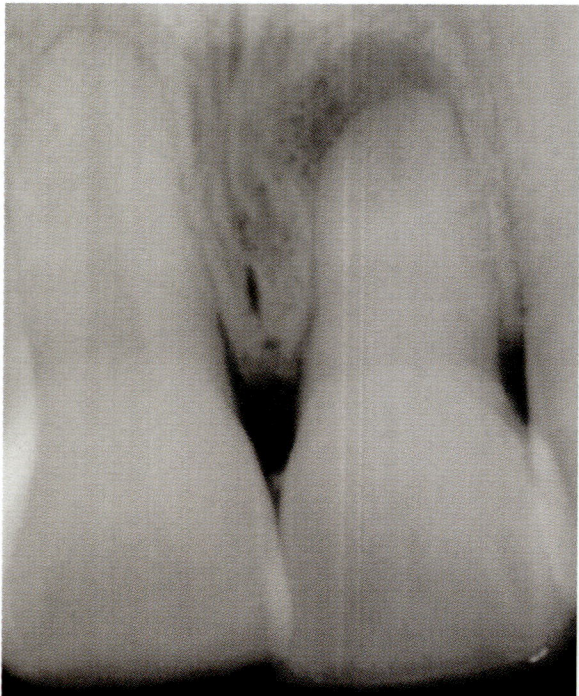

Figure 19–7B: Radiograph of a similar maxillary central incisor 10 years after a concussion injury. The pulp chamber is filled in with dentin producing the discoloration. In this case, there was pulp death years after the discoloration appeared. Because the pulp canal was obliterated, a surgical approach was used to seal the apex.

Figure 19–8A to C: *(A)* Brown staining from Terramycin. *(B)* Gray staining from Acromycin. *(C)* Tan staining from Aureomycin.

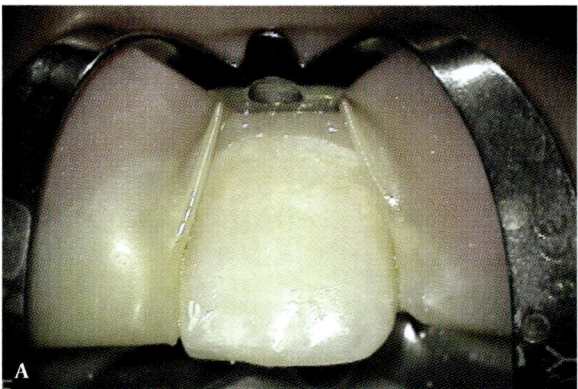 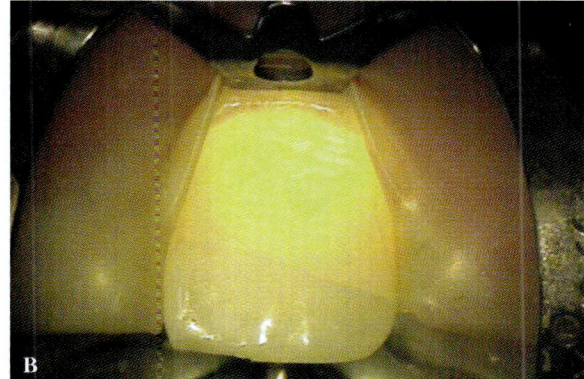

Figure 19–9A and B: *(A)* View of a maxillary central incisor tooth with overhead lighting. No fracture is visible. *(B)* Transilluminated view of the same tooth revealing the fracture line.

Heat is the least informative of the pulp tests and the most difficult to apply. Heated water applied to an individual tooth after it has been carefully isolated by a rubber dam is the most reliable method, but it is time consuming, and extreme care has to be taken so that there is no leaking under the rubber dam. It is recommended to start isolating and stimulating a tooth that is posterior to the one that is suspected to be heat sensitive and then move the rubber dam anteriorly tooth by tooth so that if there is a leak under the rubber dam, it will leak only on an already tested tooth. Heated temporary gutta-percha stopping applied to the lateral surface of a natural tooth or a metal surface of a veneer casting has been recommended, but it is difficult to control the heat, and the stopping has the tendency to stick on the tooth, causing prolonged stimuli. A rubber polishing wheel in a low-speed handpiece is an alternative also, but because it is difficult if not impossible to control the stimulus, this method is not recommended. The antiquated method of touching a tooth with a red hot burnisher should be avoided because of the risk of overheating the tooth and pulp, and there is no control over how intense the stimulus will be.

Electric Pulp Testing

Over the last 25 years, the Analytical Technology Vitality Scanner (Figure 19–13), recently renamed Kerr Vitality Scanner 2006 (KerrDental, Orange, CA), has become the standard within the endodontic community. This battery-operated device is simple, accurate, and virtually trouble free. A small amount of an electrolytic gel (toothpaste or fluoride gel) is applied to the end of the testing tip prior to its contact with the tooth. When the low-voltage

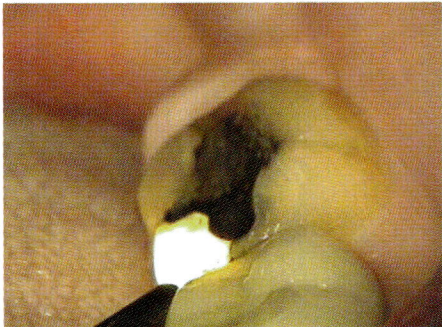 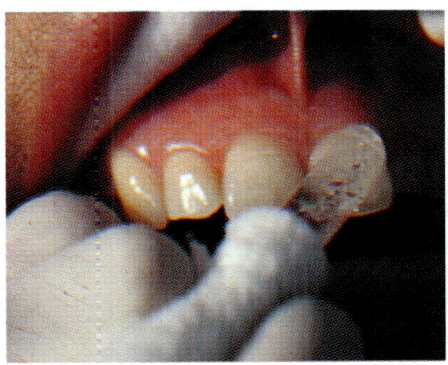

Figure 19–10: Transillumination of a mandibular second molar. The fracture lines at the mesial and lingual grooves do not allow the light to pass through.

Figure 19–11: An ice pencil being applied to a maxillary central incisor tooth.

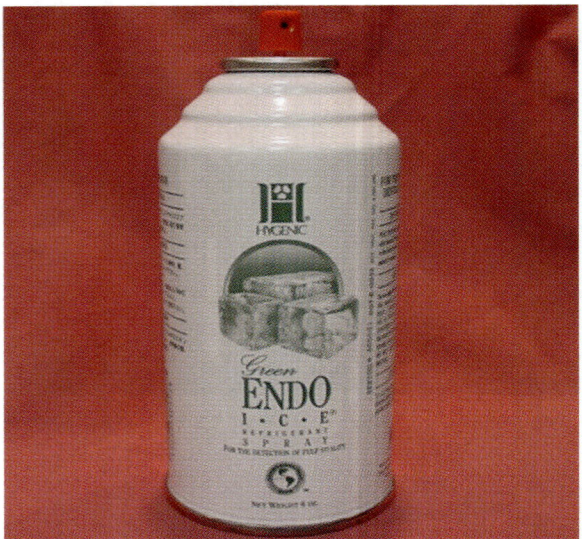

Figure 19–12: Endo-Ice (Hygenic) refrigerant.

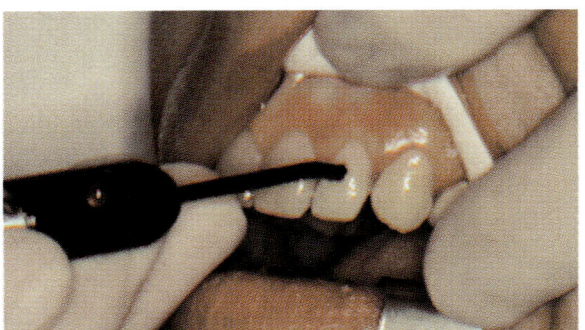

Figure 19–14: Pulp tester being applied to a dried tooth.

electrical stimulation is transmitted to the teeth (Figure 19–14), the responses can be recorded from the digital display window.

Credence should not be placed on the exactness of the numbers displayed, nor should the differential between tests of individual teeth be used to determine stages of pulpal degeneration. As previously stated, testing heavily restored teeth is difficult at best and impossible with most. It has been suggested that if root structure is exposed owing to gingival recession, the "mini-tip" that comes with the Vitality Scanner should be used (Figure 19–15). Unfortunately, this is not a very accurate method because there is a significant likelihood that the periodontal ligament would respond to the stimulus, giving the false impression that the pulp is still vital. The mini-tip, when used in conjunction with a prepared test cavity or a small opening in a cast crown (Figures 19–16A and B), is quite advantageous. This tip is placed directly through the opening and onto the exposed dentin. Care should be taken to keep the electrolyte (toothpaste or fluoride gel) from touching the metal of the casting.

If you determine that root canal therapy is indicated while the patient is still in the provisional restorations, then the endodontic needs can be addressed without disturbing the restorative margins, changing the basic shape of the prepared tooth, or disrupting the appointment schedule.

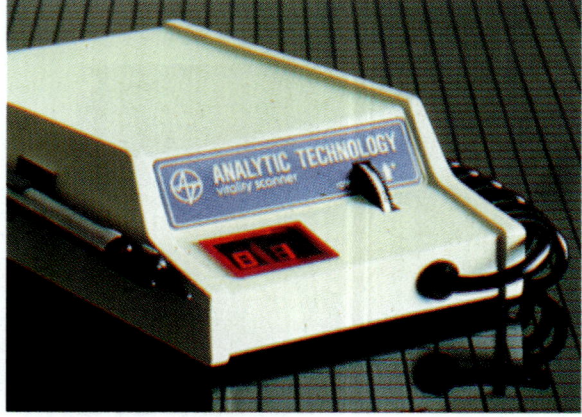

Figure 19–13: Analytical Technology Vitality Scanner Model 2005 (KerrDental).

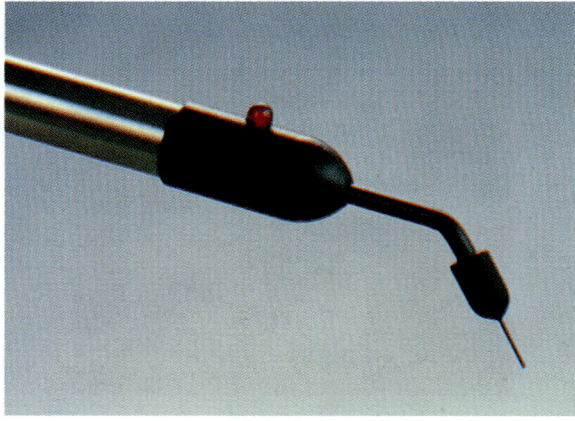

Figure 19–15: Mini-tip for the Vitality Scanner

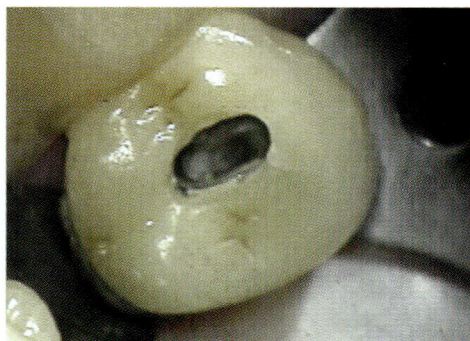

Figure 19–16A: Access through porcelain and metal to the dentin.

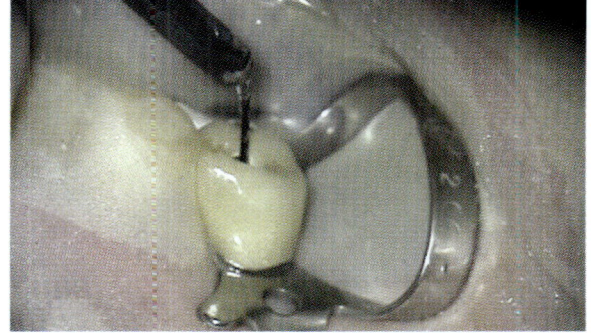

Figure 19–16B: Mini-tip placed on dentin through prepared cavity.

The patient should have been informed of such possibilities during the treatment plan discussion.

No single test should be construed as conclusive. This is particularly true when dealing with apprehensive patients. Under stress, these patients will anticipate and respond even when no stimulus exists. With these patients, the decision to treat may be based on finesse, experience, intestinal fortitude, and the intensity of pain. The option and choice of tooth should be communicated in detail. The records should indicate that the decision to continue is based on the presenting symptoms, responses (or lack thereof) to vitality tests, and emergency condition, and it is possible with the limited information gathered that the wrong tooth could be chosen. Your release form should be signed to document the discussion. In the case of an emergency, the alternative should be offered to wait until the symptoms and signs positively identify the tooth. The patient decides whether to proceed.

Cavity Tests

When tests are inconclusive with the less apprehensive patient, drilling through the crown surface and the dentin of an unanesthetized tooth is an excellent method of investigating further if the pulp is necrotic. This should be done only if the tooth has not responded to the traditional vitality tests like cold and electric pulp testing (EPT). It must be carefully explained to the patient that based on testing, it is likely that the pulp is already necrotic; therefore, he or she should not feel any pain when the tooth is drilled. If the patient reports pain or sensitivity once the cavity preparation has reached the dentin and the "normal" response has been established with a test like the EPT, then the opening is restored. If extensive caries is present, the patient is then anesthetized, and all caries and filling materials are removed prior to restoration. This will allow visual evaluation of the cavity floor and the ability to estimate the strength of the remaining core. If the patient did not report any pain or sensation, an endodontic access is cut, and appropriate endodontic therapy is initiated after all decay has been removed from the tooth.

Electric pulp testing with a "mini-tip" through a test cavity may be the key to making a diagnosis in a tooth with a radiolucency that cannot be differentiated as either of periodontal or endodontic origin.

One can suspect a necrotic pulp if the reading is negative. Endodontics would then be the treatment of choice (Figures 19–17A and B). If the reading is positive and there are no pulpal symptoms, periodontal therapy would be indicated (Figures 19–17C to E). Endodontic treatment may be required if the root apices are compromised during periodontal procedures (Figures 19–17F and G).

Periapical Tests

Percussion. Gently tapping the forefinger on the incisal or occlusal surface of a tooth may elicit a painful response (Figure 19–18). In situations when the response generated is mild or absent, a more pronounced blow should follow by percussing the tooth with a mirror handle (Figure 19–19).

A painful response usually indicates inflammatory changes in the periodontal ligament that could be caused by pulpal degeneration. When bacteria have entered the pulp, necrosis will follow. Endo-

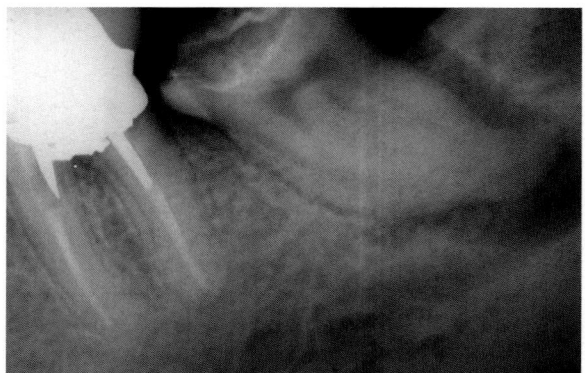

Figure 19–17A: Mandibular molar with a necrotic pulp. Root canal therapy was instituted.

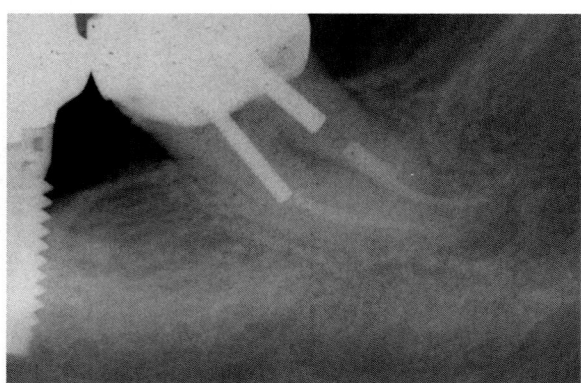

Figure 19–17B: Ten years following completion of root canal therapy there is a complete bone fill-in. No periodontal treatments were performed on this tooth.

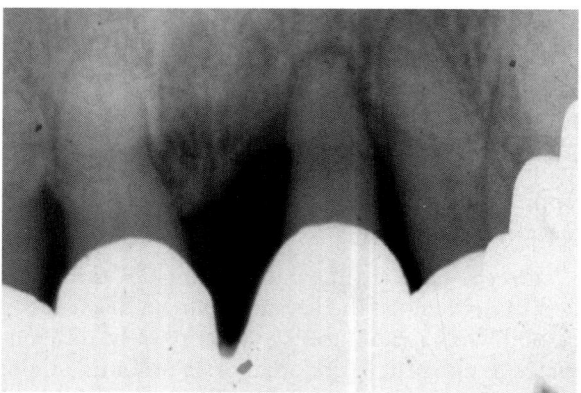

Figure 19–17C: Maxillary central incisor tooth with a vital pulp. Endodontic therapy was not indicated.

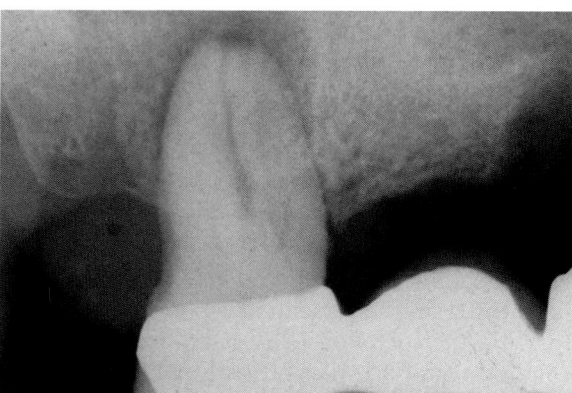

Figure 19–17D: A maxillary first molar with a periapical radiolucency.

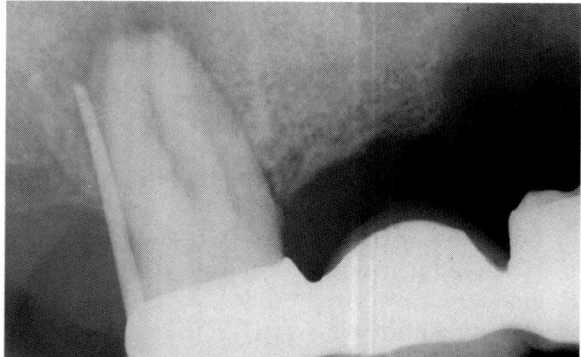

Figure 19–17E: A gutta-percha point placed in the distal pocket. Pulp testing through an occlusal opening revealed a vital pulp. The cause of the radiolucency was of periodontal origin and therapy followed that course.

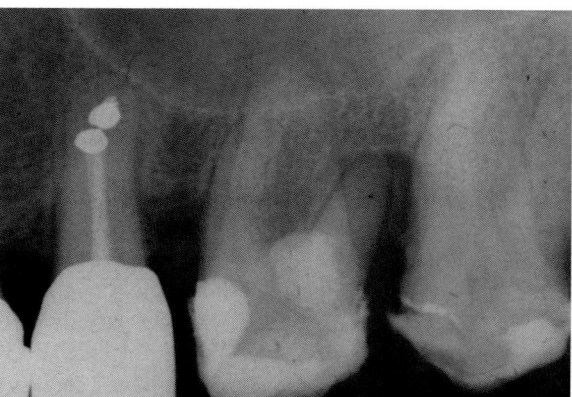

Figure 19–17F: Maxillary first molar with an uninflamed vital pulp. There was extensive bone loss surrounding the distobuccal root.

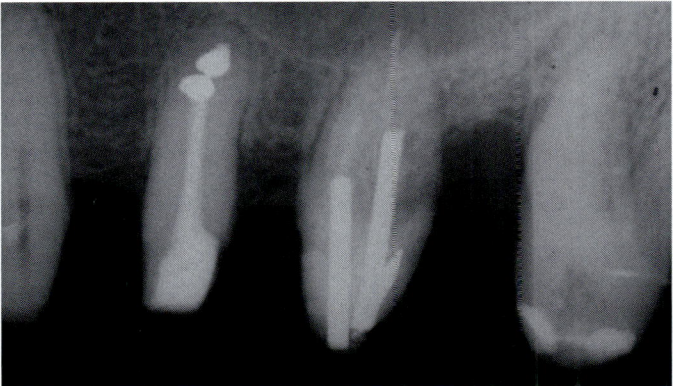

Figure 19–17G: Root canal therapy was performed to allow for the resection of the periodontally involved root.

toxins from the bacteria will eventually exit the canal and stimulate an inflammation of the periodontal tissue surrounding the apex of the tested tooth. The reaction is usually more intense when the inflammatory condition is of an endodontic rather than a periodontal origin.

Occasionally, painful responses to percussion are elicited from teeth not undergoing pulpal degeneration. Acute sinusitis often causes the maxillary posterior teeth to be painful when percussed. A careful history of the patient's respiratory experiences and allergies is essential in making the differential diagnosis. Teeth in traumatic occlusion are frequently sensitive to percussion but are also painful to cold. To exclude this possibility, a check for occlusal prematurities is indicated. A degenerative pulp does not usually respond to thermal pulp tests unless it is in its most acute stage. If a tooth is painful to both percussion and cold, one should suspect a vertical fracture. These are most frequently observed in mandibular second molars and maxillary bicuspids and occur irrespective of their restorative conditions. The use of the transilluminator or fiber-optic light is quite useful in diagnosing cracked tooth syndrome (see Fig 19–10).

Palpation. Pressure with a gloved forefinger over the apex of a suspected tooth may reveal tissue distention and elicit a painful response (Figure 19–20). This indicates the inflammatory response at the apex. The tender area may be so extensive that the teeth adjacent to the suspected tooth must also be tested. Once again, a differential diagnosis of acute sinusitis should be considered when the maxillary posterior teeth are involved. The tissues painful to palpation with sinusitis usually spread away from the dentition and extend superiorly and

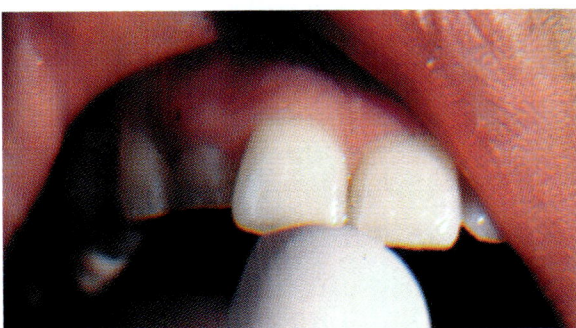

Figure 19–18: The first percussion check is a gentle tap with a gloved fingernail.

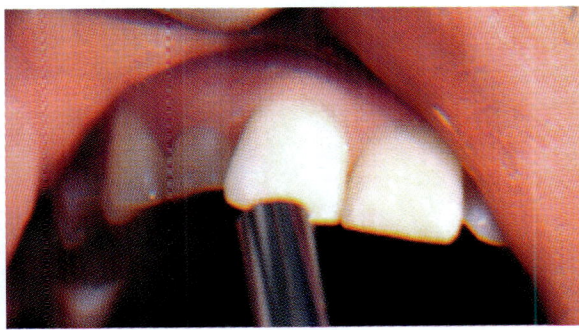

Figure 19–19: The second percussion is a gentle tap with a mirror handle.

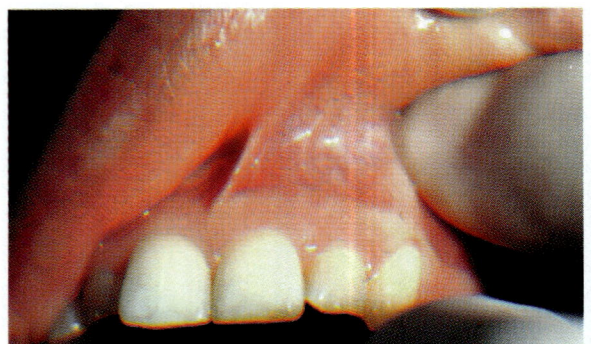

Figure 19–20: Palpation with the forefinger over a suspected tooth.

facially. Although the area of pain is usually concentrated at the zygomatic process of the maxilla, the pain may extend around the orbit and incite headaches. Pulp testing and a careful history are essential in these situations.

Bite Test

Every time that the patient's complaint is sensitivity to biting and/or chewing, it is important to investigate further which tooth and, more importantly, which part of it are sensitive to biting pressure. This is to distinguish between vertical crown/root fractures and periapical pathosis. A very convenient instrument for this investigation is the Tooth Slooth (Professional Results, Laguna Niguel, CA) (Figure 19–21). By design, this instrument has a slight depression in the biting surface, so the patient will only bite on individual cusps (Figures 19–22A and B) without adjacent cusp interference when he or she bites down. If there is a fracture in the crown, the patient is likely to report normal sensation to biting on all but the area that is fracturing. It is advisable to start with having the patient bite on the Tooth Slooth on a tooth that is not suspected of being fractured so that the patient knows what to expect. Then it is moved from tooth to tooth around the mouth as the patient exerts pressure. The patient is asked to close slowly yet exert maximum pressure. Pain on bite release is indicative of an inflamed pulp/irreversible pulpitis requiring extirpation.

A plastic saliva ejector may be used as an alternative instrument for this test (Figure 19–23).

Pretreatment Radiographs

Reconstructive planning requires a full set of well-angulated long cone–exposed films or digital images using film holders like XCP (DENTSPLY/Rinn, Elgin, IL), which enables 90-degree angulation of the x-ray beam on the film or sensor. In addition to a good angulation on the radiograph, these film holders will enable the operator to take comparable films or digital images over time, which is very important when evaluating healing or failure.

When dealing with extensive cases, panoramic film is equally essential. If the patient requires endodontic therapy and is referred for treatment, these films and a description of the goals and objectives of the referring dentist should be sent to the endodontist prior to the patient's first appoint-

Figure 19–21: Tooth Slooths, two sizes.

Endodontics and Esthetic Dentistry

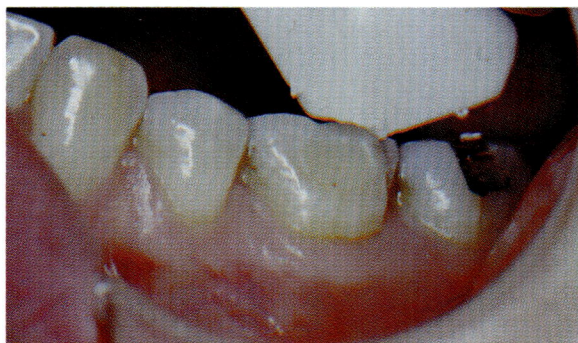

Figure 19–22A: Bite test with Tooth Slooth (Professional Results) checking DB cusp of mandibular molar.

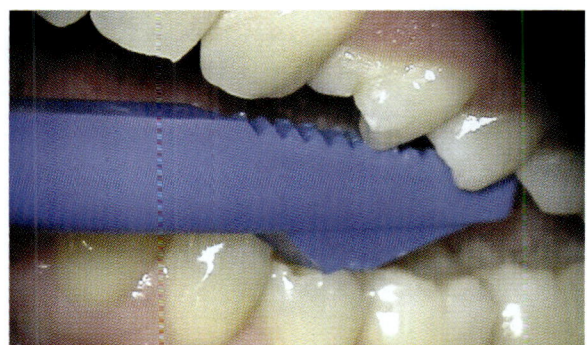

Figure 19–22B: Bite test with smaller-sized (blue) Tooth Slooth.

ment. Most endodontists will take additional films of the teeth to be treated to establish a complete record of their own.

In most cases, an endodontic procedure should not be initiated without evaluating at least two recent radiographs exposed at different horizontal angulations of the suspected tooth (Figures 19–24A and B).

Comparing varied views is essential in diagnosing the presence of additional roots, anatomic configurations, anomalies, and other unusual circumstances that may complicate the treatment.

Precementation Radiographs

Prior to cementation, Yamada (personal communication, 2001) re-radiographs the prepared teeth (Figures 19–25A and B). These images check the pulpal, periapical, and periodontal status of the teeth. Also, the radiographs, unencumbered by the presence of the metal castings, provide a chamber/canal road map record if the tooth requires endodontics in the future. This may appear pessimistic, but Arens and Chivian reported that over 40% of teeth requiring root canal therapy are crowned.[4] Prior knowledge of the size, location, and direction of the chamber and the canal will reduce the possibility of (1) crown damage during access opening, (2) lost time searching for the canal orifice, (3) perforations of the chamber or the canal because of disorientation, (4) natural core elimination by gutting, (5) crown dislodgment, and (6) sufficient destruction to alter the situation and require corrective surgery. Each of these iatrogenic possibilities reduces the prognosis and jeopardizes the tooth's reliability as an abutment.

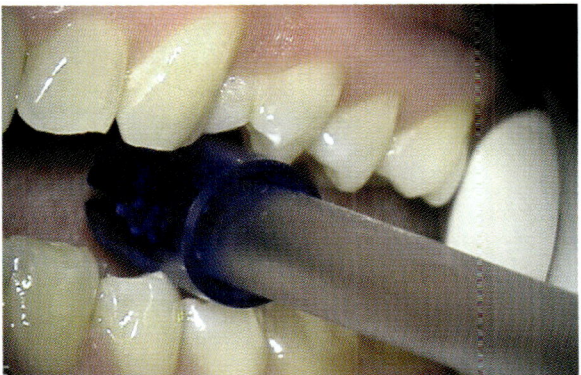

Figure 19–23: Plastic saliva ejector is useful in bite testing the entire tooth rather than an individual cusp.

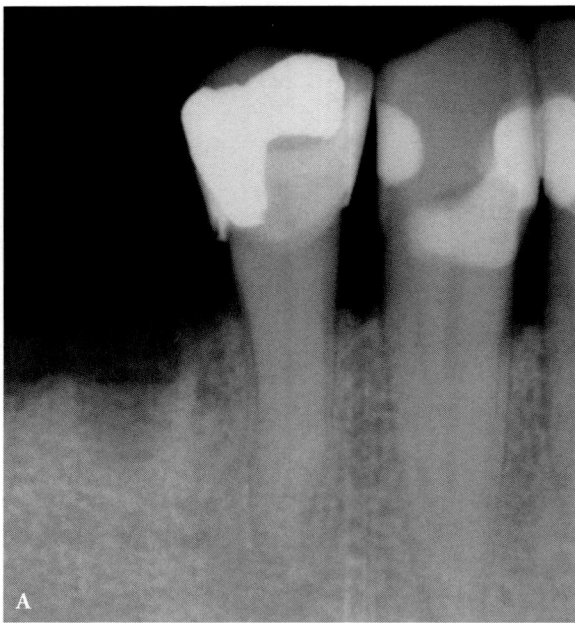
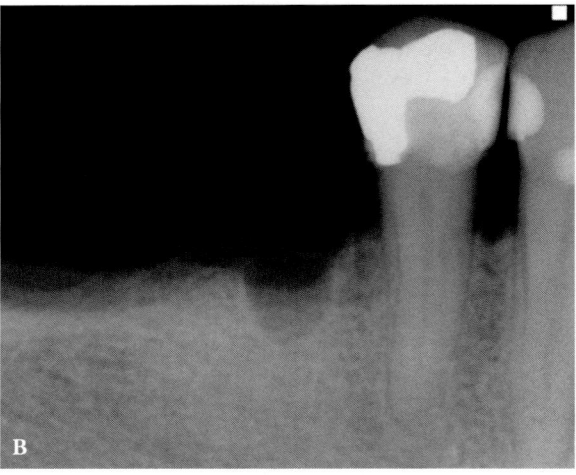

Figure 19–24A and B: *(A)* Pretreatment radiograph of a mandibular premolar shows one canal. *(B)* A second radiograph taken from an angulation of 15 degrees from the mesial discloses a second root.

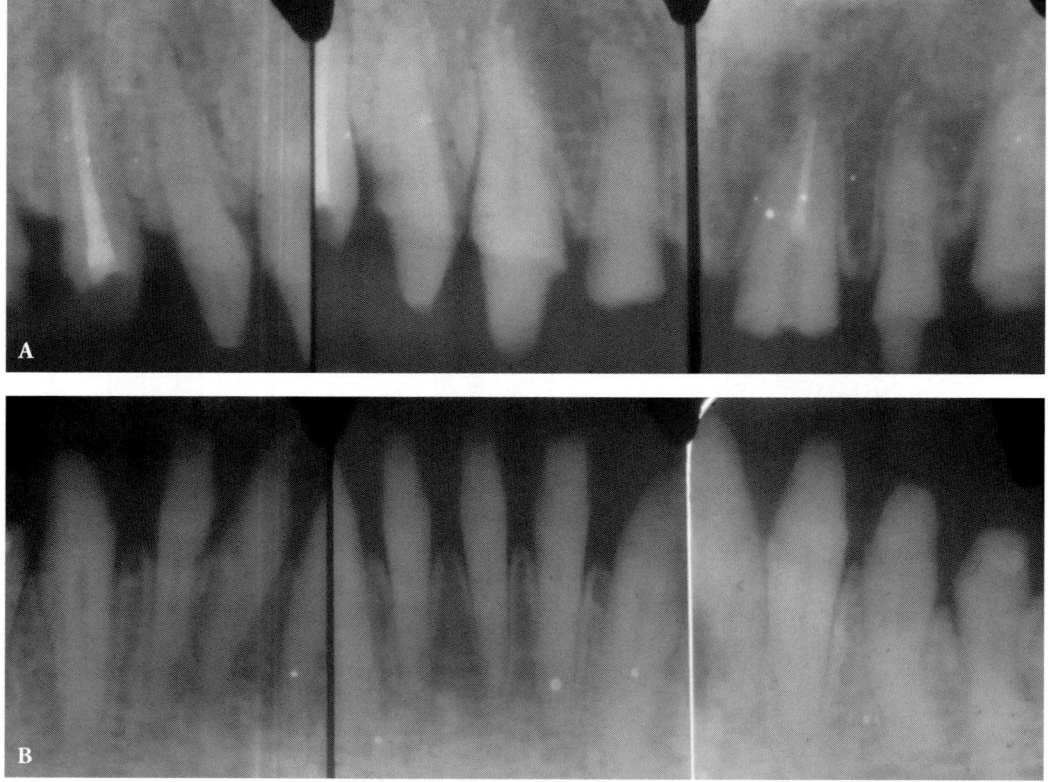

Figure 19–25A and B: Precementation radiographs provide a road map to the canals if endodontic therapy is necessary after cementation of the castings. (Radiographs courtesy of Dr. Henry Yamada.)

Diagnosis

By correlating all of the information gathered, the clinician can, within reason, determine which teeth may or may not require root canal therapy prior to the reconstructive procedures. By far the most difficult pulpal tissue status to classify is found within the confines of a previously restored tooth. For this reason, it is imperative to understand how pulps react to dental procedures.

PULPAL RESPONSE TO OPERATIVE PROCEDURES

Following caries, the single most influencing factor on the health of the pulp (Figure 19–26) is the operator. Simply modifying traumatic operative techniques could easily prevent sequelae and reduce the eventual need for iatrogenically required endodontics.

A normal tooth, when cut, responds immediately to the dentinal injury. The involved tubules are vulnerable to the heat developed during the procedure, to the air during drying, and to any of the chemicals or materials used during the restorative procedures.

Regardless of the source, the odontoblasts will react. It is only a question of degree. With tooth reduction, the equation is simple: the higher the speed of the rotating instrument, the greater the heat generated, and the greater the pulpal damage. Common sense would suggest that in response to these predictable and undesirable insults, the surface of the tooth should be reduced with high speed, and the deepest excavation and final preparation should be achieved with low speed. Adjunctively, a coolant spray should accompany all cutting, and every effort should be made to eliminate air blasts. Not only has Langeland shown that 10 seconds of air is enough to displace odontoblastic nuclei (Figure 19–27) and present a definite hazard to the viability of the pulp,[16] but Stanley's pulp studies have repeatedly demonstrated the peril of cutting fast and dry.[27]

For the above reasons, there is a definite advantage to using an alternative to the typical high-speed handpiece. Either air abrasion or a laser that cuts hard tissue, such as an erbium:YAG laser, can be much kinder to the pulp tissue.[10] Although neither of these instruments can be used for a full-crown preparation,

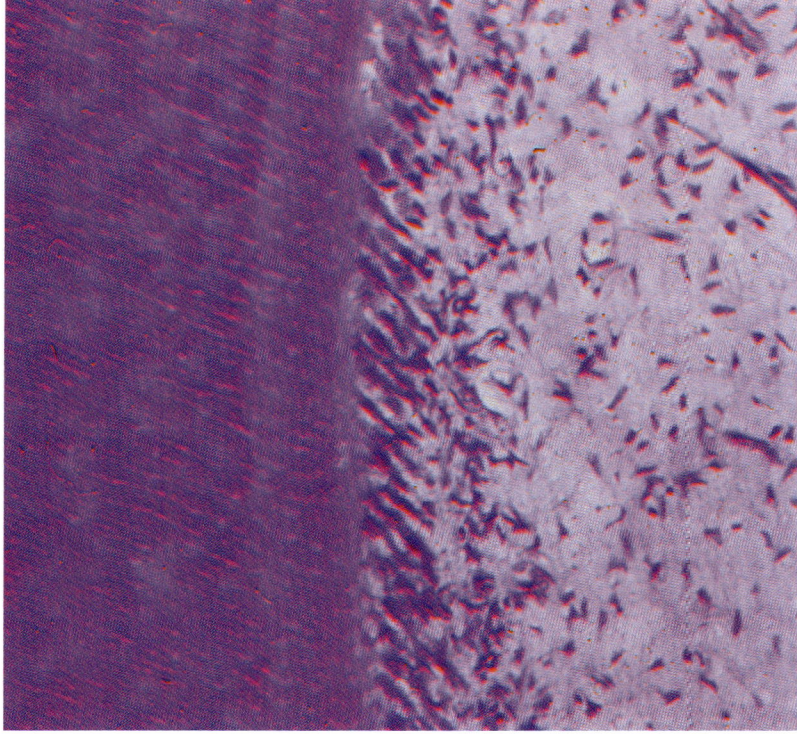

Figure 19–26: A vital healthy pulp with a typical pattern of palisading odontoblasts. (Photograph courtesy of Dr. Harold R. Stanley.)

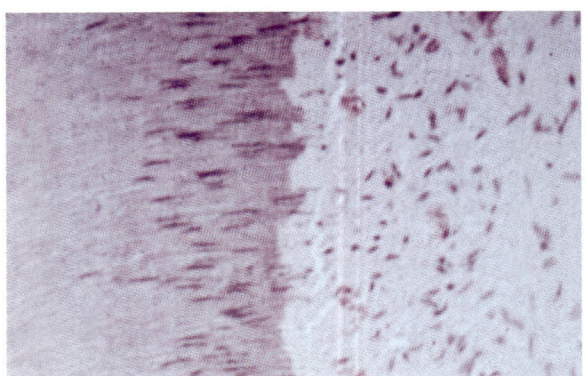

Figure 19–27: Aspiration of odontoblastic nuclei as a result of injury from cavity preparation.

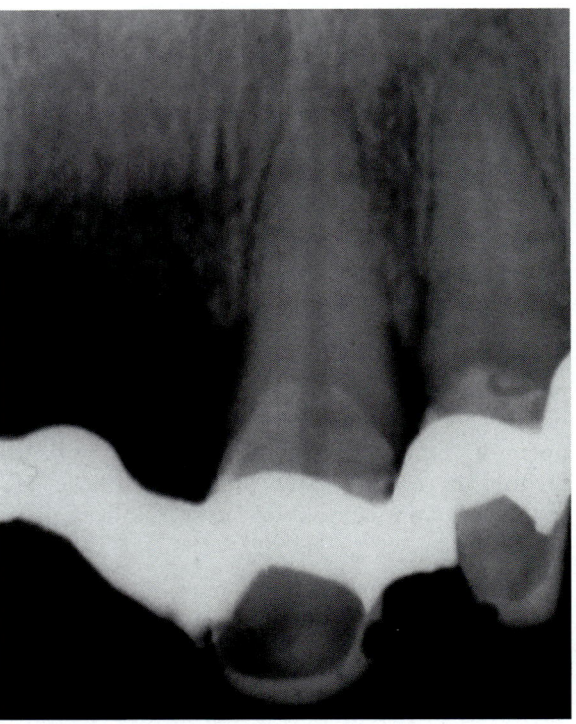

Figure 19–28: Periodontally compromised maxillary central incisor that is painful to minor temperature changes 10 weeks after deep caries excavation and crown preparation.

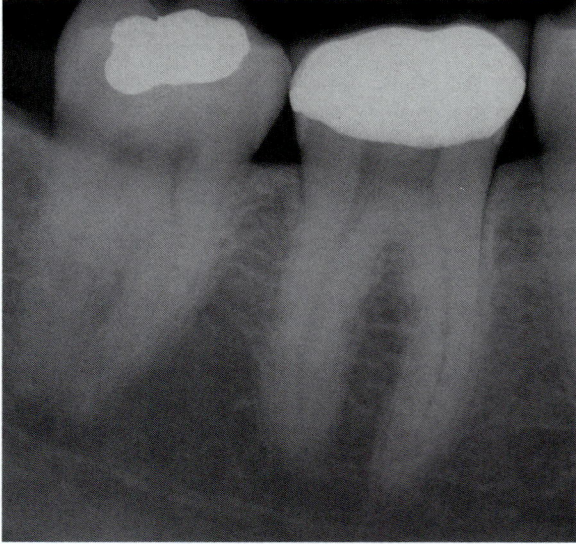

Figure 19–29: Mandibular molar with a normal radiographic appearance. However, the patient avoids using the tooth because of pain when chewing 9 months after cementation of the crown.

they may be ideal for initial cavity preparation, thereby negating potential pulp damage.

In addition, bleaching, rapid tooth movement, impression taking, temporization, and cementation are other aggressive procedures within the normal dental regimen that demand equal attention and caution.

The operator should select materials and agents that have relatively neutral pH values, create little or no heat during set, and control orthodontic forces within the physiologic tolerance of the periodontal ligament.

To ensure pulpal health and to avoid raising future diagnostic and treatment dilemmas, the pulp must be treated with the utmost care. In many situations, these problems may be avoided by careful evaluation prior to and during the restorative treatment. Examples of such situations are as follows:

1. When a tooth is exhibiting symptoms such as being exquisitely painful to cold liquids long after excavation of deep decay even with pulp protection/sedation and final restoration (Figure 19–28).

2. A patient cannot exert full biting pressure on a crown 6 to 9 months after cementation, yet the radiographs are negative (Figure 19–29).

Some postrestorative exacerbations are predisposing and unavoidable, particularly when dealing with heavily restored teeth. Such episodes of acute or chronic pulpal inflammation more often stem from a preexisting pulpal condition that has been aroused by what appeared to be a simple operative procedure. Although the healing potential of a healthy pulp following dental intervention has been well documented, the potential for complete repair has been known to decrease as the number of procedures are accumulated during a tooth's lifetime. Provided that there are no additional insults, a healthy pulp's survival with resolution of acute inflammation will usually take place within a few weeks. However, extending a patient's palliative treatment beyond that time frame is not only unjustified but also seriously threatens the patient/doctor relationship. Once that happens, further communications are diluted, and the patient usually leaves the practice. Rather, extirpation of the pulp followed by endodontic therapy should be considered early, and the patient should be warned that that might be the best treatment option if the symptoms do not resolve within a reasonable time.

Pulpal Repair

Reparative or irregular dentin is deposited to form a protective barrier for the pulp tissue and is generally localized to the injury site. This abnormal dentin forms in response to intense and aggressive pulpal irritants that have reached the limit of pulp tolerance (eg, erosion, abrasion, caries, dentinal exposure by fracture, decay or mechanical tooth reduction, traumatic injury, caustic medicaments, and harmful filling materials).

The histologic appearance of reparative dentin (Figure 19–30) demonstrates dentinal tubules that are irregular, tortuous, or even absent. The increased thickness of the total dentin is likely the reason for patients having decreased responses to cold stimuli as time passes following a dental procedure. Quantitatively, it is noted that the greater the degree of the "insult" caused by preparations and restorative materials, the greater the amount of reparative dentin that forms.

Although this calcified solid wall is considered beneficial and capable of resisting further episodes of irritation, this healing phenomenon decreases the ability of the tooth to respond to pulp testing at a later date.

Secondary Dentin

Histologically and physiologically, there is a difference between reparative and secondary dentin. Secondary dentin begins forming soon after the tooth erupts into occlusion and continues to form throughout the pulp's life. This tooth structure is deposited over the primary dentin (Figure 19–31) throughout the entire chamber and canal in response to stimuli within the limits of normal biologic function: mastication, light thermal changes, chemical irritants, and slight trauma. The newly deposited dentinal tubules are smaller, exhibit more curves, and form a protective barrier for the pulp as the size of the pulp cavity is reduced. Reparative dentin forms as a direct response to injury. Although the deposition is not uniform in thickness, this dystrophic calcification may completely occlude the canal, reduce the blood supply, necrose the tissue, and complicate the eventual endodontic therapy.

ELECTIVE ENDODONTICS FOR PULPAL REASONS

Depth of Preparation/Remaining Dentin

According to Stanley and Swerdlow, "The most important single factor in determining pulpal response to a given stimulus is the remaining dentin thickness between the floor of the cavity preparation or the surface of a crown preparation and the pulp chamber."[28] Studies have shown that a 2-mm dentin thickness between the floor of the cavity preparation and the pulp (Figure 19–32) will provide adequate insulation against the more traumatic thermogenic operative techniques in spite of intentional abuse and most restorative materials.[23] Cavity or crown preparations cut with high speed (50–200,000 rpm), air water spray, and a light touch produced minimal pathologic alteration to healthy pulps when the remaining dentin was 2 mm or more. However, Stanley stated that "Although 2 mm of primary dentin between the floor of the cavity preparation and the pulp is usually a sufficient protective barrier against cutting techniques...the effluent of cements and self-curing resins can overcome this thickness of protection."[27] To avoid such intrusions, calcium hydroxide lining materials capable of protecting the pulp tissue, when appropriately used, should be placed in all deep-seated cavity preparations prior to building a secondary protective base of cement.

If the final restoration is a one-stage procedure (ie, amalgam or composite resin), then a dentin/pulpal floor protected with a calcium

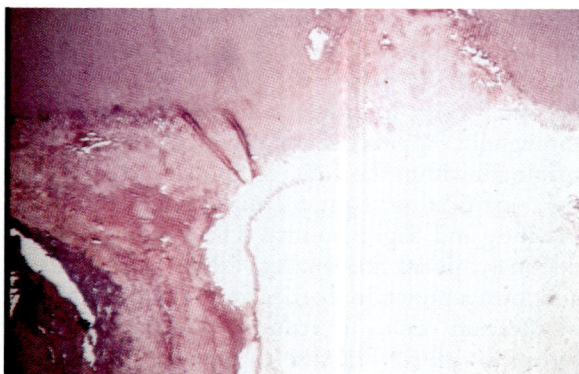

Figure 19–30: Reparative dentin is deposited at specific sites as a result of injury (ie, caries, restorative procedures, attrition, or trauma).

hydroxide dressing base can be permanently restored. The patient must be advised if there are risks involved. The records should reflect the risk condition and the discussion. The scenario differs with multistage restorations (ie, castings). If a tooth is compromised, the additional insults of impression, try-in, and cementation may exceed the pulp's ability to repair. Although judgmental, these teeth should be intentionally extirpated and endodontically treated. Success rates justify this prophylactic approach, and it is almost always unwarranted to chance discomfort, re-treatment, and repercussion.

If the requirements of the final restoration or the excavation of extensive caries result in less than 2 mm of remaining dentin, the expectation of a severe inflammatory reaction is greater. If a pink spot in the cavity or a blush on the tooth appears (Figures 19–33A and B) during or after preparation, it is obvious that the 2-mm remaining dentin barrier has been violated. The probability of complete inflammatory reversibility and healing of a noticeably hemorrhagic pulp is minimal. Considering that additional procedures are required to finish the crown, elective endodontics should be instituted before continuing. If, at any time, a patient elects to forego endodontic therapy following your recommendations, the records must indicate that the option to extirpate was strongly suggested and refused.

This presents a moral issue as to whether a patient should be allowed to dictate the final treatment when the risk of failure is involved. The dentist must realize that he or she can always refuse to continue, provide palliative but temporary treat-

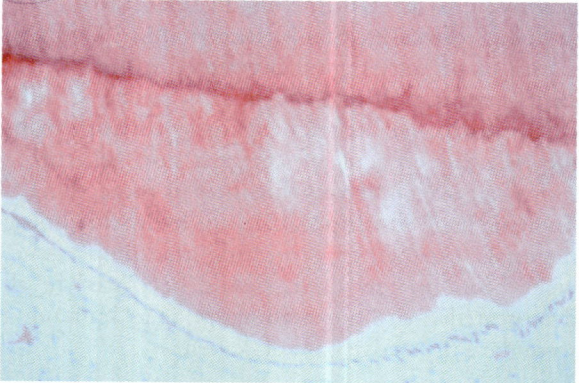

Figure 19–31: Secondary dentin represents the continuing slower circumpulpal deposition of dentin after root formation is complete.

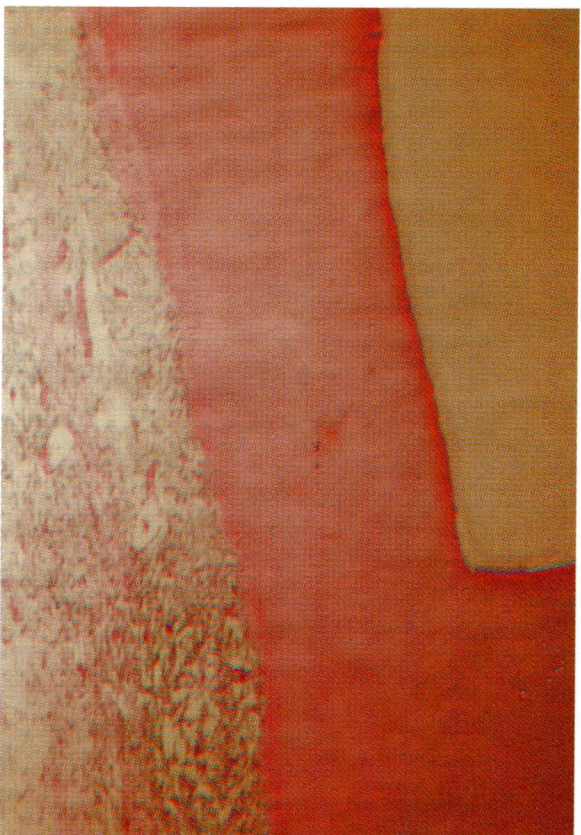

Figure 19–32: Cavity preparation with 2 mm of remaining dentin between its floor and the pulp tissue. (Photograph courtesy of Dr. Harold R. Stanley.)

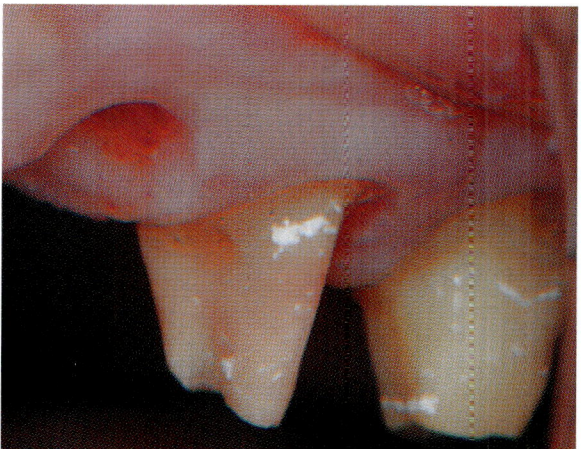

Figure 19–33A: Pink crown preparation 1 week following instrumentation.

ment to ensure comfort, and suggest that the patient see another dentist. If chosen, this decision, discussion, and referral must be recorded and witnessed. Irrespective of the remaining dentin thickness, the restoration has to be bacteria tight if the pulp is going to survive the insult. Care has to be taken to ensure the bacterial seal because if there is leakage, the bacteria will penetrate under the restoration and through the dentinal tubuli, initially cause pulpal irritation, and eventually cause pulpal necrosis if the leakage is not stopped.

Pulp Capping

Direct pulp capping in special situations has been shown to be safe, effective, and predictable. The ability of the pulp to repair when a mechanical exposure

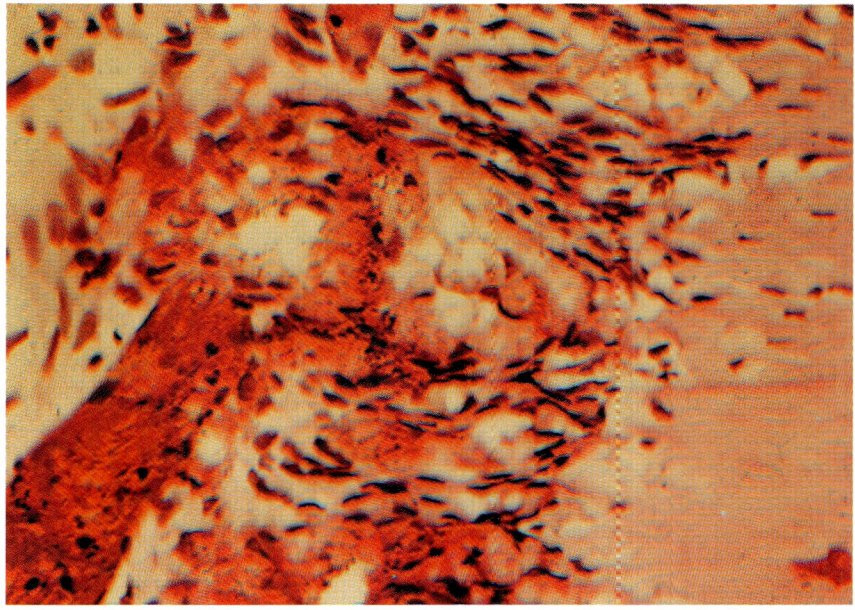

Figure 19–33B: Hemorrhagic pulp with extravasation of blood. (Photograph courtesy of Dr. Harold R. Stanley.)

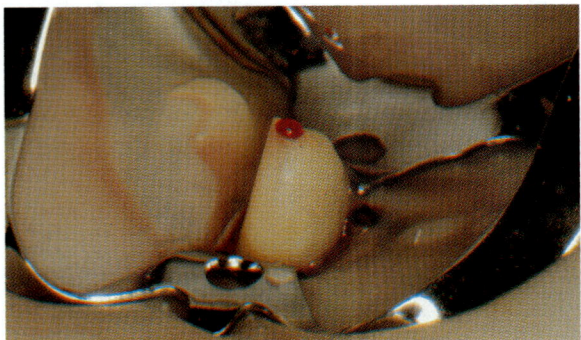

Figure 19–34: Pulp exposure during crown preparation. Pulp extirpation is indicated.

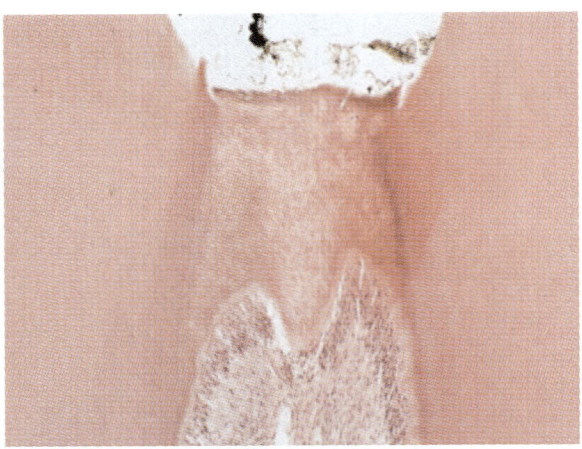

Figure 19–35: Dentin bridge following pulp capping with mineral trioxide aggregate (ProRoot MTA). Note the thickness of the bridge and the palisading odontoblastic layer. (Photograph courtesy of Dr. Mahmoud Torabinejad.)

has been dressed with calcium hydroxide is well documented. The odontoblastic layer, once stimulated, forms a matrix that leads to the bridging of new dentin. This is because if the pulp was accidentally exposed by a dental bur (Figure 19–34) or by traumatic injury, then only the surface will show reversible inflammatory changes. If the pulp exposure is under deep decay, then there is good likelihood that the inflammation has affected a large portion of the pulpal tissue and even caused partial necrosis. In a recently published study, the long-term success (over 10 years) of pulp capping of carious exposures was successful in only 13% of all cases evaluated.[6] It is also important to remember that, as a rule, pulpitis is asymptomatic,[8] so the patient might not have any history of pain even though there is a significant lesion in the pulpal chamber.

Because of the risk of leakage of bacteria into the pulp, direct pulp capping should be considered only with one-stage restorations (ie, amalgam or direct resin) and only when the patient is aware of the condition and the risk.

A thin calcium hydroxide mix of Dycal (DENTSPLY/Caulk, Milford, DE) (acid resistant) or Life (KerrDental, Orange, CA) is gently applied over the exposure. Care must be taken not to force the mix into the pulp because it could react adversely to an irritant like calcium hydroxide. However, healthy, exposed tissue, unless insulted by pressure, contaminants, or leakage of the restoration, should respond favorably to the procedure.[31] Successful pulp capping results have been reported by Ford et al. with mineral trioxide aggregate (MTA) (Figure 19–35) (ProRoot MTA, DENTSPLY/Tulsa, Tulsa, OK).[9]

Recently, pulp capping with a technique of acid etching and bonding has been advocated. This concept was based on clinical observations but has few scientific data for support. Pameijer and Stanley studied the technique in a carefully controlled experiment on primates.[22] Their results showed that pulp caps with acid etching and bonding agents produced 45% necrotic pulps, and only 25% of the specimens developed dentin bridge formation. Of the group pulp capped with calcium hydroxide, only 7% of the pulps were necrotic, and 82% of the teeth developed dentin bridge formation. Obviously, if you elect to pulp cap, calcium hydroxide and MTA are the materials of choice.

The poor long-term prognosis of pulp capping and the ease and assurance of endodontics certainly demand that the patient be offered the more predictable alternative of root canal therapy when a definite exposure is confronted. In teeth with pulp exposures for which multistage restorative procedures are contemplated (ie, inlays, crowns, bridge abutments), conventional root canal therapy is the treatment modality of choice. Performing the endodontics prior to the prosthetic delivery obviates the above-noted liabilities.

Stressed Pulp

The dental literature is replete with methods and materials that demonstrate apparent success in preserving the integrity of the pulp, including the combination of sorghum molasses and English sparrow droppings.[12] But as time passes, subtle changes take place in the pulp, creating an unhealthy and unreliable tissue to depend on as a sound foundation. This condition is often identified as "stressed pulp."

Abou-Rass considered the stressed pulp condition as an endodontic-restorative concept.[1] He felt that it was of a clinical nature and not a histologic entity. It should be considered a preexisting pulpal possibility in every restored tooth prior to subjecting the tooth to further restorative procedures. If the pulp is stressed, its ability to react favorably to the new insult will be diminished.

For example, a mandibular molar, although repeatedly filled, has remained symptomless over a long period of time. A radiographic examination of the tooth demonstrates a deep occlusal amalgam and a large buccal composite restoration, recession of the pulp chamber, and narrowing of the root canals (Figure 19–36). Another example of stressed pulps is the maxillary incisors that underwent concussion injuries and two previous crown preparations. Although there were no pulp exposures and there were minimal symptoms, intentional extirpations were performed because it was felt that the pulps would not survive another restorative procedure (Figures 19–37A to C). According to Abou-Rass's criteria, further insult to the affected (stressed) pulpal tissue would probably invite disaster. An intelligent decision would be elective endodontics, thereby intercepting potential problems.

Abou-Rass stated that the pulp's ability to recover from "stressed" pulp is relative to the type and duration of the injury, physiologic age, thickness of remaining dentin, and past trauma (impact injuries, repeated operative procedures). When all of these factors are examined and the patient's normal routine is changed because of vague symptoms, elective endodontic intervention must be considered. Another example of a stressed pulp is the patient with a maxillary anterior provisional restoration who required local anesthesia to remove the bridge 12 months after crown preparation and periodontal therapy because of pain in a maxillary central incisor tooth (Figures 19–38A and B). The combined dental procedures have created stress on the pulpal complex that have exceeded the pulp's ability to repair. No patient wants to hear why it should have been done after the fact.

Elective Endodontics for Prosthetic Reasons

No tooth or components of a tooth should be sacrificed if the prognosis of the remaining dentition can be improved by its retention. Discussing elective endodontics vis-à-vis extensive restorations, Bohannan and Abrams felt that root canal therapy should be performed for reorientation of occlusal planes, reduction of crown:root ratios, and establishment of parallelism.[7] A clinician faces many such situations when the overall esthetic and restorative results could be enhanced if the pulp was extirpated and the ideal root form was available. Unfortunately, the decision to perform the endodontics is often determined by issues other than what is beneficial to the patient (ie, economics, time, lack of skill or experience). Regardless, it is the duty of every diagnostician to evaluate and design each case with the goal of maximizing form, function, health, and esthetics. Therefore, when endodontic therapy enables the clinician to deliver the ideal restoration, why should the situation be compromised?

Endodontic Treatment Complications

An understanding of basic endodontic principles and a clearly defined restorative plan are essential prior to initiating root canal therapy. The final esthetic result should not be compromised by an inadequate approach. Therefore, various phases of endodontic treatment will be examined to see how they may enhance or preserve esthetics rather than detract from it. Although this may seem repetitious, the risk of performing endodontic procedures on restored teeth must be explained and accepted by the patient, and all discussions should be documented and recorded before a procedure is attempted.

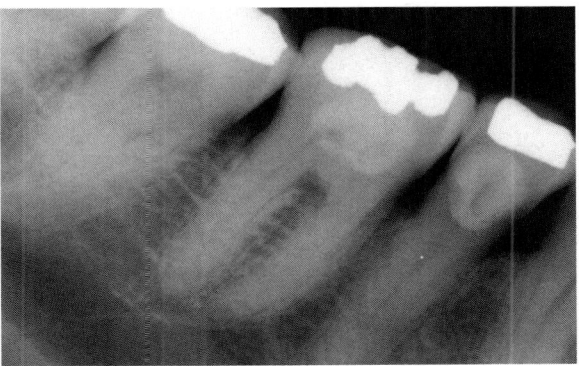

Figure 19–36: Mandibular molar with a stressed pulp.

Rubber Dam

The use of the rubber dam is regarded as mandatory in endodontics. However, isolating teeth decayed below the gingival crest or restored with all-ceramic crowns presents unique problems that invite a departure from the standard of care. It must be remembered that an untoward incident (ie, swallowing or aspirating a reamer or file when the rubber dam has not been used during therapy) leaves little doubt about legal liability.

The market offers a variety of rubber dam clamps designed to fit almost every situation. Crown lengthening prior to endodontic treatment is often required to expose sufficient tooth structure to clamp. This is not a detriment since lengthening procedures will be beneficial when the restorative dentist is establishing a finishing line for the restoration. The effect of a rubber dam clamp on porcelain or cast glass restorations can be esthetically devastating. Madison et al. studied the problem in a laboratory model.[17] The clamps were placed on the crowns and left undisturbed for 1 hour. They found that regardless of the crown margin design, all of the test samples displayed crazing of the porcelain in the area of the beaks of

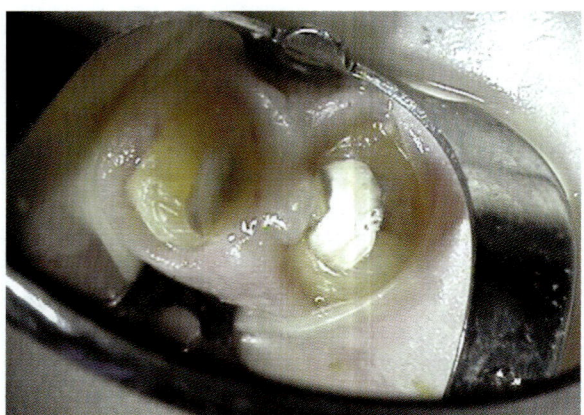

Figure 19–37A: View of maxillary central incisors following excavation of extensive caries. The pulps were not exposed.

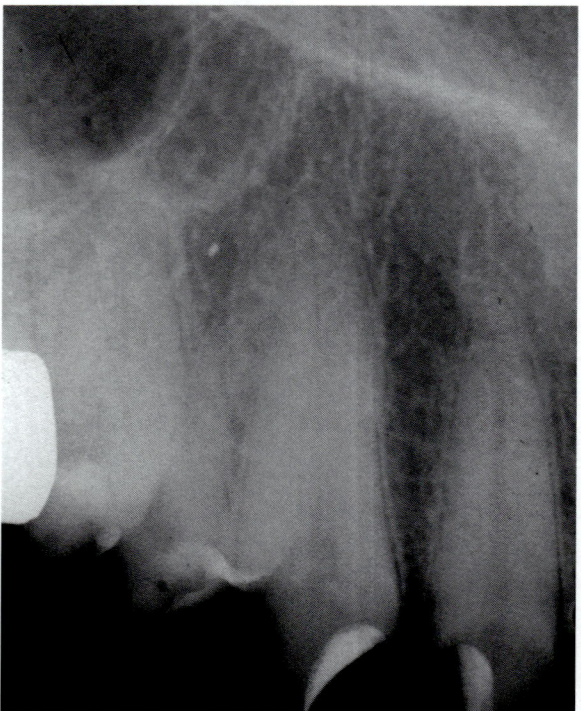

Figure 19–37B: Radiograph of the same teeth. Note the minimal thickness of dentin adjacent to the pulp chambers.

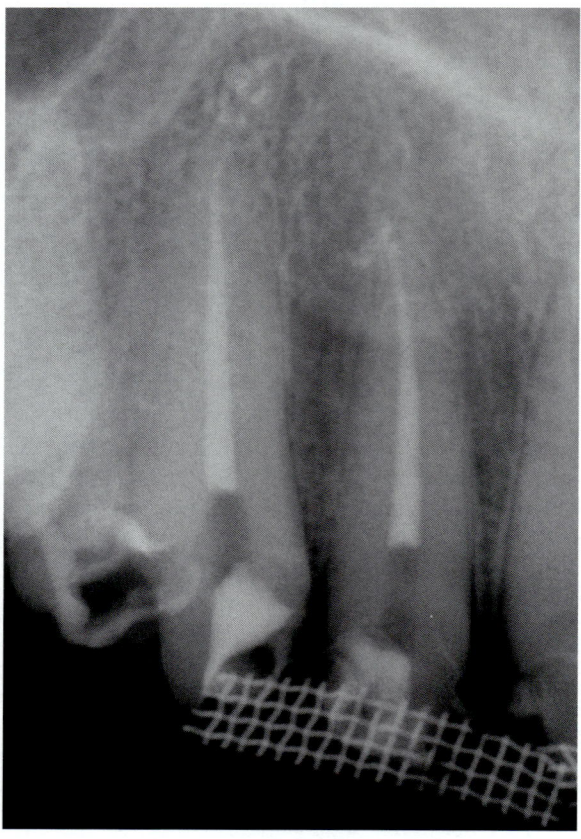

Figure 19–37C: Root canal therapy completed on the maxillary central incisors.

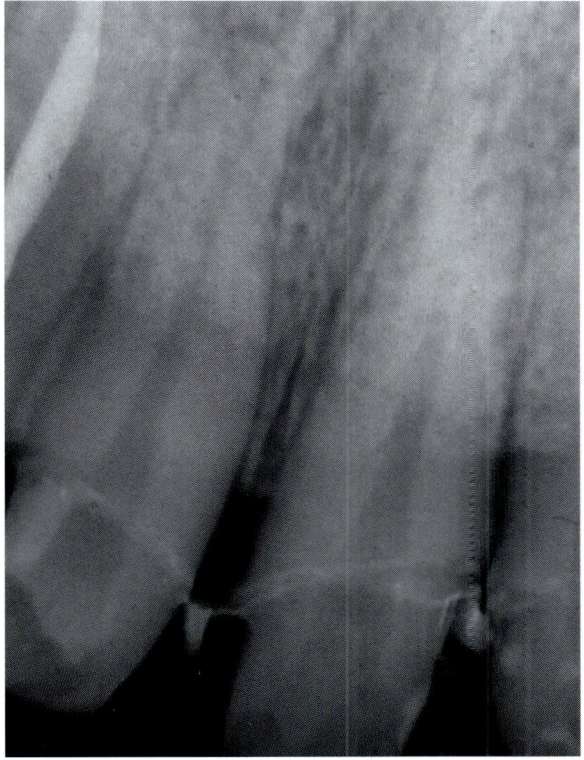

Figure 19–38A: Maxillary central incisor with a chronically inflamed (stressed) pulp.

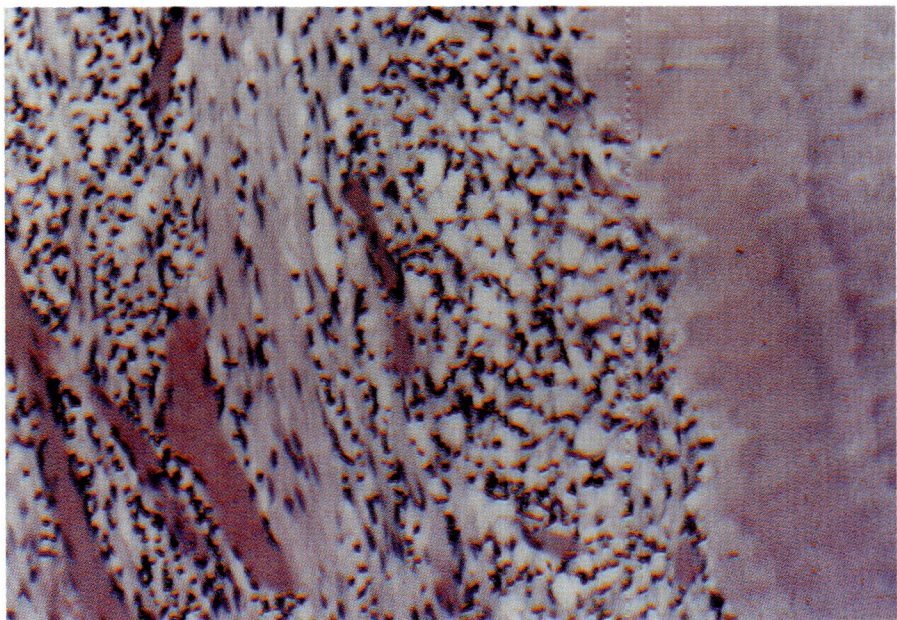

Figure 19–38B: A histologic section of chronic inflammation, irreversible pulpitis, with round cell infiltration. (Photograph courtesy of Dr. Harold R. Stanley.)

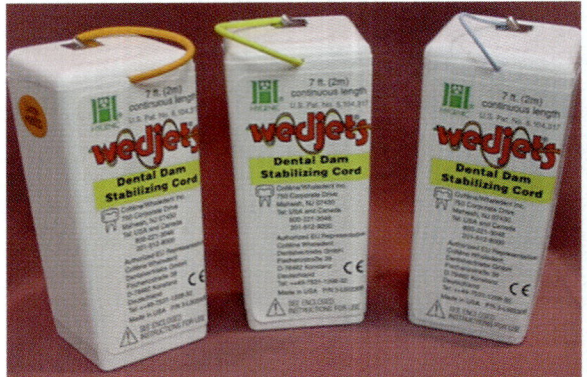

Figure 19–39A: Wedjets (Hygenic), three sizes.

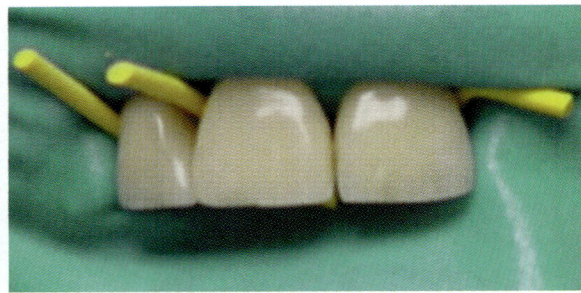

Figure 19–39B: Wedjets stabilizing the rubber dam and aiding in the isolation of a maxillary central incisor.

the clamp. Additional forces on the porcelain in clinical situations as the clamp is inadvertently moved during treatment would most certainly be destructive. As previously discussed, this problem could be eliminated if all teeth having questionable pulpal health were endodontically treated prior to cementation of the crown. The retentive value of the abutment would be increased, and damage to the porcelain would be avoided if elective endodontics preempted the crown fabrication and/or cementation.

Since over 40% of root canal treatment is performed through existing castings, the following alternative methods of rubber dam application are suggested for porcelain and cast glass crowns:

1. *Floss or rubber cord ligation.* Dental floss or Hygenic's rubber cord "Wedjets" (Figure 19–39A) can be used to retain a rubber dam when isolating a single tooth. Wedjets is a stretchable cord that is made from natural latex. The cord, available in three sizes, is placed like dental floss to hold the dam in place. Wedges can be used in conjunction with dental floss or Wedjets once the dam is in place. For convenience, it is recommended that at least one tooth on either side of the treated tooth be included in the isolation (Figure 19–39B).

2. *Multiple teeth isolation.* This technique suggests that the clamps be placed on unrestored adjacent teeth. Three or more contiguous holes are punched in the dam, and the rubber is stretched over all of the teeth to be isolated; the tooth to be treated remains unclamped, and access is unrestricted (Figures 19–40A and B).

3. *Jacoby plastic clamps.* Bay Technical Products (Freemont, CA) has introduced a series of plastic rubber dam clamps in seven of the most popular sizes, which are available through Practicon (Greenville, NC), R. Chige (Boca Raton, FL), and Sullivan-Schein (Melville, NY). The polyethylene material appears to be clinically kinder

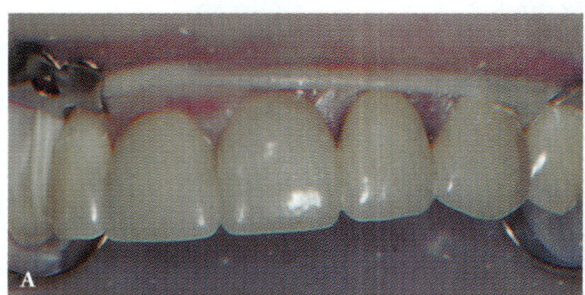
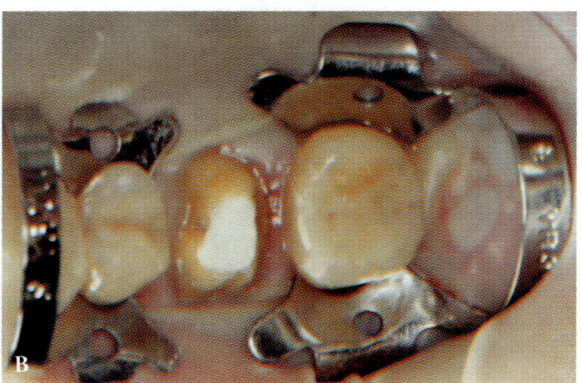

Figure 19–40A and B: Rubber dam isolation of multiple teeth.

to porcelain or cast glass and may be used in multiple teeth isolation (Figures 19–41A to C).

4. *Cushee rubber dam clamp cushions (Practicon).* Cushees are soft silicon cushions that fit over the jaws of standard steel clamps. The jaws of the

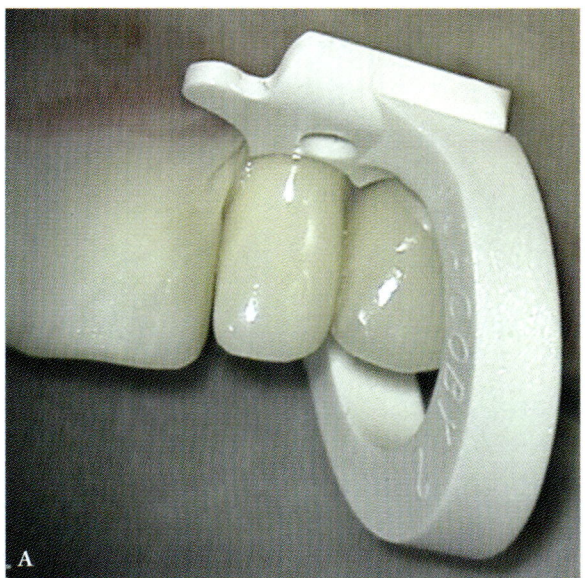
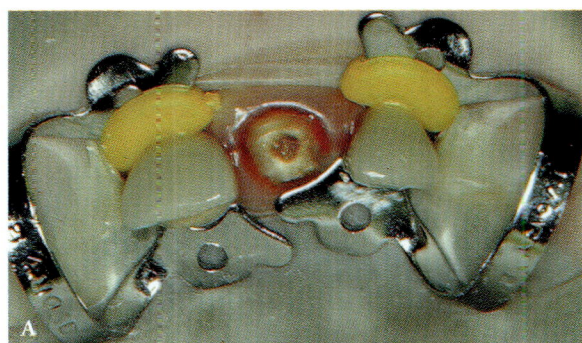
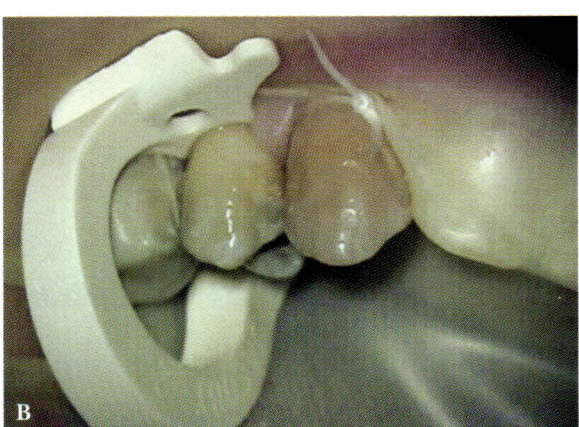
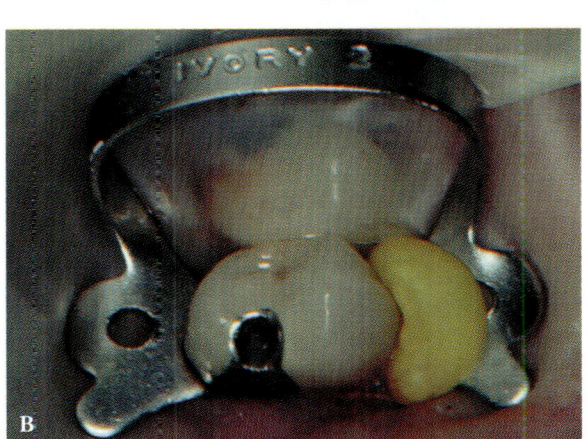
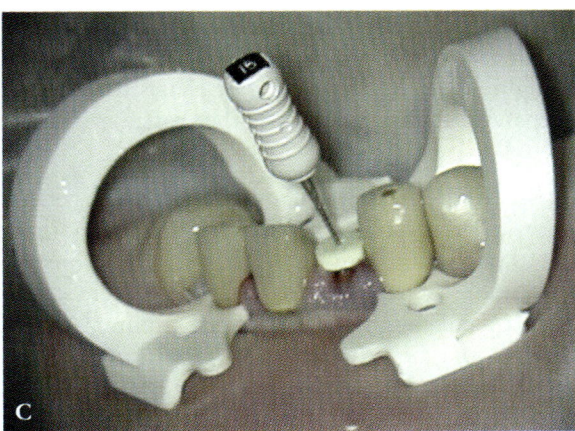
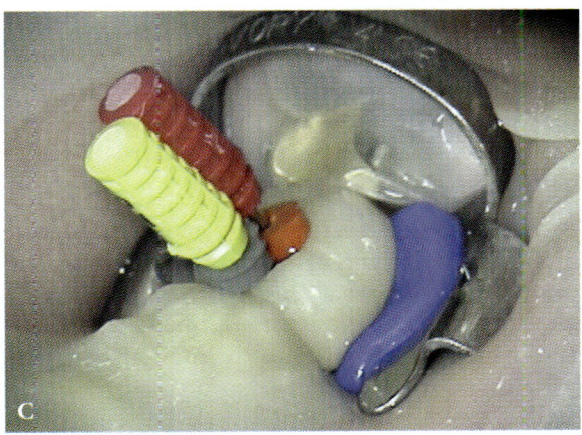

Figure 19–41A to C: Jacoby rubber dam clamps (Bay Technical Products) isolating *(A)* lateral incisor, *(B)* premolar and canine, and *(C)* multiple teeth.

Figure 19–42A to C: Cushee rubber dam clamp (Practicon) cushions isolating *(A)* multiple anterior teeth, *(B)* maxillary premolar, and *(C)* mandibular molar.

clamp do not come in contact with the gingiva, tooth structure, or restoration. Patient comfort is increased, and potential damage to porcelain and cast glass is decreased. They are available in two sizes: yellow for anterior and bicuspid clamps (Figures 19–42A and B) and blue for molar clamps (Figure 19–42C).

5. *Ingenuity*. When dealing with splinted units, ingenuity becomes part of the problem-solving equation. A triple-width hole is punched, and the teeth adjacent to the treated tooth are clamped. Once the dam is in place, Cavit (3M ESPE, St. Paul, MN), Provit (E.C. Moore, Dearborn, MI), or Oraseal Putty (Ultradent, South Jordan, UT) is compacted around the gingival margin of the crown to block off the expected leakage. When the entire arch is a porcelain-fused-to-metal or cast glass crown, you are faced with a most difficult situation and must improvise esthetic damage control. If there are individual crowns, you avoid placing rubber dam clamps on any of the anterior or first premolar teeth. Surface damage to the porcelain, when risked, should be confined to the second premolar and molar teeth, which are less visible in most situations. Cushees, Jacoby clamps, or Wedjets should be used to protect the restorations.

Again, for both contamination and patient protection, as well as medicolegal reasons, endodontic treatment should never be attempted without rubber dam isolation. Nonlatex dam is available from Hygenic for those patients with known latex allergies. Apprehensive patients may be accommodated with the use of Quick dam (Figure 19–43) from Ivoclar Vivadent (Amherst, NY). It has a built-in frame and is smaller than the standard size of a 5 × 5" rubber dam. It still affords similar protection and isolation.

Access Cavity Preparation
An access cavity must be large enough to enable proper débridement of the entire chamber and canal system yet small enough to preserve tooth structure. Discoloration from retained pulpal tissue and/or filling materials must be prevented. Therefore, chamber access must be internally widened and all pulp horns unroofed. A fine line exists between protection of existing restorations and tooth structure and a sufficiently sized access cavity to achieve the desired endodontic result.

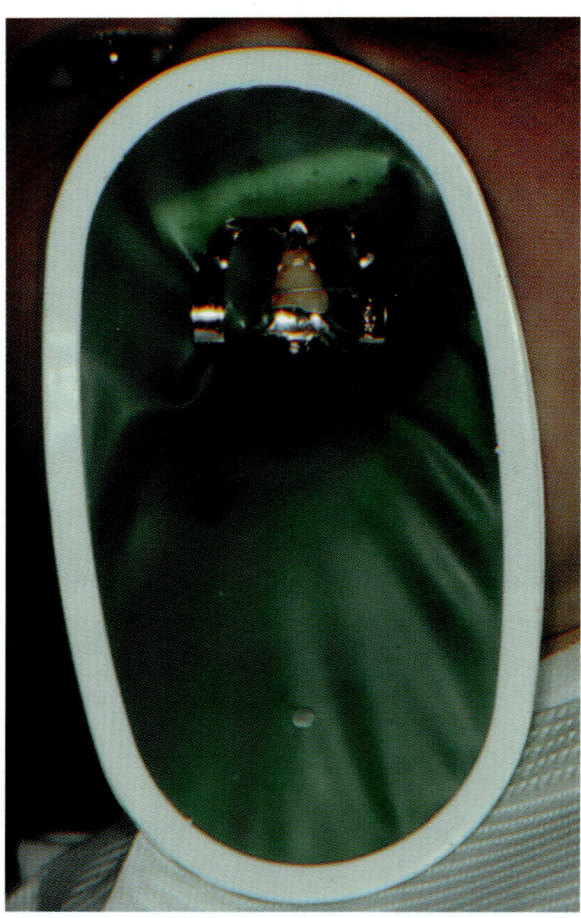

Figure 19–43: Quick dam.

A carefully planned and executed access cavity preparation should minimize weakening the tooth, provide for maximum visibility, and allow for straight line access into all root canals for optimal preparation and filling of the canal(s) (Figure 19–44).

Entering the pulp chamber requires a general knowledge of tooth morphology, the specific intricacies of the tooth in question, and proper instrumentation. Recent radiographs that were taken with a paralleling device to ensure minimal distortion should be studied prior to picking up the handpiece. It is recommended that two preoperative films be exposed from different horizontal angles to provide better information and help in visualizing the crown and root morphology (see Figures 19–24A and B).

Endodontics and Esthetic Dentistry

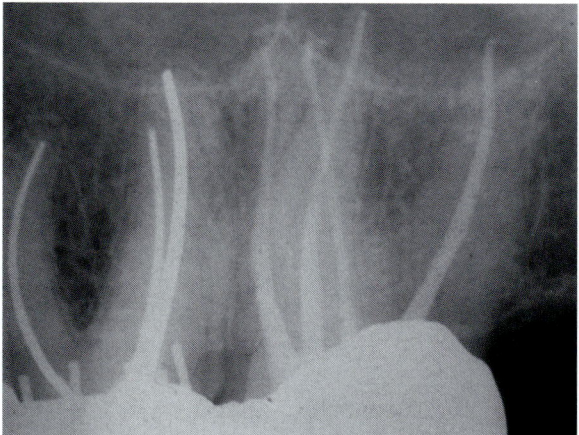

Figure 19–44: Straight line access allowed for visualization of all four canals in the maxillary second molar.

The films should depict the location of the chamber, presence or absence of calcification, number of roots and canals, and relationship of the incisal or occlusal surfaces to the axial line of the root.

Morphologically, the access cavity takes the shape of the underlying pulp chamber (Figures 19–45A to C). Variations in size and shape of the pulp chamber take place as the result of calcification resulting from caries, operative procedures, restorations, occlusal wear, abrasion, etc. Therefore, by nature, the access cavity in a youngster's nonrestored tooth (Figures 19–46A and B) would differ considerably from that of the same tooth with multiple restorations in a middle-aged person (Figures 19–47A and B).

Magnifying loupes or a dental operating microscope are necessary aids in searching for canals when calcification has obliterated the chamber. Magnification in conjunction with an auxiliary light source tends to reduce the frustration of this phase of endodontic therapy.

Procedure

If the tooth that needs an endodontic treatment has a full-coverage restoration, special care must be taken prior to cutting access preparation because in many cases, the "artificial" tooth structure could be very different from the natural tooth, both in regard to size and shape and the occlusal plane (Figure 19–48). The preoperative radiograph(s) and careful probing with a periodontal probe around the cervical area of the tooth will give some indications.

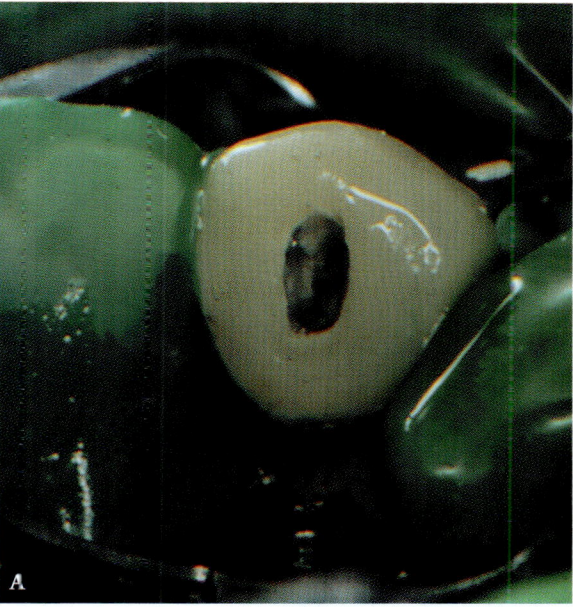
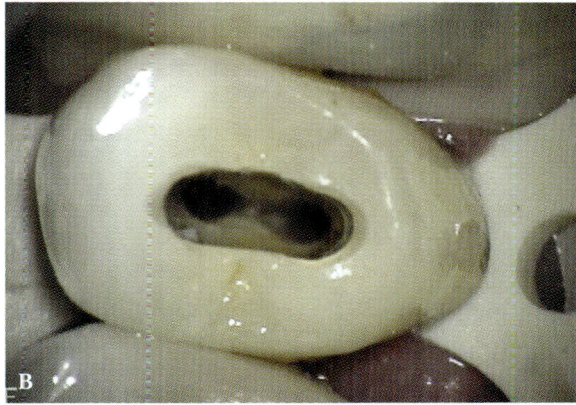
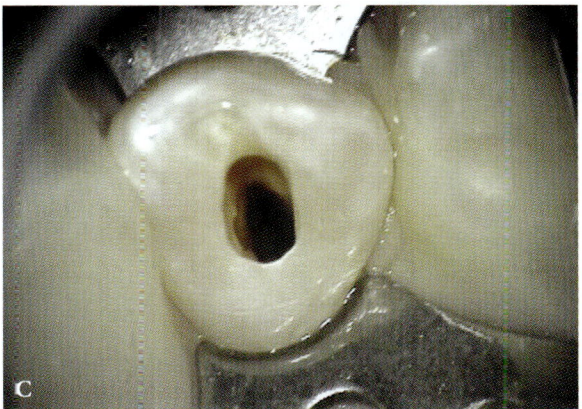

Figure 19–45A to C: Access cavity outlines reflect the shape of the pulp chambers: (A) maxillary canine, (B) maxillary premolar, and (C) mandibular premolar.

Natural tooth structure should be protected from heat. Studies have shown that deleterious crazing and cracking occur in the enamel and in the dentin when access cavities are prepared dry. Regardless of the fact that the pulp will be extirpated, water should be used to cool both the bur and the tooth during access preparation.

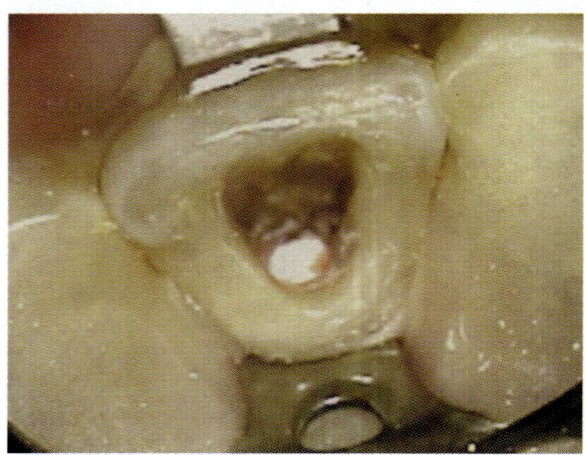

Figure 19–46A: Access cavity in a traumatized unrestored maxillary central incisor of a 16-year-old male.

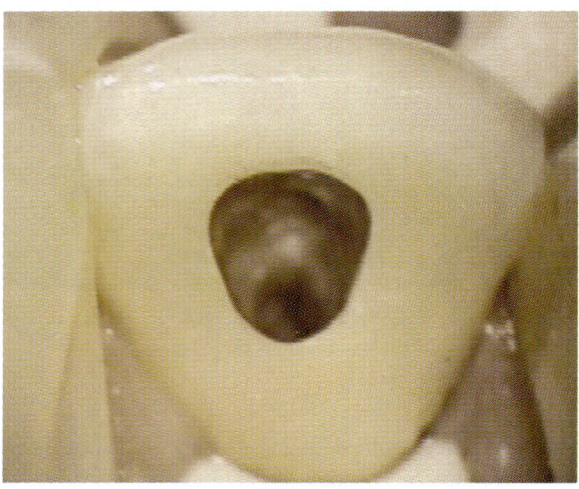

Figure 19–47A: Access cavities through porcelain-fused-to-metal crowns in a middle-aged male.

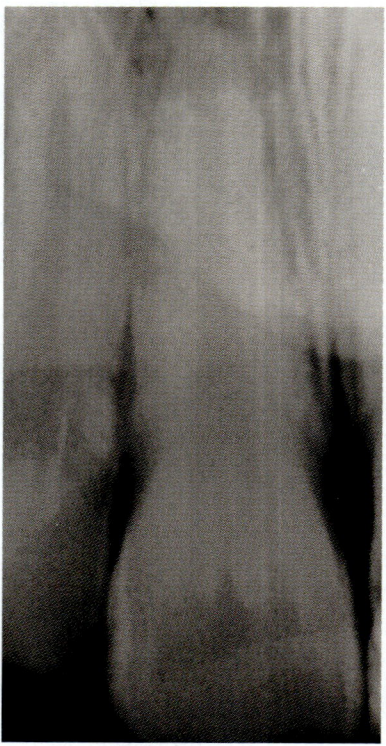

Figure 19–46B: Radiograph of the same tooth showing a large pulp chamber and root canal.

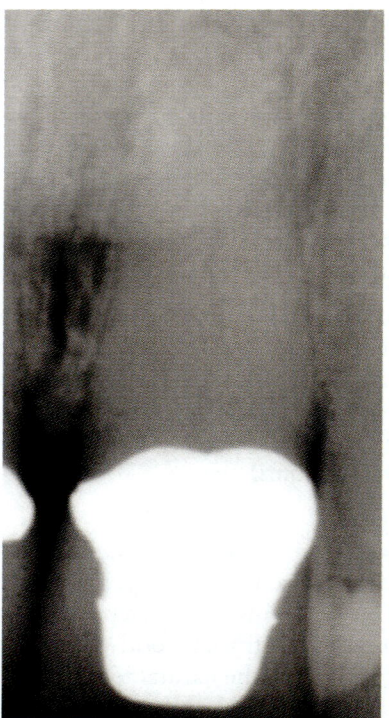

Figure 19–47B: Radiograph of the same tooth depicting a narrow root canal. The size of the access opening in the crown reflected the recession of the pulpal complex.

Burs

Penetration and funneling are the two phases of cavity preparation. This can be accomplished with a round #2 or #4 bur for penetration, followed by a #1558 or #701 fissure bur for funneling. Alternatively, the funneling could be done with an Endo-Z bur (DENTSPLY/Maillefer, Tulsa, OK), which is a specially designed bur for that task. It has a long, slightly tapered side cutting surface, but its end is blunt. The rough access, into the chamber, is then cut with a round #2 or #4 bur, and then the final outline is cut with the Endo-Z without the worry of perforating the furcation of the tooth. If decay is present in the chamber, it can be removed with a #2, #4, or #6 long-shank bur at low speed. A long-shank endodontic excavator #33L is also very useful in this process.

Removal of existing occlusal and proximal restorations should be completed prior to entering the pulp chamber. Besides providing a direct view, it also saves time and eliminates the chance that loose particles from the restoration are entering the canal, thereby preventing negotiation to full length. The only exception to this is if removing deep, but sound, proximal extension of the restoration will compromise the rubber dam seal.

Restored Teeth. To facilitate canal orientation, it may be beneficial to gain access and locate the orifices of the canals prior to placing the rubber dam because then the root eminence of the alveolar bone could be observed and used as a guide. It is important, as always, to place the rubber dam before introducing an endodontic file into the tooth to eliminate the possibility of the aspiration or ingestion of the file.

Acrylic Veneer and Full Metallic Crowns. A new #2 round or #1558 round end fissure bur is preferred when penetrating gold. The sharpness of a new bur will maximize penetration and minimize the tendency to skip or skid. As mentioned, the access opening must be large enough to allow visualization of the entire chamber, location of the root canal orifice(s), and removal of all existing decay.

Access through nonprecious metal crowns requires the use of a coarse dome-shaped cylindrical diamond bur. Stokes et al. found that the Horico 139x012 (Pfingst, South Plainfield, NJ) cut faster and lasted longer than the other burs tested on nonprecious metal.[29]

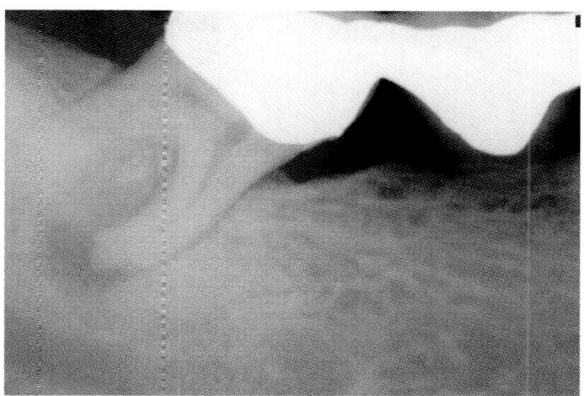

Figure 19–48: Mesially inclined mandibular second molar. Because of the tilt, the direction of the bur should be angled toward the distal to avoid a perforation during access cavity preparation.

Aluminous Porcelain. Medium- or fine-cut diamonds accompanied by a water spray should be used to cut through porcelain.[21] Carbide burs will generate incredible heat, and the cutting action of the bur will significantly increase the possibility of porcelain failure. The operator has the choice of a round diamond stone (Premier 120F, Premier Dental Products, King of Prussia, PA, or Gnathos 801-016, Gnathos Dental Products, Weston, MA), a round end fissure diamond stone (Premier 982.8, Premier Dental Products), or a pear-shaped diamond (Premier 365.4F, Premier Dental Products). Disposable diamonds are efficient when cutting porcelain or all ceramic restorations. Being new, they tend to reduce crazing or cracking in the restoration and generate less heat (eg, Gnathos 801-016).

Porcelain Fused-to-Metal Crown. A round diamond stone (Premier 120F or Gnathos 801-016) accompanied by a copious water spray is best for the porcelain entry. A classic access cavity is traced in the porcelain (Figure 19–49A). Penetration through the metal and dentin and into the pulp chamber is accomplished with a new #2 or #1558 carbide bur (Figure 19–49B). Carbide burs dull rapidly and should be discarded when they lose their cutting efficiency.

All-Ceramic Crowns. A laboratory study has shown that high-speed diamond instrumentation with water spray is efficient when cutting through Cerestore crowns (3M ESPE, St. Paul, MN).[30] The same study also indicated that carbide burs used

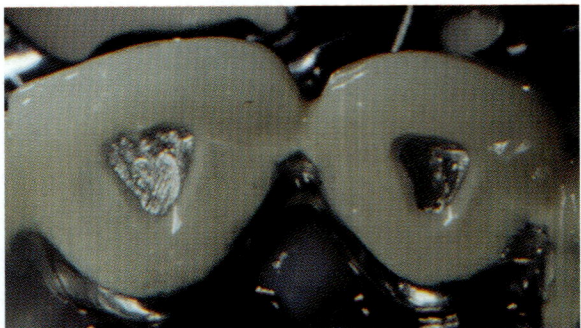

Figure 19–49A: Outline of access cavity traced through porcelain with a diamond stone.

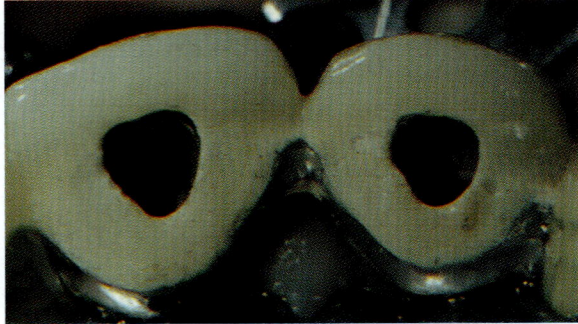

Figure 19–49B: Penetration and funneling of access cavity completed with a carbide bur.

under similar conditions were inefficient. More specifically, when preparing access cavities in cast glass crown, a diamond stone should be selected (eg, Premier 120F, Gnathos 801-016).

Porcelain Inlays and Onlays. A two-fold problem presents with these restorations vis-à-vis access preparation: fragility of the material and design of the restoration.

Fracture and dislodgment are potential sequelae when cutting into these restorations. To avoid the problem, one must be certain of the pulpal health prior to selecting these restorations. If faced with endodontic therapy through these restorations, however, the patient must be advised of the possibility of replacement. Once the risk is accepted, high-speed diamond instrumentation (Brasseler 801-016 [Brasseler, Savannah, GA], Premier 120F, Gnathos 801-016) will minimize the potential of rendering the restoration useless.

Etched Cast Bridges

Any tooth with a questionable pulp should be endodontically treated prior to placing an etched cast restoration. Frequently, this restoration is used to replace an anterior tooth that has been lost as a result of trauma. It is reasonable to assume that the adjacent teeth may have sustained injury as well. Therefore, it is imperative that the pulp and periapical status be ascertained before bonding the restoration in place. However, if faced with root canal therapy, the access cavity must be kept as small as possible. The likelihood of weakening the bond is great. In most cases, a new #2 or #1558 carbide bur and a copious water spray will minimize heat and reduce the vibration, which is the cause of debonding. Occasionally, it is more practical to prepare the access cavity through the labial surface, in particular when dealing with lower incisor teeth that are lingually inclined (Figures 19–50A to D). The distinct advantage of direct access without disturbing the casting is immeasurable. The opening can then be repaired with a light-cured composite resin. Cosmetically, the lip and smile lines should be considered before using this approach. Communicating the benefits of this approach and having the patient accept the technique before proceeding are essential.

Retentive Value After Access Preparation

In addition to esthetic compromises that occur as a result of access preparation, crown retention also becomes questionable. An in vitro study by McMullen et al. showed that the retentive value of a porcelain-fused-to-metal crown was decreased 60.17% following access cavity preparation.[19] In a follow-up study, McMullen et al. showed that the retentive value of the crown could be increased 237% over its original value if the crown was recemented with polycarboxylate cement and the access cavity was filled with amalgam.[20] However, it is rare that a crown or a bridge is removed after final cementation to allow for endodontic therapy. Unfortunately, retentive value following the filling of the access cavities with amalgam alone has not been studied. With this is mind, filling an access cavity with amalgam after endodontics may not restore it to an acceptable level. This reiterates the need to perform elective endodontics whenever a risk exists prior to the fabrication and cementation of a crown (Figure 19–51).

When faced with unusual situations (eg, occlusal rests and attachment receptacles in removable partial denture abutments), innovation enters the picture. To preserve their usefulness, attempts should be made to keep away from the attachment area. The final access preparation outline should be finished near the attachment but not encroach on it. The shape of the preparation may be decidedly atypical, but the preservation of the mechanical lock integrity will be retained.

Instrumentation/Débridement

The goal of this phase of endodontic therapy is to eliminate all microorganisms from the canal system by completely removing organic and inorganic debris. The objective is to accomplish instrumentation yet maintain the constriction of the canal apex and the flare of the coronal aspect. This canal design will accommodate condensing instruments during the gutta-percha compaction yet confine the filling materials within the canal. Thorough débridement and hemorrhage control will not only ensure endodontic success, they will also prevent discoloration of the crown. This is an extremely important esthetic consideration. Crown discoloration can stem from blood entering the dentinal tubules followed by latent red blood cell degeneration. Severe pulpal bleeding usually occurs when an acutely inflamed pulp is not entirely removed during extirpation. Once an accurate measurement is ascertained, further débridement of the canal and subsequent shaping coupled with copious irrigation with 2.5% sodium hypochlorite (NaOCl) will normally control the hemorrhage. If, on occasion, the flow continues, full-strength 5.25% NaOCl should be used as the irrigant. The solution should remain in the chamber for periods of 5 to 10 minutes.

Today's suggested medication in teeth with vital and necrotic pulps is calcium hydroxide, which does not cause tooth discoloration. However, one still encounters discolored endodontically treated teeth that have been discolored by medication, root canal cements, and paste fillings. Their removal, as well as

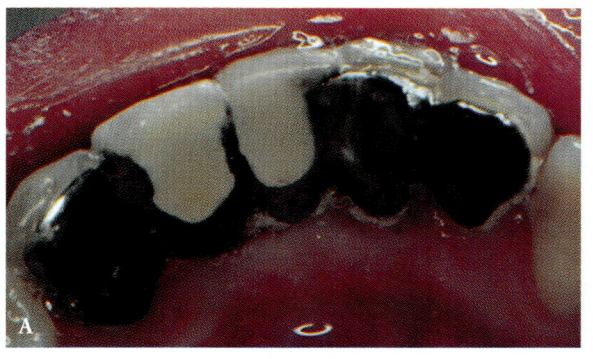
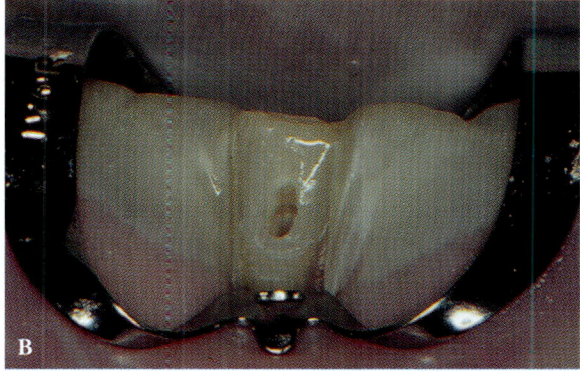
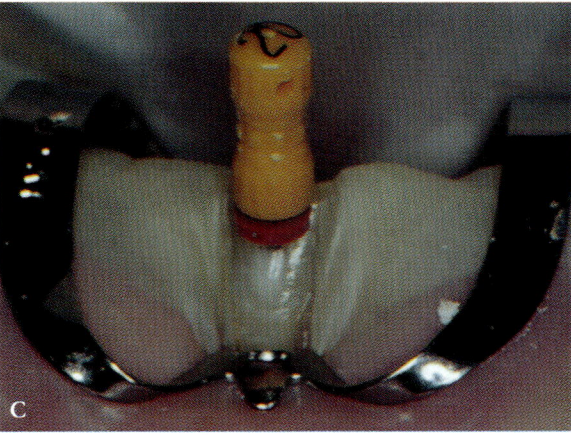
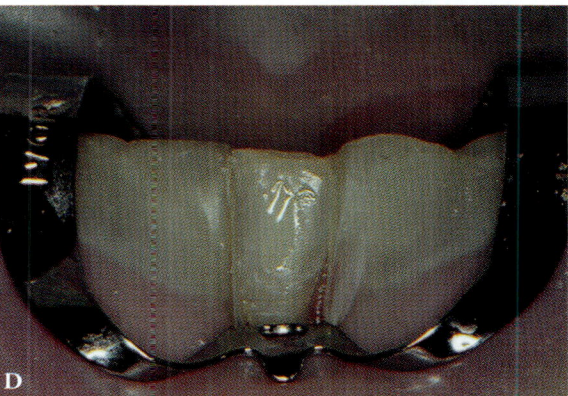

Figure 19–50A to D: Access alternative for an etched cast bridge: *(A)* five-unit bridge, *(B)* access cavity prepared on labial surface, *(C)* measurement file in place, and *(D)* composite resin repair of access cavity.

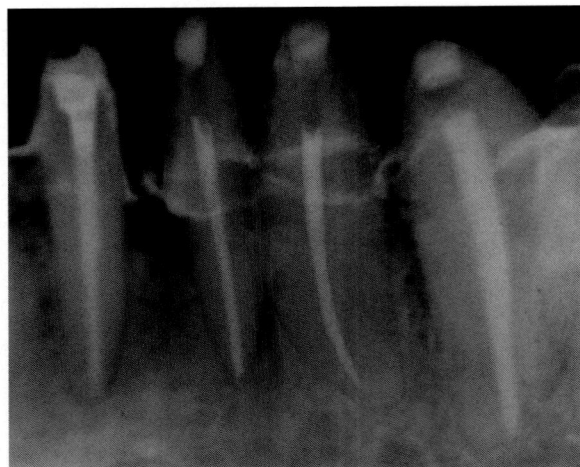

Figure 19–51: Endodontic therapy completed prior to fabrication of final castings on four mandibular anterior teeth with questionable pulpal health.

bleaching procedures, may return the crown to its optimal color, but the duration of the esthetic improvement may be short. Patients should be advised of this fact.

Sealing the Canal System

The final phase of treatment and the key to successful endodontics is the sealing of all portals of exit from the canal system. Here again, esthetic consideration revolves around discoloration of filling materials. A nonstaining root canal cement (ie, Roth 801, Roth International, Chicago, IL; U/P Root Canal Sealer, Sultan Chemists, Englewood, NJ; or Thermaseal Plus, DENTSPLY/Tulsa, Tulsa, OK) provides the necessary sealing capabilities when used in conjunction with gutta-percha. The canal walls are coated with the cement, and then gutta-percha that is deformed either by heat, pressure, or chemicals acts as a piston to drive the cement to the outer recesses of the prepared dentin walls. This results in the formation of a cement–dentin interface, which is necessary to produce successful results.

The canals should be filled completely as confirmed by radiographs. The excess gutta-percha and root canal cement should be removed 2 to 3 mm apical to the cervical line to prevent discoloration (Figure 19–52). In periodontally involved teeth where longer crowns are planned, the root-filling materials should be removed to the bone level. A 2-mm layer of white temporary stopping should be placed over the gutta-percha.[25] Remnants of the cement may be removed with alcohol. A tooth-colored restorative material (ie, composite resin or glass ionomer cement) may be used to fill the rest of the canal and chamber when a post and core are not indicated.

The coronal restoration should be placed as soon as possible after completion of the root canal treatment if it is not placed at the time when the canals are filled. There is now building evidence that the coronal restoration is as important, if not more important, in microbiologically sealing the root canal system as the root canal obturation material (Figures 19–53A and B). In a recent study, Ray and Trope evaluated the radiologic quality of both coro-

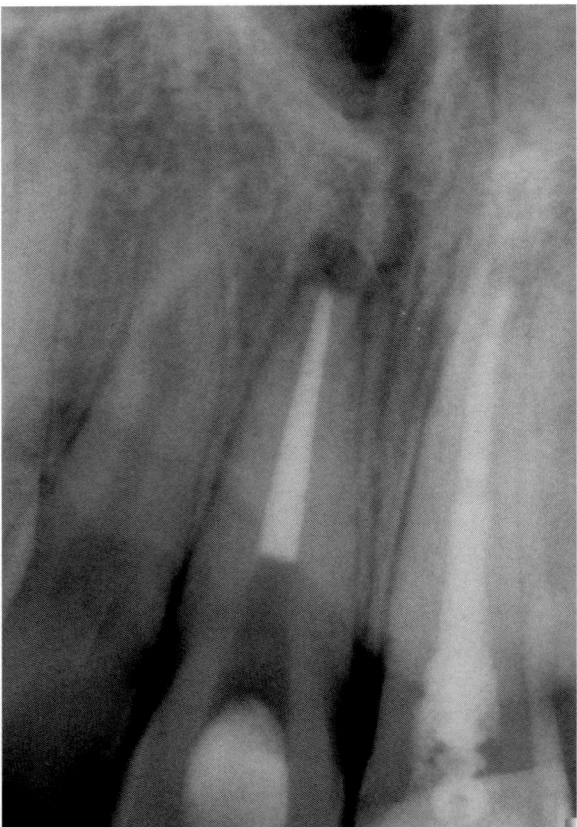

Figure 19–52: Gutta-percha root filling cut back 3 mm apical to the cervical line to prevent discoloration. Two millimeters of white temporary stopping is placed over the gutta-percha. This space will be restored with composite resin. The adjacent tooth will be restored with a crown.

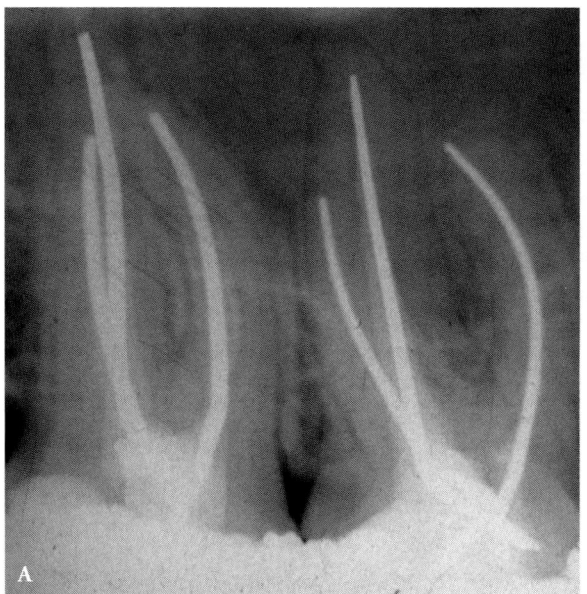
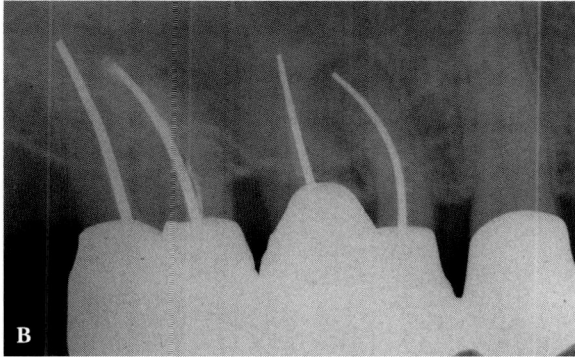

Figure 19–53A and B: (A) Thirty-five years after root canal therapy. The teeth are asymptomatic, and there are no radiographic changes. (B) Three years after distobuccal root resections and new castings. Periapical lesions developed around the mesiobuccal roots. During the extended treatment phase, the coronal ends of the silvers points were periodically exposed to saliva.

nal and canal obturations.[24] It was demonstrated that a tooth with good coronal and root seals had the best rate of absence of periapical lesions (91.4%). Good restoration resulted in significantly less incidence of periapical lesions than good endodontic filling (80% versus 75.7%). Poor restoration resulted in significantly more periapical lesions than poor endodontic fillings (48.6% versus 30.2%).

A proper finish of both the temporary and the final filling material is essential so as not to irritate the patient's tongue or soft tissue. Thirty-bladed finishing instruments (ETUF, OS 1, Brasseler) are perfectly suited to provide the smoothest margins for both the material and especially the marginal remnants of the existing restoration. Gold restorations are particularly susceptible to rough edges that need finishing with the 30-bladed instruments.

Bleaching

Bleaching endodontically treated teeth has been a successful part of the endodontic treatment armamentarium. When indicated, the procedure should be instituted at the completion of the root fillings. The results are satisfying, and the patient can readily see the change in tooth appearance.

Unfortunately, a liability associated with bleaching, external root resorption, has appeared in the literature and has been demonstrated in research studies.[32] External resorption is the result of an injury to and a subsequent reaction in the periodontal ligament. The use of 30% hydrogen peroxide (Superoxol, Sultan Chemists) and/or heat has been demonstrated to increase the probability of resorption.[18] Microscopic opening in the dentinal wall in the cervical region that is not covered by enamel or cementum may allow for the penetration of the bleaching solution to the periodontal ligament. This morphologic abnormality occurred in 5 to 10% of the teeth examined.[15] Acid etching of the chamber has been advocated prior to bleaching to allow for deeper penetration of the Superoxol. Heat, Superoxol, and acid etching of the chamber increase the probability of resorption (Figures 19–54A and B) and should be avoided, and a kinder, gentler technique should be used.

Walking Bleach Technique

A solid, well-condensed gutta-percha root filling is a prerequisite to bleaching discolored endodontically treated teeth. This should be confirmed with a radiograph. If the root filling is inadequate, it should be redone. Once it has been established that the gutta-percha filling is adequate, it should be removed 2 mm apical to the cervical line, and the reservoir that is created should be filled with a zinc oxide eugenol temporary filling material such as IRM (DENTSPLY/Caulk, Milford, DE). All rem-

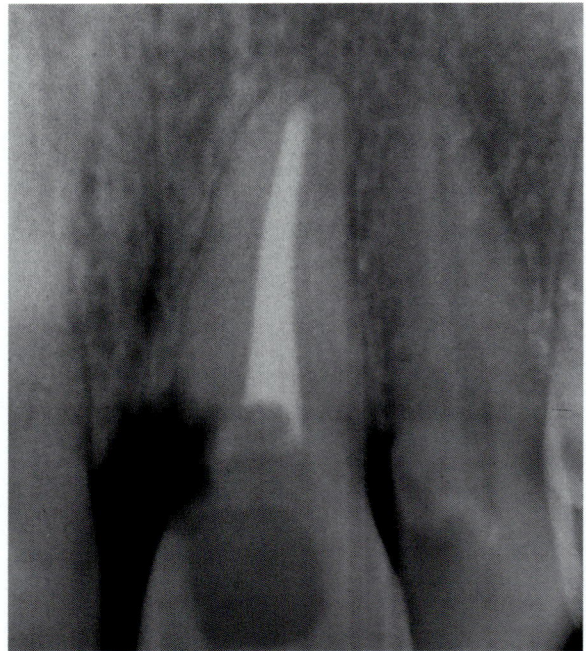

Figure 19–54A: External cervical resorption 4 years following bleaching with 30% Superoxol (Sultan Chemists) and heat.

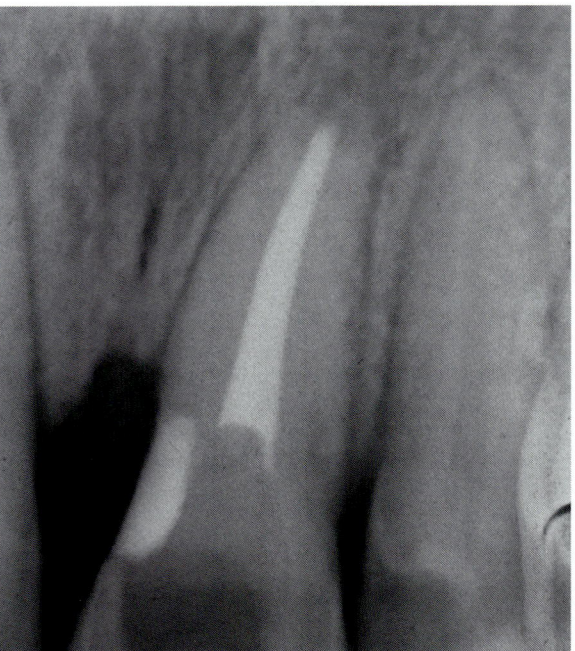

Figure 19–54B: Two years after orthodontic extrusion and a surgical approach to repair the resorptive defect.

nants of root and crown filling should be removed from the chamber. The chamber is washed with 70% alcohol. Sodium perborate powder mixed with water or 3% hydrogen peroxide to a resin-like consistency is packed into the chamber with a plastic instrument. Excess moisture is absorbed with a cotton pellet. The access cavity is closed with a good temporary filling material. An effort is made to ensure a total seal by removing the bleaching agent from the access walls. The maximum bleaching effect takes place within 48 hours (Figures 19–55A and B). The tooth is evaluated for improvement after that time. Application of the paste is repeated until an acceptable result is

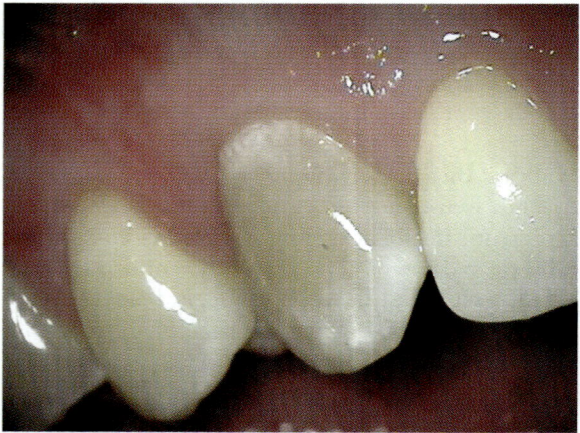

Figure 19–55A: Discolored maxillary canine with a necrotic pulp.

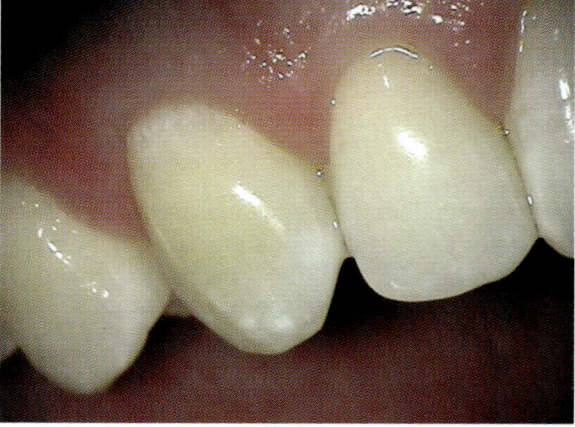

Figure 19–55B: Forty-eight hours after the completion of root canal therapy and placement of a walking bleach.

achieved, which is usually two to three applications. A case of severe discoloration could take even more applications. Rivera et al. recommended the placement of a 2-mm layer of white temporary stopping over the gutta-percha root filling following intracoronal bleaching. This is followed by a thin layer of an auto cure glass ionomer cement. The remaining access cavity is then restored with a composite resin. This approach serves two purposes: (1) prevention of microleakage and (2) prevention of iatrogenic perforation if future bleaching or re-treatment of the root canal therapy is required by providing different textures of filling materials with slight variations in shading.[25]

This walking bleach procedure was introduced by Spasser over 40 years ago.[26] The combination of sodium perborate and water apparently produces a sufficient oxygenating effect to bleach internal stains and is believed to be much gentler to the periodontal ligament.[14] In vivo and in vitro research studies have confirmed its efficacy. Its obvious advantage lies in its ability to produce the desired result without the liability of root resorption, which is associated with the use of Superoxol and heat.

TRAUMA

The era of the 1980s and 1990s and the new millennium has been one of participation, an era of sports and speed. With it came the concurrent hazard of dental injury. Any blow to a tooth, regardless of its intensity, can cause pulpal damage or pulpal necrosis. The need for endodontic treatment is predicated on the physiologic response of the pulpal tissue and periodontal ligament.[32] The esthetic interest in traumatized teeth centers more around the hard tissue damage even though the associated pulpal problems can greatly influence the treatment plan. Crown discolorations, fractured crowns, fractured roots, root displacements, and external resorption are the normal challenges. These problems and their endodontic implications will be discussed individually.

Crown Discolorations

The etiology of tooth discoloration can be congenital, chemical, metabolic, or traumatic. A tooth can absorb a blow without causing a crown or root fracture, yet the force may be sufficient enough to rupture the blood vessels of the pulp. The released blood enters the dentinal tubules, and a reddening of the crown may occur (see Figure 19–2). Treatment of this condition is immediate pulp extirpation followed by complete root canal therapy and bleaching. The sooner that treatment is initiated, the better the prognosis of the bleach. When the tooth is left untreated, the degeneration of the blood cells within the tubules and the necrotic tissue of the chamber will soon cause the crown of the tooth to turn a noticeable gray or black. Treatment is still endodontics; however, bleaching may be more difficult, and color regression after bleaching may occur within a shorter period of time. Often the pulp survives the injury but, unfortunately, undergoes a dystrophic calcification. The density of the tubular reparative dentin and its tendency to totally calcify the coronal pulp chamber cause the tooth to darken to a brownish-yellow hue (see Figure 19–7A). Owing to the obliteration of the chamber and the canal, endodontic treatment of brown-yellow discolored teeth becomes extremely difficult, and bleaching is highly unpredictable.

Crown Fractures

In the fracture of a crown that does not involve the pulp, or a so-called uncomplicated crown fracture, the pulp most often survives without further complications (Figure 19–56). Apparently, when the crown fractures, the force is dissipated and therefore is not transmitted to the root or periodontal ligament. For this reason, the internal tissues remain unharmed. When sufficient tooth structure exists to retain a crown or composite build-up, the exposed dentin is covered with calcium hydroxide and bonded with composite resin until a deferred

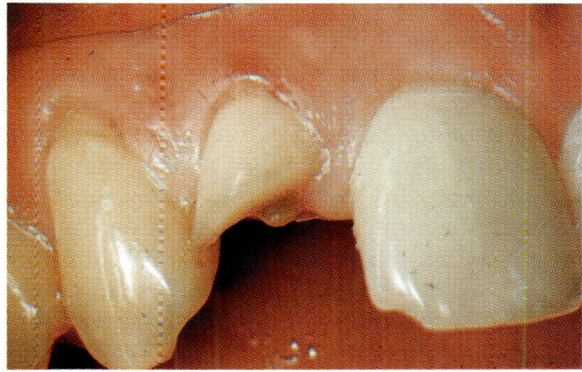

Figure 19–56: Crown fracture with no exposure; the pulp remained vital.

588 Esthetics in Dentistry

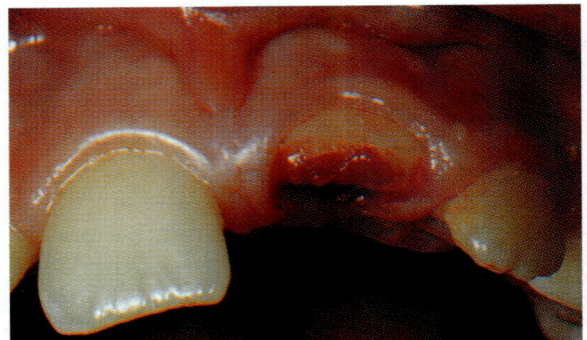

Figure 19–57: Crown fracture exposing the pulp. Root canal therapy was performed.

vitality analysis can be determined at 2, 6, and 12 weeks after the trauma. A true pulpal diagnosis may be determined at this time, and the final restoration may be safely considered.

If the remaining tooth structure is insufficient to adequately retain a restoration, the need for endodontics should be considered. Although an argument may exist to support the use of pin-retained restorations, the degree of injury of pin placement and the risk of fracture predispose elective endodontics and a full crown. The only exception would be a tooth with incomplete root apex formation. Once the root canal therapy is completed, a post and core can be fabricated to provide the ideal restorative condition. However, when the pulp is exposed, endodontic intervention is indicated (Figure 19–57): either complete root canal therapy when the root is fully formed or an apexification procedure in a tooth with an open apex.[2] Innovative solutions are required to provide for the esthetic needs of these younger patients (Figures 19–58A to C).

Root Fractures

Horizontal fractures of the root present unique problems, and the degree of difficulty is relative to the level of the break. It is very possible, and it occurs in a significant number of cases, that separation of the hard structure of a tooth can occur; however, the elasticity of soft tissue thwarts pulpal separation. For this reason, no root canal treatment is indicated and should be considered only when signs or symptoms indicate that an irreversible inflammatory reaction has occurred. When situations arise that warrant attention, the following alternatives are available.

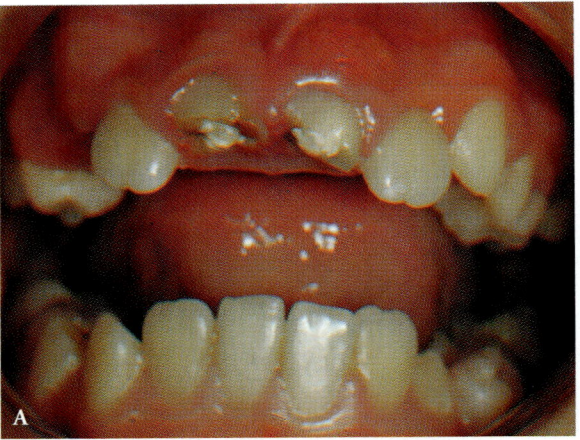
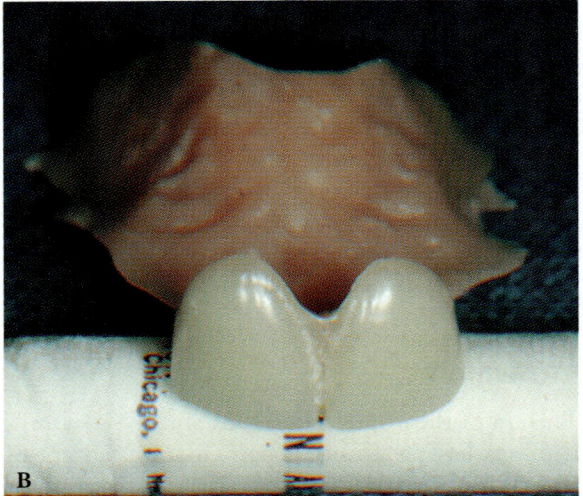
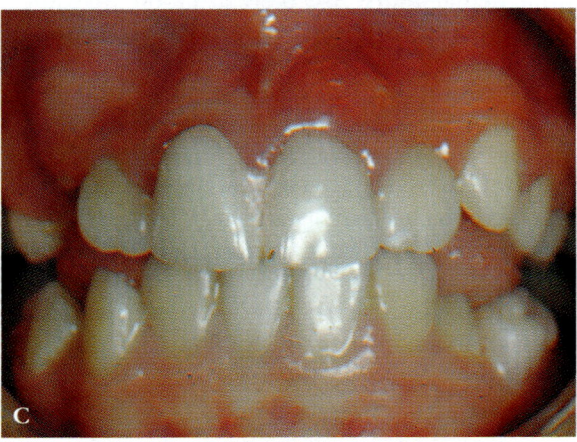

Figure 19–58A to C: Maxillary central incisor teeth: (A) crown fracture and pulp exposures requiring root pulpotomies because of immature apices, (B) a flipper was fabricated for this 9-year-old patient to satisfy the esthetic requirement, and (C) the removable denture in place.

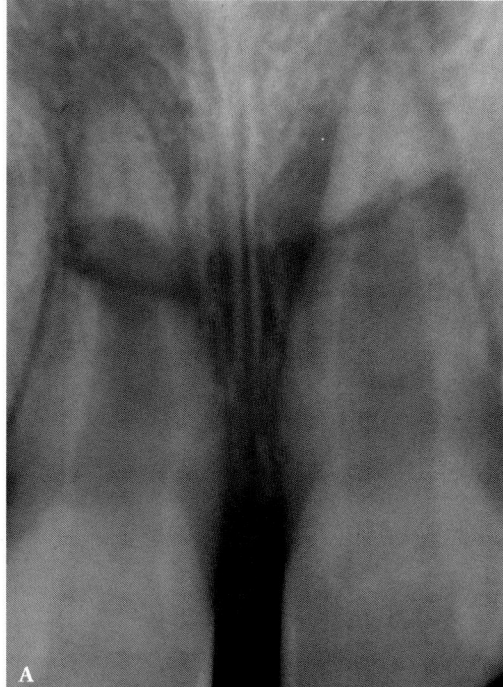 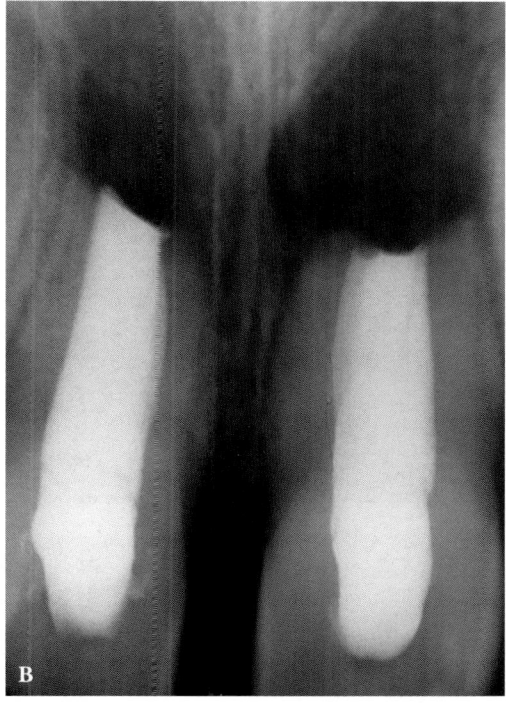

Figure 19–59A and B: Root fracture in the apical third. *(A)* Maxillary central incisors, horizontal root fractures with pulp necrosis. *(B)* Root canal therapy in the coronal segments. The apical portions of the roots were surgically removed.

For those fractures involving the apical third of the root, endodontics is performed, if the pulp necroses, to the level of the break, and the separated tip is monitored because most likely the pulpal tissue in it is healthy and does not need any treatment. In the case of a periapical lesion around the apex of the apical portion, surgical extraction is the only treatment possible (Figures 19–59A and B). As to its restorative implications, there is usually sufficient root length that adequate post preparation can be accomplished without reaching the break level and jeopardizing the seal.

Mid-root breaks create more challenging problems, the first of which is mobility. Owing to the crown:root ratio being reduced to less than one to one, stability is impaired, and a splint must be fabricated (Figures 19–60A to C). These teeth must be monitored periodically to check pulp vitality and periodontal ligament damage. Many of these teeth maintain vital pulps and a healthy periodontium and need no endodontic intervention (Figures 19–60D and E). However, if the pulp becomes necrotic, pulp extirpation is required. Endodontic options are maintaining and filling the coronal segment to the break, instrumenting both segments and uniting the segments with either gutta-percha or the more solid Vitallium (Austenal, Chicago, IL) pin, and removing the apical segment and inserting a Vitallium pin through the coronal segment and extending it to the height of the vacant apical alveolus (Figures 19–61A to C). Such endosseous stabilizers are highly successful as long as there is no communication between the pin and the oral cavity by way of the crown or the periodontium. For this reason, the pin should be reduced to a coronal level within the canal to allow the chamber to be sealed with a bonded resin filling. This obviously presents a problem when a post and core is needed to provide an adequate crown stump. Realizing that post length will be curtailed, the dentist must consider splinted units in the final treatment plan or extraction.

Root fractures that occur in the coronal third present by far the most difficult situations. The crown:root ratio is adverse, mobility is critical, and

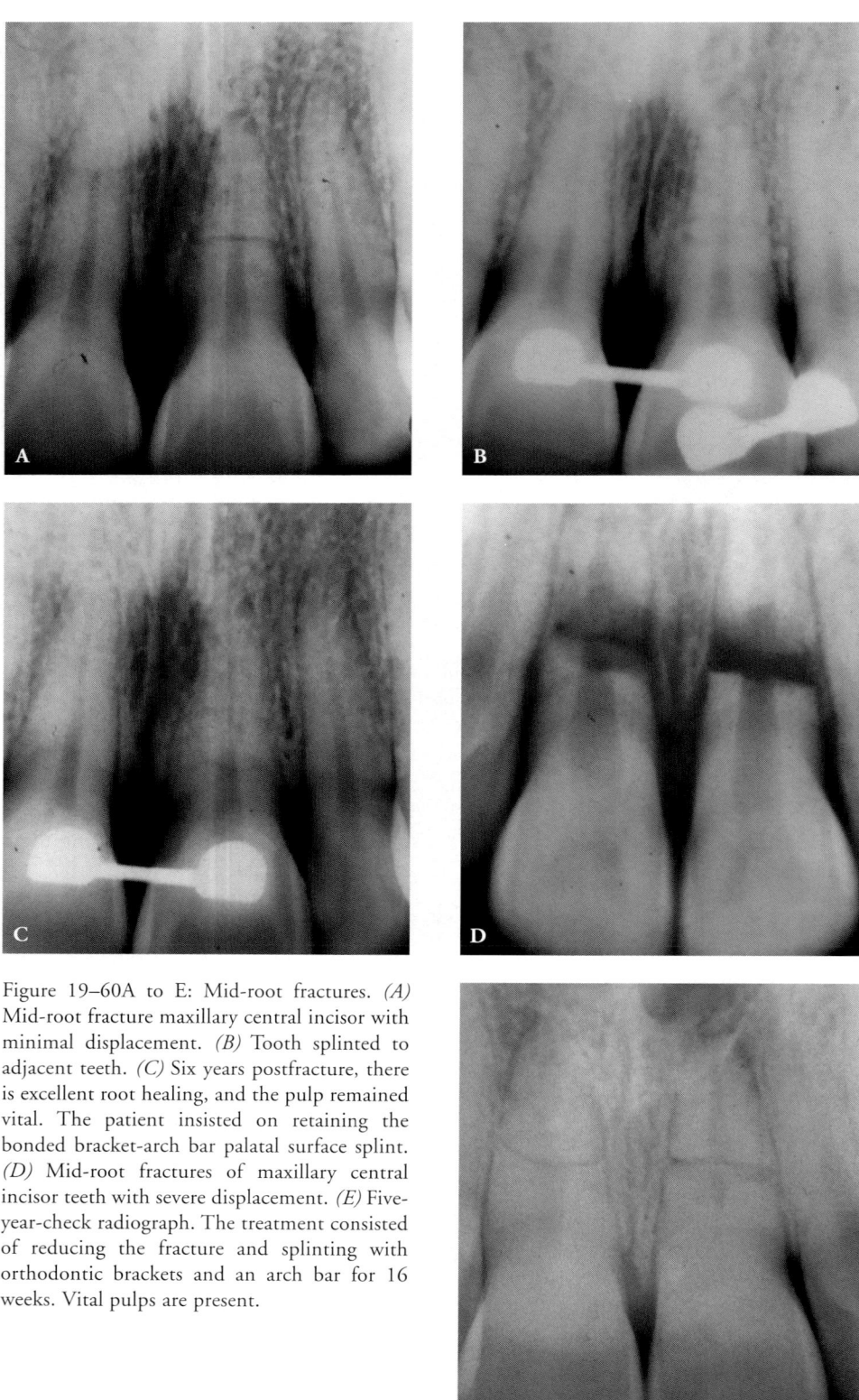

Figure 19–60A to E: Mid-root fractures. (A) Mid-root fracture maxillary central incisor with minimal displacement. (B) Tooth splinted to adjacent teeth. (C) Six years postfracture, there is excellent root healing, and the pulp remained vital. The patient insisted on retaining the bonded bracket-arch bar palatal surface splint. (D) Mid-root fractures of maxillary central incisor teeth with severe displacement. (E) Five-year-check radiograph. The treatment consisted of reducing the fracture and splinting with orthodontic brackets and an arch bar for 16 weeks. Vital pulps are present.

the prognosis is grave (Figures 19–62A and B). The coronal segment is too short to retain, and the options for the root segment are extraction followed by a single tooth implant or bridge, vertical extrusion (Figure 19–63), or embedding of the apical segment. The loss of the root would ultimately lead to the loss of the alveolar integrity and the reduction of the alveolar height. Unless ridge augmentation is performed into the vacant alveolus, an unesthetic bridge is inevitable. Endodontically treating the segment and further reducing the root coronally to a level at least 2 mm above/below the crestal height will enable bone to form across the coronal root surface. The embedded root will maintain the alveolar shape, form, and height. A fixed partial denture can then be fabricated without fear of alveolar shrinkage.

Perhaps the most favorable treatment would be extrusion of the root segment.[11] Endodontics is performed on the submerged root, and a post space is prepared to the normal depth. A stainless steel pin or post, prebent to form a hook that will extend approximately 4 mm into the oral cavity, occlusion permitting, is cemented in place. An arch wire is adapted to the labial surfaces of the two adjacent teeth on either side of the injured tooth. The wire is contoured to bend into the lingual space and create a 180-degree angle with the long axis of the root segment. The labial surfaces of the adjacent teeth are acid etched,

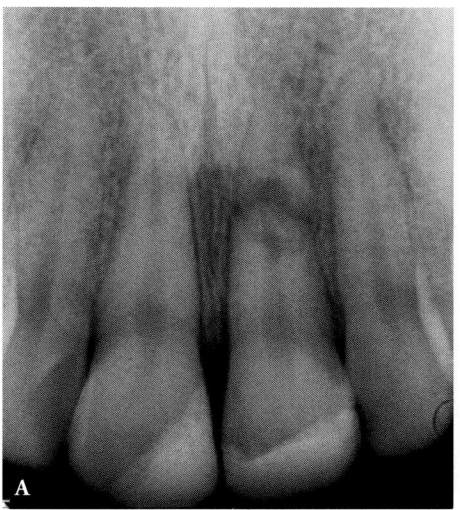
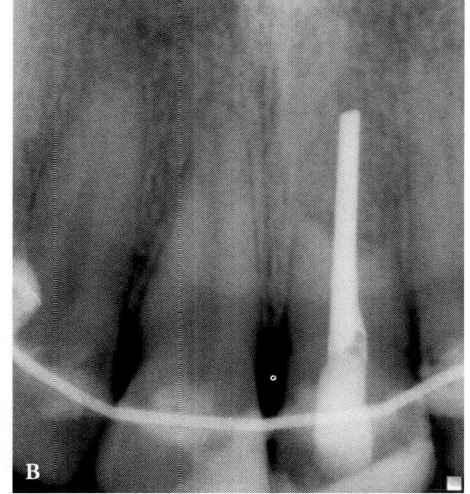
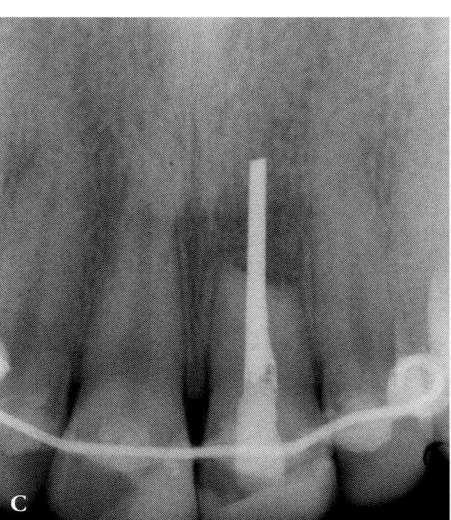

Figure 19–61A to C: *(A)* Mid-root fracture with pulp necrosis and sinus tract formation. *(B)* Treatment included pulp extirpation, Vitallium (Austenal) pin implant, bonded splint and bone graft, and guided tissue barrier. *(C)* Sixteen-month check-up shows deposition of bone in the graft area. Even though the tooth was firm, the patient insisted on retaining the splint.

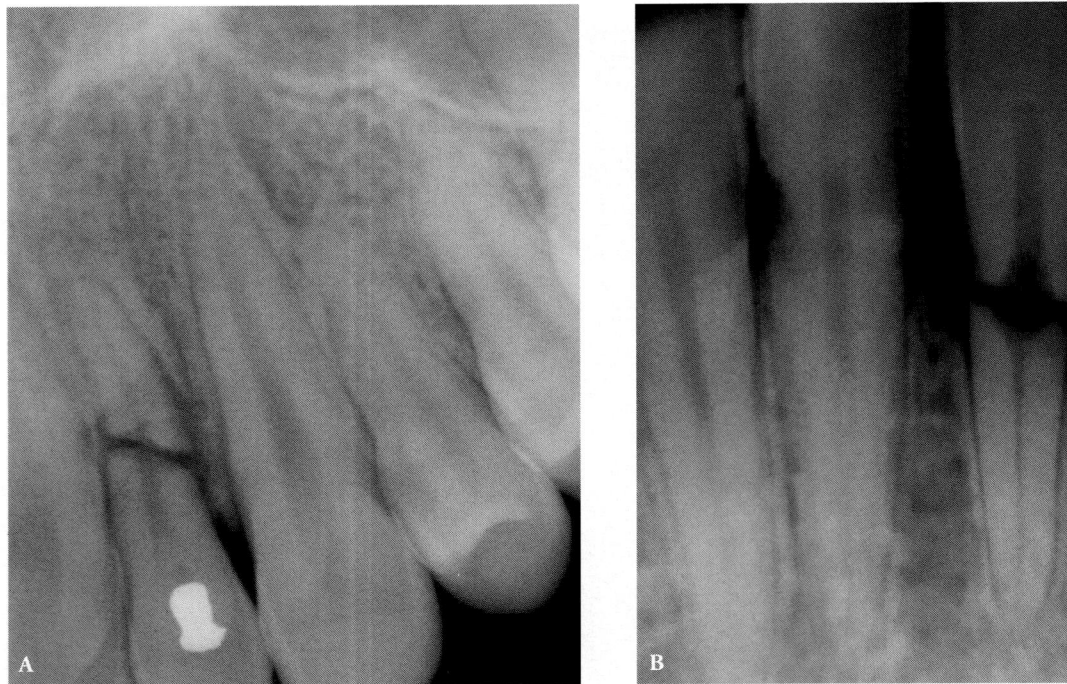

Figure 19–62A and B: Root fractures in coronal third of root requiring extraction: *(A)* maxillary lateral incisor and *(B)* mandibular lateral incisor.

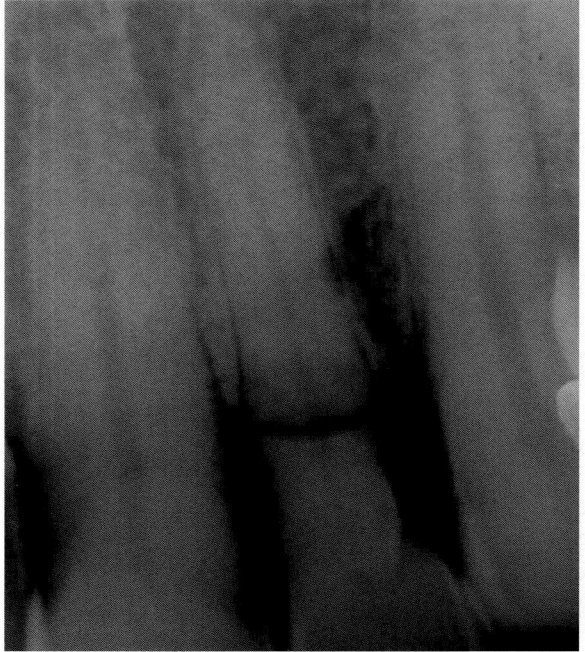

Figure 19–63: Maxillary lateral incisor with a root fracture in the coronal third. The root is long enough to consider a vertical extrusion.

and the wire is bonded in place. Ligature bands are wound around the wire and the hook. Owing to the perpendicular angle forces, the root will extrude into its predetermined position. Once the root segment is extruded to a level beyond the crest, it is prepared and impressioned. The active force is eliminated, and the root is held in a passive position for a period of 6 to 10 weeks. This enables the resistant forces of the periodontal fibers to become stable and minimize the possibility of root regression. Occasionally, postextrusion periodontal probing will reveal the need for crown lengthening. Once the dentist is confident of root stability, the final post core and crown can be fabricated with certainty.

Displaced vertical root fractures offer little hope unless the angle of the break terminates at a level that offers the options discussed for a horizontal coronal fracture.

Luxation and Avulsion

The prognosis after severe luxation and avulsion injuries has dramatically improved in the last few years because of a better understanding of how those injuries should be treated. If a tooth is replaced into its original position within a few hours after the injury, or in the case of avulsion replanted within 30 to 60 minutes after proper storage and root canal therapy is initiated 7 to 10 days later, the periodontal ligament will, in most cases, heal without any significant problems.[3] Luxated or avulsed teeth that were not properly treated or that suffered a massive injury to the periodontal ligament could present atypical problems created by subsequent ankylosis and root resorption.

Ankylosis without excessive resorption is not a serious problem unless the tooth fuses to bone in a location that creates an esthetic problem. Such is the possibility when the tooth is replanted on a child before the maxilla has had the opportunity to complete its growth. The maxilla continues to develop to adulthood, at which time the injured tooth is superior and labial to the adjacent uninjured incisors. When extracted, ridge augmentation and grafting are required to close the labial mucosa and reconstruct an esthetic alveolar ridge level. Currently, there is no treatment known to arrest ankylosis once it has started. In most cases, root canal treatment will not have any effect on the process because it is caused and maintained by the damage to the periodontal ligament.

Inflammatory root resorption presents a somewhat different situation. The endodontic objectives are centered on the arrest of the inflammatory processes that were initiated by damage to the periodontal ligament, which are being maintained by irritation from an infected root canal system and dentinal tubules. Presently, treatment consists of periodic applications of calcium hydroxide dressings within the cleansed canals. If successfully arrested, the normal periodontal ligament will establish itself again over some period, and the endodontic seal can be completed. When there is extensive damage that is so bad that it has broken into the canal space from the root surface, additional repair is attempted by surgically exposing the defect, preparing a Class I cavity preparation, and filling the defect with a nondiscoloring material. The choice of material depends on the location of the problem; however, a resin-modified glass ionomer cement (Figures 19–64A to E) (ie, Geristore, DEN-MAT, Santa Monica, CA) and MTA are presently the materials of choice. When the defect extends deep beneath the gingival crest, the crown shoulder may need to be prepared within the repair. This is not a desirable situation, but it is often the only alternative.

ENDODONTIC SURGERY

Although the technological advancements in endodontics have improved the rate of success, the demands of the populace to save teeth present degrees of difficulty that test the best of conventional therapy. In an effort to satisfy these demands, we are often called on to overcome anatomic, dentistogenic, or traumatic complications by intervening surgically. Sealing portals of exit surgically, for example, post perforations (Figures 19–65A and B), root resorption lesions (see Figures 19–64A to D), and inadequate root fillings where nonsurgical treatment is not practical (Figures 19–66A to C) constitute an extension of endodontic therapy and are alternatives to extraction.

Within the endodontic community, there is an emphasis on re-treating wherever possible and feasible rather than resorting to surgery as the first treatment option. The advent of sophisticated techniques, equipment, and materials allows for the nonsurgical retreatment of teeth that were heretofore candidates for extraction (Figures 19–67A to C).

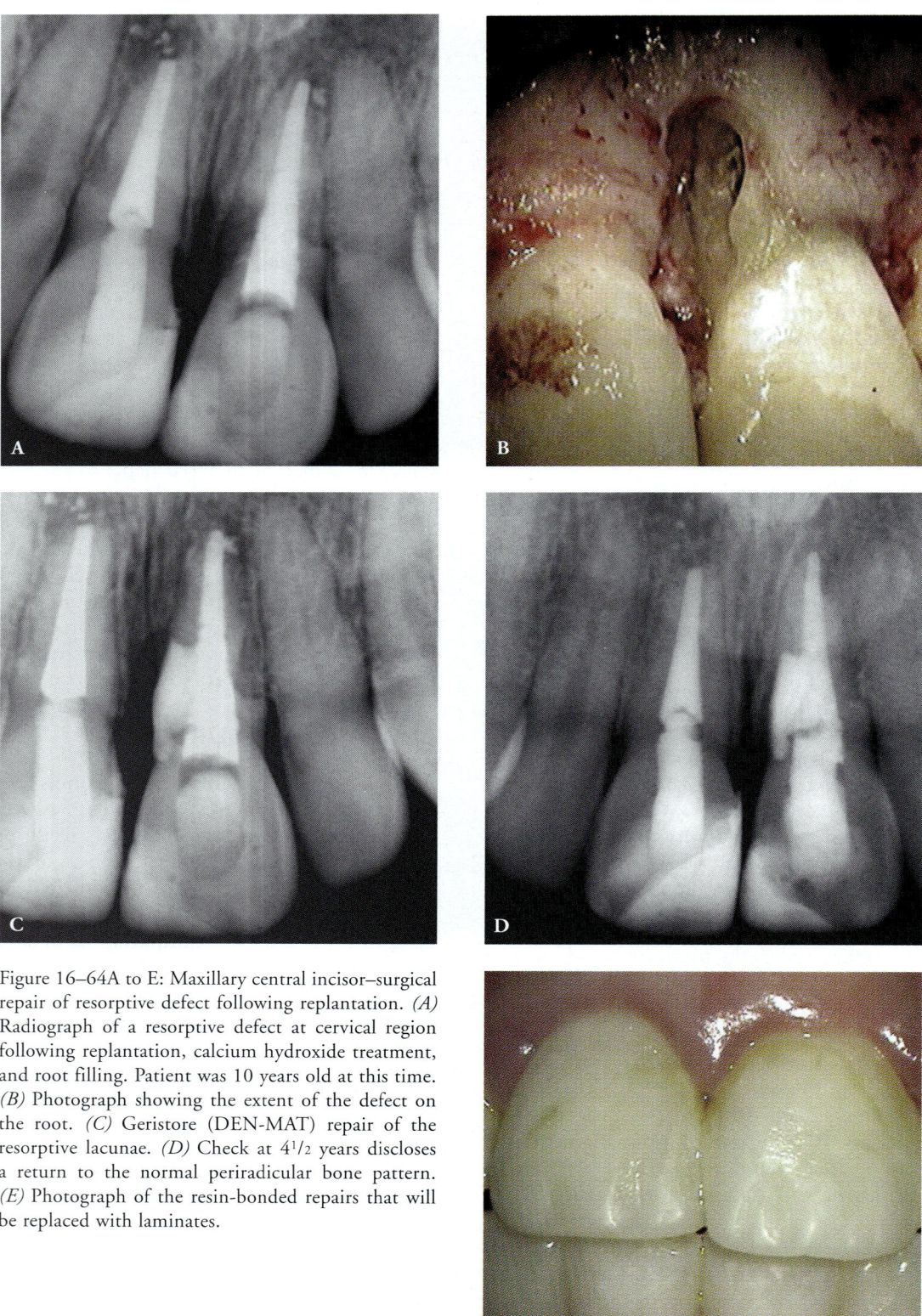

Figure 16–64A to E: Maxillary central incisor–surgical repair of resorptive defect following replantation. *(A)* Radiograph of a resorptive defect at cervical region following replantation, calcium hydroxide treatment, and root filling. Patient was 10 years old at this time. *(B)* Photograph showing the extent of the defect on the root. *(C)* Geristore (DEN-MAT) repair of the resorptive lacunae. *(D)* Check at 4$^{1}/_{2}$ years discloses a return to the normal periradicular bone pattern. *(E)* Photograph of the resin-bonded repairs that will be replaced with laminates.

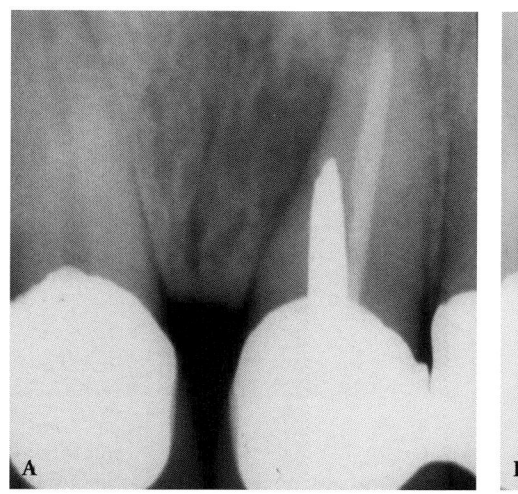
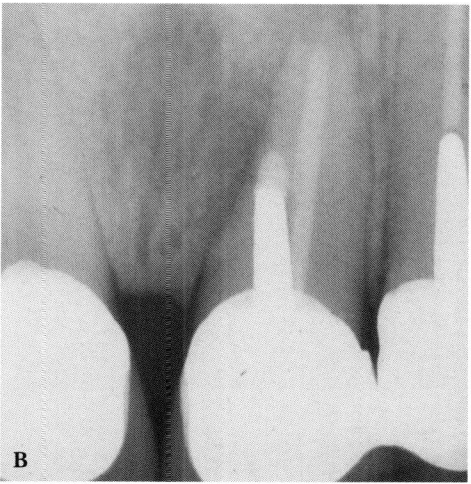

Figure 19–65A and B: Post perforation repair: *(A)* post perforation maxillary central incisor tooth and *(B)* 5 years after the surgical repair of the defect with IRM (DENTSPLY/Caulk).

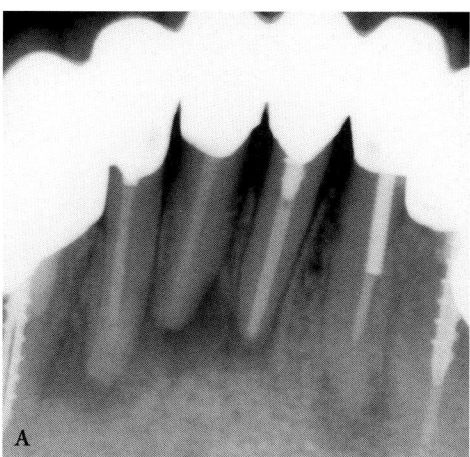
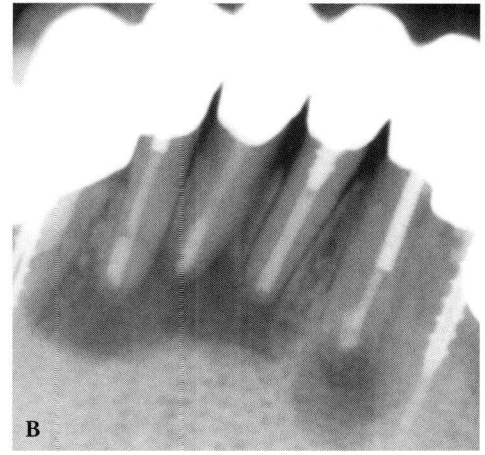
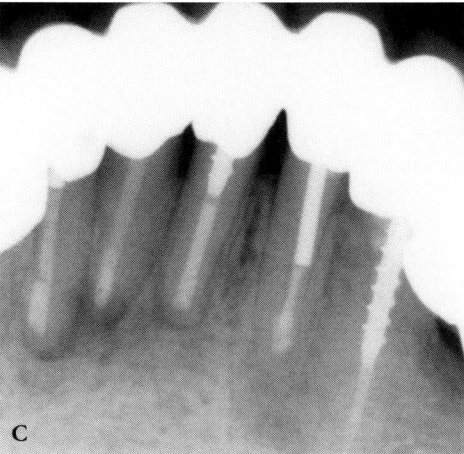

Figure 19–66A to C: Surgical re-treatment of mandibular anterior teeth: *(A)* preoperative radiograph, *(B)* mineral trioxide aggregate seals of the mandibular central and lateral incisors, and *(C)* 18-month check-up radiograph shows evidence of bone deposition.

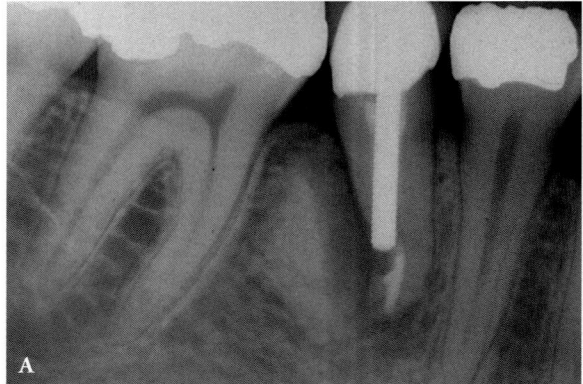
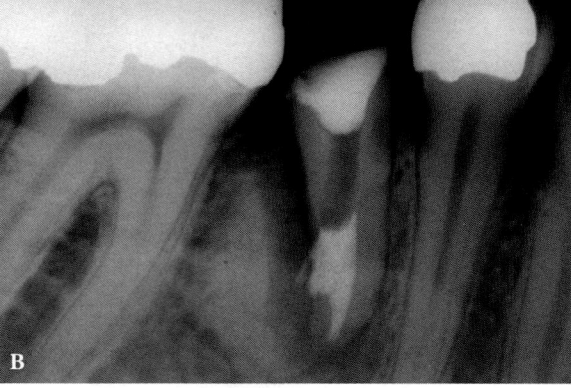
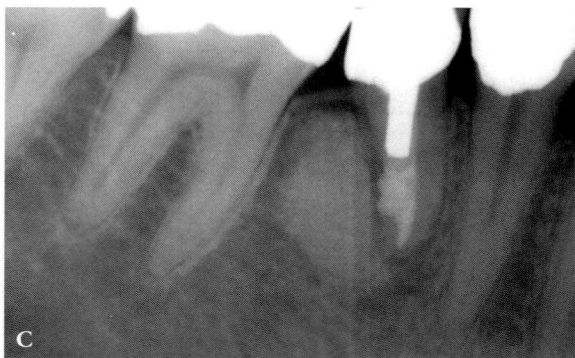

Figure 19–67A to C: Nonsurgical repair of a post perforation. *(A)* Preoperative radiograph of a mandibular premolar tooth. The position of the strip perforation on the distal surface obviates the possibility of surgical repair. *(B)* The crown, core build-up, and post were removed. The perforation was sealed with MTA. The tooth was restored with a cast post and a porcelain-fused-to-metal crown. *(C)* Six years later, the tooth is asymptomatic, and there is complete bone regeneration of the bone in the defect site.

Since endodontic surgery requires incising and elevating the soft tissue from bone, the obvious esthetic consequences can be recession and scarring. For these reasons, the choice and location of the surgical flap must be carefully evaluated before a scalpel ever touches tissue.[5] There are several major flap designs that could be used, depending on existing restorations and anatomic factors.

TISSUE DISCOLORATION (TATTOO)

In the past, silver amalgam was the material of choice for retrofilling teeth when nonsurgical therapy could not be accomplished. The same material was indicated for the repair of perforations and resorptions. In a tissue environment, this material is notorious for its discoloring effect. Once the black tattoo occurs, corrective treatment requires removal of the cause, excising the tattoo, and grafting tissue across the defect. Such treatment can now be avoided by using either zinc oxide- and eugenol-based filling material (Super EBA, H.J. Bosworth, Skokie, IL, or IRM, DENTSPLY/Caulk), composite resin, glass ionomer cements (Geristore), or MTA because not only do they seal better than amalgam, they also do not cause the staining that is associated with the amalgam.

SUMMARY

Endodontic therapy may be the key to long-term maintenance of esthetic restorations. It is essential that the patient is aware of this fact from the outset. This way, there will be no misunderstanding about "fault" if pain should arise. Thus, a well-informed patient will continue to be a trusting patient who values these services throughout the life of the dental procedures.

References

1. Abou-Rass M. The stressed pulp condition: an endodontic-restorative diagnostic concept. J Prosthet Dent 1982;48:264.

2. Andreasen JO, Andreasen FM. Essentials of traumatic injuries to teeth. Copenhagen: Munksgaard, 1990.

3. Andreasen JO, Borum MK, Jacobsen HL, Andreasen FM. Replantation of 400 avulsed permanent incisors. 4. Factors related to periodontal ligament healing. Endodont Dent Traumat 1995;11:76–89.

4. Arens DE, Chivian N. Endodontic contributions to esthetic dentistry. Annual Meeting American Academy of Esthetic Dentistry, Los Angeles, CA, 1993.

5. Arens DE, Torabinejad M, Chivian N, Rubinstein R. Practical lessons in endodontic surgery. 3rd edn. Carol Stream, IL: Quintessence, 1998.

6. Barthel CR, Rosenkranz B, Lwuenberg A, Roulet JF. Pulp capping of carious exposures: treatment outcome after 5 and 10 years: a retrospective study. J Endodont 2000;26:525–8.

7. Bohannan H, Abrams L. Intentional vital extirpation in periodontal prosthesis. J Prosthet Dent 1961;11:781–9.

8. Dummer PMH, Hicks R, Huws D. Clinical signs and symptoms in pulpal disease. Int Endod J 1980;13:27–35.

9. Ford TR, Torabinejad M, Abedi HR, et al. Using mineral trioxide aggregate as a pulp-capping material. J Am Dent Assoc 1996;127:1491–4.

10. Glockner K, Rumpler J, Ebeleseder K, Stadtler P. Intrapulpal temperature during preparation with the er: YAG laser compared to the conventional bur: an in vitro study. J Clin Laser Med Surg 1998;16:153–7.

11. Heithersay GS. Combined endodontic-orthodontic treatment of transverse root fractures in the region of the alveolar crest. Oral Surg 1973;3:404.

12. Hunter FA. Saving pulps. A queer process. Dent Item Int 1883;5:352.

13. Ingram TA, Peters DD. Evaluation of the effects of carbon dioxide used as a pulpal test. Part 2: in vivo effect on canine enamel and pulpal tissues. J Endodont 1983;9:296–303.

14. Jimenez-Rubio A, Segura JJ. The effect of the bleaching agent sodium perborate on macrophage adhesion in vitro: implications in external cervical root resorption. J Endodont 1998;24:229–32.

15. Lado EA, Stanley HR, Weissman MI. Cervical resorption in bleached teeth. Oral Surg 1983;55:78.

16. Langeland K. Prevention of pulpal damage. Dent Clin North Am 1972;16:709–32.

17. Madison S, Jordan RD, Krell KV. The effects of rubber dam retainers on porcelain fused-to-metal restorations. J Endodont 1986;12:183–6.

18. Madison S, Walton R. Cervical root resorption following bleaching of endodontically treated teeth. J Endodont 1990;16:570–4.

19. McMuller AF, Himmel VT, Sarkar NK. An in vitro study of the effect endodontic access preparation has upon the retention of porcelain fused to metal crowns of maxillary central incisors. J Endodont 1989;15:4.

20. McMuller AF, Himmel VT, Sarkar NK. An in vitro study of the effect endodontic preparation and amalgam restoration have upon incisor crown retention. J Endodont 1990;16:4.

21. Michanowicz AE, Michanowicz JP. Endodontic access to the pulp chamber via porcelain jacket crowns. Oral Surg 1962;15(Suppl 2):S1483–8.

22. Pameijer CH, Stanley HR. The disastrous effects of the "total etch" technique in vital pulp capping in primates. Am J Dent 1998;11:S45–54.

23. Peters D, Lorton L, Mader C, et al. Evaluation of the effects of carbon dioxide used as a pulpal test. Part I: in vitro effect of human enamel. J Endodont 1983;9:219–27.

24. Ray HA, Trope M. Periapical status of endodontically treated teeth in relation to the technical quality of the root filling and the coronal restoration. Int Endo J 1995;28:12–8.

25. Rivera EM, Vargas M, Ricks-Williamson L. Considerations for the aesthetic restoration of endodontically treated teeth following intracoronal bleaching. Pract Periodont Aesthet Dent 1997;9:117–28.

26. Spasser HF. A simple bleaching technique using sodium perborate. N Y State Dent J 1961;27:332–4.

27. Stanley HR. Human pulp response to restorative dental procedures. Gainesville, FL: University of Florida College of Dentistry, 1981.

28. Stanley HR, Swerdlow H. Reaction of the human pulp to cavity preparation: results produced by eight different operative techniques. J Am Dent Assoc 1959;58:49.

29. Stokes AN, Tidmarsh BG. A comparison of diamond and tungsten carbide burs for preparing endodontic access cavities through crowns. J Endodont 1988;14:11.

30. Teplitsky PE, Sutherland JK. Endodontic access of Cerestore crowns. J Endodont 1985;11:12.

31. Torabinejad M, Chivian N. Clinical applications of mineral trioxide aggregate. J Endodont 1999;25:3.

32. Trope M, Chivian N, Sigurdsson A. Trauma. In: Pathways of the pulp. 8th edn. St. Louis: Mosby, 2001: 603–49.

CHAPTER 20

ORAL HABITS

Ronald E. Goldstein, DDS, James W. Curtis Jr., DMD, Beverley A. Farley, DMD

Habits can, and all too frequently do, cause esthetic and/or functional problems in the mouth. For this reason, destructive habits need to be diagnosed and corrected as early as possible. Many patients are unaware that they have habits involving their mouths, particularly unconscious behaviors such as bruxism. Most have no idea that simple behaviors such as "occasionally" holding their glasses in their mouth or chewing ice can cause permanent problems. Adequate diagnosis of damaging habits requires a thorough evaluation of each patient's stomatognathic state. This must include examination of the form and function of the teeth and the status of the temporomandibular joints and related musculature.

Oral habits should be foremost in the examination and diagnosis of pediatric patients. Later in life, the permanent teeth and mouth should be carefully examined for changes related to oral habits that

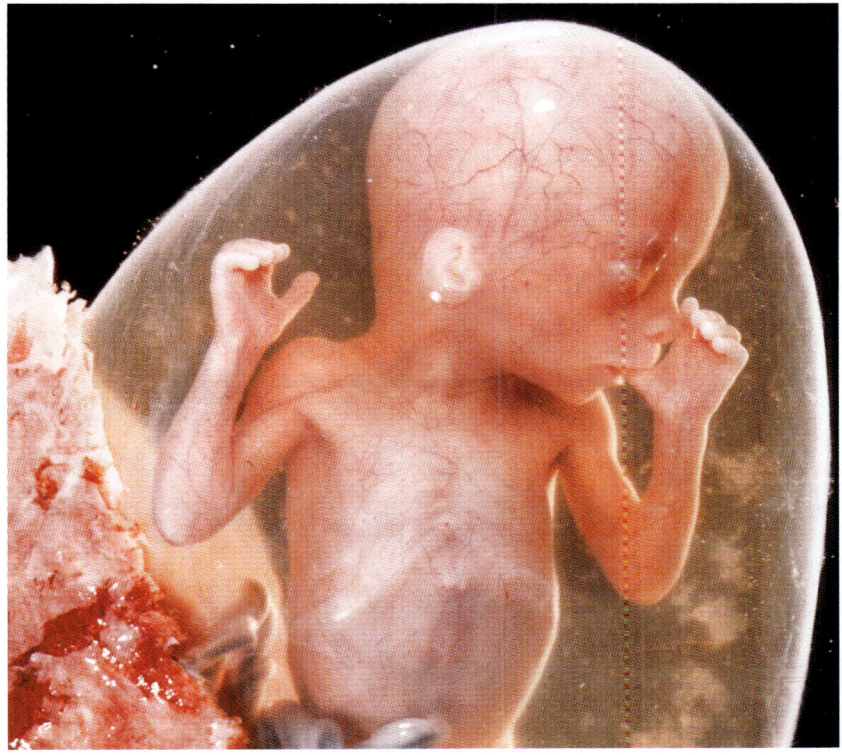

Figure 20–1: This unusual photograph demonstrates the early age (18-week-old fetus) at which thumb sucking may be manifested. Whereas many habits may be acquired, some seem to be genetically inbred as evidenced in this magnificent photograph. (Reproduced with permission from Nilsson L. A child is born. Stockholm: Albert Bonniers, 1976:125.)

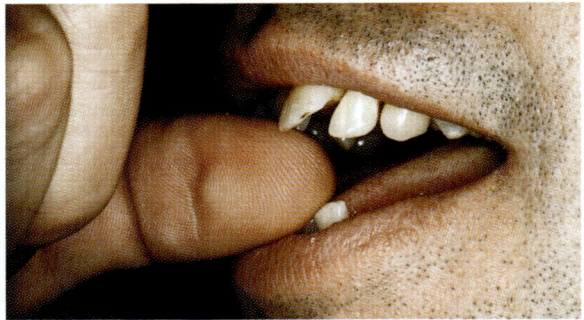

Figure 20–2A: This 33-year-old education director told of sucking his thumb as a child, which graduated into a finger-biting habit. Note the position of the thumb during the biting habit.

often occur in response to stress. Hygienists can play a key role in initially detecting wear patterns in teeth that could be arrested. Most people are surprised, but pleased, that their destructive habits can be stopped or the damage from them controlled. Dental procedures and corrective behavioral techniques may be helpful in breaking such oral habits. However, unless these habits are totally discontinued, treatment will inevitably serve as only a stopgap measure.

DIGIT SUCKING

Digit sucking is a habit that usually begins and ends in childhood (Figure 20–1). Failure to stop this behavior can result in adult arch deformities that make correction more difficult (Figures 20–2A to C).

It is estimated that roughly 4 of 10 children between the ages of birth and 16 years of age engage in digit sucking at some time during their lives. This habit may also involve several digits or fist sucking as well. Chandler, in 1878, was among the first dentists to correlate thumb- and finger-sucking habits with specific facial deformities.[13] He felt that displacement of teeth, as well as frequent elongation and narrowing of the bones of the nose, resulted from this habit. Much attention has been given to this widespread habit and the adverse dental effects that prolonged frequent digit sucking can produce. Digit sucking may damage the primary dentition and contribute to an atypical resorption pattern of maxillary primary central incisors.[22,82] Detailed reviews of the effects of prolonged thumb and finger sucking on the dental, soft-tissue, and skeletal structures have been written by numerous authors.[36,45–48,52,86] These orofacial malformations are usually unesthetic and may cause malocclusion and speech dysfunction. What is striking about the anomalies described in such abundance in the pediatric dentistry and orthodontic literature is the frequency with which some self-correction occurs if the behavior can be stopped.

For example, Larsson has presented the results of longitudinal studies of children using lateral cephalometric radiographs and observation of the occlusion.[45–47] In the younger children, thumb sucking increased the incidence of open bite with proclined and protruded maxillary incisors, a lengthened maxillary dental arch, and anteriorly displaced maxillary base. He found that finger sucking frequently caused a unilateral abnormal molar relationship on the sucking side of the mouth when the child consistently sucked a

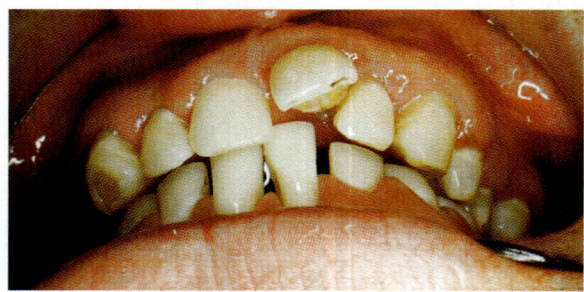

Figure 20–2B: Both maxillary and mandibular left central incisors are in labioversion as a result of the finger-biting habit.

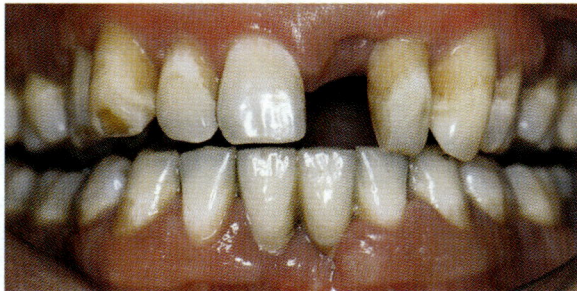

Figure 20–2C: Treatment in this type of habit sometimes consists of orthodontics and/or prosthodontics, depending on whether bone loss is present. Since there was considerable bone loss in this patient, treatment consisted of extraction of maxillary and mandibular left central incisors, plus additional periodontal therapy. Maxillary and mandibular resin bonded fixed partial dentures followed.

thumb. Finger sucking was also an important etiologic factor in the development of a posterior crossbite in the primary dentition. However, if the children stopped thumb sucking, these malocclusions were somewhat corrected by increased growth of the alveolar process and the eruption of the incisors. Similarly, others have found a tendency to an open bite and an elongated maxillary arch length among children with strong sucking habits between ages 7 and 16 years.[61,81,86] The dental effects of the thumb sucking were primarily in the anterior region of the mouth, with 80% of the children shoving the tongue over the lower incisors during swallowing. Eliminating the sucking habit tended to produce spontaneous closure of the open bite and cessation of the tongue thrust.

Bowden found yet other disturbances in persistent thumb suckers: significant increases in the proportion of the protrusive maxillary dental base relationships, tongue thrust activities, tongue-to-lip resting positions, and open bite tendencies.[10] Haryett and colleagues noted crowding of the mandibular incisors and facial asymmetries resulting from tooth interferences in the molar area because of maxillary contraction from sucking.[31] Infante's study of preschool children found posterior lingual crossbite and protrusive position of the maxillary molars relative to the mandibular molars to be more prevalent and pronounced among those children who were thumb suckers.[35] Popovich and Thompson concluded that, as the habit persisted, the probability increased that a child would develop a Class II malocclusion.[63] In each of these studies, the problems appeared to diminish in prevalence and severity as digit sucking declined, usually occurring naturally as the child grew older.

Massler believes that some of these displacements can be self-corrected by the molding action of normal labial and lingual musculature once thumb sucking is discontinued. For example, the continued and forceful placement of the thumb against the long axis of the erupting tooth may temporarily displace the erupting anterior teeth.[56] Massler suggested that more marked protrusions probably have a genetic basis. Although this protrusive tendency can be maximized by thumb-sucking behaviors, it can also manifest itself in children who have never been habitual digit suckers.

In addition to the orofacial effects caused by digit sucking, other injuries may arise as a result of this habit. Rayan and Turner described hand complications that may develop from prolonged digit sucking.[65]

Because thumb sucking is such an obvious oral habit, and perhaps because it occurs at a time when parental attention is most focused on the child, the general public has taken part in a sometimes acrimonious open debate over the possible permanent effect of the habit. The debate extends to when, or even if, the parent and/or dentist should intervene. In the 1930s and 1940s, pediatricians, pediatric dentists, and parents were frequently united in their battle against thumb sucking to prevent malocclusion. Infants were sometimes wrapped in elbow cuffs or had the sleeves of their nightgowns tied to prevent fingers from reaching their mouth. However, as Massler described, the result was "that we now are treating a generation of tongue suckers with anterior open bites and lip suckers with the so-called mentalis habit."[56] These habits, he pointed out, persist much longer than thumb sucking and are considerably more difficult to discontinue.

The accepted wisdom of our own age is that most children give up sucking by the age of 3 to 7 years. Until a child passes this age, it is just as well, and much simpler, to avoid intervention. There is much agreement that digit-sucking habits are unlikely to produce permanent damage to the orofacial structures if the habits are abandoned by 4 to 5 years of age. Beyond this period, the likelihood of harmful effects is increased. At that time, the help of a behavioral therapist or psychiatrist may be warranted. Techniques available for eliminating the habit include (1) prevention of the habit, (2) positive reinforcement, and (3) aversive conditioning methods.

Management of the habit should involve enlisting the parent and child in a cooperative effort to stop the digit sucking.[23,25,57] Treatment may require the insertion of a fixed intraoral appliance to stop the sucking activity. For example, a palatal crib appliance blocks the habitual placement of the thumb, alleviates the suction stimuli, and works to restrain the tongue from thrusting against the incisors.

HABITS IN ADULT LIFE

None of us outgrows the need for oral gratification. Few adults lack some type of learned oral habit to meet these needs. Levitas explains that an action repeated constantly becomes a habit.[49] Usually, the original stimulus or cause quickly becomes lost in the unconscious. Because the need for oral gratification never quite disappears, even as adults, the most common of the unconscious habits center in and around the mouth.

It is the dentist's responsibility to detect habits that are destructive. Unlike children, adult patients seldom make your task easier by displaying the action. Most often, you cannot look for the habit itself but rather only the product of the habit. Unfortunately, by the time the problems are visible, the chances are that the habit has been present for a long time and is fairly ingrained. This is even more reason for vigilance in detection.

HOW TO DETECT EVIDENCE OF DESTRUCTIVE HABIT PATTERNS

The following are signs that may help discover destructive occlusal habit patterns:

1. Loss of enamel contour, especially on the incisal edges of the anterior teeth.

2. A change in the smile line over the years. This can be observed by asking the patient for earlier photographs beginning at age 13 or 14 years and studying the progressive facial changes. An 8× loop should magnify photographs enough to see these changes.

3. Changes in vertical dimension showing facial collapse.

4. Wear facets that are destroying the natural esthetic contour of the teeth. In particular, any change in the canine's silhouette form should be noted.

5. Newly apparent spaces in the mouth or the enlargement of previously existing spaces.

6. Newly flared, erupted, or submerged teeth.

7. Ridges, lumps, or masses in the tissue of the tongue, lips, or inside the mouth.

Evaluate the patient's stomatognathic state, including examination of the teeth in form and function and the temporomandibular joints and related musculature.

BRUXISM

The most damaging, most frequently seen, and most frequently missed of all of the destructive oral habits is bruxism, which can destroy the form and integrity of the incisal edges of the anterior teeth (Figure 20–3A)

Esthetic treatment of the ravages of bruxism first involves habit correction or control. Second, if possible, restore the lost tooth form with bonding, laminating, or crowning combined with cosmetic contouring (Figure 20–3B) of the opposing teeth.[5,7,8,64] This usually consists of beveling the opposing teeth and replacement of the worn tooth structure. Sinuocclusal pathways must remain the same; try not to contour areas that are involved in excursive movement. If it is not possible to restore missing tooth structure, it may be possible to

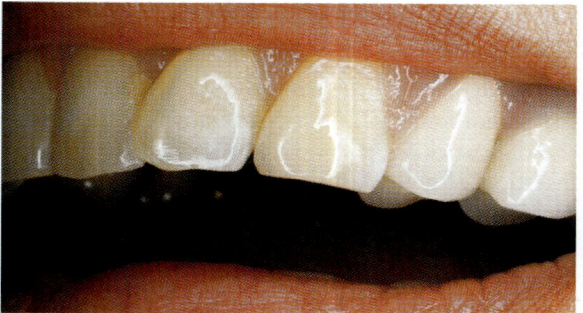

Figure 20–3A: This 30-year-old teacher had worn her left canine flat due to bruxism.

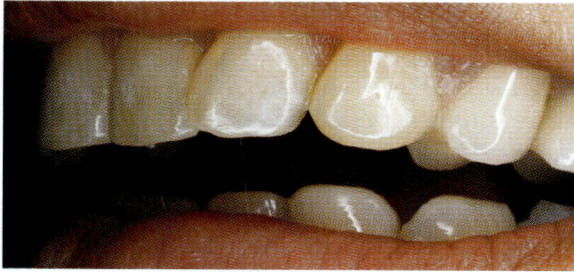

Figure 20–3B: After treatment for the condition, which consisted of appliance therapy, the anteriors were cosmetically contoured rather than adding to the tooth surface. In cases like this, it is important for the patient to wear an appliance afterward to make certain that additional bruxism will no longer destroy enamel.

restore esthetics through cosmetic contouring. Also, if the anterior teeth have worn evenly, reshape the laterals to create more interincisal distance. This technique can be effective in achieving an illusion of greater incisal length, thus providing enhanced esthetics.

Bruxism may be a learned behavior that is a reaction to stress associated with various dental or medical conditions, such as malocclusions, missing or rough teeth, infections, malnutrition, and allergies.[16,19,20,33,34,37] These conditions may contribute to the extent to which bruxism is manifested (Figures 20–4A and B). Studies by Hicks and colleagues showing an increase in bruxism among college students implicated stress as a major etiologic factor.[32,33] Cigarette smoking has been shown to exacerbate nocturnal bruxism.[48,54] Numerous reports have shown bruxism to be related to sleep disorders and sleep apnea.[3,53,62,90]

Bruxism can sometimes begin after orthodontic treatment for crowded teeth. After incisors are realigned, the patient can develop a habit of clinching and grinding in the anterior region that can eventually destroy incisal anatomy.

BRUXISM WITH TEMPOROMANDIBULAR JOINT PAIN

Esthetic destruction of the patient's teeth can be sufficient to enable us to recognize the disease process of temporomandibular joint pain long before the patient actually begins treatment.[1,41,51,60,73,77,83–85]

The following case illustrates this position. A young woman had been treated without success by several physicians for headaches, dizzy spells, and neck, back, and shoulder pain (Figures 20–5A to E). Her problems with pain, as well as with the destruction of her teeth, appeared to be related to her bruxism. When asked to open her mouth, she deviated sharply to one side. The intraoral muscles (pterygoid and masseter) and ligaments were in acute spasm and tender to palpitation. Treatment began with insertion of a maxillary bruxing appliance. (With bruxism patients, it is important to obtain study casts to determine if there are wear facets, where they are located, and why they occurred.) The bruxing appliance was constructed to help stop the incisal wear. The patient's teeth were then reshaped to improve the smile line. Most pain and headaches stopped within a period of 3 to 6 weeks after the insertion of this appliance, together with muscle therapy to the affected areas.

The patient must realize the importance of continuing to wear the bruxing appliance to maintain the esthetic correction and to avoid reintroducing temporomandibular joint pain and dysfunction.[91]

CHEWING HABITS

The use of smokeless tobacco is another habit that causes excessive wear on the dentition, in addition to the potential of causing oral cancer.[11,55,71] The lingual cusps of maxillary teeth and buccal cusps of mandibular teeth are the most affected, often worn to the gingival margin. Staining of exposed dentin is also readily apparent.

Dark brown/black stains on the teeth, marked abrasion of anterior teeth, and pathologic changes of the oral mucosa are seen in many Eastern countries, such as India, Malaysia, and Thailand, in

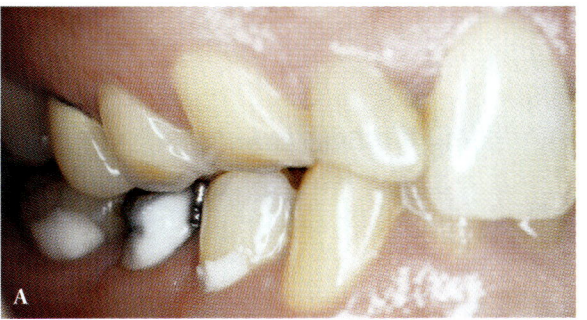
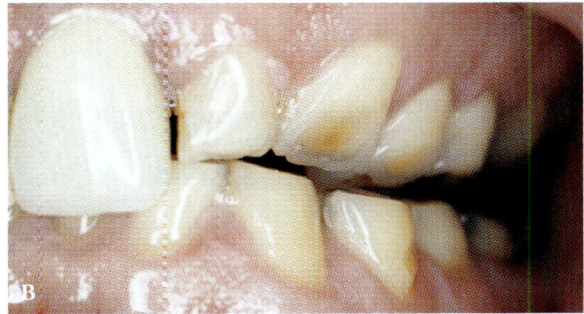

Figure 20–4A and B: This 50-year-old man was completely unaware of his nocturnal bruxism. In fact, during waking hours, it was difficult for him to get his teeth to fit together in the excentric position.

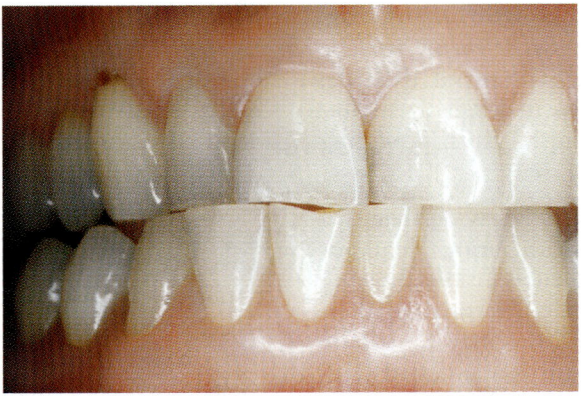

Figure 20–5A: Bruxism was the chief cause of wear for this 31 year old.

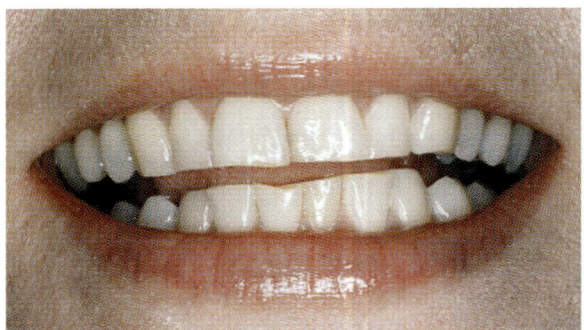

Figure 20–5B: Note how she would unconsciously put the tongue behind the front teeth to hide the space that shows a jagged outline. In addition to poor esthetics, the patient also suffered constant headaches and neck and back discomfort because of further temporomandibular joint dysfunction.

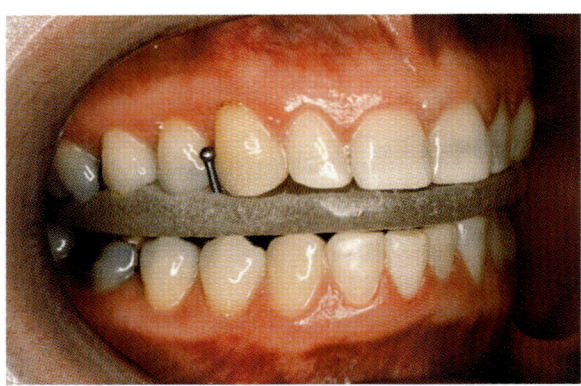

Figure 20–5C: A removable appliance was made to correct the temporomandibular joint dysfunction and prevent teeth from further wearing away. Following 3 months of temporomandibular joint treatment to cure the symptoms and relax the muscles, the patient wore the appliance only at night.

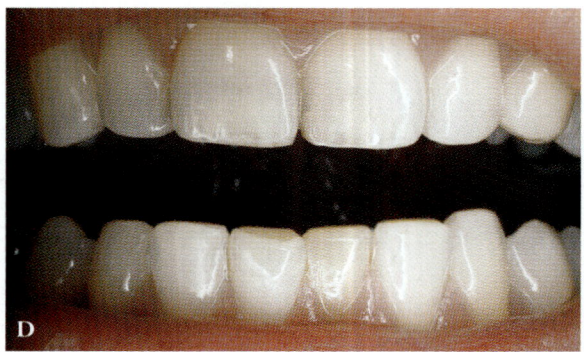

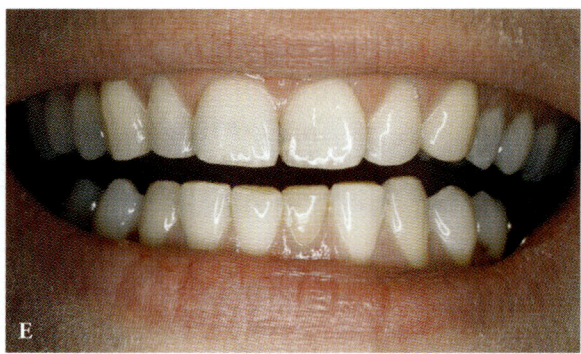

Figure 20–5D and E: After several months of appliance therapy, the square, masculine-looking upper and lower teeth were cosmetically contoured to produce a more feminine and prettier smile.

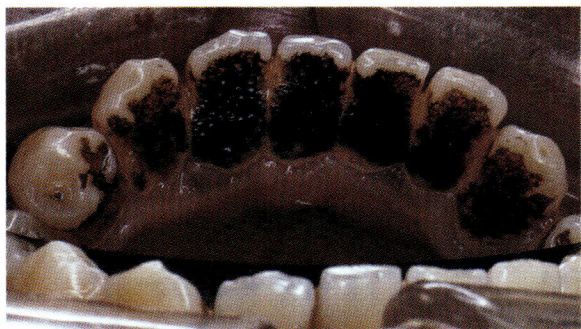

Figure 20–6: This 35-year-old male had the habit of placing betel nuts under his tongue, which helped to produce black stain as shown.

those who chew betel nuts for medicinal and/or psychological purposes[67,92,93] (Figure 20–6). Patients who refuse or cannot stop the habit should be on monthly "cosmetic" cleanings. This type of prophylaxis is most readily accomplished using a high-powered, mildly abrasive spray. These patients should be warned that the sharp edges of the betel nut may cut the gingiva, leading to ulceration. In addition, the betel nut contains carcinogens that can lead to the development of oral cancer in habitual users. Coca leaf chewing was shown to cause similar effects on the dentition in ancient cultures.[44]

TONGUE HABITS

The tongue is one of the strongest muscles in the human body. The most frequent signs of tongue thrust are protrusion of the tongue against or between the anterior teeth and excessive circumoral muscle activity during swallowing. Although pushing the tongue against teeth, particularly between spaces in the teeth, does not invariably cause harm, it is certainly a potential cause of damage. Either maxillary or mandibular teeth can become involved (Figure 20–7). Indentations in the tongue have been reported to provide an indication of clenching.[75] Gellin, however, feels that anterior tongue positioning does improve with time, and the continual growth and development of the lower face allow for diminishing anterior tongue positioning.[23] Various studies showed the relationship between tongue thrust and malocclusion.[2,58,59]

There are clinicians who have observed a large number of patients with malocclusions who demonstrate a protrusive tongue tip pattern against or between the anterior teeth while speaking or swallowing. This group suggests that tongue thrusting is one of the primary etiologic factors in open bite and incisor protrusion. There is also much controversy concerning the use of removable appliances in the treatment of tongue twisting.

The beautiful young woman in Figures 20–8A and B would like to advance her modeling career, but a space between her teeth appears as a black hole in photographs. Consequently, she poses with her tongue pressed behind the space in her teeth in an attempt to hide the darkness. This trick helps with the photographic illusion, but if she presses her tongue too much in a labial direction, the space can increase over the years. The habit of putting the tongue between the teeth to disguise a space will almost certainly cause the space to increase with time (Figure 20–8C). Treatment of spaces between the teeth is usually best handled through orthodontic care and possibly myofunctional therapy to promote a more positive resting and swallowing tongue position. However, some patients may not mind, and may even prefer their teeth with a space. Although no space should be corrected without approval from the patient, even these patients need to be referred to an orthodontist for monitoring and control of any further widening that might have functional implications.

For those patients who desire closure of the diastema, referral to an orthodontist can determine if repositioning of the teeth is appropriate. In discussing the referral with the patient, make certain that it is understood that orthodontics does not need to be a matter of metal brackets. One of the most common solutions to gaps is the construction

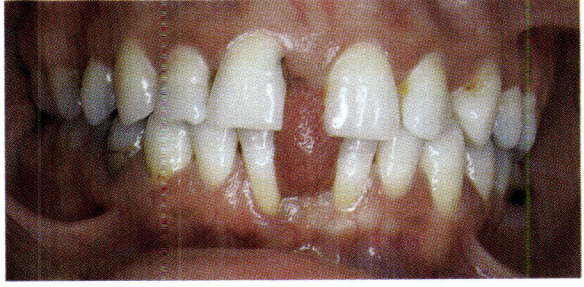

Figure 20–7: This 47-year-old teacher developed a habit of forcing her tongue between her maxillary and mandibular incisors. Note the large space created as a result of years of tongue pressure.

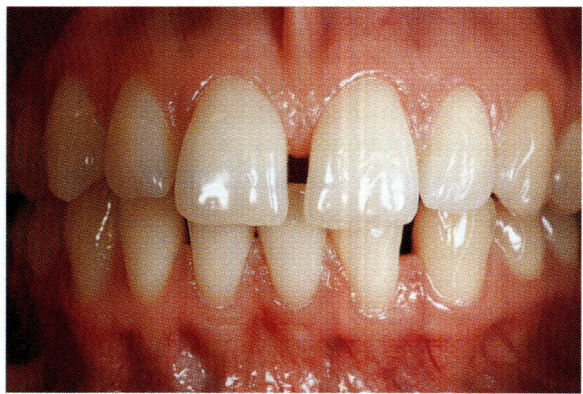

Figure 20–8A: This 23-year-old model had a diastema between the maxillary central incisors.

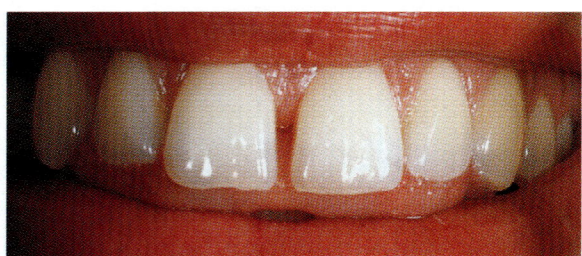

Figure 20–8B: When smiling, she would place her tongue behind the two front teeth to hide the space, which would otherwise show up dark. Note how the tongue creates a pink filler similar to gingival tissue. Many models unconsciously develop similar habits, which can create additional space because of the tongue pressure if done over a long period of time. It is much wiser to either close these spaces orthodontically or compromise with restorative means.

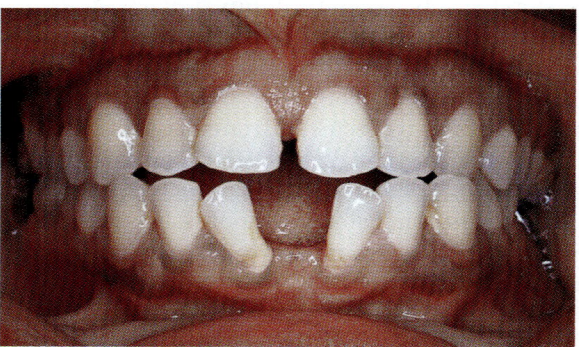

Figure 20–8C: The habit of placing the tongue between the teeth to disguise a space will almost certainly cause the space to increase with time.

of a retainer that the patient wears at night. After the teeth have stabilized, the retainer can be worn a few nights each week to maintain tooth position and prevent reopening the space.

An alternative or compromise treatment consists of bonding composite resin to close the spaces. Crowns and porcelain veneers can also serve this function, but bonding has the advantage of reversibility. The patient could later elect to have orthodontic treatment, especially if the spaces continue to widen.

Sometimes, orthodontics may not be the patient's choice, and the following case illustrates an alternative, restorative means of treatment. The young man shown in Figures 20–9A to H was extremely self-conscious about a space between his central incisors caused by a tongue thrust. He was referred for orthodontics, both to correct the space and to correct his destructive habit. However, the appliance needed to correct the spacing between this young man's teeth gave him what he considered a freakish appearance, and he asked for an alternative treatment. Treatment was then planned using composite resins, which, although not permanent, produce immediate results.

LIP OR CHEEK BITING

The signs of lip or cheek biting are usually telltale marks from the teeth (Figures 20–10A and B). Glass and Maize have described the appearance of

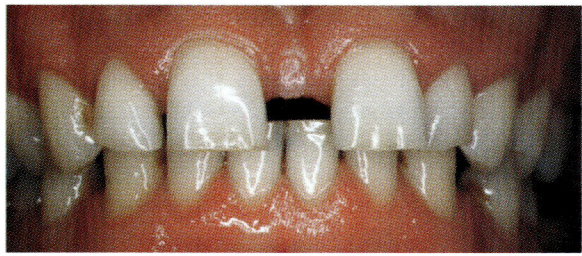

Figure 20–9A: This 32-year-old was self-conscious about a space between his front teeth that was originally caused by tongue thrusting.

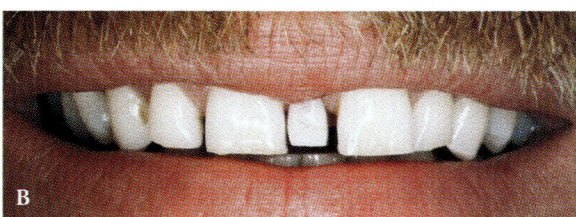

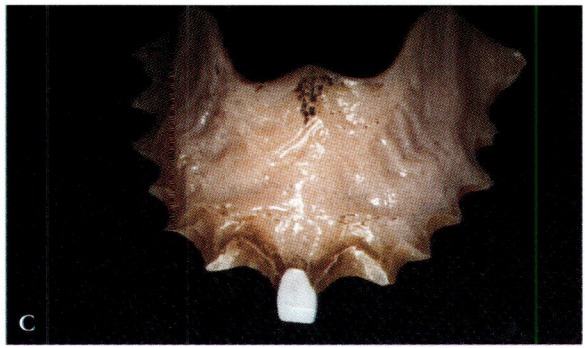

Figure 20–9B and C: He felt that people were noticing his smile, and since he did public speaking, he wanted to improve his appearance. This replacement had been in the mouth for 16 years.

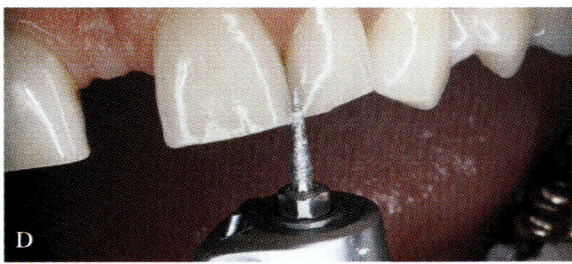

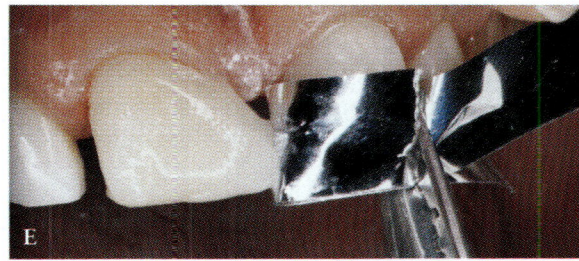

Figure 20–9D and E: The patient was referred for orthodontic consultation but elected to have composite resin bonding as a compromise treatment.

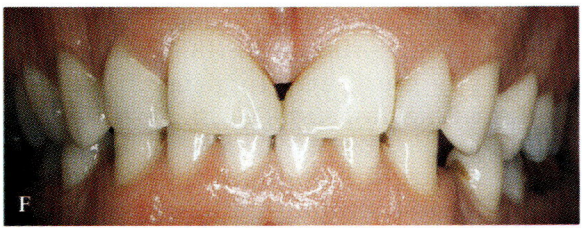

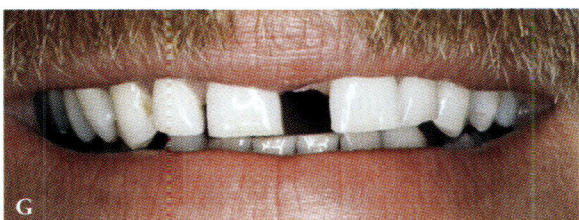

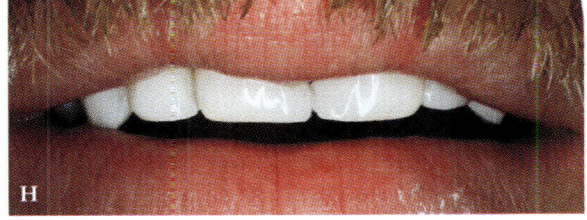

Figure 20–9F to H: Although closing the space created a disproportionate overbuilding of the two central incisors, through judicious carving of the finished bonded restorations, a more proportionate and not unattractive arrangement can be achieved. This consisted of opening the incisal embrasures, as well as creating a greater interincisal distance.

oral tissues that have been chewed or bitten over a period of time.[24] This results in the appearance of hard fibrous knots or masses known as morsicatio buccarum et labiorum. Sometimes, the patient uses the teeth to suck or knead the altered tissue. If the habit continues over an extended period of time, it can also cause tooth abnormalities by enlarging any small diastema or interdental space. The more a patient chews or sucks, the more pressure is created between the teeth and the wider the space.

Other lip habits such as lip wetting or lip sucking and a swallowing pattern that includes a hyperactive mentalis muscle can cause damage to developing orofacial structures in children. Lip wetting is frequently unnoticed by the average dental practitioner. Clinically, the entire lip looks soft and moist and does not have a sharply demarcated vermilion border.

Cheek biting is one of the most frequently seen destructive oral habits and can reflect a circular pattern (Figure 20–10C). Sometimes, loss of part of a tooth or an entire tooth can initiate cheek biting. The presence of resulting fibrous tissue may cause the patient to pull the knot of tissue between the teeth and begin to suck. Diagnosis of cheek biting can be made by examining the inside border of the cheek for a flickered, sometimes white fibrous ridge midway between the arches.

Treatment of lip biters and cheek biters consists of several steps. The first usually involves reshaping the teeth to round, smooth, and polish any sharp edges. It is also important in working with such patients to find out if there has been any recent crowning, lengthening, or shortening of the teeth or other changes that might have induced this habit. If so, they may need to be modified.

The second part of treatment usually involves creating an appliance to prevent the patient from biting the lip or cheek (Figures 20–10D and E).[89] This should be as thick as feasible and rounded on the labial surface. As a temporary measure, a removable acrylic interdental spacer or a vacuform matrix can be used to prevent the patient from biting or sucking (Figures 20–11A to C).

One of the added advantages of such devices, which are worn around the clock during the early phases of treatment, is that they make the patient more aware of the intensity and frequency of such habits and the circumstances under which they most often manifest themselves. Many patients are not aware that they bite or suck their lips or cheeks, especially in relation to stress. Once the patient stops biting the lip, the use of the appliance can be reduced to evenings only. Most patients will require between 3 and 6 months to correct the problem (Figures 20–12A to D).

Finally, any space between the teeth can be corrected via orthodontics or the application of composite resin bonding or porcelain veneers to close the diastema (see Figure 20–11C). The use of full crowns would be a third choice to close the space.

MOUTH BREATHING

Common in childhood, mouth breathing is the habit of using the mouth instead of the nose for respiration regardless of whether the nose is obstructed. However, there are often specific reasons for mouth breathing, such as allergies, enlarged nasopharyngeal lymphoid tissues, and asthma.[6,14,50,87] The prevailing hypothesis is that prolonged mouth breathing during certain critical growth periods in childhood causes a sequence of events that results in dental and skeletal changes. Excessive eruption of the molars is almost always a constant feature of chronic mouth breathing. This molar eruption causes clockwise rotation of the mandible during growth, with a resultant increase in lower facial height. The increased lower facial height is often associated with retrognathia and anterior open bites. Low tongue posture is seen with mouth breathing and impedes the lateral expansion and anterior development of the maxilla.[15,18,26–28,30,39,40,42,78,80,88] The dentofacial effects that develop in children persist into adulthood, and the mouth-breathing and tongue-thrusting behavior may continue. Barber has found that mouth breathing can lead to dryness and irritation of the throat, mouth, and lips, as well as chronic marginal gingivitis.[4] Also, it is strongly associated with both lip-biting and lip-wetting habits. It may be necessary to treat the mouth-breathing habit prior to or in conjunction with the treatment of the lip habit.

EATING DISORDERS AND POOR DIETARY HABITS

Anorexia nervosa and bulimia are psychosomatic eating disorders that have associated oral symp-

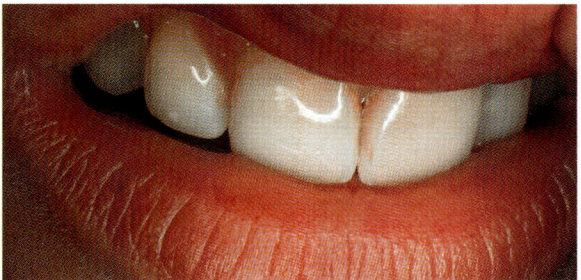

Figure 20–10A: This 29-year-old woman felt that her upper teeth were "growing down more" and irritating her lower lip. She was told to let us know exactly when she closed her lip and felt that it was fitting tightly into the teeth.

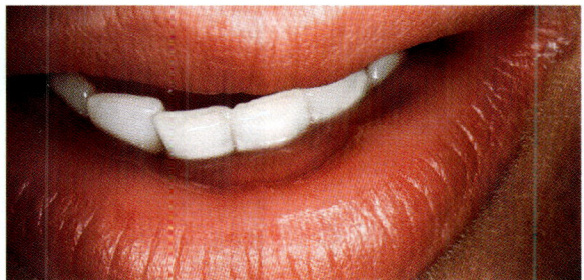

Figure 20–10B: During her next appointment, she stated that she realized that she is both sucking and biting down on her lip at the same time.

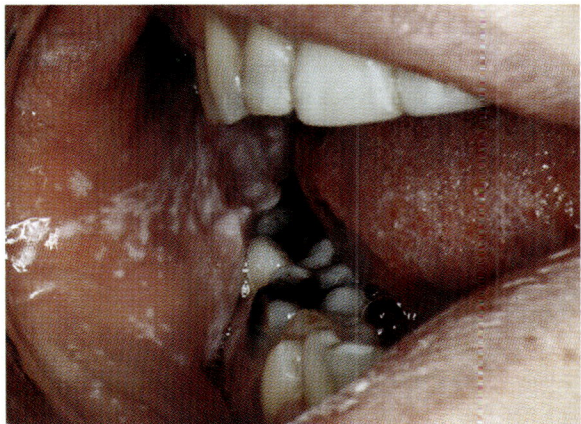

Figure 20–10C: This 50-year-old woman had a habit of biting her cheek. Note the pattern of white fibrous tissue.

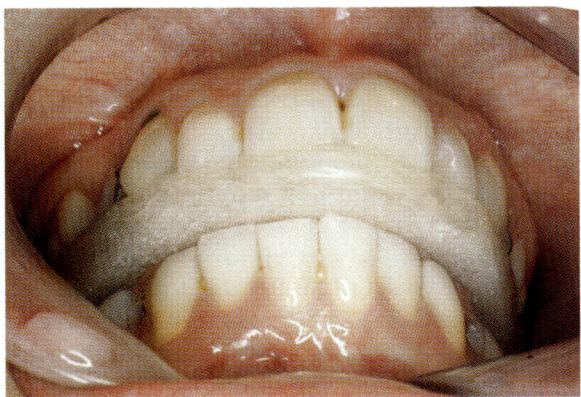

Figure 20–10D: Since her external pterygoid muscles were in spasm, it was also felt that she could be grinding her teeth, so an upper temporomandibular joint appliance was constructed, rounding the labial incisal angle in particular.

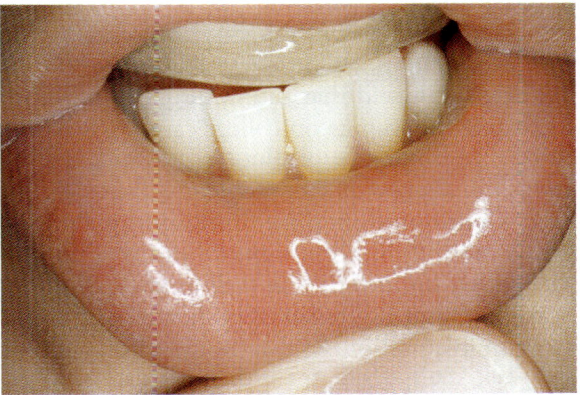

Figure 20–10E: After 5 months of wearing the appliance, at first all of the time and then at night only, the patient's tissue returned to normal. In addition, her muscle spasms disappeared, and all other symptoms subsided.

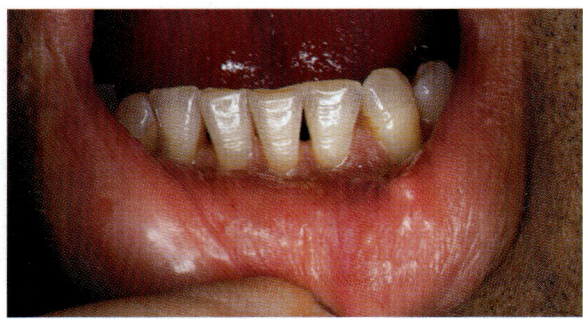

Figure 20–11A: This 50-year-old man had been sucking the lower left lip into an open interdental space between the mandibular left central and lateral. Note the lesion created on the lower left inner border of the lip due to the patient's sucking habit.

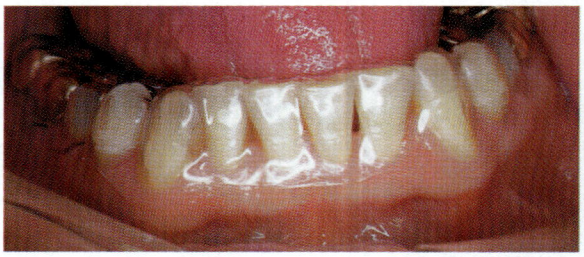

Figure 20–11B: A vacuform matrix was made to close up this area to see if the patient could break the sucking habit. Unfortunately, the only time the patient could eliminate the habit of sucking was when the appliance was being worn.

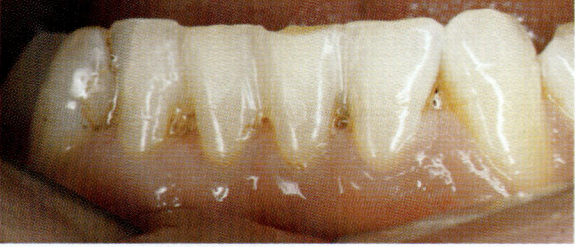

Figure 20–11C: It was decided to bond the mandibular incisors to eliminate space and thereby help to eliminate his sucking habit. Had the patient been able to alleviate the habit with the matrix, it would have been possible to eliminate the need for closure of this space.

toms. The exact prevalence of these eating disorders is unknown. However, they are most frequently seen in young women, ranging from adolescence into early adulthood. In some studies,[21,38,68,76] it has been estimated that eating disorders affect up to 20% of the women on college campuses. As our culture continues to emphasize outward appearance, it is likely that this problem will not resolve soon. Dentists are often the first health care professionals to recognize the signs of eating disorders, particularly bulimia. It may well be that the obsession to improve outward appearances that drives some individuals to develop eating disorders may also fuel their desire for esthetic dental services. Thus, practices that have a strong emphasis on esthetic care should be diligent in assessing their patients, especially young women, for signs of eating disorders.

The bulimic patient ingests large amounts of food, followed by voluntary or involuntary purging. The purging may occur with the use of high doses of laxatives or induced vomiting. In those bulimics who purge by vomiting, the pH of the gastric acid is low enough to initiate dissolution of the enamel. Further compounding the problem is the frequent vigorous tooth brushing that is used to rid the mouth of the taste and telltale odor of the vomitus. Brushing the teeth immediately after they have been exposed to gastric acids will accelerate the loss of enamel. Numerous studies show that a high percentage of patients seen with bulimia exhibit lingual erosion of the maxillary anterior teeth caused by regurgitation of gastric acids (Figures 20–13A to D).[9,12,70,72,74] If the disorder persists, the erosion will eventually affect the occlusal surfaces of the molars and premolars. If the bulimia is not controlled, the entire

Oral Habits 611

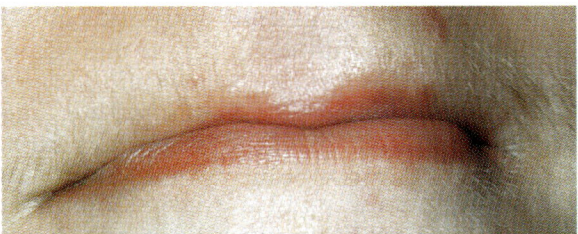

Figure 20–12A: This young lady developed a habit of sucking her upper lip.

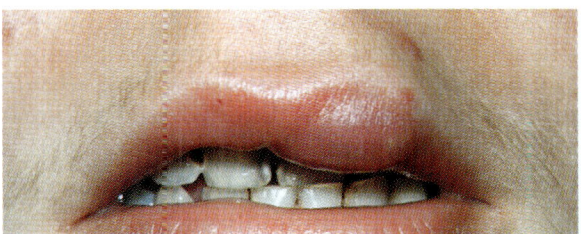

Figure 20–12B: A bulbous lesion was the result of the constant suction action that prompted the patient to seek treatment only for the lip but not the obvious caries. (Reproduced with permission from Goldstein RE. Change your smile. 3rd edn. Carol Stream, IL: Quintessence, 1997:287.)

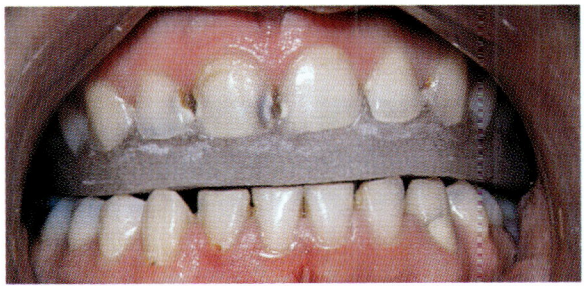

Figure 20–12C: A removable maxillary appliance was made for the patient to wear full time until she completely broke the habit. Note also advanced caries, which needed to be treated.

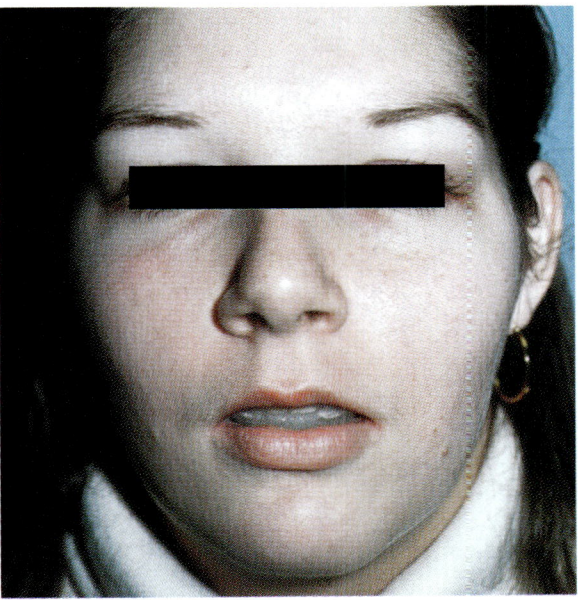

Figure 20–12D: It required only several weeks for the patient to gain back her normal-appearing lip. Then the patient could focus her attention on her other dental treatment.

dentition may be destroyed, necessitating complete dental rehabilitation with full-coverage restorations. Unfortunately, if the habit persists after the rehabilitation, these patients are likely to develop recurrent caries around the margins of the crowns.

Patients with anorexia nervosa pose an entirely different set of problems. Although bulimia and anorexia are disorders that involve a severely altered self-perception, individuals with anorexia may tend to fully lose self-esteem and fall into a state of total oral neglect. In its severest form, patients with anorexia may present with rampant caries and notably dry mucosa (Figures 20–14A to C). They are very prone to the effects of metabolic imbalance and should be treated cautiously in the dental office.

In addition to the intraoral ravages of bulimia and anorexia, outwardly visible signs of these disorders can be seen. Figure 20–15 shows a 35-year-old female who suffered from both bulimia and anorexia. Notice the swelling of the parotid gland, clearly seen at the angle of the mandible. This hypertrophy of the gland is commonly seen in bulimics. It is caused by repeated vomiting and is present bilaterally. Also, on close examination of the photograph, a fine, downy facial hair can be detected. This facial hair is called lanugo and may be found in anorexics.

The dental manifestations of eating disorders can be treated immediately, but treatment must be limited to emergency, preventive, and/or tempo-

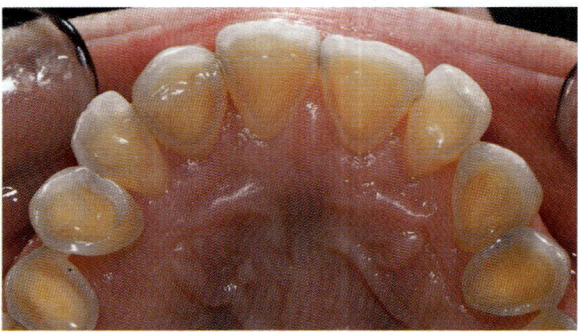

Figure 20–13A: Preoperative upper anterior palatal view of a bulimic patient shows extreme erosion of the lingual and occlusal surfaces. (Courtesy of Dr. Vincent Celenza.)

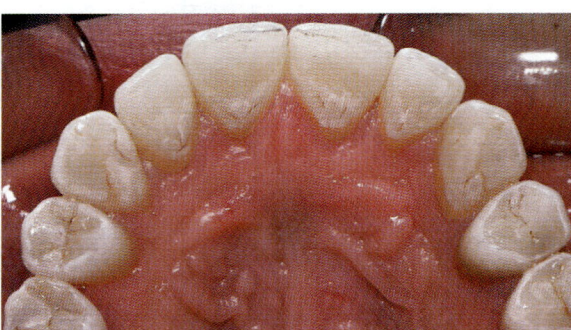

Figure 20–13B: Final restorations in place. (Courtesy of Dr. Vincent Celenza.)

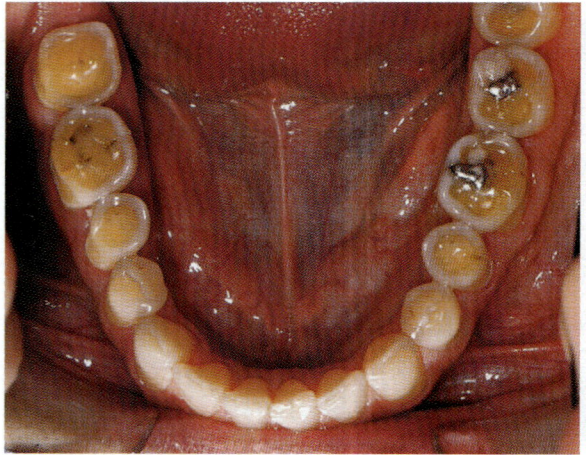

Figure 20–13C: Preoperative occlusal view of the lower arch showing extreme occlusal acid erosion. (Courtesy of Dr. Vincent Celenza.)

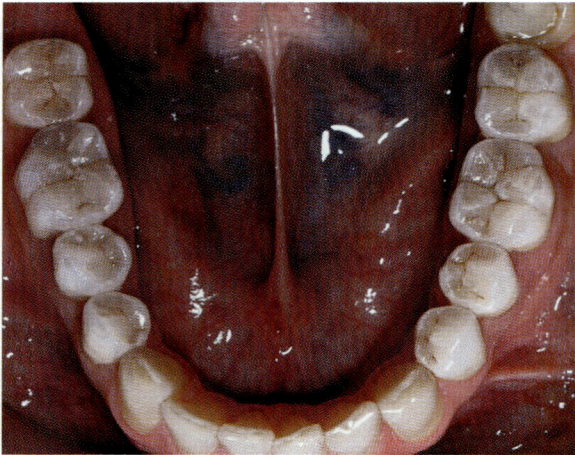

Figure 20–13D: Full arch view, 2$^{1}/_{2}$ years after placement. (Courtesy of Dr. Vincent Celenza.)

rary measures until the disorder is brought under control. Preventive measures to reduce the damaging effects of gastric acids can be immediately employed. The first measure is to have the individual refrain from brushing the teeth after vomiting. Second, oral rinses to reduce the pH in the mouth can be extremely helpful. Water can be used to rid the mouth of the acids that are present. If available, sodium bicarbonate (baking soda) rinses can neutralize the acidity in the mouth following an episode of vomiting. Various topical fluoride preparations will aid in minimizing the acidic destruction of the enamel and dentin. Because of the psychosomatic nature of anorexia and bulimia, it is imperative for the dentist to approach these patients in a factual, nonconfrontational, concerned manner that will encourage them to seek proper medical attention.

People who habitually eat or suck on lemons or drink large amounts of lemon-flavored water may exhibit acid erosion (Figures 20–16A and B). This erosion is seen on the labial surfaces of the anterior teeth if they suck the fruit or the lingual surfaces if they chew it. Those who actually eat lemons may present with lingual erosion that mimics that of bulimia. Excessive consumption of fruits and drinks with high acid content can cause decalcification of enamel and dissolution of dental tissues (refer to Chapter 17).

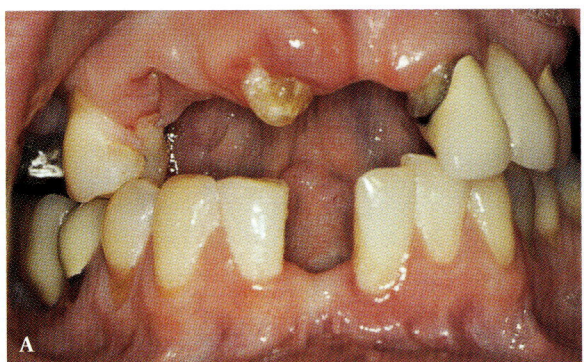
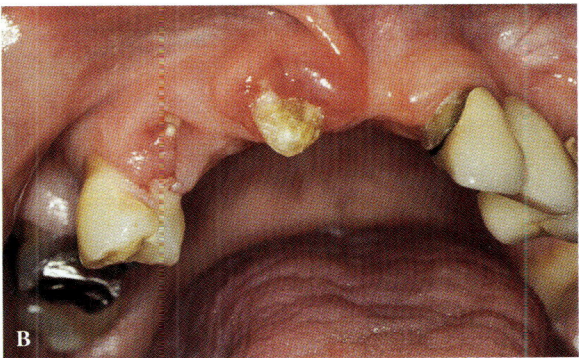

Figure 20–14A and B: This 28-year-old female had been anorexic since age 17. She had unsuccessfully participated in numerous counseling programs, and her self-image continued to be extremely poor. Although she weighed only 92 pounds, she perceived herself to be grossly overweight. She was so focused on her body's appearance that she totally neglected her oral health. Note the loss of teeth and decay.

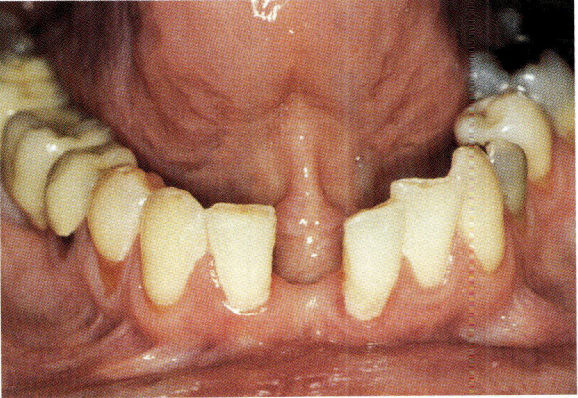

Figure 20–14C: Although not completely visible, this photograph illustrates drying and atrophy of the oral mucosa as seen on the lateral and ventral surfaces of the tongue.

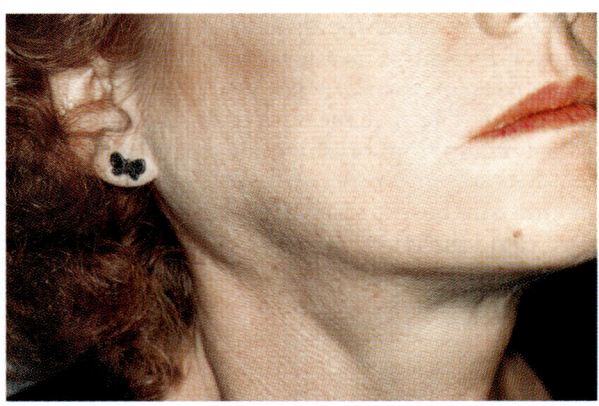

Figure 20–15: Bulimia and anorexia can occur in the same patient. This 35-year-old female initially manifested her eating disorder as bulimia when she was about 15 years old. Over the years, she has continued her purging and while in college began to exhibit behavior characteristic of anorexia. She is now firmly entrenched in both bulimia and anorexia. Her parotid hypertrophy is a manifestation of her bulimia. The lanugo (fine facial hair) is a sign sometimes seen in anorexics.

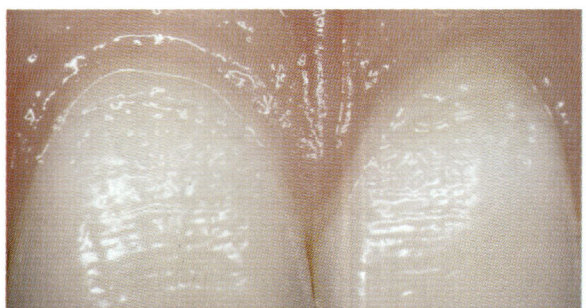

Figure 20–16A: People who have a habit of sucking lemons seldom are aware of the potential for damage to their enamel. This patient was diagnosed early in her habit, so a minimum of damage was done.

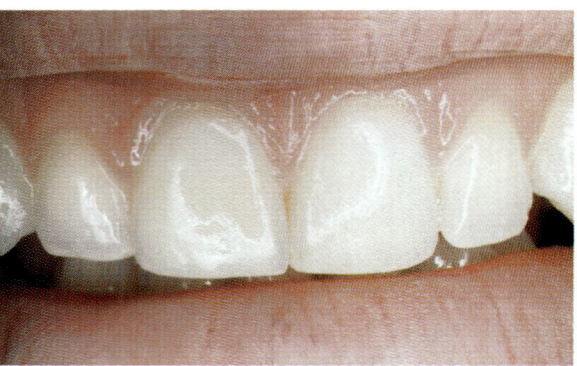

Figure 20–16B: Composite resin bonding was the treatment of choice.

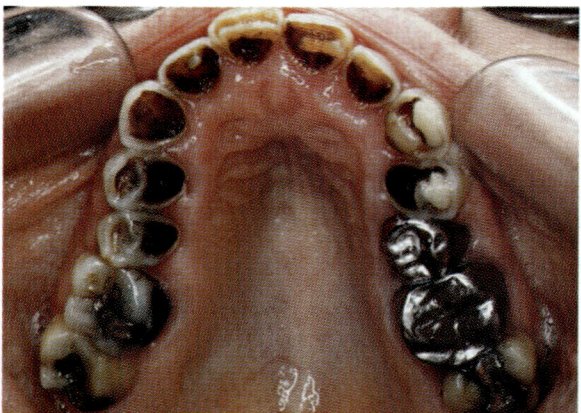

Figure 20–16C: This 63 year old had a habit of sucking one pack of Lifesavers candy daily. In addition, she ingested two tablespoons of vinegar and 500 mg of vitamin C. Her maxillary teeth showed considerable damage due to caries and erosion. Treatment included full-mouth restoration with full crowns on the maxillary teeth.

In cases of dental erosion, the teeth first exhibit a diminished luster. As continual erosion leads to smoothing of enamel pits, the eroded areas eventually appear smooth and polished. Advancing erosion results in exposed dentin that wears down rapidly and often exhibits extensive sensitivity.

Early detection of erosive lesions and identification of patients at high risk for developing erosion are most important. If you detect erosion, it is essential to ask if the patient has changed his or her eating habits or diet recently.

Caries is frequently seen in patients who have a habit of sucking hard citrus-flavored candies with high sugar content (Figure 20–16C). Thus, rebuilding the lost tooth structure offers only palliative therapy. Dietary changes must be made in these patients who insist on continuing with this habit pattern. Dental management of patients with these disorders should be conservative. Bonded composite resin or glass ionomer materials may reduce sensitivity and prevent the erosion from progressing. Any extensive dental treatment, such as crown and bridge, should be postponed until the disorder/habit itself is controlled or stabilized. Otherwise, dental treatment may not be effective.

ALCOHOL AND DRUG ABUSE

Chronic alcoholism is another disorder that has oral implications (Figure 20–17). Case studies describe patients with a history of chronic alcoholism that have extensive wear of the teeth.[29,69,79] All had loss of lingual and incisal surfaces of the maxillary anterior teeth consistent with regurgitation erosion. This regurgitation results from a gastritis that is produced by ingestion of excessive amounts of alcohol.

Abuse of specific drugs has been shown to have adverse effects on the dentition. Individuals who regularly use methylenedioxy-methamphetamine ("Ecstasy") may have excessive wear of the teeth.[17,66] This occurs through a dual mechanism of decreased salivation and hyperactivity of the muscles of mastication. In essence, this drug evokes a form of bruxism that occurs in a dry mouth. Although not reported, other amphetamines may cause similar conditions. Cocaine has been reported to cause dental erosions because of its acidic nature.[43] Some abusers obtain their high by wetting the tip of their finger, dipping it into the cocaine, and wiping the drug into the buccal vestibule or onto the gingival tissues. When the acidic drug comes in contact with the tooth surface, erosive lesions can develop.

FOREIGN OBJECTS IN THE MOUTH

Another habit that can produce permanent damage to the dentition relates to placing foreign objects in the mouth. The resultant damage is caused by abrasion, which is a term used to describe wear or defects in tooth tissues resulting from contact with a foreign object. The following are some of the more common types of habits that can cause this damage.

Fingernails

Since the fingernail is an extension of the finger, one may wonder if the common practice of placing

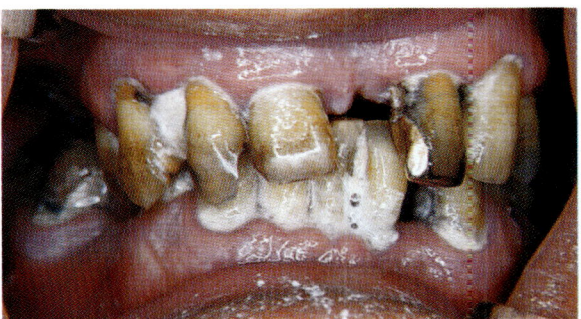

Figure 20–17: Chronic alcoholism is a habit that can produce various intraoral problems. This retired gentleman is a good example of how loss of self-respect can lead to greater oral disease. He quit caring about his appearance and completely gave up oral hygiene as evidenced in the above picture.

the fingernails between the teeth is a continuation of a previous thumb- or finger-sucking habit. It may also begin suddenly, well into adult life, because of a chipped or spaced tooth or some roughness in the mouth that acts like a magnet for some people, perhaps in an effort to smooth out the roughness.

The most destructive of the fingernail habits involves the patient's wedging the fingernail in an interdental area that eventually becomes a space (Figures 20–18A to D). Treatment involves closure of the space. It is important that the patient be aware that continuation of this habit can quickly reopen the space. In some cases, it may be necessary to restrain the individual by constructing a vacuform matrix to cover the entire arch or an orthodontic retaining appliance (see Figures 20–18C and D). The patient should wear this appliance full time for 6 weeks. Closure of the space during this period, together with a 3-month retaining period, should be sufficient to break the habit. You can help ensure that the habit does not recur by cosmetically contouring the teeth to remove any rough or sharp edges.

Nail biting is also a learned habit that may provide a physical mechanism for stress relief. Encourage your patients to have short, well-manicured nails. Rough edges in the nail may cause the patient to smooth the nail unconsciously by rubbing it in the incisal embrasure. Also, advise the nail biter to carry a fingernail clipper at all times so that "nervous energy" can be converted into self-manicuring the nails when a possible urge to bite the nails exists. Behavioral techniques to reduce stress levels will aid in eliminating this type of habit.

Pins Placed between the Teeth

Placing various types of pins, needles, or even bobby pins in one's mouth is not an uncommon habit, particularly among people who knit and sew. People suffering tooth deformity from this habit usually hold the pin or needle between their anterior teeth (Figures 20–19A to D). Diagnosis can often be made by checking the patient's protrusive end-to-end relationship to see if a perfect matching groove is present. It is helpful to ask patients about their work and hobbies. Taking a thorough habit history, such as the one in Figure 20–20, is helpful. Treatment follows the pattern of other habits described

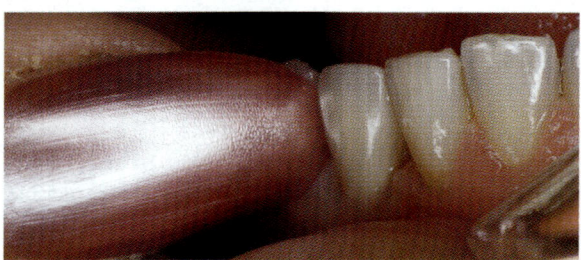

Figure 20–18A: This 30 year old developed a habit of putting her nail between her lower incisors.

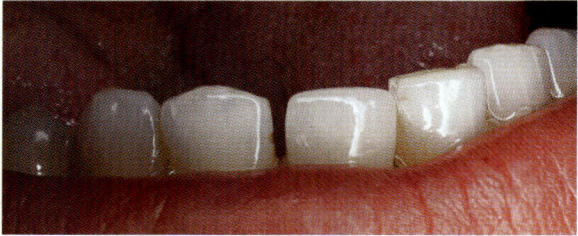

Figure 20–18B: Note the space created between the lateral and central incisors on the lower right side due to fingernail pressure.

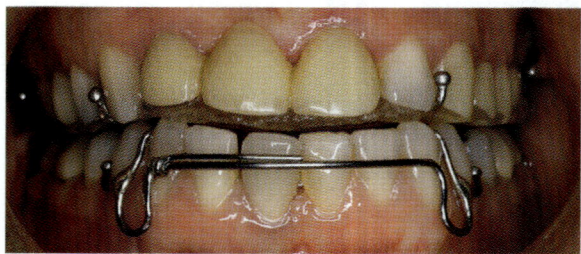

Figure 20–18C: A removable Hawley-type orthodontic appliance was constructed to reposition the lower anteriors. Because of the nature of this appliance, it also helped the patient to break the habit since she could not put the fingernail into the same space.

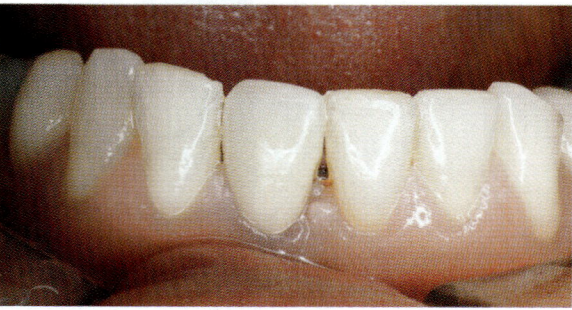

Figure 20–18D: The final result after approximately 6 months of treatment.

in this section, that is, appearance is restored and whatever appliances and means necessary to discourage continuance of the habit are used. With this problem, it is also useful to tell the patient to at least vary the location where the pins are held.

Thread Biting
Thread biting may produce notches in the incisal edges of anterior teeth. This is an occupational habit. Patients who are seamstresses should be warned against this behavior. Sharp edges of enamel that produce irritation should be eliminated by careful rounding or restorative treatment (Figures 20–21A and B).

Stimudents or Toothpicks Used as Wedges
Toothpicks or Stimudents can provide an effective means of cleaning tooth surfaces. If the object is forced between the teeth, however, it can create unwanted spaces. Patients should be told to use the toothpick or Stimudent like a soft brush to clean plaque or debris from the smooth surface of the tooth (Figures 20–22A and B).

Incorrect Use of Dental Floss and Toothbrush
Abnormal tooth wear may result from improper oral hygiene procedures. Misuse of dental floss may cause abnormal tooth wear. Excessive and strenuous use of dental floss apical to the cementoenamel

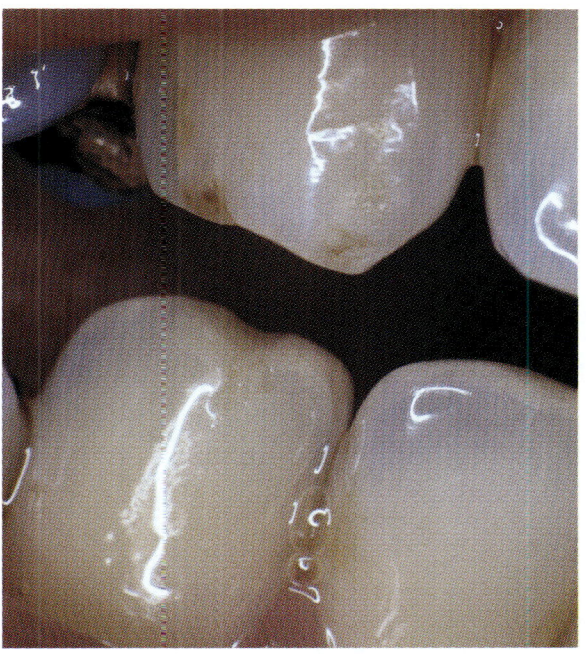

Figure 20–19B: The patient had actually worn a small groove in the biting edge of the teeth that exactly fit the sewing needle she used. In addition to cosmetic contouring or composite resin bonding to add to the worn spot, be sure to have the patient avoid consistently placing any foreign objects between the teeth.

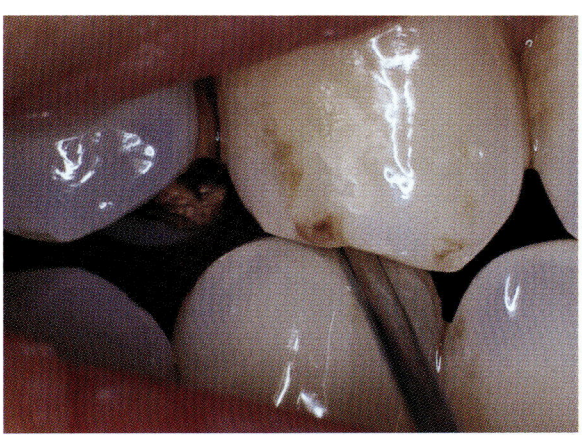

Figure 20–19A: This 39-year-old interior designer had a habit of holding sewing needles and pins between her cuspids.

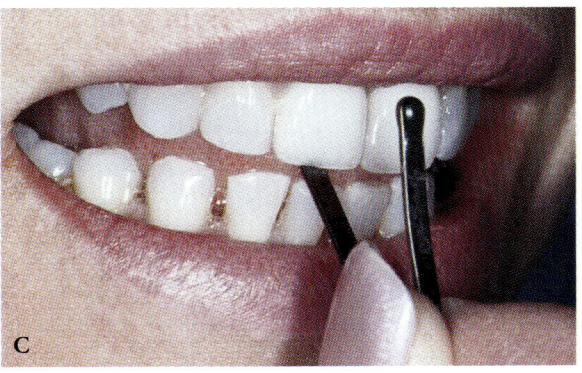

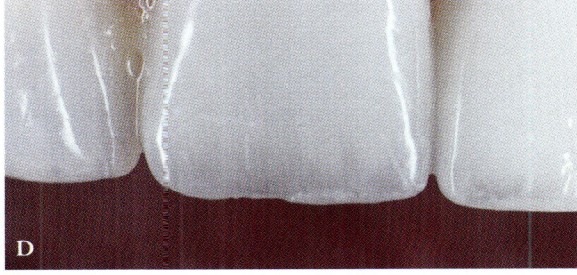

Figure 20–19C and D: This patient wore a small groove in her tooth from constant use of bobby pins.

junction may result in notching of the root surfaces. In addition, tooth abrasion may occur from incorrect use of a toothbrush. Toothbrush abrasion can be extreme, particularly if related to obsessive or compulsive behavior (Figures 20–23A to C).

Finally, incorrect use of dental floss can lead to abnormal loss of interdental space. Figures 20–24A to D show a patient who has had bonding of her anterior teeth and unfortunately developed an incorrect method of flossing.

Pen/Pencil Chewing

This habit became considerably more destructive when pencils changed from wood to the newer plastic types (Figures 20–25A to E). It is not uncommon to see this habit in business people who spend a great deal of time at their desks working figures. Treatment involves wearing an appliance that prevents the patient from placing the pen or pencil between the teeth.

Pipe Smoking

Any kind of smoking creates its own unesthetic results, staining the teeth and affecting the health of the oral soft tissues. Pipe smoking has the most potential for changing tooth relationships. Continually holding a pipe in one location may cause large notches in several teeth. The problem is that the patient usually places the pipe stem in the same position, most often the premolar area. These teeth then become worn or submerged (Figures 20–26A and B).

Treatment involves correcting the deformity and helping the patient break the habit. In this case, it

---

Habit Questionnaire
Does Your Habit Affect Your Smile?

(Please check the appropriate space)
Do you now or did you ever

	Yes	No
1. Chew your lips or cheeks?		
2. Suck your fingers, thumbs, or lemons?		
3. Chew ice?		
4. Bite your fingernails?		
5. Hold pins or needles in your mouth?		
6. Chew pencils or plastic pens?		
7. Chew or hold your glasses in your mouth?		
8. Crack nuts or ice with your teeth?		
9. Play a musical instrument that requires you to hold the instrument with your teeth?		
10. Smoke a pipe, cigar, or cigarettes?		
11. Bite or suck your lips?		
12. Use Stimudents or toothpicks?		
13. Keep your tongue pressed against the upper teeth?		
14. Place your tongue in a space between your teeth?		
15. Grind or clench your teeth?		

If you answer "yes" to two or more of the above questions, you may have a habit problem. Ask your dentist to see if your habit or habits are causing potential damage to your teeth.

Figure 20–20: The first step in either preventing or stopping a destructive oral habit is to help patients to discover their habits. (Reproduced with permission from Goldstein RE. Change your smile. 3rd edn. Carol Stream, IL: Quintessence, 1997:284.)

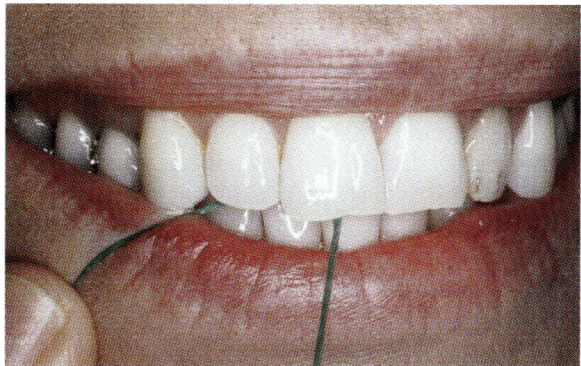

Figure 20–21A: This 55-year-old woman developed a habit of cutting sewing thread with her incisors.

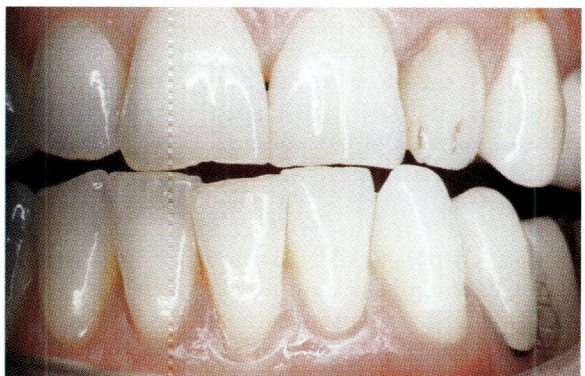

Figure 20–21B: The patient eventually wore a groove in the maxillary right central incisor.

may be easier to teach the patient to change the pattern of holding the pipe rather than give up the habit altogether. At the very least, this would make certain that the occlusal forces are distributed among many teeth. Although the submerged teeth can usually be orthodontically repositioned, restorative means may provide an easier solution. However, some tooth structure would probably have to be removed so that the bonded restoration could be attached using the etched occlusal surface enamel.

Eyeglasses or Other Objects Placed between the Teeth

Most persons who consistently place eyeglasses, plastic swizzle sticks, or other objects in their mouths are not aware of the habit, much less the resulting functional and esthetic deformity (Figures 20–27A and B). Treatment is the same as noted above.

Ice Chewing

Patients seldom realize the damage that chewing ice, a seemingly innocuous habit, can cause. Chewing ice can fracture teeth and can also produce microcracks in the enamel. The microcracks themselves are usually not visible to the eye, but they stain much more readily than normal, especially with coffee, tea, and soy sauce. If the person chewing ice has defective restorations, a sliver of ice can also act as a wedge that can split the tooth.

Nut Cracking

Using teeth to open the shell of a nut may be the handiest way to reach the nutmeat, but it may also

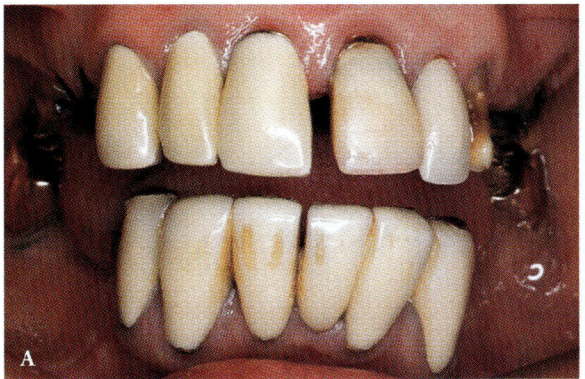

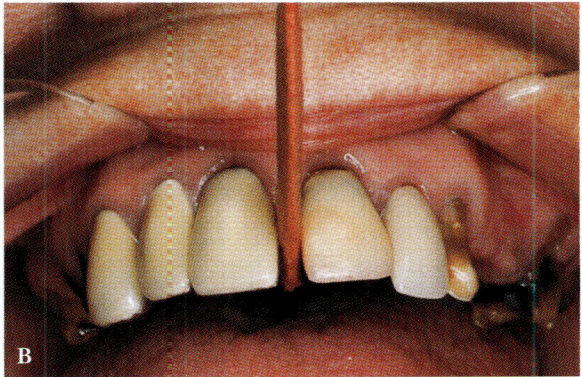

Figure 20–22A and B: These photographs show a patient who constantly placed Stim-udents between her front teeth. Although these teeth were originally together with no spaces, the patient quickly separated the teeth to create a space. Her goal was to expand her arch to give more fullness to her face. She had previously been referred for orthodontic treatment but rejected this treatment plan.

be the quickest way to break a tooth. A common offender is the pistachio nut. In general, the harder the nut is, the more chance there is of a fractured tooth. The only preventive measure you can take is to warn patients of the potential damage, particularly if any incisal edge has been bonded with composite resin.

This chapter could continue for pages with examples of habits of a similar nature, but the principles of diagnosis and treatment are similar. The first and most important of these principles is that *early diagnosis means preventive esthetics.*

The second principle to remember is that *treating the signs of oral habits is only a temporary measure if the patient continues the habit.* Helping patients break these habits may well be the most difficult part. Important keys include (1) precise diagnosis of the exact nature of the habit, (2) helping the patient recognize the habit and the tactful suggestion that the patient learn through counseling or other methods to better deal with stress and tension, and (3) correction of damage caused by the habit so that rough edges, open gaps, tissue changes, or other signs do not contribute to resumption of the habit that caused them. Appliances to physically prevent the habit may also be useful in making the patient more aware of the tendency and be a turning point in breaking the cycle of habit-sign-habit.

The treatment of children's oral habits, particularly digit sucking, is somewhat easier because there is usually an adoring adult to reinforce changed

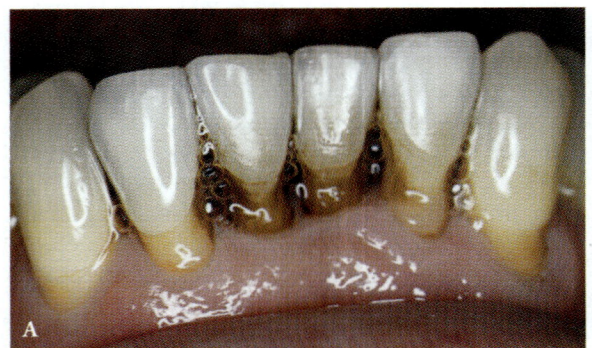
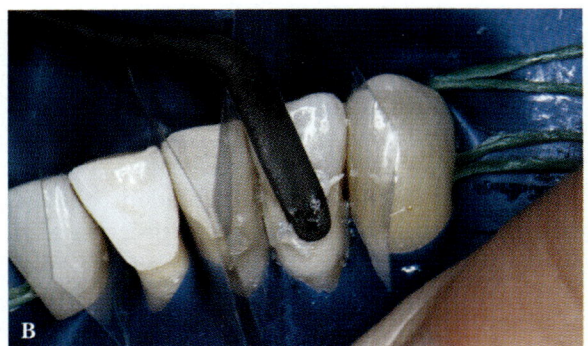
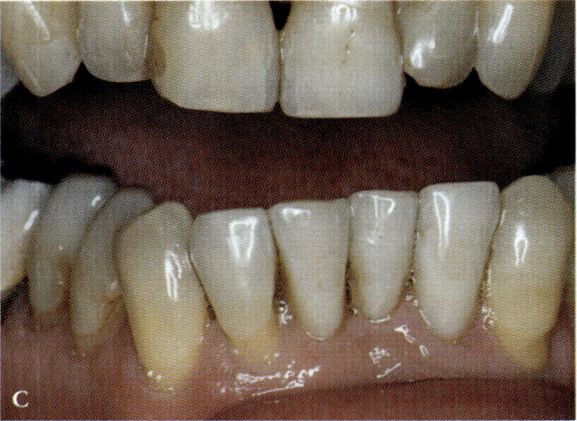

Figure 20–23A to C: This is severe toothbrush abrasion and gingival recession seen in a 37-year-old male with a known obsessive-compulsive disorder. The aggressive brushing of his teeth was one of his extreme habits (see also Chapter 17, Figures 17–9A and B). Composite resin bonding was done to restore the cervical deformities.

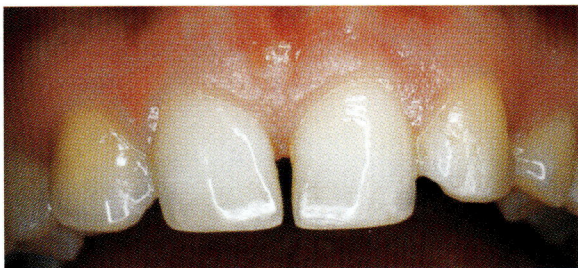

Figure 20–24A: This 25 year old originally presented with a maxillary diastema.

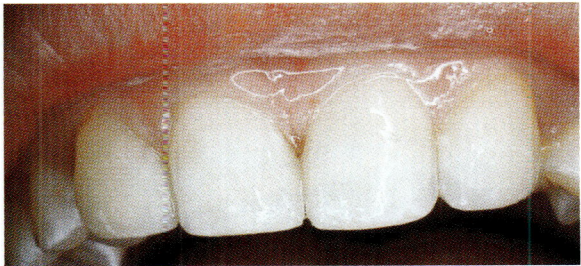

Figure 20–24B: Composite resin bonding was chosen to close the space between the central incisors and convert her canines into laterals. Note that the interdental space looks good between the central incisors.

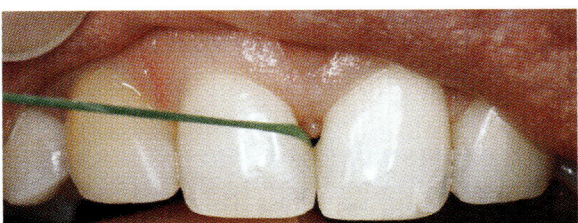

Figure 20–24C: After questioning the patient about habits, she was requested to demonstrate exactly how she flossed her teeth. What she was doing was pushing the floss into the teeth on one side and then going straight across to the other side without coming back into the contact area; thus, she was "guillotining" her interdental papilla away.

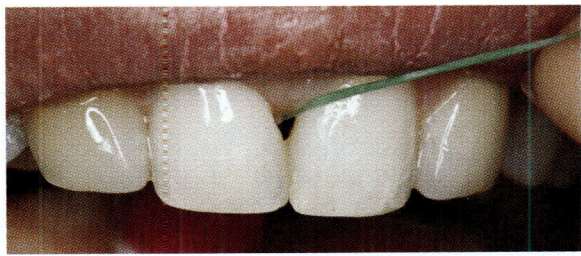

Figure 20–24D: Treatment involved new oral care instructions to prevent further tissue loss and provide an opportunity for the gingiva to regenerate and fill in the interdental space.

behavior. The therapists who participated in a convention of speech pathologists concerned with such behavior almost uniformly suggested methods that require commitment on the part of the patient, removal of guilt about the habit, and a willingness of the parent to give the child some extra attention as the habit is relinquished. Charts with checkmarks or gold stars are often used as reinforcement, as are kisses and praises.[25]

Adults can modify these methods for their own habits:

1. An extremely precise diagnosis of the problem is an essential first step since many adults may not realize that they have a destructive habit.

2. Once the patient has become aware of the habit, he or she can monitor the behavior, writing down when, how intensely, and under what circumstances it occurs. This will reinforce the patient's awareness of the habit, provide some clues as to what evokes it (such as cheek biting occurring most often in stressful situations or when tired), and provide many occasions in which not using the habit can be reinforced. Suggest to your patient that he or she enlist the assistance of someone else to help identify various aspects of the habit. A colleague would be a good source if the habit occurs primarily during working hours. Spouses, relatives, or friends may provide assistance if the habit takes place during nonworking hours.

3. Some behavioral scientists believe that one habit replaces another. Certainly, it is easier to create a habit than to break one, so it could be suggested to patients that they attempt to temporarily replace the destructive oral habit with a less destructive one such as chewing sugarless gum.

4. Finally, the use of orthodontic devices such as those described in this chapter will help the patient recognize and break this habit.

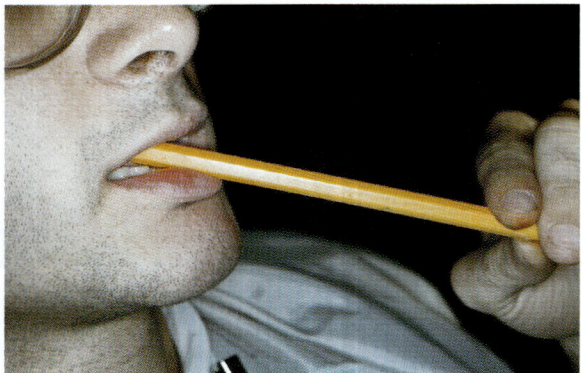

Figure 20–25A: This 21 year old developed a habit of chewing pencils.

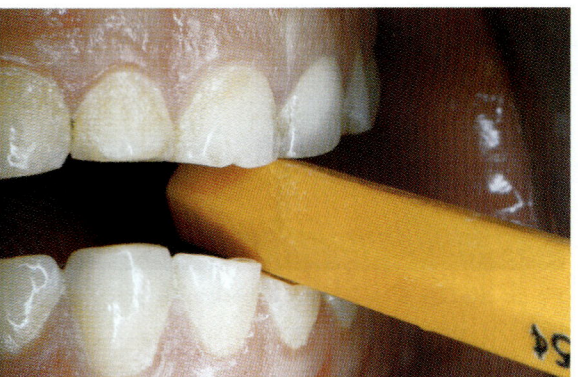

Figure 20–25B: Eventually, wooden pencils were replaced with plastic ones, which he began to turn with his fingers, causing incisal wear.

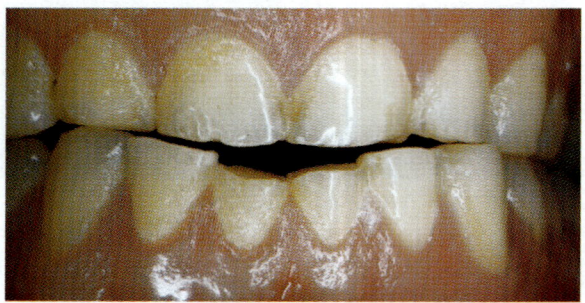

Figure 20–25C: Note the amount of damage caused by the pencil chewing. Composite resin bonding was used as an economic and immediate esthetic replacement for the missing tooth structure. The patient was also given a plastic bite appliance for the maxillary arch that he would wear anytime he felt the need to put a pencil in his mouth.

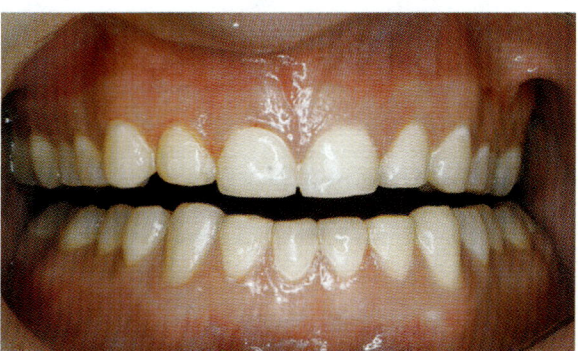

Figure 20–25D: He successfully broke the habit, and the bonding held up for approximately 12 years, when, unfortunately, the patient restarted his previous habit.

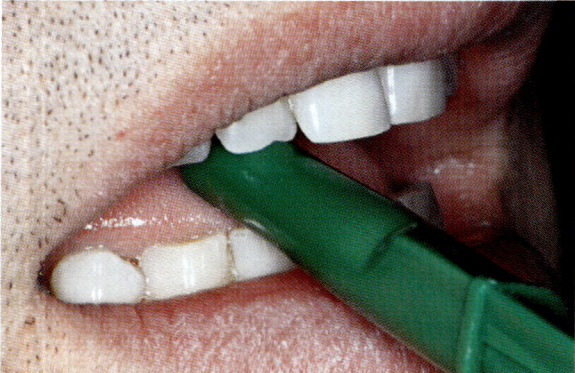

Figure 20–25E: This 46-year-old man had an unconscious habit of not only placing plastic pens in his mouth but also sliding the pen in and out. This wore a groove in the center of the incisal edge.

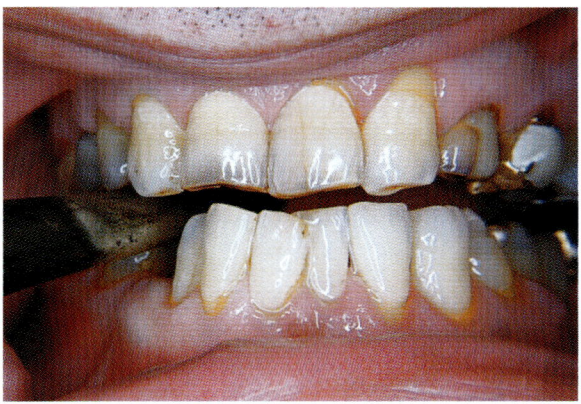

Figure 20–26A: This 56 year old had a long-standing habit of pipe smoking.

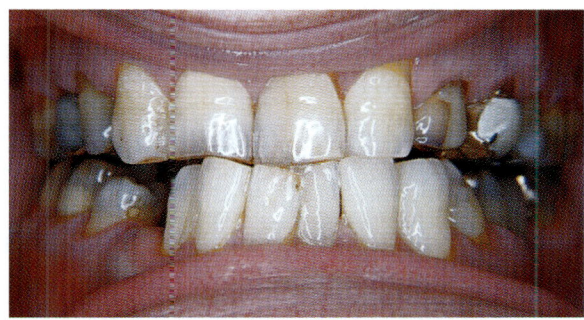

Figure 20–26B: After the pipe was removed, and the patient bit down, the amount of damage caused by the pipe being held in the premolar positions was evident. Particularly note how he favored the right side, which showed a greater amount of abnormal space.

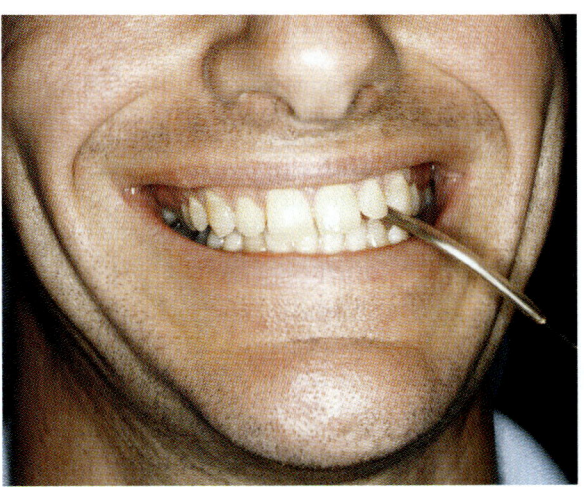

Figure 20–27A: This 31 year old had a habit of holding his eyeglasses with his teeth.

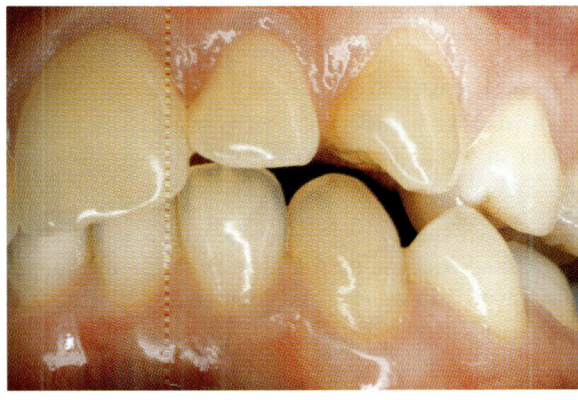

Figure 20–27B: He always held them in the same position, causing the left canine to flare out, thus creating an unattractive and unnecessary space between his front teeth. Patients should always be advised never to hold anything but food between their teeth.

An important part of treatment, as well as the record of each new patient, should be a completed thorough habit questionnaire, such as the one in Figure 20–20. The patient can fill this out unless he or she is so young that a parent or guardian would be a more appropriate source of information. This questionnaire should be updated as regularly as a patient's medical history. Destructive habits can start anytime, and it is the dentist's responsibility—and opportunity as a professional with diagnostic ability and an inquisitive nature—to identify these habits and stop them before more damage is done.

References

1. Allen JD, Rivera-Morales WC, Zwemer JD. Occurrence of temporomandibular disorder symptoms in healthy young adults with and without evidence of bruxism. Cranio 1990;8:312–8.

2. Andrianopoulos MV, Hanson ML. Tongue-thrust and the stability of overjet correction. Angle Orthod 1987;57:121–35.

3. Bailey DR. Tension headache and bruxism in the sleep disordered patient. Cranio 1990;8:174–82.

4. Barber TK. Lip habits in preventive orthodontics. J Prev Dent 1978;5:30–6.

5. Bartlett DW, Ricketts DN, Fisher NL. Management of the short clinical crown by indirect restorations. Dent Update 1997;24:431–6.

6. Bayardo RE, Mejia JJ, Orozco S, Montoya K. Etiology of oral habits. ASDC J Dent Child 1996;63:350–3.

7. Becker W, Ochsenbein C, Becker BE. Crown lengthening: the periodontal-restorative connection. Compend Cont Educ Dent 1998;19:239–40, 242, 244–6.

8. Bishop K, Bell M, Briggs P, Kelleher M. Restoration of a worn dentition using a double-veneer technique. Br Dent J 1996;180:26–9.

9. Bouquot JE, Seime RJ. Bulimia nervosa: dental perspectives. Pract Periodont Aesthet Dent 1997;9:655–63.

10. Bowden BD. A longitudinal study of the effects of digit- and dummy-sucking. Am J Orthod 1966;52:887–901.

11. Bowles WH, Wilkinson MR, Wagner MJ, Woody RD. Abrasive particles in tobacco products: a possible factor in dental attrition. J Am Dent Assoc 1995;126:327–31.

12. Brown S, Bonifazi DZ. An overview of anorexia and bulimia nervosa, and the impact of eating disorders on the oral cavity. Compend Cont Educ Dent 1993;14:1594, 1596–1602, 1604–8.

13. Chandler TH. Thumbsucking in childhood as a cause of subsequent irregularity of the teeth. Boston Med Surg J 1878;99:204–8.

14. Coccaro PJ, Coccaro PJ Jr. Dental development and the pharyngeal lymphoid tissue. Otolaryngol Clin North Am 1987;20:241–57.

15. Cooper BC. Nasorespiratory function and orofacial development. Otolaryngol Clin North Am 1989;22:413–41.

16. da Silva AM, Oakley DA, Hemmings KW, et al. Psychosocial factors and tooth wear with a significant component of attrition. Eur J Prosthodont Restor Dent 1997;5:51–5.

17. Duxbury AJ. Ecstasy—dental implications. Br Dent J 1993;175:38.

18. Ellingsen R, Vandevanter C, Shapiro P, Shapiro G. Temporal variation in nasal and oral breathing in children. Am J Orthod Dentofac Orthop 1995;107:411–7.

19. Faulkner KD. Bruxism: a review of the literature. Part I. Aust Dent J 1991;35:266–76.

20. Faulkner KD. Bruxism: a review of the literature. Part II. Aust Dent J 1991;36:355–61.

21. Fombonne E. Increased rates of psychosocial disorders in youth. Eur Arch Psychiatry Clin Neurosci 1998;248:14–21.

22. Fukuta O, Braham RL, Yokoi K, Kurosu K. Damage to the primary dentition resulting from thumb and finger (digit) sucking. ASDC J Dent Child 1996;63:403–7.

23. Gellin ME. Digit sucking and tongue thrusting in children. Dent Clin North Am 1978;22:603–18.

24. Glass LF, Maize JC. Morsicatio buccarum et labiorum (excessive cheek and lip biting). Am J Dermatopathol 1991;13:271–4.

25. Greenly L. Suggestions for combating digit sucking as offered by members at the 1982 I.A.O.M. Convention. Int J Orofac Myol 1982;8:22–3.

26. Gross AM, Kellum GD, Franz D, et al. A longitudinal evaluation of open mouth posture and maxillary arch width in children. Angle Orthod 1994;64:419–24.

27. Gross AM, Kellum GD, Michas K, et al. Open-mouth posture and maxillary arch width in young children: a three-year evaluation. Am J Orthod Dentofac Orthop 1994;106:635–40.

28. Gross AM, Kellum GD, Morris T, et al. Rhinometry and open-mouth posture in young children. Am J Orthod Dentofac Orthop 1993;103:526–9.

29. Harris CK, Warnakulasuriya KA, Johnson NW, et al. Oral health in alcohol misusers. Community Dent Health 1996;13:199–203.

30. Hartgerink DV, Vig PS. Lower anterior face height and lip incompetence do not predict nasal airway obstruction. Angle Orthod 1989;59:17–23.

31. Haryett RD, Hansen FC, Davidson PO, Sandilands ML. Chronic thumb sucking: the psychologic effects and the relative effectiveness of various methods of treatment. Am J Orthod 1967;53:569–85.

32. Hicks RA, Conti PA. Changes in the incidence of nocturnal bruxism in college students: 1966–1989. Percept Mot Skills 1989;69:481–2.

33. Hicks RA, Conti PA, Bragg HR. Increases in nocturnal bruxism among college students implicate stress. Med Hypotheses 1990;33:239–40.

34. Hublin C, Kaprio J, Partinen M, Koskenvuo M. Sleep bruxism based on self-report in a nationwide twin cohort. J Sleep Res 1998;7:61–7.

35. Infante PF. An epidemiological study of finger habits in preschool children as related to malocclusion, socioeconomic status, race, sex, and size of community. J Dent Child 1976;43:33–8.

36. Johnson ED, Larson BE. Thumb-sucking: literature review. ASDC J Dent Child 1993;60:385–91.

37. Kampe T, Edman G, Bader G, et al. Personality traits in a group of subjects with long-standing bruxing behaviour. J Oral Rehabil 1997;24:588–93.

38. Keel PK, Mitchell JE. Outcome in bulimia nervosa. Am J Psychiatry 1997;154:313–21.

39. Kellum GD, Gross AM, Walker M, et al. Open mouth posture and cross-sectional nasal area in young children. Int J Orofac Myol 1993;19:25–8.

40. Kerr WJ, McWilliam JS, Linder-Aronson S. Mandibular form and position related to changed mode of breathing—a five-year longitudinal study. Angle Orthod 1989;59:91–6.

41. Kieser JA, Groeneveld HT. Relationship between juvenile bruxing and craniomandibular dysfunction. J Oral Rehabil 1998;25:662–5.

42. Klein JC. Nasal respiratory function and craniofacial growth. Arch Otolaryngol Head Neck Surg 1986;112:843–9.

43. Krutchkoff DJ, Eisenberg E, O'Brien JE, Ponzillo JJ. Cocaine-induced dental erosions. N Engl J Med 1990;322:408.

44. Langsjoen OM. Dental effects of diet and coca-leaf chewing on two prehistoric cultures of northern Chile. Am J Phys Anthropol 1996;101:475–89.

45. Larsson E. Dummy- and finger-sucking habits with special attention to their significance for facial growth and occlusion. Swed Dent J 1978;2:23–33.

46. Larsson E. The effect of finger-sucking on the occlusion: a review. Eur J Orthod 1987;9:279–82.

47. Larsson E. Artificial sucking habits: etiology, prevalence and effect on occlusion. Int J Orofac Myol 1994;20:10–21.

48. Lavigne GL, Lobbezoo F, Rompe PH, et al. Cigarette smoking as a risk factor or an exacerbating factor for restless legs syndrome and sleep bruxism. Sleep 1997;20:290–3.

49. Levitas TC. Examine the habit—evaluate the treatment. ASDC J Dent Child 1970;37:122–3.

50. Linder-Aronson S, Woodside DG, Lundstrom A. Mandibular growth direction following adenoidectomy. Am J Orthod 1986;89:272–84.

51. Lobbezoo F, Lavigne GJ. Do bruxism and temporomandibular disorders have a cause-and-effect relationship? J Orofac Pain 1997;11:15–23.

52. Luke LS, Howard L. The effects of thumb sucking on orofacial structures and speech: a review. Compend Cont Educ Dent 1983;4:575–9.

53. Macaluso GM, Guerra P, Di Giovanni G, et al. Sleep bruxism is a disorder related to periodic arousals during sleep. J Dent Res 1998;77:565–72.

54. Madrid G, Madrid S, Vranesh JG, Hicks RA. Cigarette smoking and bruxism. Percept Mot Skills 1998;87:898.

55. Magnusson T. Is snuff a potential risk factor in occlusal wear? Swed Dent J 1991;15:125–32.

56. Massler M. Oral habits: development and management. J Pedod 1983;7:109–19.

57. McSherry PF. Aetiology and treatment of anterior open bite. J Irish Dent Assoc 1996;42:20–6.

58. Melsen B, Attina L, Santuari M, Attina A. Relationships between swallowing pattern, mode of respiration, and development of malocclusion. Angle Orthod 1987;57:113–20.

59. Mikell B. Recognizing tongue related malocclusion. Int J Orthod 1935;23:4–7.

60. Molina OF, dos Santos J Jr, Nelson SJ, Grossman E. Prevalence of modalities of headaches and bruxism among patients with craniomandibular disorders. Cranio 1997;15 14–25.

61. Ngan P, Fields HW. Open bite: a review of etiology and management. Pediatr Dent 1997;19:91–8.

62. Okeson JP, Phillips BA, Berry DT, et al. Nocturnal bruxing events in subjects with sleep-disordered breathing and control subjects. J Craniomandib Disord 1991;5:258–64.

63. Popovich F, Thompson GW. Thumb and finger-sucking—its relation to malocclusion. Am J Orthod 1973;63:148–55.

64. Quinn JH. Mandibular exercises to control bruxism and deviation. Cranio 1995;13:30–4.

65. Rayan GM, Turner WT. Hand complications in children from digit sucking. J Hand Surg 1989;14:933–6.

66. Redfearn PJ, Agrawal N, Mair LH. An association between the regular use of 3,4 methylenedioxymethamphetamine (Ecstasy) and excessive wear of the teeth. Addiction 1998;93:745–8.

67. Reichart PA, Phillipsen HP. Betel chewer's mucosa—a review. J Oral Pathol Med 1998;27:239–242.

68. Ressler A. "A body to die for": eating disorders and body-image distortion in women. Int J Fertil Womens Med 1998;43:133–8.

69. Robb ND, Smith BG. Prevalence of pathological tooth wear in patients with chronic alcoholism. Br Dent J 1990;169:367–9.

70. Roberts MW, Li SH. Oral findings in anorexia nervosa and bulimia nervosa: a study of 47 cases. J Am Dent Assoc 1987;115:407–10.

71. Robertson PB, DeRouen TA, Ernster V, et al. Smokeless tobacco use: how it affects the performance of major league baseball players. J Am Dent Assoc 1995;126:1115–21.

72. Ruffs JC, Koch MO, Perkins S. Bulimia: dentomedical complications. Gen Dent 1992;40:22–5.

73. Rugh JD, Harlan J. Nocturnal bruxism and temporomandibular disorders. Adv Neurol 1988;49:329–41.

74. Rytomaa I, Jarvinen V, Kanerva R, Heinonen OP. Bulimia and tooth erosion. Acta Odontol Scand 1998;56:36–40.

75. Sapiro SM. Tongue indentations as an indicator of clenching. Clin Prev Dent 1992;14:21–4.

76. Schwitzer AM, Bergholtz K, Dore T, Salimi L. Eating disorders among college women: prevention, education, and treatment responses. J Am Coll Health 1998;46:199–207.

77. Seligman DA, Pullinger AG. A multiple stepwise logistic regression analysis of trauma history and 16 other history and dental cofactors in females with temporomandibular disorders. J Orofac Pain 1996;10:351–61.

78. Shapiro PA. Effects of nasal obstruction on facial development. J Allergy Clin Immunol 1988;81:967–71.

79. Smith BGN, Robb ND. Dental erosion in patients with chronic alcoholism. J Dent 1989;17:219–21.

80. Stokes N, Della Mattia D. A student research review of the mouthbreathing habit: discussing measurement methods, manifestations and treatment of the mouthbreathing habit. Probe 1996;30:212–4.

81. Subtelny JD, Subtelny J. Oral habits—studies in form, function and therapy. Angle Orthod 1973;43:349–83.

82. Taylor MH, Peterson DS. Effect of digit-sucking habits on root morphology in primary incisors. Pediatr Dent 1983;5:61–3.

83. Tsolka P, Walter JD, Wilson RF, Preiskel HW. Occlusal variable, bruxism and temporomandibular disorders: a clinical and kinesiographic assessment. J Oral Rehabil 1995;22:849–56.

84. Vanderas AP. Relationship between craniomandibular dysfunction and oral parafunctions in Caucasian children with and without unpleasant life events. J Oral Rehabil 1995;22:289–94.

85. Vanderas AP, Manetas KJ. Relationship between malocclusion and bruxism in children and adolescents: a review. Pediatr Dent 1995;17:7–12.

86. Van Norman RA. Digit-sucking: a review of the literature, clinical observations and treatment recommendations. Int J Orofac Mycol 1997;23:14–34.

87. Venetikidou A. Incidence of malocclusion in asthmatic children. J Clin Pediatr Dent 1993;17:89–94.

88. Vickers PD. Respiratory obstruction and its role in long face syndrome. Northwest Dent 1998;77:19–22.

89. Walker RS, Rogers WA. Modified maxillary occlusal splint for prevention of cheek biting: a clinical report. J Prosthet Dent 1992;67:581–2.

90. Weideman CL, Bush DL, Yan-Go FL, et al. The incidence of parasomnias in child bruxers versus nonbruxers. Pediatr Dent 1996;18:456–60.

91. Yustin D, Neff P, Rieger MR, Hurst T. Characterization of 86 bruxing patients with long-term study of their management with occlusal devices and other forms of therapy. J Orofac Pain 1993;7:54–60.

92. Zain RB, Gupta PC, Warnakulasuriya S, et al. Oral lesions associated with betel quid and tobacco chewing habits. Oral Dis 1997;3:204–5.

93. Zain RB, Ikeda N, Gupta PC, et al. Oral mucosal lesions associated with betel quid, areca nut and tobacco chewing habits: consensus from a workshop held in Kuala Lumpur, Malaysia, November 25–27, 1996. J Oral Pathol Med 1999;28:1–4.

Additional Resources

Aanestad S, Poulsen S. Oral conditions related to use of the lip plug (ndonya) among the Makonde tribe in Tanzania. Acta Odontol Scand 1996;54:362–4.

Abreu Tabarini HS. Dental attrition of Mayan Tzutujil children—a study based on longitudinal materials. Bull Tokyo Med Dent Univ 1995;42:31–50.

al-Hiyasat AS, Saunders WP, Sharkey SW, Smith GM. The effect of a carbonated beverage on the wear of human enamel and dental ceramics. J Prosthodont 1998;7:2–12.

al-Hiyasat AS, Saunders WP, Sharkey SW, et al. The abrasive effect of glazed, unglazed, and polished porcelain on the wear of human enamel, and the influence of carbonated soft drinks on the rate of wear. Int J Prosthodont 1997;10:269–82.

al-Hiyasat AS, Saunders WP, Sharkey SW, et al. Investigation of human enamel wear against four dental ceramics and gold. J Dent 1998;26:487–95.

Altshuler BD. Eating disorder patients. Recognition and intervention. J Dent Hyg 1990;64:119–25.

Attanasio R. Nocturnal bruxism and its clinical management. Dent Clin North Am 1991;35:245–52.

Attin T, Zirkel C, Hellwig, E. Brushing abrasion of eroded dentin after application of sodium fluoride solutions. Caries Res 1998;32:344–50.

Bader GG, Kampe T, Tagdae T, et al. Descriptive physiological data on a sleep bruxism population. Sleep 1997;20:982–90.

Bader JD, McClure F, Scurria MS, et al. Case-control study of non-carious cervical lesions. Community Dent Oral Epidemiol 1996;24:286–91.

Bartlett DW. The causes of dental erosion. Oral Dis 1997;3:209–11.

Bartlett DW, Coward PY, Nikkah C, Wilson RF. The prevalence of tooth wear in a cluster sample of adolescent schoolchildren and its relationship with potential explanatory factors. Br Dent J 1998;184:125–9.

Bartlett DW, Evans DF, Smith BG. The relationship between gastro-oesophageal reflux disease and dental erosion. J Oral Rehabil 1996;23:289–97.

Bartlett D, Smith B. Clinical investigations of gastro-oesophageal reflux: part 1. Dent Update 1996;23:205–8.

Bartlett DW, Smith BG. The dental impact of eating disorders. Dent Update 1994;21:404–7.

Bauer W, van den Hoven F, Diedrich P. Wear in the upper and lower incisors in relation to incisal and condylar guidance. J Orofac Orthop 1997;58:306–19.

Beckett H. Dental abrasion caused by a cobalt-chromium denture base. Eur J Prosthodont Restor Dent 1995;3:209–10.

Beckett H, Buxey-Softley G, Gilmour AG, Smith N. Occupational tooth abrasion in a dental technician: loss of tooth surface resulting from exposure to porcelain powder—a case report. Quintessence Int 1995;26:217–20.

Behlfelt K. Enlarged tonsils and the effect of tonsillectomy. Characteristics of the dentition and facial skeleton. Posture of the head, hyoid bone and tongue. Mode of breathing. Swed Dent J Suppl 1990;72:1–35.

Berge M, Johannessen G, Silness J. Relationship between alignment conditions of teeth in anterior segments and incisal wear. J Oral Rehabil 1996;23:717–21.

Bigenzahn W, Fischman L, Mayrhofer-Krammel U. Myofunctional therapy in patients with orofacial dysfunctions affecting speech. Folia Phoniatr 1992;44:238–44.

Bishop K, Kelleher M, Briggs P, Joshi R. Wear now? An update on the etiology of tooth wear. Quintessence Int 1997;28:305–13.

Blair FM, Thomason JM, Smith DG. The traumatic anterior overbite. Dent Update 1997;24:144–52.

Bohmer CJ, Klinkenberg-Knol EC, Niezen-de Boer MC, et al. Dental erosions and gastro-oesophageal reflux disease in institutionalized intellectually disabled individuals. Oral Dis 1997;3:272–5.

Brenchley ML. Is digit sucking of significance? Br Dent J 1992;171:357–62.

Burke FJ, Whitehead SA, McCaughey AD. Contemporary concepts in the pathogenesis of the Class V noncarious lesion. Dent Update 1995;22:28–32.

Carlson-Mann LD. Recognition and management of occlusal disease from a hygienist's perspective. Probe 1996;30:196–7.

Cash RC. Bruxism in children: a review of the literature. J Pedodont 1988;12:107–12.

Champagne M. Upper airway compromise (UAC) and the long face syndrome. J Gen Orthod 1991;2:18–25.

Cook DA. Using crayons to educate patients about front-tooth wear patterns. J Am Dent Assoc 1998;129:1149–50.

de Cuegas JO. Nonsurgical treatment of a skeletal vertical discrepancy with a significant open bite. Am J Orthod Dentofac Orthop 1997;112:124–31.

Delcanho R. Screening for temporomandibular disorders in dental practice. Aust Dent J 1994;39:222–7.

Djemal S, Darbar UR, Hemmings KW. Case report: tooth wear associated with an unusual habit. Eur J Prosthodont Restor Dent 1998;6:29–32.

Dodds AP, King D. Gastroesophageal reflux and dental erosion: case report. Pediatr Dent 1997;19:409–12.

Donachie MA, Walls AW. Assessment of tooth wear in an ageing population. J Dent 1995;23:157–64.

Douglas WH. Form, function and strength in the restored dentition. Ann R Austr Coll Dent Surg 1996; 13:35–46.

Edwards M, Ashwood RA, Littlewood SJ, et al. A videofluoroscopic comparison of straw and cup drinking: the potential influence on dental erosion. Br Dent J 1998; 185:244–9.

Ehrlich J, Hochman N, Yaffe A. Contribution of oral habits to dental disorders. Cranio 1992;10:144–7.

Evans RD. Orthodontics and the creation of localised inter-occlusal space in cases of anterior tooth wear. Eur J Prosthodont Restor Dent 1997;5:69–73.

Evans RD, Briggs PF. Tooth-surface loss related to pregnancy-induced vomiting. Prim Dent Care 1994;1: 24–6.

Formicola V. Interproximal grooving: different appearances, different etiologies. Am J Phys Anthropol 1991;86:85–7.

Frayer DW. On the etiology of interproximal grooves. Am J Phys Anthropol 1991;85:299–304.

Friman PC, Schmitt BD. Thumb sucking: pediatrician's guidelines. Clin Pediatr 1989;28:438–40.

Gilmour AG, Beckett HA. The voluntary reflux phenomenon. Br Dent J 1993;175:368–72.

Goldstein RE. Esthetics in dentistry. J Am Dent Assoc 1982;104:301–2.

Goldstein RE. Diagnostic dilemma: to bond, laminate, or crown? Int J Periodont Restor Dent 1987;87(5):9–30.

Goldstein RE. The difficult patient stress syndrome: Part 1. J Esthet Dent 1993;5:86–7.

Goldstein RE. Change your smile. 3rd edn. Carol Stream, IL: Quintessence, 1997.

Goldstein RE, Garber DA, Schwartz CG, Goldstein CE. Patient maintenance of esthetic restorations. J Am Dent Assoc 1992;123:61–6.

Goldstein RE, Parkins F. Air-abrasive technology: its new role in restorative dentistry. J Am Dent Assoc 1994;125:551–7.

Gregory-Head B, Curtis DA. Erosion caused by gastroesophageal reflux: diagnostic considerations. J Prosthodont 1997;6:278–85.

Grippo JO. Abfractions: a new classification of hard tissue lesions of teeth. J Esthet Dent 1991;3:14–9.

Grippo JO. Noncarious cervical lesions: the decision to ignore or restore. J Esthet Dent 1992;4(Suppl):55–64.

Hacker CH, Wagner WC, Razzoog ME. An in vitro investigation of the wear of enamel on porcelain and gold in saliva. J Prosthet Dent 1996;75:14–7.

Harris EF, Butler ML. Patterns of incisor root resorption before and after orthodontic correction in cases with anterior open bites. Am J Orthod Dentofac Orthop 1992;101:112–9.

Hazelton LR, Faine MP. Diagnosis and dental management of eating disorder patients. Int J Prosthodont 1996;9:65–73.

Hertzberg J, Nakisbendi L, Needleman HL, Pober B. Williams syndrome—oral presentation of 45 cases. Pediatr Dent 1994;16:262–7.

Heymann HO, Sturdevant JR, Bayne S, et al. Examining tooth flexure effects on cervical restorations: a two year clinical study. J Am Dent Assoc 1991;122:41–7.

Hicks RA, Conti P. Nocturnal bruxism and self reports of stress-related symptoms. Percept Mot Skills 1991; 72:1182.

Hicks RA, Lucero-Gorman K, Bautista J, Hicks GJ. Ethnicity and bruxism. Percept Mot Skills 1999;88:240–1.

Horsted-Bindslev P, Knudsen J, Baelum V. 3-year clinical evaluation of modified Gluma adhesive systems in cervical abrasion/erosion lesions. Am J Dent 1996;9:22–6.

Hsu LK. Epidemiology of the eating disorders. Psychiatr Clin North Am 1996;19:681–700.

Hudson JD, Goldstein GR, Georgescu M. Enamel wear caused by three different restorative materials. J Prosthet Dent 1995;74:647–54.

Hugoson A, Ekfeldt A, Koch G, Hallonsten AL. Incisal and occlusal tooth wear in children and adolescents in a Swedish population. Acta Odontol Scand 1996;54:263–70.

Ikeda T, Nishigawa K, Kondo K, et al. Criteria for the detection of sleep-associated bruxism in humans. J Orofac Pain 1996;10:270–82.

Imfeld T. Dental erosion. Definition, classification and links. Eur J Oral Sci 1996;104:151–4.

Imfeld T. Prevention of progression of dental erosion by professional and individual prophylactic measures. Eur J Oral Sci 1996;104:215–20.

Ingleby J, Mackie IC. Case report: an unusual cause of toothwear. Dent Update 1995;22:434–5.

Jagger DC, Harrison A. An in vitro investigation into the wear effects of selected restorative materials on enamel. J Oral Rehabil 1995;22:275–81.

Jagger DC, Harrison A. An in vitro investigation into the wear effects of selected restorative materials on dentine. J Oral Rehabil 1995;22:349–54.

Jarvinen VK, Rytomaa II, Heinonen OP. Risk factors in dental erosion. J Dent Res 1991;70:942–7.

Johansson A. A cross-cultural study of occlusal tooth wear. Swed Dent J Suppl 1992;86:1–59.

Josell SD. Habits affecting dental and maxillofacial growth and development. Dent Clin North Am 1995;39:851–60.

Josephson CA. Restoration of mandibular incisors with advanced wear. J Dent Assoc S Afr 1992;47:419–20.

Kaidonis JA, Richards LC, Townsend GC, Tansley GD. Wear of human enamel: a quantitative in vitro assessment. J Dent Res 1998;77:1983–90.

Kampe T, Hannerz H, Strom P. Ten-year follow-up study of signs and symptoms of craniomandibular disorders in adults with intact and restored dentitions. J Oral Rehabil 1996;23:416–23.

Kelleher M, Bishop K. The aetiology and clinical appearance of tooth wear. Eur J Prosthodont Restor Dent 1997;5:157–60.

Khan F, Young WG, Daley TJ. Dental erosion and bruxism. A tooth wear analysis from south east Queensland. Aust Dent J 1998;43:117–27.

Kidd EA, Smith BG. Toothwear histories: a sensitive issue. Dent Update 1993;20:174–8.

Kiliaridis S, Johansson A, Haraldson T, et al. Craniofacial morphology, occlusal traits, and bite force in persons with advanced occlusal tooth wear. Am J Orthodont Dentofac Orthop 1995;107:286–92.

Kleinberg I. Bruxism: aetiology, clinical signs and symptoms. Aust Prosthodont J 1994;8:9–17.

Knight DJ, Leroux BG, Zhu C, et al. A longitudinal study of tooth wear in orthodontically treated patients. Am J Orthod Dentofacial Orthop 1997;112:194–202.

Kokich VG. Esthetics and vertical tooth position: orthodontic possibilities. Compend Cont Educ Dent 1997;18:1225–31.

Lambrechts P, van Meerbeek B, Perdigao J, et al. Restorative therapy for erosive lesions. Eur J Oral Sci 1996;104:229–40.

Lavigne GL, Rompre PH, Montplaisir JY. Sleep bruxism: validity of clinical research diagnostic criteria in a controlled polysomnographic study. J Dent Res 1996;75:546–52.

Lee CL, Eakle WS. Possible role of tensile stress in the etiology of cervical erosive lesions of teeth. J Prosthet Dent 1984;52:374–80.

Lee CL, Eakle WS. Stress-induced cervical lesions: review of advances in the past 10 years. J Prosthet Dent 1996;75:487–94.

Leinfelder KF, Yarnell G. Occlusion and restorative materials. Dent Clin North Am 1995;39:355–61.

Leung AK, Robson WL. Thumb sucking. Am Fam Physician 1991;44:1724–8.

Levine RS. Briefing paper: oral aspects of dummy and digit sucking. Br Dent J 1999;186:108.

Lussi A. Dental erosion clinical diagnosis and case history taking. Eur J Oral Sci 1996;104:191–8.

Lussi A, Portmann P, Burhop B. Erosion on abraded dental hard tissues by acid lozenges: an in situ study. Clin Oral Investig 1997;1:191–4.

Mair LH, Stolarski TA, Vowles RW, Lloyd CH. Wear: mechanisms, manifestations and measurement. Report of a workshop. J Dent 1996;24:141–8.

Marchesan IQ, Krakauer LR. The importance of respiratory activity in myofunctional therapy. Int J Orofac Myol 1996;22:23–7.

Maron FS. Enamel erosion resulting from hydrochloride acid tablets. J Am Dent Assoc 1996;127:781–4.

Matis BA, Cochran M, Carlson T. Longevity of glass-ionomer restorative materials: results of a 10-year evaluation. Quintessence Int 1996;27:373–82.

McCoy G. The etiology of gingival erosion. J Oral Implantol 1982;10:361–2.

McCoy G. On the longevity of teeth. J Oral Implantol 1983;11:248–67.

McIntyre JM. Erosion. Aust Prosthodont J 1992;6:17–25.

Mehler PS, Gray MC, Schulte M. Medical complications of anorexia nervosa. J Womens Health 1997;6:533–41.

Menapace SE, Rinchuse DJ, Zullo T, et al. The dentofacial morphology of bruxers versus non-bruxers. Angle Orthod 1994;64:43–52.

Mercado MD. The prevalence and aetiology of craniomandibular disorders among completely edentulous patients. Aust Prosthodont J 1993;7:27–9.

Mercado MD, Faulkner KD. The prevalence of craniomandibular disorders in completely edentulous denture-wearing subjects. J Oral Rehabil 1991;18:231–42.

Metaxas A. Oral habits and malocclusion. A case report. Ont Dent 1996;73:27.

Millward A, Shaw L, Smith AJ. Dental erosion in four-year-old children from differing socioeconomic backgrounds. ASDC J Dent Child 1994;61:263–366.

Millward A, Shaw L, Smith AJ, et al. The distribution and severity of tooth wear and the relationship between erosion and dietary constituents in a group of children. Int J Paediatr Dent 1994;4:151–7.

Milosevic A. Tooth wear: an aetiological and diagnostic problem. Eur J Prosthodont Restor Dent 1993;1:173–8.

Milosevic A, Brodie DA, Slade PD. Dental erosion, oral hygiene, and nutrition in eating disorders. Int J Eat Disord 1997;21:195–9.

Milosevic A, Dawson LJ. Salivary factors in vomiting bulimics with and without pathological tooth wear. Caries Res 1996;30:361–6.

Milosevic A, Lennon MA, Fear SC. Risk factors associated with tooth wear in teenagers: a case control study. Community Dent Health 1997;14:143–7.

Morley J. The esthetics of anterior tooth aging. Curr Opin Cosmet Dent 1997;4:35–9.

Moses AJ. Thumb sucking or thumb propping? CDS Rev 1987;80:40–2.

Moss RA, Lombardo TW, Villarosa GA, et al. Oral habits and TMJ dysfunction in facial pain and non-pain subjects. J Oral Rehabil 1995;22:79–81.

Murray CG, Sanson GD. Thegosis—a critical review. Aust Dent J 1998;43:192–8.

Nel JC, Bester SP, Snyman WD. Bruxism threshold: an explanation for successful treatment of multifactorial aetiology of bruxism. Aust Prosthodont J 1995;9:33–7.

Nel JC, Marais JT, van Vuuren PA. Various methods of achieving restoration of tooth structure loss due to bruxism. J Esthet Dent 1996;8:183–8.

Nemcovsky CE, Artzi Z. Erosion-abrasion lesions revisited. Compend Cont Educ Dent 1996;17:416–8.

Neo J, Chew CL. Direct tooth-colored materials for noncarious lesions: a 3-year clinical report. Quintessence Int 1995;27:183–8.

Neo J, Chew CL, Yap A, Sidhu S. Clinical evaluation of tooth-colored materials in cervical lesions. Am J Dent 1996;9:15–8.

Nunn JH. Prevalence of dental erosion and the implications for oral health. Eur J Oral Sci 1996;104:156–61.

Nunn J, Shaw L, Smith A. Tooth wear—dental erosion. Br Dent J 1996;180:349–52.

Nystrom M, Kononen M, Alaluusua S, et al. Development of horizontal tooth wear in maxillary anterior teeth from five to 18 years of age. J Dent Res 1990;69:1765–70.

Okeson JP. Occlusion and functional disorders of the masticatory system. Dent Clin North Am 1995;39:285–300.

Osborne-Smith KL, Burke FJ, Farlane TM, Wilson NH. Effect of restored and unrestored non-carious cervical lesions on the fracture resistance of previously restored maxillary premolar teeth. J Dent 1998;26:427–33.

O'Sullivan EA, Curzon ME, Roberts GJ, et al. Gastroesophageal reflux in children and its relationship to erosion of primary and permanent teeth. Eur J Oral Sci 1998;106:765–9.

Owens BM, Gallien GS. Noncarious dental "abfraction" lesions in an aging population. Compend Cont Educ Dent 1995;16:552–62.

Paterson AJ, Watson IB. Case report: prolonged match chewing: an unusual case of tooth wear. Eur J Prosthodont Restor Dent 1995;3:131–4.

Pavone BW. Bruxism and its effect on the natural teeth. J Prosthet Dent 1985;53:692–6.

Pierce CJ, Chrisman K, Bennett ME, Close JM. Stress, anticipatory stress, and psychologic measures related to sleep bruxism. J Orofac Pain 1995;9:51–6.

Pintado MR, Anderson GC, DeLong R, Douglas WH. Variation in tooth wear in young adults over a two-year period. J Prosthet Dent 1997;77:313–20.

Powell LV, Johnson GH, Gordon GE. Factors associated with clinical success of cervical abrasion/erosion restorations. Oper Dent 1995;20:7–13.

Principato JJ. Upper airway obstruction and craniomandibular morphology. Otolaryngol Head Neck Surg 1991;104:881–90.

Ramp MH, Suzuki S, Cox CF, et al. Evaluation of wear: enamel opposing three ceramic materials and a gold alloy. J Prosthet Dent 1997;77:523–30.

Ribeiro RA, Romano AR, Birman EG, Mayer MP. Oral manifestations of Rett syndrome: a study of 17 cases. Pediatr Dent 1997;19:349–52.

Ritchard A, Welsh AH, Donnelly C. The association between occlusion and attrition. Aust Orthod J 1992;12:138–42

Rivera-Morales WC, McCall WD Jr. Reliability of a portable electromyographic unit to measure bruxism. J Prosthet Dent 1995;73:184–9.

Robb ND, Cruwys E, Smith BG. Regurgitation erosion as a possible cause of tooth wear in ancient British populations. Arch Oral Biol 1991;36:595–602.

Rogers GM, Poore MH, Ferko BL, et al. In vitro effects of an acidic by-product feed on bovine teeth. Am J Vet Res 1997;58:498–503.

Schmidt U, Treasure J. Eating disorders and the dental practitioner. Eur J Prosthodont Restor Dent 1997;5:161–7.

Schneider PE. Oral habits—harmful and helpful. Update Pediatr Dent 1991;4:1–4, 6–8.

Schwartz JH, Brauer J, Gordon-Larsen P. Brief communication: Tigaran (Point Hope, Alaska) tooth drilling. Am J Phys Anthropol 1995;97:77–82.

Seligman DA, Pullinger AG. The degree to which dental attrition in modern society is a function of age and of canine contact. J Orofac Pain 1995;9:266–75.

Seow WK. Clinical diagnosis of enamel defects: pitfalls and practical guidelines. Int Dent J 1997;47:173–82.

Sherfudin H, Abdullah A, Shaik H, Johansson A. Some aspects of dental health in young adult Indian vegetarians. A pilot study. Acta Odontol Scand 1996;54:44–8.

Silness J, Berge M, Johannessen G. A 2-year follow-up study of incisal tooth wear in dental students. Acta Odontol Scand 1995;53:331–3.

Silness J, Berge M, Johannessen G. Longitudinal study of incisal tooth wear in children and adolescents. Eur J Oral Sci 1995;103:90–4.

Silness J, Berge M, Johannessen G. Re-examination of incisal tooth wear in children and adolescents. J Oral Rehabil 1997;24:405–9.

Smith BG, Bartlett DW, Robb ND. The prevalence, etiology and management of tooth wear in the United Kingdom. J Prosthet Dent 1997;78:367–72.

Smith BG, Robb ND. The prevalence of toothwear in 1007 dental patients. J Oral Rehabil 1996;23:232–9.

Sognnaes RF, Wolcott RB, Xhonga FA. Dental erosion I. Erosion-like patterns occurring in association with other dental conditions. J Am Dent Assoc 1972;84:571–6.

Speer JA. Bulimia: full stomach, empty lives. Dent Assist 1991;60:28–30.

Spranger H. Investigation into the genesis of angular lesions at the cervical region of teeth. Quintessence Int 1995;26:183–8.

Steiner H, Lock J. Anorexia nervosa and bulimia nervosa in children and adolescents: a review of the past 10 years. J Am Acad Child Adolesc Psychiatry 1998;37:352–9.

Stewart B. Restoration of the severely worn dentition using a systematized approach for a predictable prognosis. Int J Periodont Restor Dent 1998;18:46–57.

Suzuki S, Suzuki SH, Cox CF. Evaluating the antagonistic wear of restorative materials when placed against human enamel. J Am Dent Assoc 1996;127:74–80.

Taylor G, Taylor S, Abrams R, Mueller W. Dental erosion associated with asymptomatic gastroesophageal reflux. ASDC J Dent Child 1992;59:182–5.

Teaford MF, Lytle JD. Brief communication: diet-induced changes in the rates of human tooth microwear: a case study involving stone-ground maize. Am J Phys Anthropol 1996;100:143–7.

Teo C, Young WG, Daley TJ, Sauer H. Prior fluoridation in childhood affects dental caries and tooth wear in a south east Queensland population. Aust Dent J 1997;42:92–102.

Thompson BA, Blount BW, Krumholz TS. Treatment approaches to bruxism. Am Fam Physician 1994;49:1617–22.

Timms DJ, Trenouth MJ. A quantified comparison of craniofacial form with nasal respiratory function. Am J Orthod Dentofac Orthop 1988;94:216–21.

Touyz LZ. The acidity (pH) and buffering capacity of Canadian fruit juice and dental implications. J Can Dent Assoc 1994;60:448–54.

Turp JC, Gobetti JP. The cracked tooth syndrome: an elusive diagnosis. J Am Dent Assoc 1996;127:1502–7.

Tyas MJ. The Class V lesion – aetilogy and restoration. Aust Dent J 1995;40:167–70.

Ung N, Koenig J, Shapiro PA, et al. A quantitative assessment of respiratory patterns and their effects on dentofacial development. Am J Orthod Dentofac Orthop 1990;98:523–32.

Villa G, Giacobini G. Subvertical grooves of interproximal facets in Neandertal posterior teeth. Am J Phys Anthropol 1995;96:51–62.

Waterman ET, Koltai PJ, Downey JC, Cacace AT. Swallowing disorders in a population of children with cerebral palsy. Int J Pediatr Otorhinolaryngol 1992;24:63–71.

West NX, Maxwell A, Hughes JA, et al. A method to measure clinical erosion: the effect of orange juice consumption on erosion of enamel. J Dent 1998;26:329–35.

Westergaard J, Moe D, Pallesen U, Holmen L. Exaggerated abrasion/erosion of human dental enamel surfaces: a case report. Scand J Dent Res 1993;101:265–9.

Woodside DG, Linder-Aronson S, Lundstrom A, McWilliam J. Mandibular and maxillary growth after changed mode of breathing. Am J Orthod Dentofac Orthop 1991;100:1–18.

Yaacob HB, Park AW. Dental abrasion pattern in a selected group of Malaysians. J Nihon Univ Sch Dent 1990;32:175–80.

Yamaguchi H, Tanaka Y, Sueishi K, et al. Changes in oral functions and muscular behavior due to surgical orthodontic treatment. Bull Tokyo Dent Coll 1994;35:41–9.

Young DV, Rinchuse DJ, Pierce CJ, Zullo T. The craniofacial morphology of bruxers versus nonbruxers. Angle Orthod 1999;69:14–8.

Part 4

Esthetic Problems of Missing Teeth

CHAPTER 21

FIXED REPLACEMENT OF MISSING TEETH

Steven K. Nelson, DMD, F. Michael Gardner, DDS, MA, Ronald E. Goldstein, DDS

With the development of many new metal alloy systems, porcelains to fire to these alloys, all-ceramic crown materials, porcelain margins for metal-ceramic restorations, porcelain veneers, and much stronger bonding and cementing systems, both functional and esthetic results may be obtained today that were unthought of in the past. However, with the evolution of such varied choices in materials and techniques, the requirements for selecting the correct combinations for success become ever more difficult.

Once a patient decides to have a lost tooth replaced with a fixed partial denture, it must be remembered that regardless of how skillfully the biomechanical requirements have been met, the patient will judge his or her result primarily on the basis of esthetics, especially if the prosthesis is in the anterior region. Today's patient is more aware of the interrelationship between teeth and facial appearance and is entitled to the dentist's best artistic efforts.

Prior to choosing a fixed partial denture as the restoration of choice for a given edentulous situation, a logical sequence of diagnosis and treatment planning must be followed to achieve a successful outcome. A thorough diagnostic work-up should be performed, which will provide the restoring dentist with all of the information needed to determine the best treatment plan for the patient.[3,5,20] This diagnostic information is best gathered through a systematic approach such as the one outlined below.

DIAGNOSIS

Medical and Dental History
The starting point for any patient care begins with thorough medical and dental histories. Information gathered on the written history sheet and expanded verbally can provide the restoring dentist with data pertinent to successful prosthodontic treatment. Noting prior dental experiences and the patient's attitude toward treatment is of extreme importance in developing a rapport with the patient. The patient's chief complaint should be ascertained, and if it is esthetic in nature, specific esthetic desires and needs should be assessed, as well as any esthetic shortcomings with previous prostheses. Once these facts have been established and a good working relationship exists between the dentist and the patient, the correct treatment for that patient can be pursued.

Intraoral Examination
A comprehensive intraoral examination should be performed on all patients. The charting of preexisting restorations and any new pathoses should be a routine procedure. All diagnoses should be documented, such as missing teeth, periodontal status, pulpal pathosis, caries, fractures, wear, unesthetic restorations, muscle and temporomandibular joint pathosis, and neoplasm. All data should be recorded, and the patient should be treatment planned as a total entity, rather than only addressing the specific edentulous area and adjacent tooth structure. Often, steps for developing comprehensive treatment plans are overlooked, and the treatment starts before a diagnosis is made. Proper work-up procedures help achieve a sound prosthodontic outcome.

The intraoral examination can be enhanced by using an intraoral camera (see Figures 2–7A to C, Chapter 2, *Esthetics in Dentistry,* Volume 1, 2nd Edition)[16,18] or surgical microscope (Figure 21–1).[21] Revelations such as hidden microcracks, defective restoration margins, and other tooth and tissue defects can determine a choice of single or multiple retainers when weakened teeth thought to be in

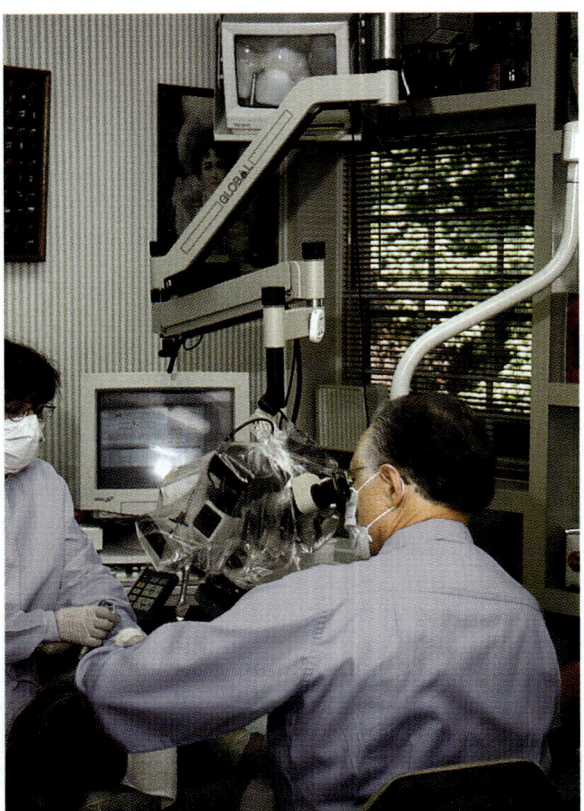

Figure 21–1: The surgical microscope, due to the extremely bright field and high magnification, provides the ultimate in intraoral diagnosis.

good condition are discovered. Each tooth should be manually recorded in the chart and/or electronically in the computer for diagnostic and legal purposes.

Extraoral Examination
The extraoral examination should include assessment of symmetry, muscle hypertrophy, possible loss of vertical dimension of occlusion, and a smile analysis that determines the amount of each tooth that will be seen while smiling, speaking, etc. (see Chapter 2, *Esthetics in Dentistry,* Volume 1, 2nd Edition).

Radiographs
A full-mouth series of radiographs or a panoramic radiograph with selected periapical radiographs of the proposed abutment teeth is necessary in the evaluation for treatment with a fixed partial denture. The primary purpose of radiographs is to disclose hidden areas and structures such as the root morphology, pulpal outline, periodontal ligament space, and the extent of present and past caries.[30] In addition to the intraoral examination, the radiographs can provide the restoring dentist with information such as pulpal pathosis, crown-to-root ratio, and quality of remaining bone and aid in determining the tilt of teeth.

Computerized radiographs[37,42] can also be a helpful way to communicate with the patient. The ability to colorize the findings plus isolate and enlarge segments of the root or crown in question, while producing a greatly reduced amount of radiation, provides an avenue to enhance patient-doctor relationships.

Diagnostic Casts
Diagnostic casts are imperative in diagnosis and treatment planning. The casts are used as an educational aid for the patient and to provide the dentist with the preexisting condition of the patient. Casts mounted on a suitable articulator, at the treatment position, will enable the restoring dentist to evaluate the condition of the patient's mouth. Clinical crown length, tipped or rotated teeth, ridge form, and the span of the edentulous area can all be evaluated, thereby helping the dentist in the decision-making process. The interarch space and the occlusal plane can be evaluated on the diagnostic casts, which may lead to the diagnosis of lost interocclusal space or supraeruption of a segment of the dentition. The treatment, therefore, may involve crown lengthening, ridge reduction, endodontic therapy, repositioning of teeth, segmental osteotomy, or extraction. Properly mounted, accurate diagnostic casts are a very important element of the diagnosis and treatment planning of a fixed partial denture.

Diagnostic Waxing
A diagnostic waxing of the proposed fixed partial denture can be invaluable in determining the esthetic criteria for a treatment plan. It allows for the opportunity to observe the abutment tooth–pontic relationship and the pontic–ridge relationship. The diagnostic waxing also allows the dentist to evaluate and work within the exact space of the edentulous area. The edentulous area itself may be badly resorbed and require surgical correction with grafting of bone, soft tissue, or both. Often, other treatment issues or necessary modifications become evident at this point in the planning process.[39] Frequently, orthodontic treatment is the best solution for limited space and rotated,

tipped, or malposed teeth. This may be done in place of or prior to fabrication of a fixed partial denture. In some situations, the diagnostic waxing will indicate the need for endodontic treatment when tooth preparation will involve the pulp of slightly malposed or tipped teeth.

Esthetic Considerations
A prime part of diagnosis is ascertaining the requirements relating to esthetics, especially from the patient's perspective. Communication with the patient provides a general sense of what his or her expectations are and therefore provides information that may dictate, for example, the type of retainer margin, retainer margin placement in relation to the gingiva, or whether porcelain occlusal surfaces are indicated. The dentist should know what the patient expects esthetically before treatment begins to avoid esthetic disasters.

For example, although the maxillary anterior region is usually the most demanding due to its easy visibility, certain patients will place just as much demand for exact shade duplication in the posterior region.

The arch in which the prosthesis is to be placed, the restoration's position in that arch, the amount of display of the prosthesis, and the patient's esthetic awareness all have to be considered when designing the elements of an esthetic fixed partial denture. These elements include retainer type, material and amount of coverage of the teeth, margin location and material, ceramic–metal junction location on metal-ceramic crowns, and pontic design. These esthetic considerations must be coupled with biologic and functional considerations such as span length, need for splinting, periodontal support, soft-tissue management, the use of provisionals, and the need for adjunctive care such as orthodontics, endodontics, periodontics, and oral and maxillofacial surgery.

The anterior fixed prosthesis often presents the most difficult esthetic problem. The choice of tooth form, shade, and arrangement used for complete dentures is not usually available for the fabrication of a fixed prosthesis. Artistic skill is required to obtain a pleasing result. Correct occlusal function is difficult, if not impossible, without correct form. They are inseparable qualities.

Pleasing esthetics can best be achieved when restorations blend inconspicuously with the patient's remaining natural dentition. An exception to this rule is when the entire dentition is changed. In addition, existing facial features should always be evaluated during the diagnostic period before any treatment is instituted. In other words, all "pieces to the puzzle" should be evaluated during diagnosis.

Computer-generated analyses and imaging can also be used as an adjunct when considering esthetic requirements.[13,14] One of the greatest advantages of this technique is the ability to evaluate proposed tooth sizes and shapes before the final restoration is constructed. This imaging will not only assist in the planning of the restoration but also in the actual construction of a provisional fixed partial denture.

Functional Considerations
Functional considerations, by their nature, are most intimately tied to esthetic values. The type and number of abutments used requires functional considerations, and the choice can affect the esthetic result. The use of intracoronal or extracoronal retainers depends on the length of the space to be restored, the functional stresses that will be placed on the prosthesis, and the age of the patient. If extracoronal retainers are chosen, the same considerations apply to the choice of either complete- or partial-coverage crowns that apply to intracoronal retainers.

Patients with deep vertical overlap or who have severe bruxism or clenching, especially in protrusive movements, can be at risk for restoration fracture. The best solution is to improve the occlusal relationship through orthodontic treatment (Figures 21–2A to F).

Interdisciplinary Consultations
Interdisciplinary consultations and treatment referrals are important to providing comprehensive care. Multiple treatment modalities and all treatment options for the patient should be investigated and presented during the treatment planning phase.[17]

Once the diagnostic process has been completed, treatment options may be selected from the following choices:

I. Retainers
   A. Partial coverage
      1. Cemented
      2. Resin bonded
      3. Porcelain veneers

638 Esthetics in Dentistry

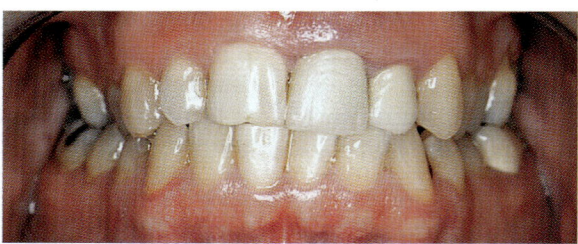

Figure 21–2A: This 50-year-old man had a habit of grinding in a protrusive excursion, continuously chipping his anterior teeth.

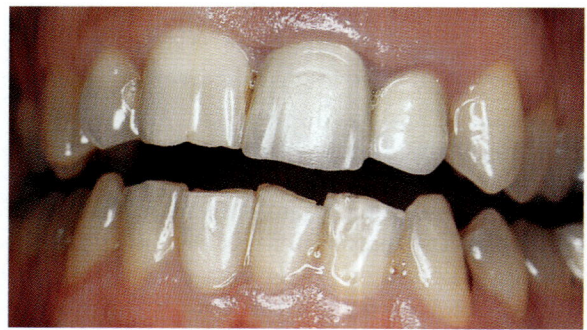

Figure 21–2B: In addition to the chipped anteriors, the left central incisor had advanced periodontal disease, requiring extraction.

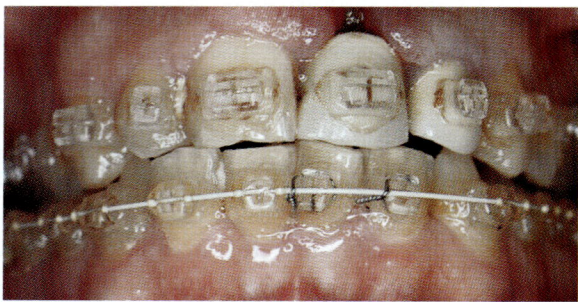

Figure 21–2C: Orthodontic treatment was suggested to improve the occlusion and provide a more favorable protrusive excursion. Unfortunately, the patient lost the left central incisor because of a nonrestorative root fracture.

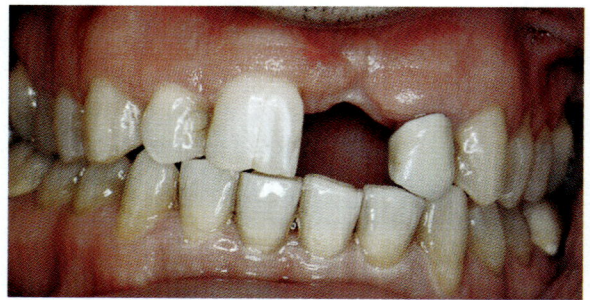

Figure 21–2D: After orthodontic treatment, the occlusion is now in a much more favorable relationship.

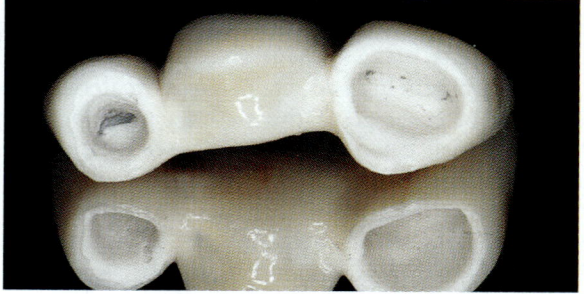

Figure 21–2E: A three-unit all-ceramic (Inceram, Vident, Brea, CA) fixed partial denture was constructed.

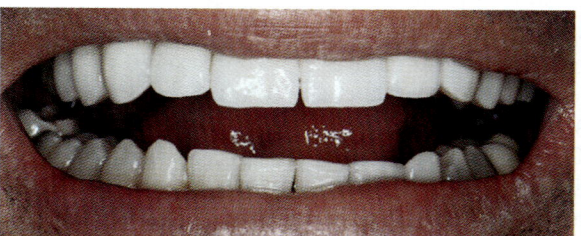

Figure 21–2F: The after smile shows how larger central incisors enhance the esthetics.

B. Complete coverage
   1. All metal
   2. All ceramic
   3. Metal ceramic
      a. Margins
         - Location
         - Material
         - Metal collar margin
         - Disappearing metal margin
         - Porcelain margin
      b. Porcelain–metal junction
C. Other considerations
   1. Cantilever fixed partial denture
   2. Implants
   3. Splinting
   4. Use of telescoping crowns as abutments
II. Pontics
   A. Design
   B. Edentulous ridge form
   C. Material

RETAINERS

When selecting appropriate retainers for a fixed partial denture, esthetics is only one of three important factors to be considered. The other two are biologic considerations and functional or mechanical considerations. Unfortunately, some of the most esthetically advantageous retainers can be the poorest from a mechanical standpoint, and other very esthetic retainers can be the most biologically invasive. Some of these biologic and mechanical considerations are the size of the abutment tooth; the amount of remaining tooth structure; the size and type of restorative material in the tooth; the size, age, and status of the pulp; the clinical crown length; the location of the tooth in the mouth; the type of occlusal load; the interocclusal space; the opposing dentition or prostheses; the edentulous span length; and, especially, the consideration of the insertion path (Figures 21–3A and B). It does the patient little good to have a beautifully esthetic restoration that fails because the biologic and functional issues are not treated correctly.

Fixed partial denture retainers can be separated broadly into two categories, partial- and complete-coverage retainers. Usually, the most esthetic material the restoring dentist can choose to match the patient's existing dentition is natural tooth structure. This display of natural tooth structure in the esthetic zone is accomplished by using partial-veneer restorations.

Partial-Coverage Retainers

The oldest, and now probably least used, of the partial-coverage retainer designs is the metal inlay, onlay, or three-quarter crown. These are usually made of a relatively soft gold alloy and cemented with traditional, mechanically retentive cements (Figures 21–4A to D). Due to the buttressing, retention, and resistance form necessary to make these retainers functionally successful, it is virtually impossible to avoid some show of metal at the proximal and incisal or occlusal line angles. Because of this show of metal, this retainer is unacceptable in the anterior region of the mouth for the esthetically conscious patient. It can be used very acceptably, however, in less esthetically critical areas of the mouth. Its best application is for use on

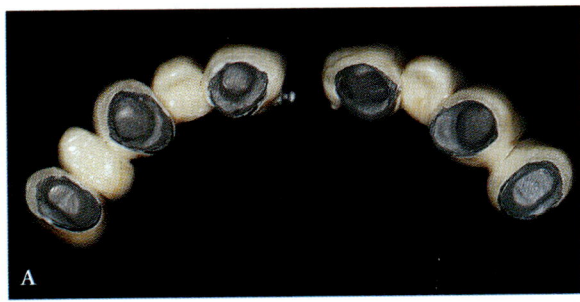 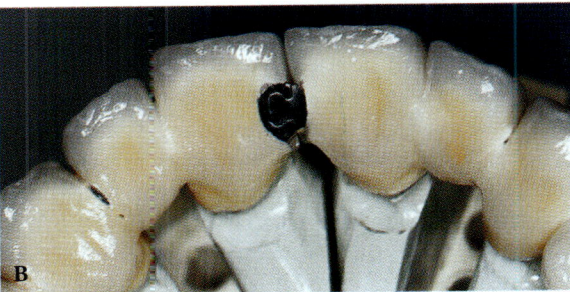

Figures 21–3A and B: When patients have lost considerable bone support, resulting in extremely divergent roots, linking two fixed partial denture segments together with attachments may be a treatment option.

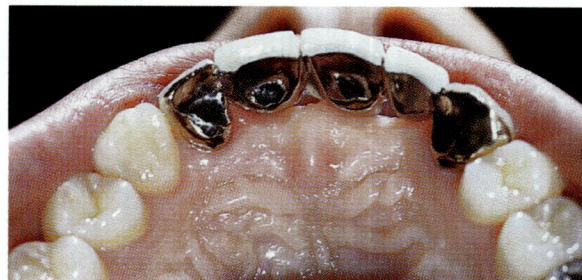

Figure 21–4A: Although the three-quarter crown can be a functionally sound retainer, it is esthetically difficult to avoid showing metal at the proximal, incisal, or occlusal line angles.

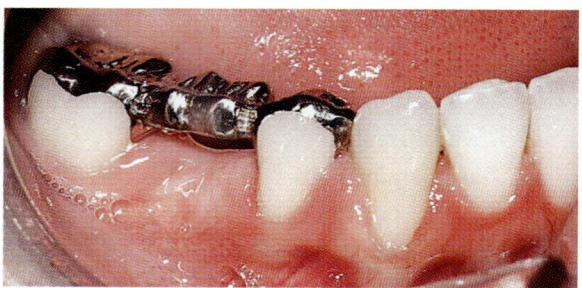

Figure 21–4B: This conservative, economical, three-unit hygienic pontic fixed partial denture is supported with gold onlays and can be esthetically acceptable for some patients.

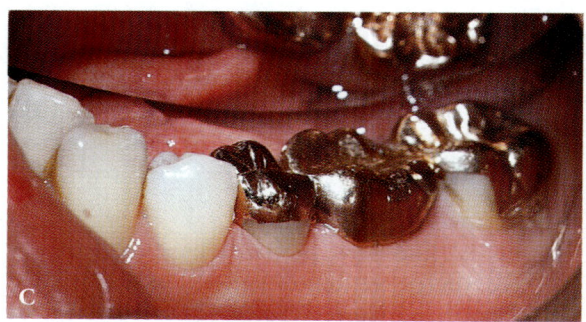
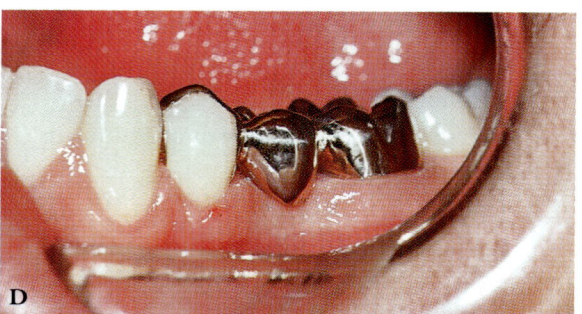

Figure 21–4C and D: These two versions of three-quarter and full-crown abutments supporting all-gold pontics were esthetically acceptable for the patients.

large, relatively unrestored second premolars and first molars in the maxillary arch.

Currently, the most widely used partial-coverage retainer is the resin-bonded retainer (Figures 21–5A to E). In its original form, it was described as the "prepless bridge."[19,32,41] The preparation design was overly conservative, lacked resistance form, and relied almost entirely on the resin bond to enamel for retention. The documented success rates for these early restorations varied widely and left much room for improvement. Gradually, the preparation design for resin-bonded retainers has evolved to look much like the classic three-quarter crown preparation. It is now advocated that parallel grooves be used for resistance; that retention be augmented with pins, potholes, or ledges; and that a definite finish line be created (Figures 21–6A to C).[8,10,28,33] The only concession for the sake of esthetics is the lack of the incisal offset and proximal metal display seen in the classic three-quarter crown preparation. This is compensated for by the use of base metal alloys that are relatively rigid in thin sections and micromechanical retention potential between the cement and metal and the cement and tooth enamel. The current preparation design is technically difficult to perform and requires a great deal of attention to detail. For this reason, properly constructed resin-bonded fixed partial dentures may fall from favor with the dental profession much as traditional partial-coverage retainers have.

Resin-bonded partial-veneer fixed partial dentures would be the restoration of choice, particularly in the anterior part of the mouth if the following conditions are met: the abutment teeth are esthetically acceptable to the patient in their present size, form, and color; the teeth are free of restorations or have only minimal restoration that does not involve the crown margins; and the abutment teeth are of adequate length to afford preparation resistance and retention and of adequate thickness to prevent metal shadowing from the lingual surface. For the best results, the resin-bonded partial-veneer retained prosthesis should only replace one tooth. The teeth should have only normal mobility. Failure rates rise rapidly with increased numbers of pontics and with mobile abutment teeth. The pontic space must be of the ideal width since little widening or narrowing of the edentulous space can be accomplished with partial-veneer retainers. One of the most frequently seen esthetic problems with this type of retainer is the difficulty of perfect shade matching. If the adjacent retainers are metal, light translucency of the abutment teeth is diminished, resulting in possible shade variance.

A third type of partial-coverage restoration made from traditional crown materials and cemented or bonded to tooth structure is the porcelain veneer. It is, no doubt, one of the most esthetic of all partial-

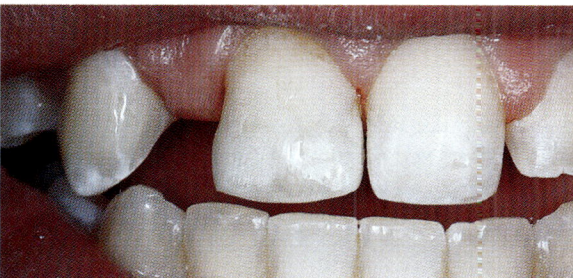

Figure 21–5A: This 17-year-old male is missing his maxillary right lateral incisor.

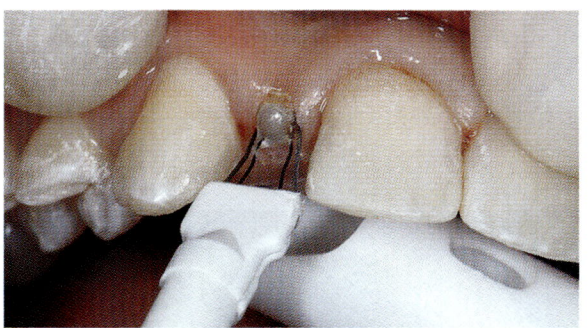

Figure 21–5B: To make a proper pontic site, tissue surgery was accomplished with electrosurgery.

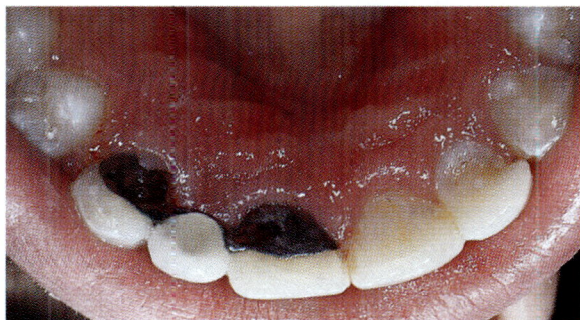

Figure 21–5C: The conventional resin-bonded fixed partial denture is made of thin metal linguals on each of the retainers.

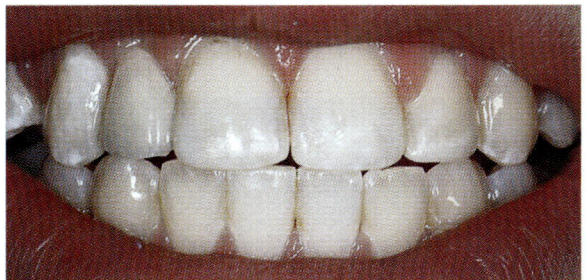

Figure 21–5D: The final result shows a natural-appearing tooth replacement due to a favorably shaped tissue site and the use of the ovate pontic.

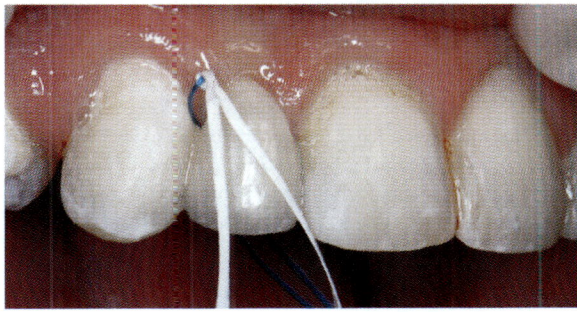

Figure 21–5E: An adequate space must be provided for the use of a floss threader to maintain optimal oral health.

coverage restorations but has limited advocacy as a fixed partial denture retainer. The porcelain veneer that fits and is bonded to the tooth correctly has adequate strength to survive most clinical conditions as a single tooth restoration. The problem of survivability is greatly magnified when porcelain pontics are attached to porcelain veneers with porcelain connectors. For this type of restoration to succeed, two requirements are necessary: minimal or no occlusion force and patient compliance in avoiding biting or occluding on hard foods or objects. In addition, the patient should be advised to wear an occlusal splint (Figures 21–7A to H).

Complete-Coverage Retainers

Full-veneer retainers are the most popular and the most universally used of all retainers for fixed partial dentures. They generally fall into three categories: all-metal, all-ceramic, and metal-ceramic retainers.

All metal crowns are not particularly esthetic and therefore should be used only in patients who have low esthetic demands. Typically, they are placed in areas of the mouth that virtually cannot be viewed by observers or the patient. They are ideal for maxillary and mandibular second and third molar abutments and for the occasional maxillary first molar in patients with acceptable esthetic smile lines that do not expose this tooth. It is fortunate that these areas of the mouth lend themselves to all-metal crowns since it is rare to find a second or third molar, particularly mandibular, that has sufficient gingivo-occlusal height to allow preparation reduction sufficient for porcelain occlusal coverage. The major advantages of all metal retainers are minimal tooth reduction in comparison with the metal-ceramic or all-ceramic crown preparation, ease of fabrication, and lack of wear of the opposing dentition. The chief disadvantage beyond the lack of esthetics is high thermal conductivity.

The use of all-ceramic restorations as retainers for fixed partial dentures is experimental and is unsupported by any long-term clinical studies. The all-ceramic fixed partial denture should, at best, be used with extreme caution and limited to one-tooth anterior replacements in patients with less than normal occlusal force (see Figures 21–2A to F). The inferior mechanical properties related to the strength of all-ceramic connectors should be fully explained to the patient, as well as other more traditional alternatives, before selecting this unproven choice. Maximum esthetics rather than longevity must be the overriding consideration in the use of all-ceramic fixed prostheses (Figures 21–8A to M).

By far the most commonly used retainer for fixed partial dentures is the metal-ceramic crown. During

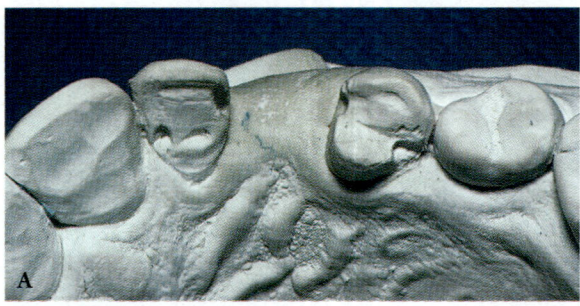
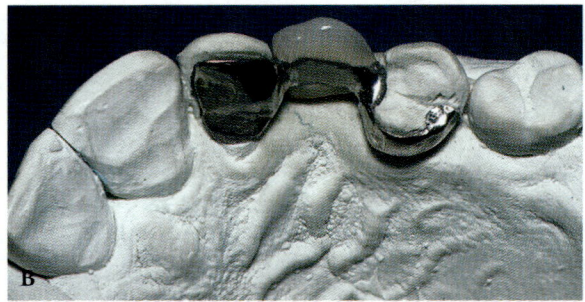
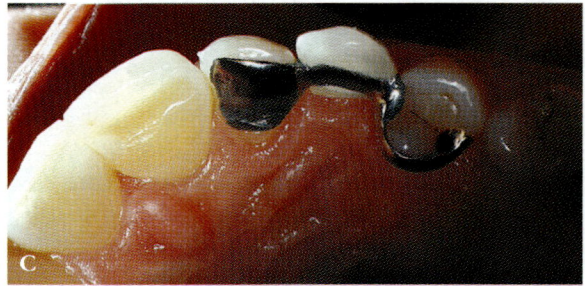

Figure 21–6A to C: The best design for long-term results with a resin-bonded fixed partial denture is to include parallel groves to aid retention and resistance form, in addition to the possible use of potholes, pins, or ledges and a well-defined finish line.

Fixed Replacement of Missing Teeth 643

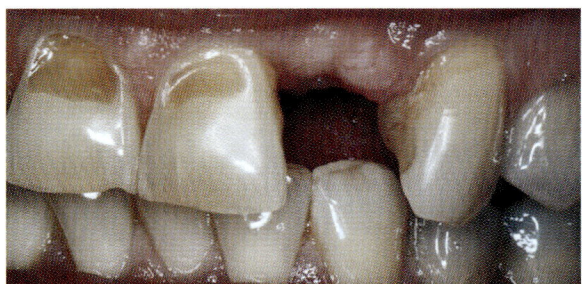

Figure 21–7A: This 52-year-old lady is missing her maxillary left lateral incisor and has severely eroded central incisors.

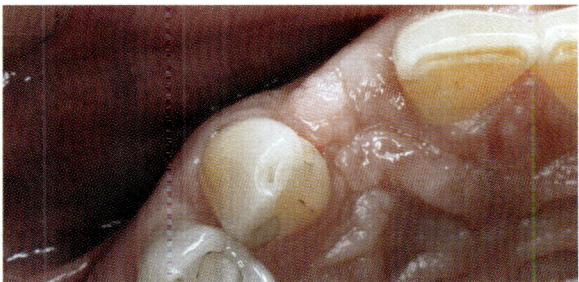

Figure 21–7B: Note the linguoincisal wear on the left central incisor.

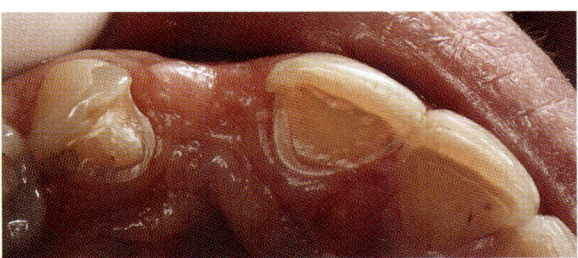

Figure 21–7C: The lingual surfaces are prepared for a resin-bonded bridge. Note the retentive ledges placed.

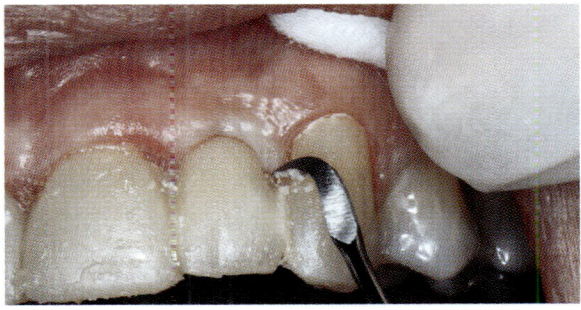

Figure 21–7D: A three-unit all-ceramic (Inceram, Vident) fixed partial denture is placed, and the resin cement is trimmed with the Novatek 12 (Hu-Friedy, Chicago, IL).

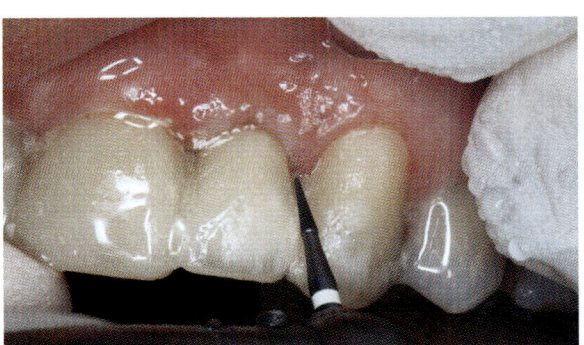

Figure 21–7E: After removing the excess cement, the interproximal margins are carefully polished with a 30-blade carbide (ETUF4, Brasseler, Savannah, GA).

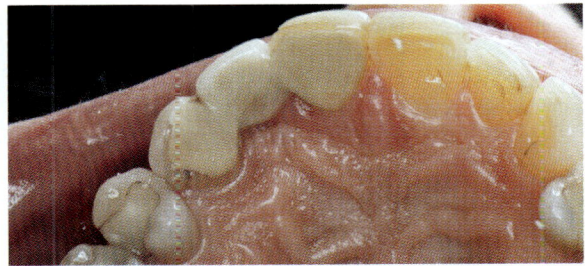

Figure 21–7F: The main advantage for using the all-ceramic retainer is to avoid abutment tooth discoloration.

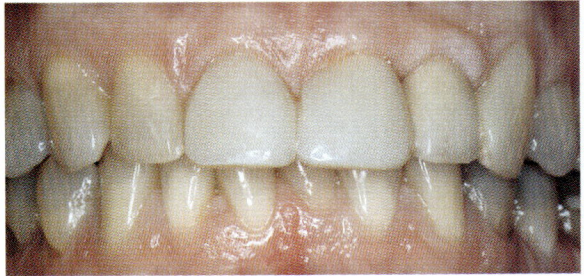

Figure 21–7G: Labial view of the final restoration, which also shows composite resin bonding of the two central incisors.

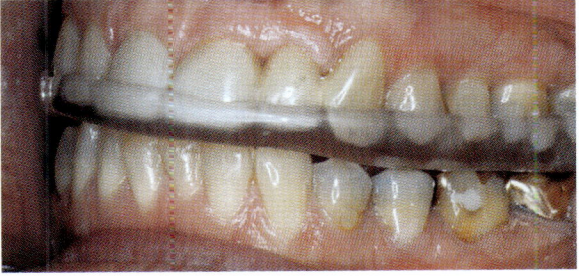

Figure 21–7H: It is essential that the patient be required to wear a well-fitting occlusal night guard.

644 Esthetics in Dentistry

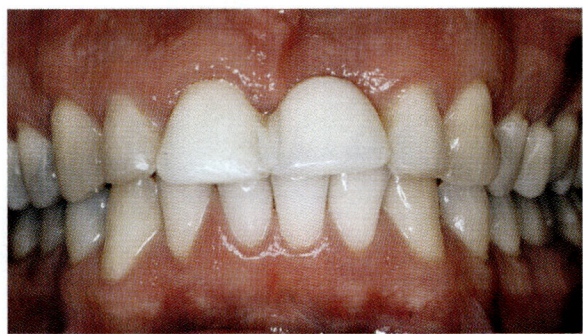

Figure 21–8A: This 33-year-old dentist wanted to improve the appearance of his front teeth.

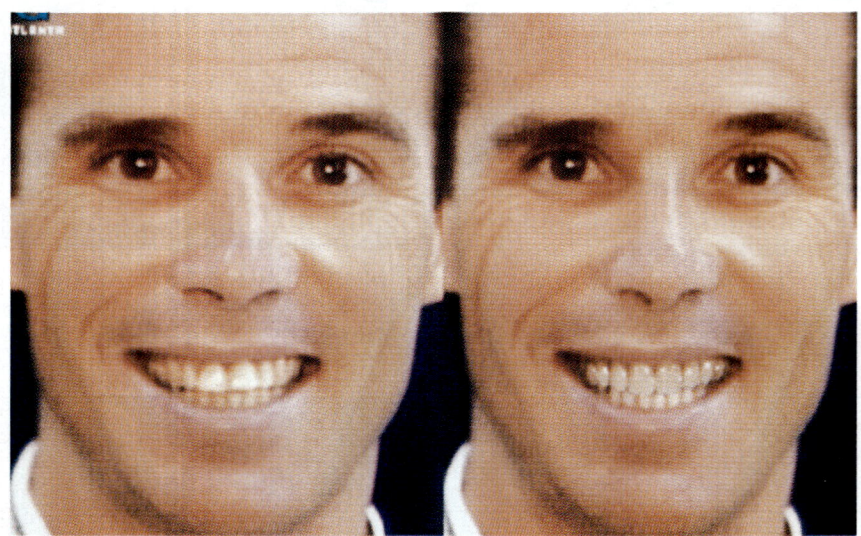

Figure 21–8B: Other than improving the color of his smile, the main problem was the lack of proportion of the two central incisors with the rest of the anterior teeth. Esthetic imaging shows the improvements that would be gained with better-proportioned teeth.

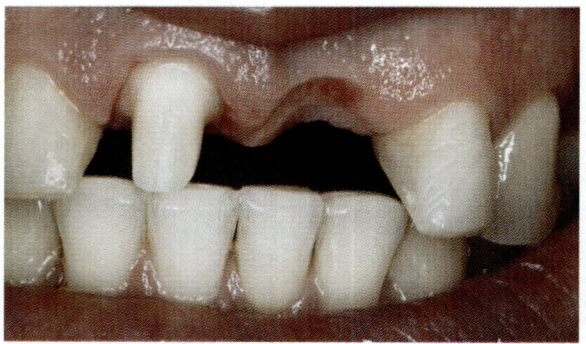

Figure 21–8C: After diagnosis and treatment planning, the next step was to remove the too-wide existing cantilever fixed partial denture.

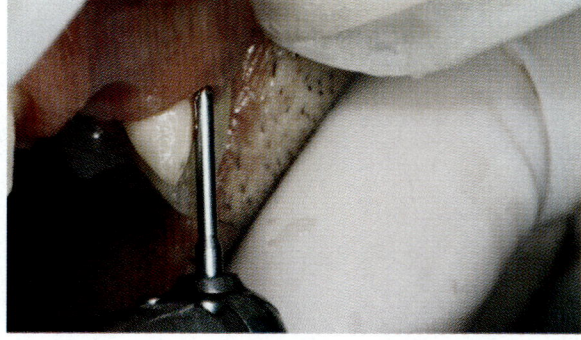

Figure 21–8D: After an all-ceramic three-unit fixed partial denture was selected, a full-shoulder margin on the left lateral incisor is finished with a diamond bur.

the last 30 to 40 years, this restoration has proven to be a very satisfactory compromise between functional success and esthetics. The acceptance of this retainer has fostered many variations and choices that impact on esthetics, as well as biologic acceptance, functional success, ease of predictable fabrication, and economics. Some of the variables that should be considered with metal-ceramic retainers are the location of the margins in relation to the gingiva, the materials used for margin fabrication, and the location of the porcelain–metal junction in relation to the occlusal surface of the retainer.

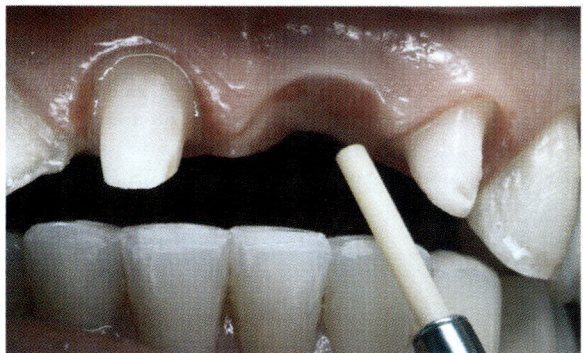

Figure 21–8E: The pontic site is enhanced using a CO_2 laser to prepare the tissue for an ovate pontic.

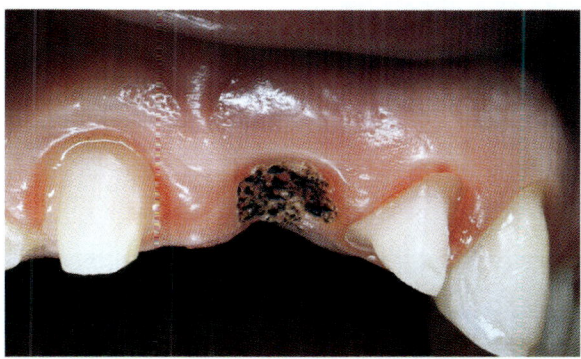

Figure 21–8F: Note the lack of bleeding directly after laser surgery.

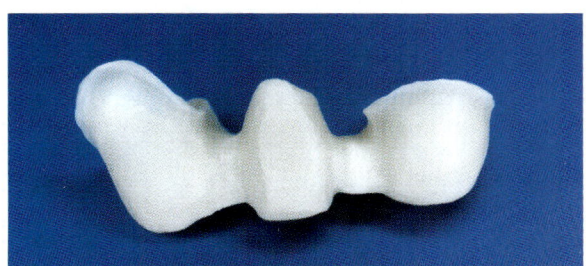

Figure 21–8G: The three-unit all-ceramic core structure (Inceram, Vident) provides the strength for the all-ceramic fixed partial denture.

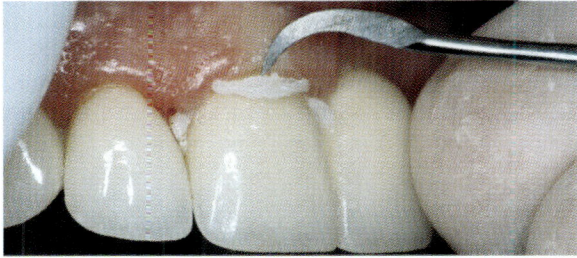

Figure 21–8H: The three-unit all-ceramic fixed partial denture is cemented with a resin cement containing fluoride for both strength and caries protection. The excess cement is trimmed with a double-ended, heavy-duty, cement-removing instrument.

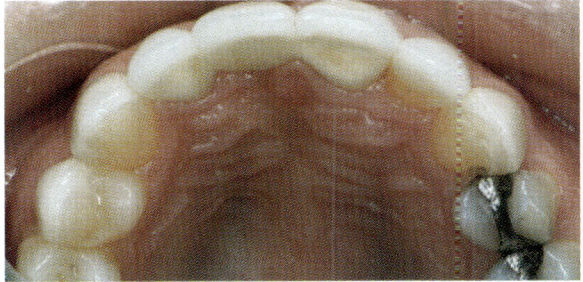

Figure 21–8I: The color and proportion were further enhanced by placing porcelain laminate veneers on the opposing lateral incisor, both canines, and the left first premolar.

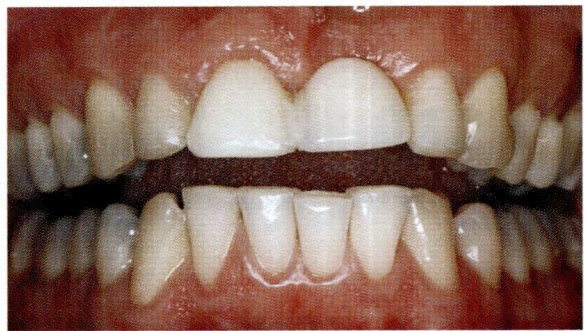

Figure 21–8J: This picture shows the maxillary discolored and disproportionate teeth and the crowded mandibular incisors.

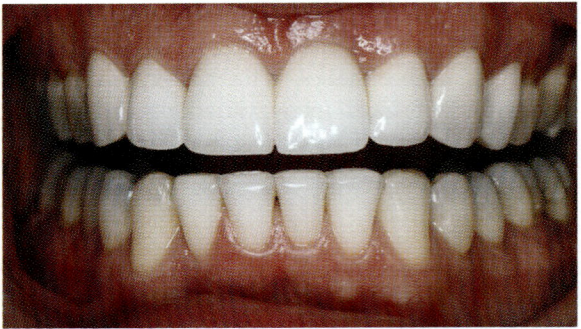

Figure 21–8K: Note the esthetic improvement of the mandibular incisors following esthetic contouring of these teeth. Eventually, it may be necessary to treat the cervical erosion on the maxillary posterior teeth.

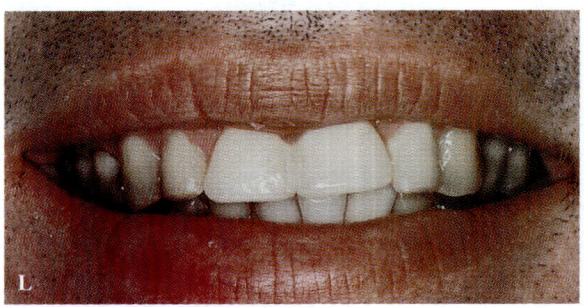

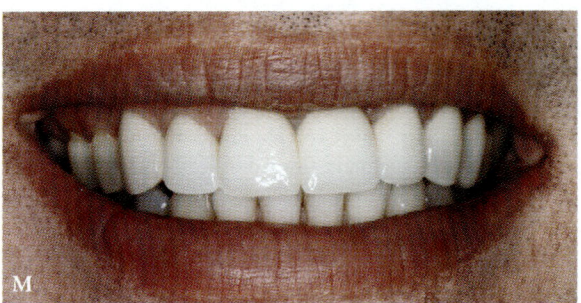

Figure 21–8L and M: The comparison of the before and after smile. Maximum esthetics rather than longevity was the overriding consideration in the choice of an all-ceramic fixed prosthesis. Because this patient is a dentist, he is well aware of occlusal limitations, especially in excursive movements.

Margin Location

Studies have shown that with respect to biologic acceptance of an artificial crown by the gingival apparatus, the situation is generally healthier when the artificial material remains supragingival.[38] Supragingival margins are also easier to prepare, impress, and evaluate for fit (Figures 21–9A and B). Although it has been shown that soft-tissue health can be maintained in the presence of subgingival margins,[31] the general consensus is that margins should only be placed into the gingival sulcus for reasons of esthetics, wall height for resistance and retention, or extension beyond existing caries or restorations.[25] If subgingival margins are chosen solely for esthetics, they should be limited to areas in which the gingival margins are visible to observers of the patient in normal and extreme facial movement. It was shown that less than 50% of the population observed in one study revealed the gingival area of any of their mandibular teeth during movements of facial expression (without manually pulling down their lower lips).[7] Further, a smaller percentage in the same study did not reveal their maxillary gingival margins during facial muscle use. It has been the author's observations that many patients do not show their gingival margin areas of maxillary molars. In general, when the patient permits, subgingival metal-ceramic margins should be limited to a patient's visible esthetic zone. This may require some prior education by the restoring dentist so that the patient will understand that what is visible with mirrors, cheek retractors, and fingers in the mouth is not necessarily visible in normal circumstances. However, patients whose primary concern is esthetics will often only agree to subgingival metal margins (Figures 21–10A to D). With these situations, the porcelain shoulder butt margin design prepared supragingivally should also

Fixed Replacement of Missing Teeth 647

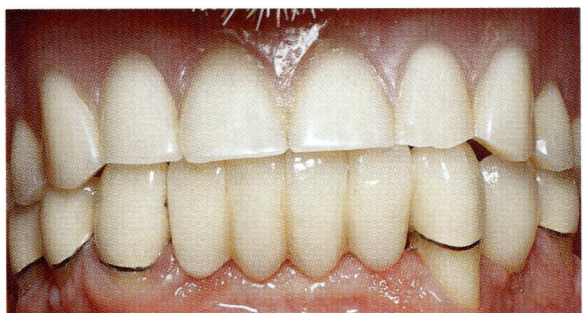

Figure 21-9A: Supragingival margins with exposed metal will generally not be an esthetic problem if the lip line is favorable.

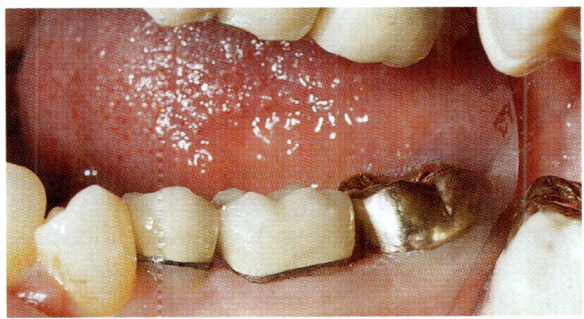

Figure 21-9B: A complete metal crown can be the longest-lasting retainer of choice anytime esthetics permit.

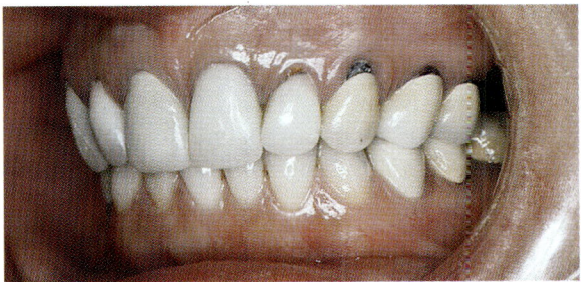

Figure 21-10A: This patient was extremely dissatisfied with the recession of maxillary gingival exposing metal margins.

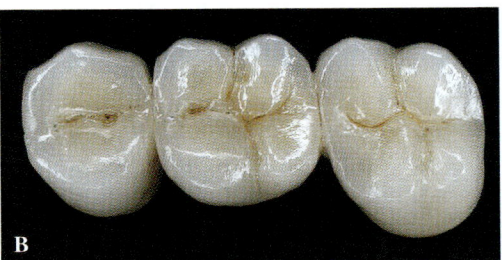
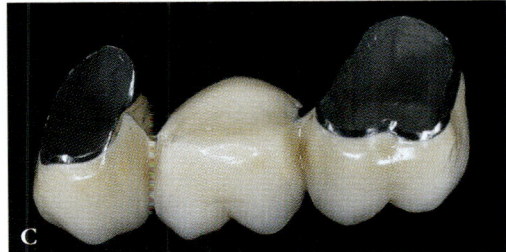

Figure 21-10B and C: A three-unit fixed partial denture replacement was constructed using concealed metal-ceramic margins.

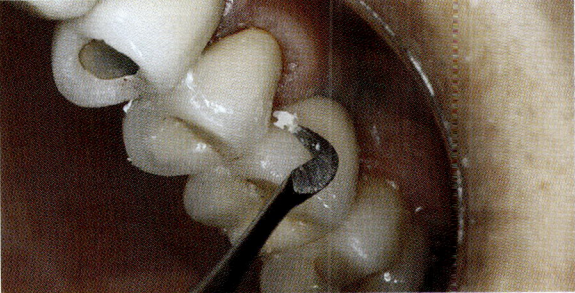

Figure 21-10D: Since caries was present, the fixed partial denture had to be redone and the adjacent Class V area esthetically repaired.

be considered either 180 or 360 degrees (Figures 21–11A and B) (see also *Esthetics in Dentistry,* Volume 1, 2nd Edition, Figure 15–11).

Margin Materials

Certain subgingival margins are not completely natural and esthetic in appearance. This is usually because the restorative material shows through the thin gingival sulcular tissue or there is too much artificial crown material subgingivally either in the form of overcontouring, overextension, or both (Figure 21–12). This unesthetic subgingival material has led to three different approaches to metal-ceramic crown margins. The first is the classic metal collar margin, in which a small band of metal creates the terminus for the crown with no porcelain overlaying it. The metal collar margin was the technique for all early metal-ceramic crowns and is currently used for a large proportion of them. Many metal collars have been placed subgingivally with good esthetic results. This requires a superior technical approach to margin preparation, retraction, and impression techniques and soft-tissue management in the interim phase. However, the results are often less than predictable.

This unpredictability of consistently hiding the metal collar subgingivally led to the second approach to metal-ceramic crown margins. This is a compromise variously named the metal-porcelain margin, the covered metal margin, or the disappearing metal margin. This is a technique in which the technician creates the metal collar as thin as possible without opening or shortening the crown margin and then overlays this thin metal with porcelain, also as thin as possible, to completely hide the metal margin. In other words, both metal and porcelain end precisely at the crown margin (Figures 21–13A to D). This compromise, unfortunately, has several severe drawbacks. Because the metal is extremely thin at the margin and is chemically bonded to the porcelain, the marginal metal often distorts more

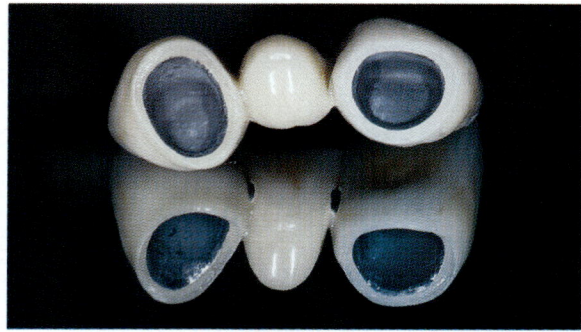

Figure 21–11B: This three-unit metal-ceramic fixed partial denture features a 360-degree all-porcelain margin.

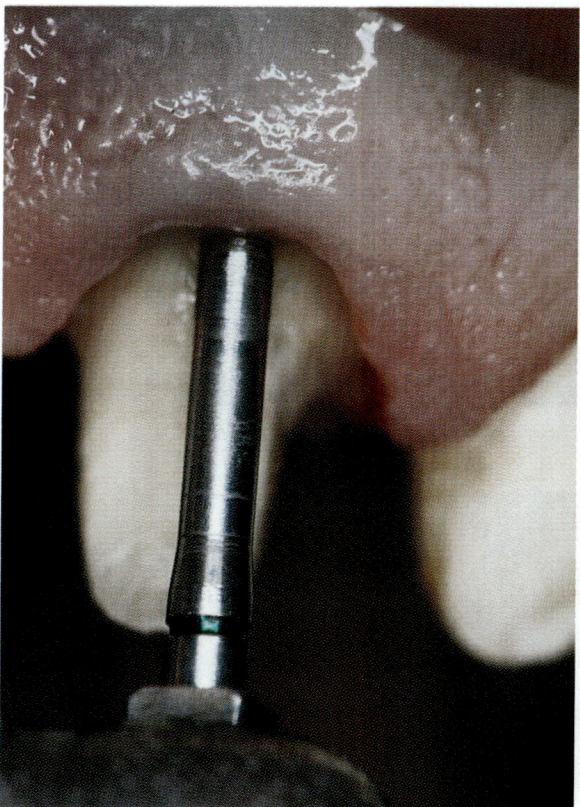

Figure 21–11A: A tissue-protective end-cutting diamond can be used to prepare a 360-degree full-shoulder margin.

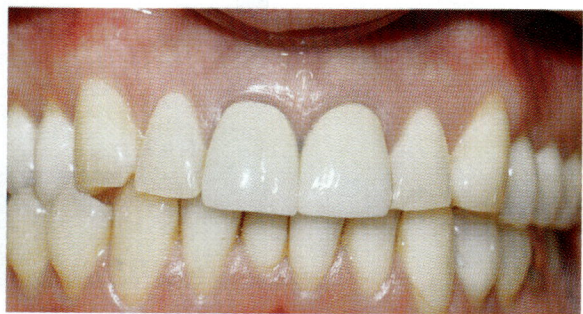

Figure 21–12: Thin, transparent gingiva may not be thick enough to fully mask a subgingival metal margin.

than the traditional metal collar during the porcelain firing cycles.36 Because of the extreme thinness of the porcelain overlying this metal, it is almost purely opaque porcelain (the first coat applied in the firing cycle). This opaque porcelain is virtually unglazable and unpolishable, resulting in a very rough marginal surface. Since there are two layers of restorative material attempting to end at the same finite finish line, the porcelain portion must be external to the normal contour of the tooth prior to preparation, thus creating a potentially rough, open, overcontoured margin. Even the best attempts to hide the metal margin are questionable because the overlying porcelain is often too thin to truly mask the metal color. The margin is still apparent as an off-color area of porcelain even though it is preferable to a shiny silver metal collar.

The third approach to achieving esthetics in the margin area of metal-ceramic crowns is the all-ceramic margin. This is accomplished by removing all metal back to the internal line angle of the shoulder of the preparation as far proximally as is possibly visible and replacing it with a special higher-fusing shoulder porcelain of the same shade as the body or gingival porcelain. Some techniques also remove the metal to some distance up the facial surface of the metal coping.22 It was originally thought that this technique would not yield sufficiently accurate marginal adaptation to be clinically acceptable. Several studies have shown that margins of equal clinical acceptability with metal margins can be created by many different porcelain application techniques.2,4,44 As technicians become more comfortable with these various techniques, clinically acceptable margins may be produced more often. This is due to the virtually infinite ability to repair or correct porcelain margins, a characteristic not possible with cast metal margins. Initially, ceramic margins were not expected to be strong enough to

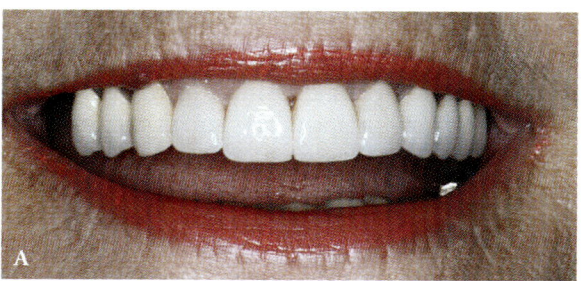
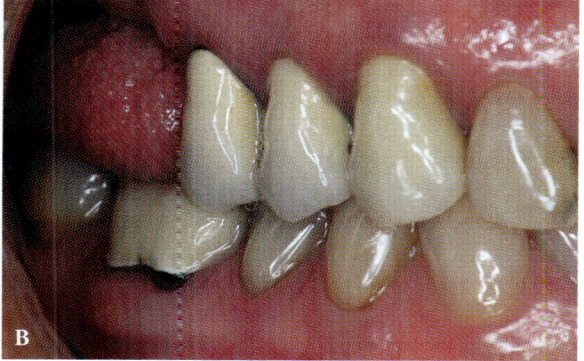

Figure 21–13A and B: This patient was embarrassed to smile fully due to the darkness caused by her missing molars.

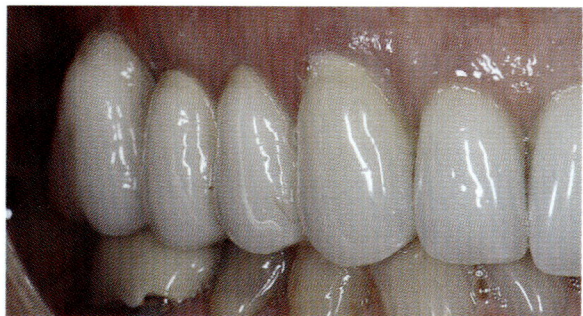
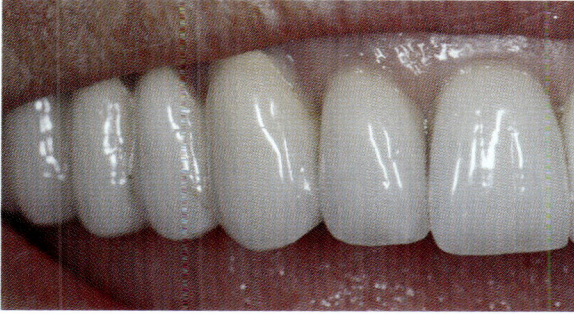

Figure 21–13C: Since she was not a candidate for implants because of advanced bone loss and a large maxillary sinus, this patient elected to have distal extensions for both esthetics and function.

Figure 21–13D: Note how effectively the distal cantilever masks the spaces even with a wide smile.

withstand clinical loads. However, research has indicated that once cemented to the abutment teeth, all-ceramic margins have equal or possibly greater strength than metal collar margins.[12]

The authors' recommendation for margin selection for metal-ceramic retainers is to use metal collar margins in esthetically noncritical areas. These are the ones previously outlined where supragingival margins are esthetically acceptable. All-ceramic margins should be used in the patient's esthetic zone or for patients with higher esthetic demands, and the combination metal-porcelain margin should be avoided whenever possible.

Porcelain–Metal Junction
The last area to consider in the relative esthetics of the metal-ceramic crown is the location of the porcelain–metal junction. Obviously, the most esthetic choice is to cover the entire metal coping with porcelain in all areas of the mouth where the abutment retainer is visible. As long as the underlying metal coping is of sufficient thickness and shape to protect and support the overlying porcelain and the porcelain is of adequate and equal thickness throughout, this design produces no functional problems. If inadequate occlusal reduction occurs in the preparations for porcelain overlying metal, this will usually lead to poor esthetics of the porcelain and often to fracture of the ceramic under functional load. However, in certain patients and certain occlusal schemes, these all-porcelain occlusal surfaces can have disastrous results on the opposing dentition, particularly if the restorations will occlude with natural tooth structure or metal alloy. Nevertheless, all of these rules are negated if the patient expects or demands no metal showing even if he or she has to pull the cheek back to view it.

The most esthetically necessary area for complete-porcelain coverage is the mandibular premolars and first molar (Figure 21–14). This is because the occlusal and lingual surfaces of these teeth are readily visible when the mouth is open. In some patients, even the mandibular second molar is visible. However, except for public performers, who are observed by audiences or cameras from below, rarely are the maxillary posterior occlusal surfaces visible, even in wide open movements. Therefore, from a functional and esthetic perspective, these retainers can usually have porcelain–metal junctions that end on the lingual slope of the bucco-occlusal surfaces (Figure 21–15). The exception to this is when the maxillary fixed prostheses are opposed by all-porcelain occlusal coverage in the mandibular arch. In this case, complete-porcelain coverage of the maxillary restorations is advisable to prevent excessive wear by the opposing porcelain. It does little good to use this buccal-only porcelain coverage in the previously mentioned area of the mandibular premolars and molars since this area of these teeth is covered by the cheek when the mouth is opened and the metal occlusal surface will still be visible (see Figure 21–9B). The delicate balance of porcelain occlusal coverage for esthetics and prevention of wear of the opposing dentition may be compensated for in the posterior occlusion if the patient has anterior or mutually protected occlusion in lateral and protrusive excursive movements. If the patient does not have or cannot be restored to an anterior disclusive occlusal scheme, then the problem of porcelain wear of the opposing dentition must be addressed much as it would in a bruxer or other parafunctional patient with some sort of protective occlusal splint prescription.

The decision of the location of the porcelain–metal junction for maxillary anterior crowns for Angle Class I patients is an entirely different matter. The location of the junction is of little consequence esthetically since the lingual surface of maxillary anterior teeth is never visible. Some clinicians feel that having the intercuspal contact in metal on the maxillary anterior prosthesis will preclude wear. This is not entirely true since all of these patients

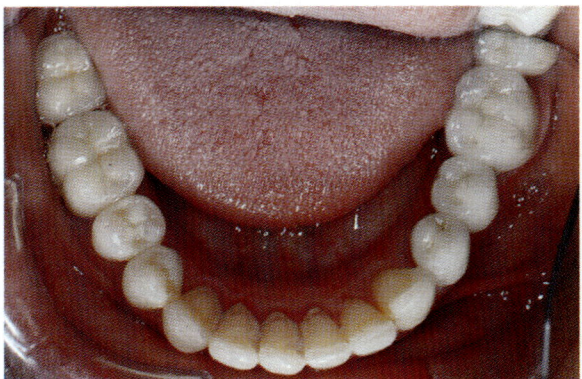

Figure 21–14: The most esthetically necessary use of complete-coverage porcelain is with the mandibular premolar and even the mandibular molars when patients demand them.

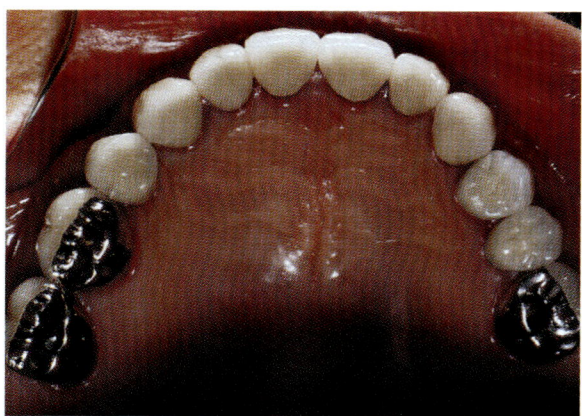

Figure 21–15: This patient was happy with metal occlusal surfaces because he recognized that, under ordinary circumstances, they would not show.

will still function to some degree in excursive movements on porcelain of the lingual surface of these crowns incisively to the porcelain–metal junction. Since porcelain contact in lateral and protrusive movements with the opposing mandibular incisors and canines is unavoidable, the best solution is careful re-creation of the patient's natural incisal guidance in the porcelain prosthesis. This means avoiding creating a new, steeper incisal guide angle or longer incisal guide path. If the patient shows tendencies of parafunction, splint protection should be prescribed. If wear of the opposing mandibular anterior teeth continues, restoration with porcelain of similar hardness may be a last resort. For many patients, the porcelain–metal junction location on mandibular anterior restorations is rarely of importance either esthetically or functionally. Biologically, owing to the small size of mandibular anterior teeth, overcontouring of the lingual surface of the restorations is best avoided by locating the junction as far incisively as esthetics allows.

OTHER CONSIDERATIONS

Anterior Restorations Involving One Missing Tooth

Cantilever Fixed Partial Denture. The ideal choice for the single missing tooth is the single-tooth implant. However, there are times when an implant may not be possible or practical. A conservative alternative would be the cantilever fixed partial denture involving one or more abutment teeth.

The cantilevered restoration is highly desirable esthetically (especially in areas adjacent to sound, attractive teeth), and the final result, using a cantilevered retainer, can be natural looking and quite attractive (Figures 21–16A to G).

For esthetic reasons, it may be necessary to cantilever a posterior abutment. For example, if the patient's smile line shows the missing molar, then this tooth can be replaced as a posterior cantilever (see Figure 21–13).

Implants. It has become the standard of care to also evaluate each patient possessing an edentulous space for the possibility of replacing that space with an implant. The patient has a right to know the potential functional and esthetic success associated with the placement of an implant instead of a fixed or removable prosthesis.

The question of whether to select an implant prosthesis rather than a tooth-borne fixed partial denture is generally decided by the dentist and the patient after a thorough analysis of the advantages and disadvantages, both esthetically and functionally, of each treatment. A frank discussion must include an honest analysis of the longevity, costs, and esthetic appearance of each proposed treatment. Although computer imaging can usually demonstrate the esthetic appearance of the proposed final result, the esthetic difference may be too subtle to see on the computer screen. Instead, a diagnostic waxing may be necessary to reveal the difference, especially if it involves soft-tissue issues. The form of the lip line will help to determine the treatment choice. Further, when a tissue recession problem exists, a periodontal procedure may be necessary regardless of whether an implant or fixed partial denture is chosen.

Splinting. Esthetically, it is much better not to splint the incisors to achieve individuality between teeth. Either separation or the appearance of separation helps to make a missing tooth replacement appear natural. In addition, the lack of splinting will promote easier maintenance and good oral care. However, the issue of splinting is determined by mobility patterns of teeth, and esthetic compromises will necessarily have to be made when functional requirements indicate splinting.

To achieve a natural appearance, restorations should appear bilaterally symmetric. There should

652   Esthetics in Dentistry

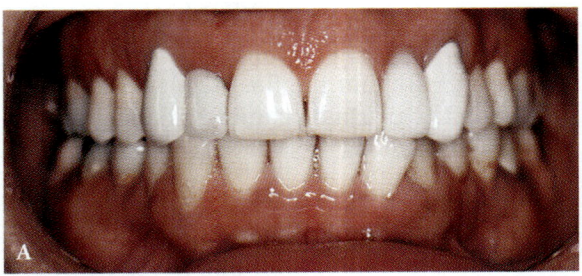 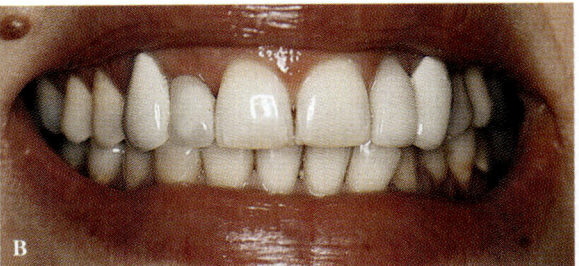

Figure 21–16A and B: This lady, who was congenitally missing her maxillary lateral incisors, was unhappy with the appearance of the replacement fixed cantilever partial dentures.

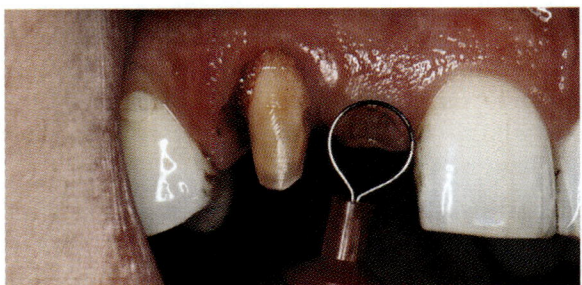 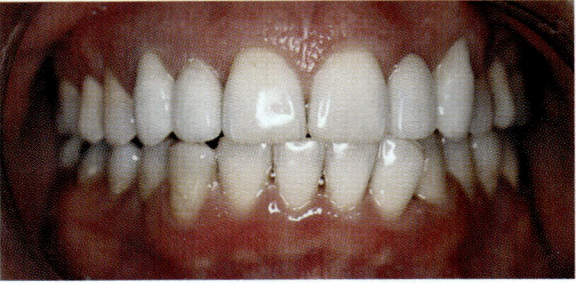

Figure 21–16C: Electrosurgery was used to contour the tissue for the ovate pontic.

Figure 21–16D: The final replacement has a more harmonious gingival relationship between the pontic and the abutment.

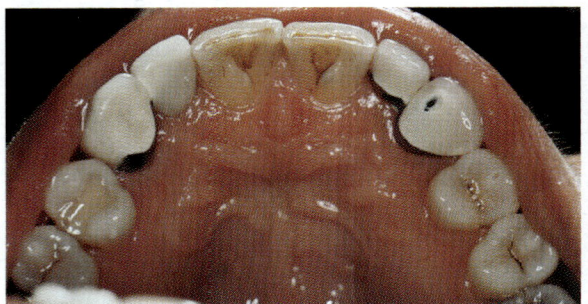 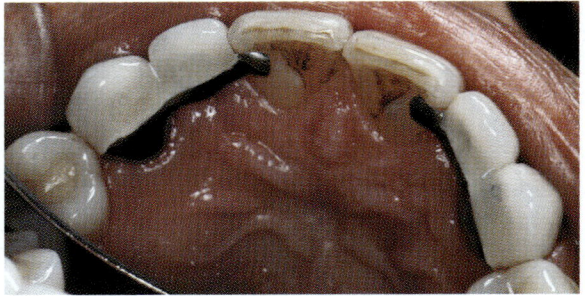

Figure 21–16E: Note that the previous cantilever fixed partial denture had no lingual rest on the lateral incisor.

Figure 21–16F: The new bridges were strengthened by adding lingual rests. Note also the severe stain produced by the patient's continued smoking habit.

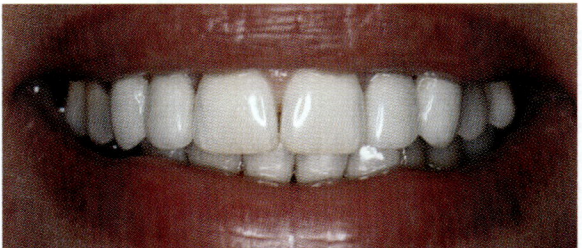

Figure 21–16G: The patient's after smile shows improved shade match, proportion, and fixed partial denture contours.

also be harmony in both gingival contour and incisal levels to prevent a "replacement" look.

Use of Telescoping Crowns as Abutments
Advantages. Telescoping restorations offer certain benefits but are not without problems. One advantage of telescoping crowns is that the preparations do not have to conform to a common path of insertion.[24] Only the functional surfaces of the copings require waxing to a common path. Another advantage is the ability to link different segments of fixed partial dentures while still keeping the span small. This is particularly useful when using a metal-ceramic prosthesis where a long span may produce excessive flexure and, subsequently, the possibility of fracture. It allows the smaller spans to be removed in the event of acrylic resin wear, porcelain fracture, or need for access to the pulp chambers if endodontic procedures become necessary. The flexibility of telescoping procedures permits alterations in design that may not require making the entire restoration. For example, in the event of the loss of a posterior abutment, the superstructure may be able to be redesigned without remaking the entire prosthesis. Depending on how the coping linkage is designed, a great deal of latitude is thus provided.

Building the teeth anterior to the ridge to gain more space should be avoided. This will alter the occlusal relationship, and if the patient has a high or medium lip line, unattractive spaces can result. If extractions are contemplated, the patient's natural teeth should be noted. If they are crowded, they can be restored with crowded or straight teeth. Since crowding indicates a space problem, the patient and the dentist need to understand the esthetic problem and alternative solutions. This situation was treated successfully in a patient who wanted his natural teeth to be copied in the final restoration (Figures 21–17A to G). It is interesting to note that even during the provisional stage, the patient could not enunciate properly until the crowded teeth were simulated.

Figure 21–17C shows the use of four copings splinted to serve as abutments for two possible superstructure combinations. Inserting the six-unit anterior segment separately achieves splinting (Figure 21–17D). The use of the interlock attachments distally on the canines aids retention of two future planned implants. If this were not successful, an alternative plan provides for use of an attachment removable partial denture retained by the remaining copings and interlocks. Figure 21–17E shows the extra superstructure crowns in place with flexibility to be used in either capacity.

The use of telescopic procedures to splint mobile teeth is seen in Figures 21–18A to C. Figure 21–18A shows the copings in place. Note the soldered joints between the canine-lateral incisor on the left side and the canine-premolar on the right side. Figure 21–18B shows the posterior metal-ceramic superstructure in place, and Figure 21–18C shows how the anterior segment completes the splinting using porcelain occlusal surfaces. The copings are cemented with a definitive cement and the superstructure with a provisional cement. If the restoration is to be removed, the superstructure should be designed with exposed metal at the connector site so that a reverse hammer can be used to tap off the superstructure without fracturing the porcelain.

Disadvantages. The main disadvantage in telescoping is twofold. First, bulk is created by an extra layer of metal, which can be a problem unless there is adequate room for preparation. To avoid producing additional stress, the buccolingual diameter of the superstructure should not be increased. Therefore, using telescoping crowns in small, flat teeth should be avoided. Another disadvantage with the coping and telescope procedure is the need for an extra-long gold collar. This may create an esthetic problem at the gingiva unless there is enough space to hide or mask the metal. A compromise coping can be constructed for anterior teeth by not covering the gingival half of the tooth, making crosslinkage possible without loss of esthetics.[26,27]

Copings are especially useful in the patient with a low lip line. The patient should be shown that during normal conversation, laughing, or smiling, the gingival portion of the tooth will not be seen.

Because of increased bulk, metal occlusal surfaces should be used whenever possible for coping procedures. A compromise can be made in the anterior section for esthetic purposes (Figures 21–19A to C). Cross-arch splinting is accomplished by using soldered copings and a three-segment superstructure.

An alternative in the posterior region, where vertical height is severely restricted, is the open-telescopic technique. The occlusal surface of the

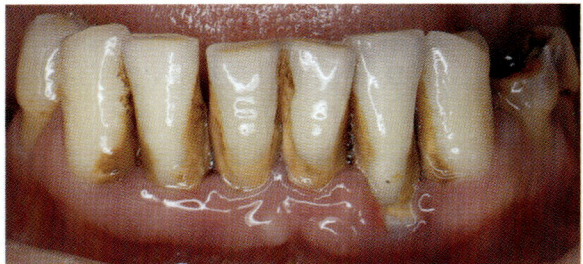

Figure 21–17A: This man had to lose his mandibular incisors due to periodontal disease; he insisted that the replacements copy the look of his natural teeth.

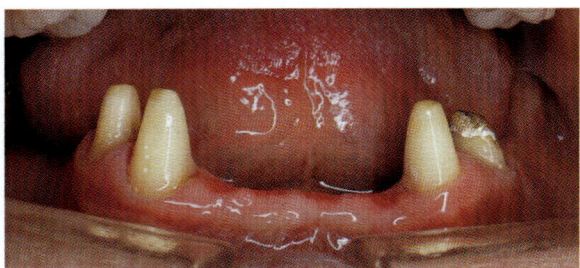

Figure 21–17B: After extraction, even in the provisional stage, the patient could not enunciate correctly until the crowded teeth were simulated.

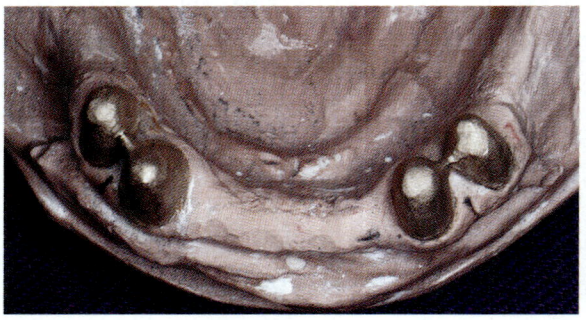

Figure 21–17C: Four copings crosslinked to serve as abutments for two possible superstructure combinations.

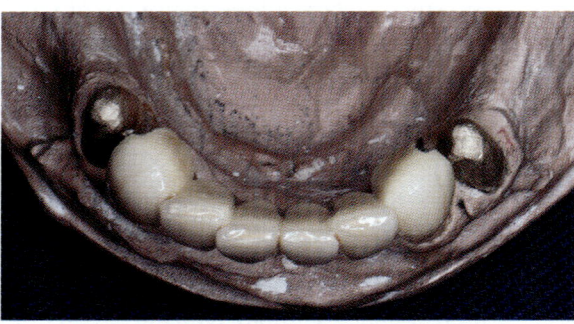

Figure 21–17D: This shows the anterior segment in place.

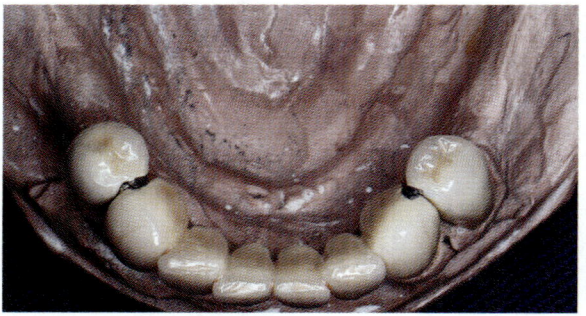

Figure 21–17E: The two premolar crowns can be removed for an attachment removable partial denture in the future.

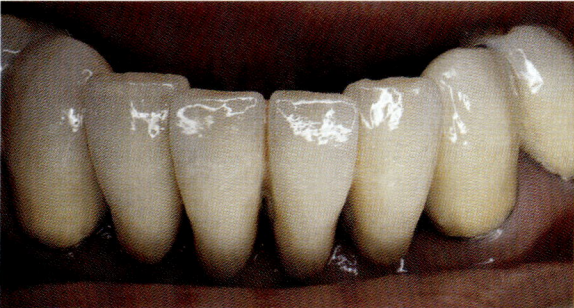

Figure 21–17F: Note how the final metal-ceramic fixed prosthesis accurately simulates his natural dentition.

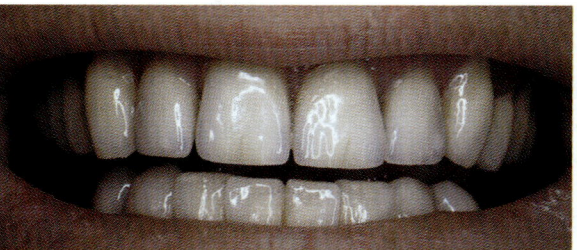

Figure 21–17G: The final smile shows the maxillary denture occluding against the new mandibular prosthesis.

Fixed Replacement of Missing Teeth 655

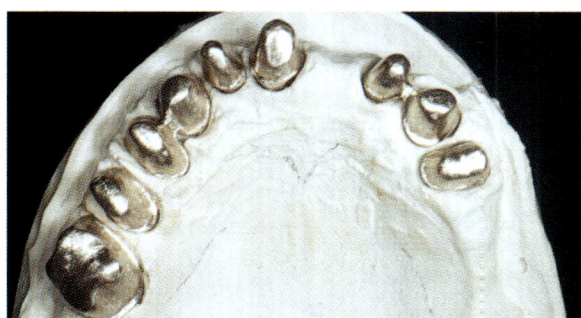

Figure 21–18A: Copings are in place with soldered joints between the canine-lateral incisor on the left side and the canine-premolar on the right side.

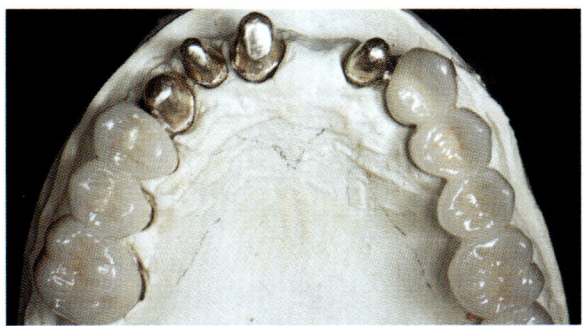

Figure 21–18B: The posterior metal-ceramic superstructure in place.

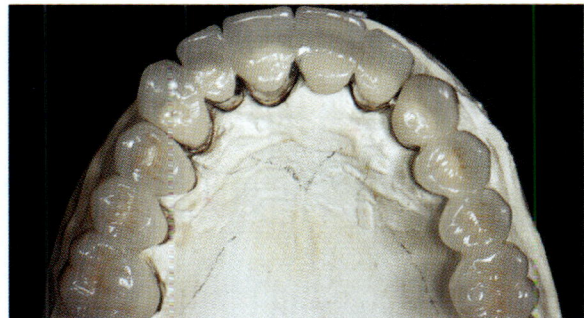

Figure 21–18C The anterior segment completes the crossarch splinting using porcelain occlusal surfaces.

restoration is wholly or partially a part of the inner coping, and the outer crown fits around the inner coping. Provision must be made for occlusal seating by incorporating a shoulder in the coping. Anteriorly, it is possible for the facing material to be on either the coping or the superstructure (Seymour M, personal communication, 1974).

The necessity and advantages of the telescoping procedure should be re-emphasized in a letter to the patient documenting why the procedure is being used.

Use of Precision Attachments

Where advantages outweigh the disadvantages, copings should be used with full-arch procedures if space and economic factors permit. When full-arch copings cannot be used, it is wise to interlock at strategic positions with the use of four copings. These copings can then be splinted together, and three segments can be made. If this is not feasible, an interlocking type of matrix-patrix attachment can be used. It is preferable to use precision attachments that allow either segment to be removed at will. Other types of interlocking devices may require that both segments be removed together to remove the matrix portion. This means more chance for porcelain fracture and is therefore not as convenient a device for cross-arch splinting.

Semiprecision or precision internal attachments in fixed partial dentures may improve the quality of the prosthesis significantly. Their two primary uses are to eliminate problems of parallelism and to interlock smaller segments, which avoids lengthy spans of porcelain to metal.

PONTICS

Pontic Design

The overall esthetic objective in pontic design is to make the missing tooth replacement look like a real tooth. A tooth substitute should be in harmony with the abutment teeth and the remaining dentition. Concealing the fact that the pontic is an artificial replacement is accomplished by the outline form, size, alignment, contour, surface texture, and color. In addition, it must function with the opposing occlusion and provide comfort and support to the adjacent tissues and continuity to food flow patterns; it must have contours that are easy to keep clean.

There are several pontic designs available for fixed partial dentures. The choices include ridge lap, modified ridge lap, conical or bullet, hygienic, modified hygienic, and the ovate pontic (Figure 21–20). Esthetics, edentulous ridge anatomy, and the patient's ability to maintain adequate hygiene must be considered during pontic design selection. Due to the inability of the patient to maintain adequate hygiene under the ridge lap pontic, the authors do not recommend the use of this type of pontic design.

To optimize esthetics, the modified ridge lap described by Stein[40] and the ovate pontic (Figures 21–21A to C)[9,11] are considered the pontics of choice. These two pontic designs work well because a natural-appearing emergence profile can be achieved, leading to a more esthetic result. However, certain requirements are necessary to accomplish a favorable esthetic outcome. The pontic must have the proper incisogingival or occlusogingival length in relation to the abutment teeth. Excessively open

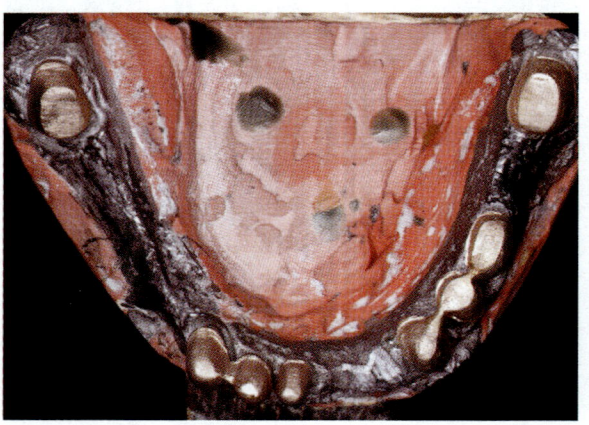

Figure 21–19A: Splinted copings are in place to permit the superstructure to be inserted in three sections.

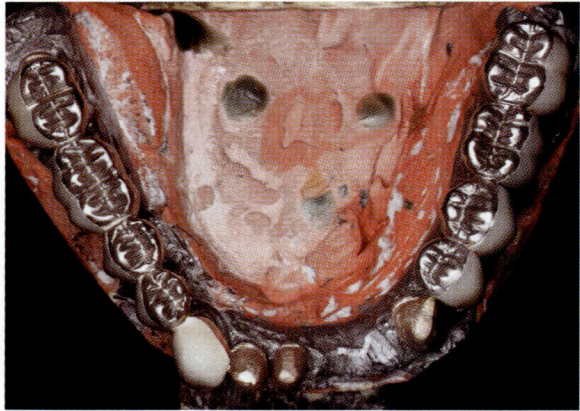

Figure 21–19B: Metal occlusal surfaces were used because this patient had insufficient vertical space for porcelain.

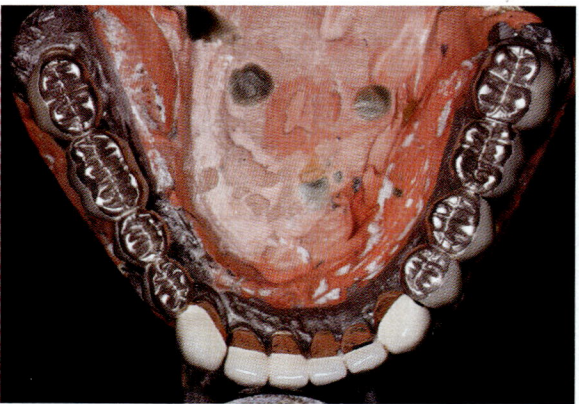

Figure 21–19C: A compromise can usually be obtained anteriorly so that ceramic material can be used.

Fixed Replacement of Missing Teeth 657

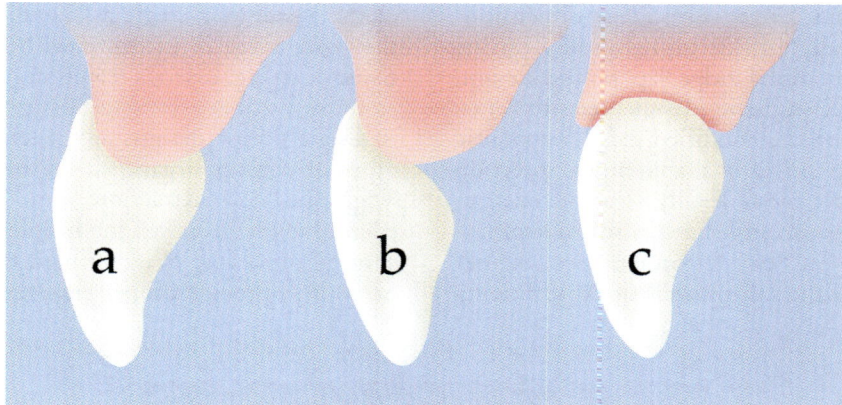

Figure 21–20: Pontic design. *(A)* Total ridge lap. *(B)* Modified ridge lap. *(C)* Ovate.

interproximal embrasures or "black triangles" must be avoided in the anterior region, and a proper labiolingual or buccolingual relationship with the abutment teeth should be obtained, creating a proper emergence profile. To accomplish these three requirements, proper edentulous ridge tissue form is imperative. Preprosthetic surgery is often needed to enhance the edentulous area to achieve the desired esthetic results (Figures 21–22A to E).

Preparation of Tissue

A diagnostic waxing of the fixed partial denture will aid in assessing the pontic–ridge relationship to determine if the three design requirements will be met. If the relationship reveals that an esthetic result would be enhanced through modification of the edentulous ridge area, then further adjunctive therapy should be considered to correct the pontic-tissue site.

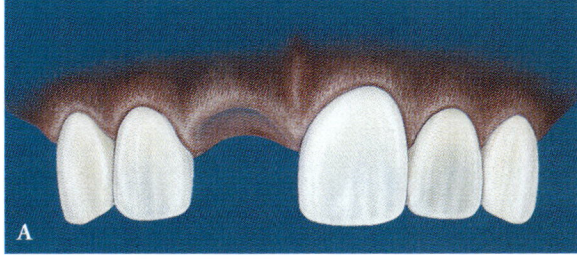

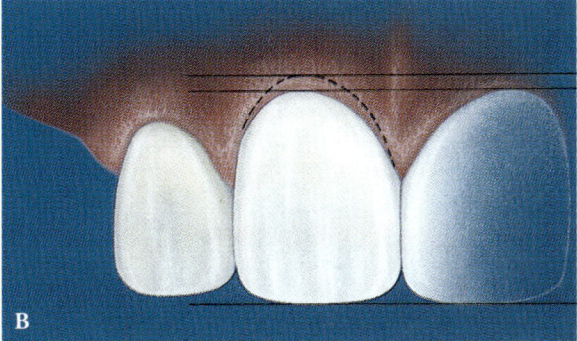

Figure 21–21A and B: The ovate pontic has become one of the most desired forms for maximum esthetics and function.

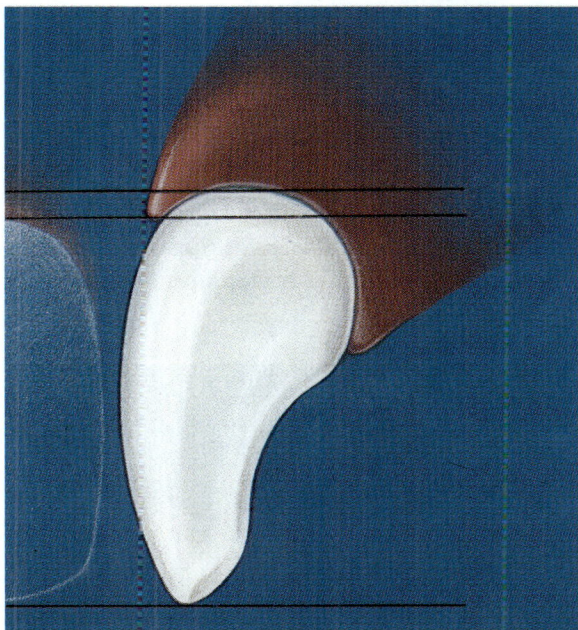

Figure 21–21C: The shape of the pontic, as seen in sagittal section, is conducive to effective cleaning with dental floss.

The edentulous ridge with ideal dimensions both buccolingually and occlusogingivally can be treated with a modified ridge lap pontic design, meeting all three esthetic design requirements. Ridge contour for the modified ridge-lap pontic should be slightly convex in a labiolingual direction and gently concave mesiodistally.[1] For the edentulous ridge that has excessive hard or soft tissue, surgical reduction can be performed (see Figures 21–5D and E). If the soft tissue is thick, scalloping of the tissue may create a favorable pontic site. If the hard tissue is excessive with a minimal soft-tissue covering, osseous resection may be necessary.

Ovate pontic designs are generally used in two types of clinical situations: the healed edentulous ridge and new extraction sites. When a healed edentulous ridge exists, the recipient site requires a surgical procedure of either hard tissue, soft tissue, or both to provide proper emergence from the tis-

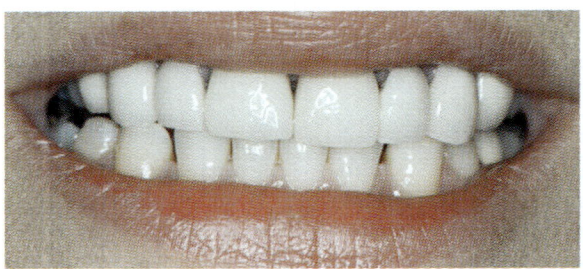

Figure 21–22A: This patient was unhappy with the unnatural-looking "black triangles" caused by loss of interdental tissue.

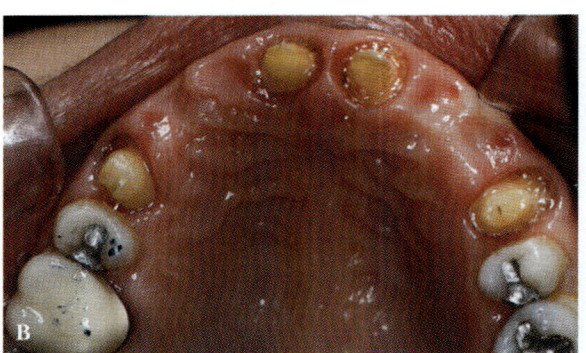
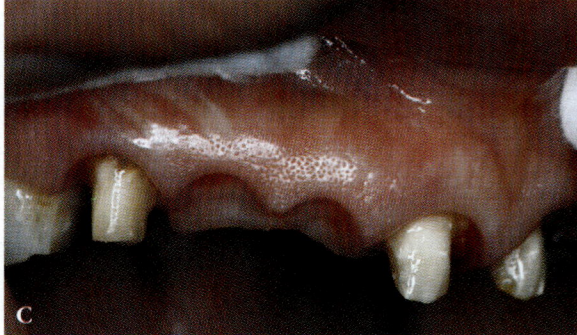

Figure 21–22B and C: Ridge augmentation plus sculpting for ovate pontics was done during the interim phase.

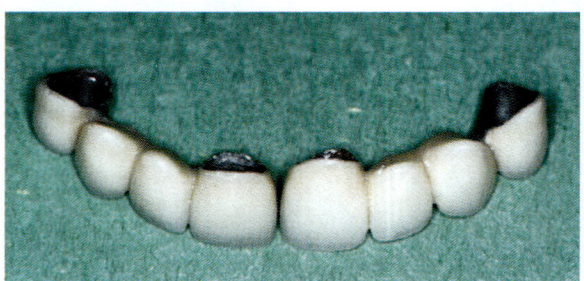
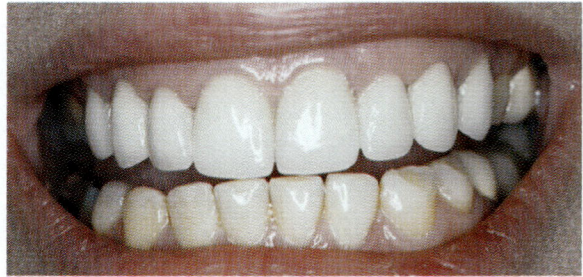

Figure 21–22D: Two four-unit fixed partial dentures were fabricated with ovate pontics.

Figure 21–22E: This patient was extremely pleased that her widest smile did not give a hint of missing teeth.

sue. However, with a new extraction site, at the time of extraction, the abutment teeth can be prepared and the fixed partial denture provisional fabricated; then, the ovate pontic provisional can be placed so that it emerges from the extraction site. This type of procedure quite often leads to a highly acceptable esthetic effect. However, be aware that, occasionally, to enhance esthetics, a surgical procedure may be necessary once the extraction site heals around the pontic. Ridge anatomy for the ovate pontic requires a wider labiolingual ridge dimension (see Figures 21–21A to C).[29]

Adjunctive Tissue Treatment

Frequently, adjunctive treatment involves a deficient edentulous ridge. Deficient pontic areas may occur as a result of trauma, developmental defects, or disease. The edentulous area may be deficient in height, width, or both, depending on the individual situation. Seibert classified the deficient ridge based on the dimension of the defect as follows: (1) buccolingual loss of tissue with normal ridge height (Class I), (2) apicocoronal loss of tissue with normal ridge width (Class II), or (3) combined loss of ridge contour in both the buccolingual and apicocoronal dimensions (Class III).[35] For the deficient ridge, adjunctive treatment involves surgical site augmentation, which can be accomplished using an autogenous or allogenic graft of hard or soft tissues, an alloplastic graft, or a combination of these grafts depending on the amount of augmentation needed. The volume of donor tissue needed to repair the defect and the availability of such tissue will have a bearing on the source of graft material.[15] Larger augmentations quite often involve multiple surgeries to achieve optimal results. However, for sites that can be augmented with soft tissue alone, esthetic results can often be obtained with one surgical grafting procedure. If the deficient site cannot be augmented, for reasons that may include cost, medical history, or too severe a defect, another modality such as a removable partial denture should be considered.

The goal of the pontic site tissue preparation procedure is to provide a ridge in which the pontic looks natural in its emergence. To achieve this, proper soft-tissue thickness must be generated. Although the hard tissue gives the augmented site the necessary support, modifying the thickened-ridge soft tissue helps to eliminate the "black triangles"; then, a proper emergence from the ridge area can be generated.

Tissue thickness over edentulous ridge areas can vary depending on the location. In Stein's study of 50 anterior ridges and 50 posterior ridges, he found that, regardless of the degree of ridge atrophy, the mean tissue thickness of the posterior regions was 2.05 mm. The mandibular anterior region was similar to the posterior regions, whereas the maxillary anterior regions showed a mean tissue thickness of 4.13 mm. This study and many others have shown that pontic placement against the underlying ridge can cause a chronic inflammatory reaction. A certain thickness of tissue needs to be maintained, and encroachment on the tissue leads to an inflammatory process. If additional tissue thickness is generated over the ridge, soft-tissue modification can be performed.[40] Class I category defects can be treated with a soft-tissue augmentation procedure buccally to improve esthetics. This is a highly successful and fairly predictable procedure. Class II and Class III defects are much less predictable and quite often require multiple surgeries to increase the likelihood of a successful result.

The potential pontic site often has a nonrestorable root that needs to be extracted prior to fabrication of the fixed partial denture. Another alternative to the ovate pontic fabricated to the extraction site is orthodontic extrusion of the root, which manipulates "hopeless" teeth to modify local defect areas.[34] Orthodontic extrusion before extraction can modify the ridge to help in controlling pontic site design by also erupting the bone as the tooth erupts.

Prosthodontic preparation prior to ridge augmentation can follow this protocol. Prior to ridge augmentation, the abutments are prepared, and a provisional acrylic resin fixed partial denture is fabricated. The proper form and function of the prosthesis are created in the provisional, and the pontic intaglio surface (the surface that approximates the ridge tissue) is designed to simulate the position and contour desired in the final prostheses. At the surgical appointment, the provisional is removed, and the ridge is augmented. The surgeon uses the intaglio surface of the pontic as a reference point for the amount of augmentation, making sure to compensate for tissue shrinkage. The intaglio surface of the pontic is then modified prior to recementation, ensuring no tissue contact. The surgical site is allowed to heal for 6 to 8 weeks, depending on the location (longer period for anterior esthetic areas). Once adequate healing has occurred, the provisional fixed partial denture is removed, and the pontic intaglio surface is modified by forming acrylic resin to the ideal shape. At this time, the soft tissue is modified either by electrosurgery, a surgical blade, laser surgery, or rotary instrumentation to a contour adaptive to the provisional. The highly polished provisional is again provisionally cemented, and the area is allowed to heal for an additional 6 to 8 weeks prior to making the final impression for the definitive prosthesis. "Scalloping" the soft-tissue site and adapting the fabricated provisional to the scalloped site affords the clinician the opportunity to shape the tissue, creating an esthetic prosthesis. The tissue scalloping allows the pontic to closely mimic the emergence of the abutment teeth. The pontic-ridge relationship will look natural, and the three requirements for an esthetic pontic/edentulous ridge will be met.

If attempts at surgery are unsuccessful or even only moderately successful, resulting in small black triangles, then esthetic masking must take place in the fabrication of the prosthesis. This can take the form of either fixed or removable tissue inserts. The fixed tissue insert can be fabricated from tissue-colored ceramic or composite resin material. Greater longevity if ceramics are used to replace the interdental tissue should be expected (Figures 21–23A to F and 21–24A to C).

As an alternative, some patients use a removable tissue insert fabricated from acrylic resin. Certain patients prefer these, particularly for photographic or social occasions (Figures 21–25A to E).

Pontic Materials

The type of material used to fabricate the pontic also depends on the esthetic result required. Pontic material types can be all metal, metal ceramic, all ceramic, or metal with acrylic resin. Porcelain covering all visible areas is the selection of choice for an esthetic situation. As mentioned earlier, all-ceramic fixed partial dentures should be avoided due to the inherent lack of strength. Metal with acrylic resin is occasionally used today in the posterior regions when

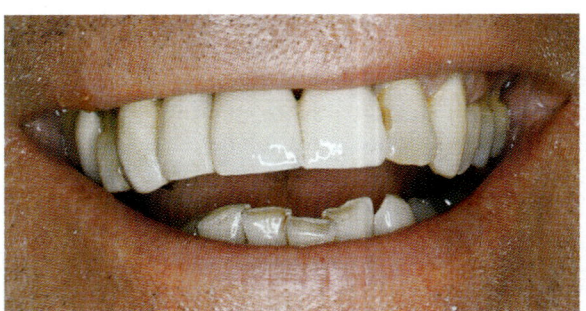

Figure 21–23A: This patient wanted to improve his fixed partial denture without implants or tissue surgery.

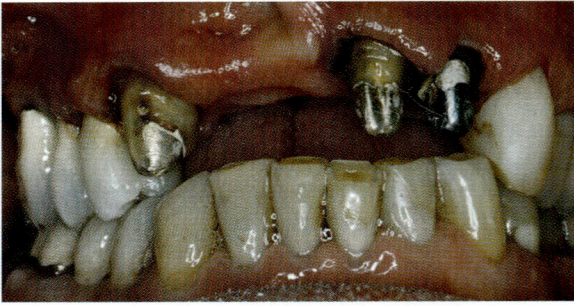

Figure 21–23B: The old fixed partial denture was removed and the abutments reprepared.

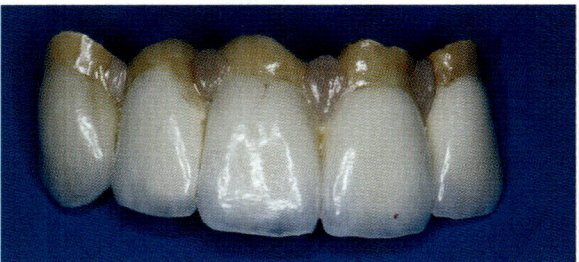

Figure 21–23C: The new five-unit fixed partial denture included fixed pink porcelain to resemble gingival papilla to mask the interdental space.

Fixed Replacement of Missing Teeth 661

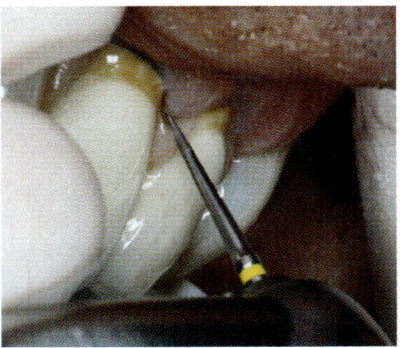

Figure 21–23D: A diamond bur is used to carefully create sufficient space for a floss threader.

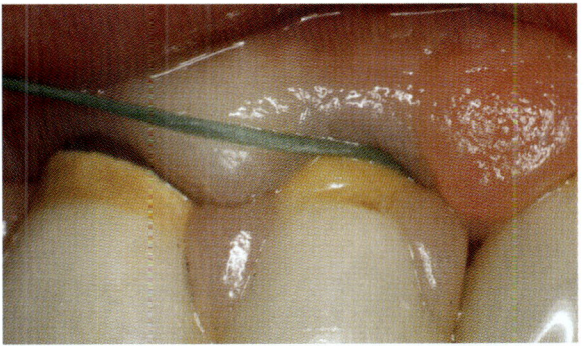

Figure 21–23E: The space allows the floss to effectively clean below the pontic.

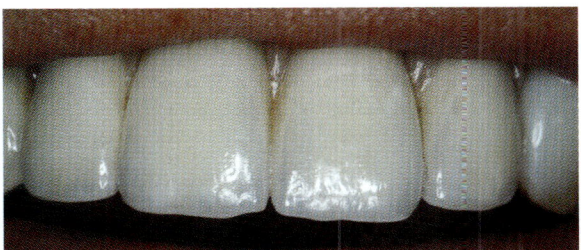

Figure 21–23F: A maximum smile reveals an esthetic result.

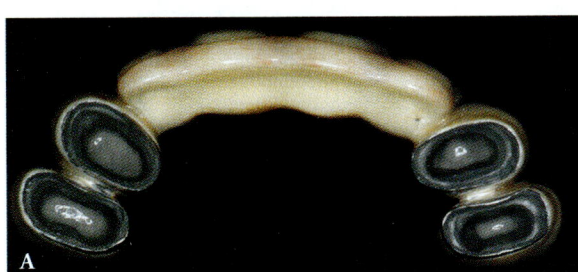

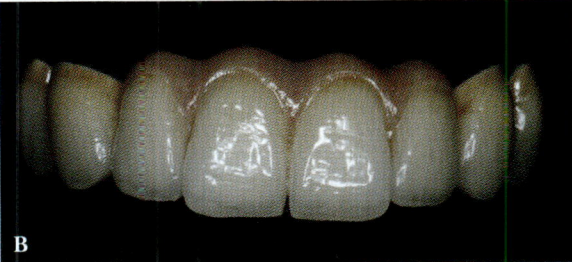

Figure 21–24A and B: This eight-unit fixed partial denture featured four anterior pontics. Note how a pink porcelain fixed-tissue insert was constructed to blend in with this patient's tissue.

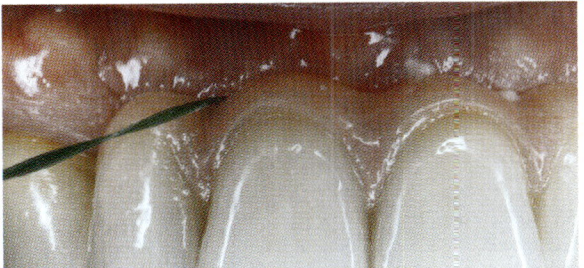

Figure 21–24C: The dental floss can effectively clean above this well-fitting tissue insert.

retainer design dictates Type III gold, but more often than not the esthetic pontic is fabricated as a metal-ceramic prosthesis. The length of span of a fixed partial denture can influence material choice. Many failures associated with the fixed partial denture can be related to the choice of materials.[43] For longer-span fixed partial dentures, the more rigid (higher modulus of elasticity) predominantly base metal alloy such as Rexillium III (Jeneric/Pentron, Wallingford, CT) may be the alloy of choice to minimize flexure.

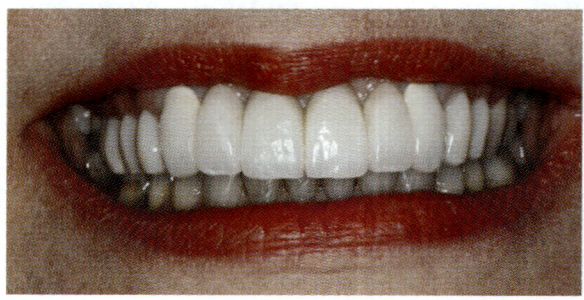

Figure 21–25A: This high fashion model wanted to mask the length of her anterior fixed partial denture so that she could do photographic modeling.

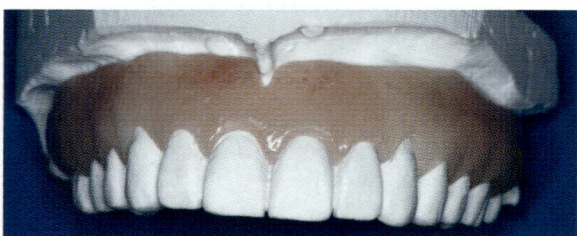

Figure 21–25B: An impression is made of the seated maxillary fixed partial denture. It is then poured and the laboratory waxes, invests, and cures the insert in pink acrylic resin. A slightly flexible removable tissue insert is fabricated that will then lock into her premolars and molars.

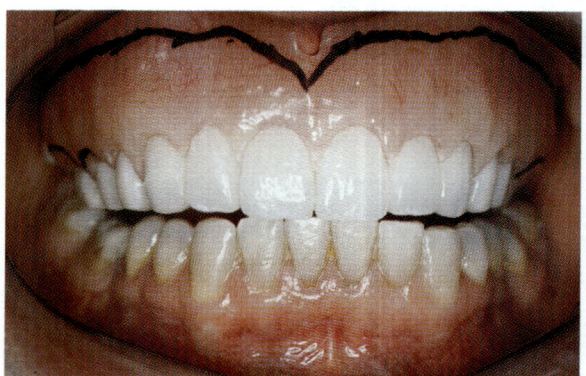

Figure 21–25C: The removable tissue insert is tried in and marked approximately where the flange will be trimmed.

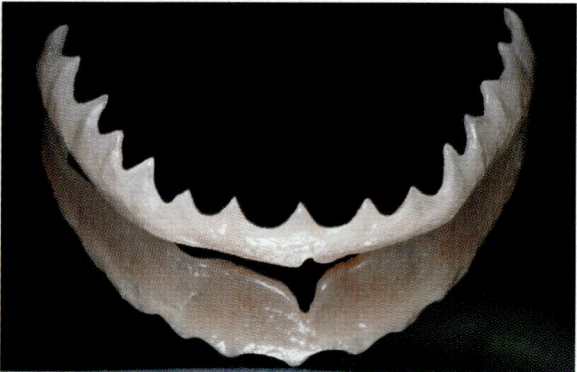

Figure 21–25D: The trimmed and polished, slightly flexible removable insert is photographed on a mirror to view both aspects.

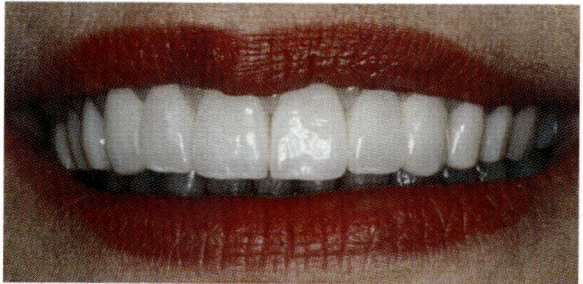

Figure 21–25E: The removable tissue insert camouflages the uneven and excessively long teeth, resulting in an attractive smile.

Proper pontic-tissue contours and surface finish are the key to healthy tissue response. Pontic design has been found to be the foremost factor in obtaining inflammatory-free pontic–ridge relationships. According to Stein, the ideal pontic design is the modified ridge lap with a pinpoint contact on the facial slope of the residual ridge. Surface smoothness and a fine finish are prerequisites; there is no observable distinguishing advantage with porcelain, acrylic resin, or gold. However, Stein also found that modification of the pontic outline form without attention to the surface smoothness did not prevent gingival inflammation.[40] Other studies have found that from a hygienic perspective, glazed porcelain and highly polished gold are preferable choices at this time for tissue contact.[6,23]

CONCLUSION

Although the field of fixed prosthodontics has been greatly enhanced by the emerging field of implant dentistry, patients will continue to desire nonsurgical fixed prosthetics. The future will, no doubt, be influenced by further improvements in the science of dental materials.

References

1. Abrams L. Augmentation of the deformed residual edentulous ridge for fixed prosthetics. Compend Cont Educ Dent 1980;3:205–14.

2. Belser UC, MacEntee MI, Richter WA. Fit of three porcelain-fused-to-metal margin designs in vivo: a scanning electron microscope study. J Prosthet Dent 1985; 53:24–9.

3. Bowley JF, Stockstill JW, Attanasio R. A preliminary diagnostic and treatment protocol. Dent Clin North Am 1992;36:551–68.

4. Boyle JJ Jr, Naylor WP, Blackman RB. Marginal accuracy of metal ceramic restorations with porcelain facial margins. J Prosthet Dent 1993;69:19–27.

5. Brehm TW. Diagnosis and treatment planning for fixed prosthodontics. J Prosthet Dent 1973;30:876–81.

6. Cavazos E Jr. Tissue response to fixed partial denture pontics. J Prosthet Dent 1968;20:143–53.

7. Crispin B, Watson J. Margin placement of esthetic veneer crowns. Part 1: anterior tooth visibility. J Prosthet Dent 1981;45:278–82.

8. De Karter RJ, Creugers NH, Verzijden CW, Van't Hof MA. A five-year multi-practice clinical study on posterior resin-bonded bridges. J Dent Res 1998;77: 609–14.

9. Dewey KW, Zugsmith R. An experimental study of tissue reactions about porcelain roots. J Dent Res 1933;13:459–72.

10. El Salam Shakal MA, Pfeiffer P, Hilgers RD. Effect of tooth preparation on bond strengths of resin-bonded prostheses: a pilot study. J Prosthet Dent 1997;77:243–9.

11. Garber DA, Rosenberg ES. The edentulous ridge in fixed prosthodontics. Compend Cont Educ Dent 1981;2:212–23.

12. Gardner FM, Tillman-McCombs KW, Gaston ML, Runyan DA. In-vitro failure load of metal-collar margins compared with porcelain facial margins of metal-ceramic crowns. J Prosthet Dent 1997;78:1–4.

13. Goldstein CE, Goldstein RE, Garber DA. Computer imaging: an aid to treatment planning. J Calif Dent Assoc 1991;19:47–51.

14. Goldstein RE, Miller MC. High technology in esthetic dentistry. Curr Opin Cosmet Dent 1993;1:5–11.

15. Johnson GK, Leary JM. Pontic design and localized ridge augmentation in fixed partial denture design. Dent Clin North Am 1992;36:591–605.

16. Johnson LA. A systemic evaluation of intraoral cameras. J Calif Dent Assoc 1994;22:34–42, 44–7.

17. Johnson PF, Taybos GM, Grisius RJ. Prosthodontics; diagnostic, treatment planning, and prognostic considerations. Dent Clin North Am 1986;30:503–18.

18. Levin RP. Building your practice with an intraoral video camera. Compendium 1990;11:52, 54, 56.

19. Livaditis GJ. Cast metal resin-bonded retainers for posterior teeth. J Am Dent Assoc 1980;110:926–9.

20. McCracken WL. Differential diagnosis: fixed or removable partial dentures? J Am Dent Assoc 1961;63: 767–75.

21. Musikant BL, Cohen BI, Deutsch AS. The surgical microscope, not just for the specialist. N Y State Dent J 1996;62:33–5.

22. O'Boyle KH, Norling BK, Cagna DR, Phoenix RD. An investigation of new metal framework design for metal ceramic restorations. J Prosthet Dent 1997; 78:295–301.

23. Podshadley AG. Gingival response to pontics. J Prosthet Dent 1968;19:51–7.

24. Preiskel H. Telescopic prosthesis. Israel J Dent 1969;18:12.

25. Preston JD. Rational approach to tooth preparation for ceramo-metal restorations. Dent Clin North Am 1977;21:683–98.

26. Prichard JP. Advanced periodontal diseases. 2nd edn. Philadelphia: WB Saunders, 1972.

27. Prichard JF, Feder M. A modern adaptation of the telescopic principle in periodontal prosthesis. J Periodont 1962;33:360.

28. Priest G. An 11-year reevaluation of resin-bonded fixed partial dentures. Int J Periodont Restor Dent 1995;15:238–47.

29. Reel DC. Establishing esthetic contours of the partially edentulous ridge. Quintessence Int 1988;19:301–10.

30. Reynolds MJ. Abutment selection for fixed prosthetics. J Prosthet Dent 1968;19:483–8.

31. Richter WA, Ueno H. Relationship of crown margin placement to gingival inflammation. J Prosthet Dent 1973;30:156–61.

32. Rochette AL. Attachment of a splint to enamel of lower anterior teeth. J Prosthet Dent 1973; 30:418–23.

33. Saad AA, Claffey N, Byrne D, Hussey D. Effects of groove placement on retention/resistance of maxillary anterior resin-bonded retainers. J Prosthet Dent 1995; 74:133–9.

34. Salama H, Salama M. The role of orthodontic extrusive remodeling in the enhancement of soft and hard tissue profiles prior to implant placement: a systematic approach to the management of extraction site defects. Int J Periodont Restor Dent 1993;13:313–33.

35. Seibert JS. Reconstruction of deformed, partially edentulous ridges, using full thickness onlay grafts. Part I. Technique and wound healing. Compend Cont Educ Dent 1983;4:437–53.

36. Shillingburg HT, Hobo S, Fisher DW. Preparation design and margin distortion in porcelain-fused-to-metal restorations. J Prosthet Dent 1973;29:276–84.

37. Shrout MK, Russell CM, Potter BJ, et al. Digital enhancement of radiographs: can it improve caries diagnosis? J Am Dent Assoc 1996;127:469–73.

38. Silness J. Periodontal conditions in patients treated with dental bridges. 2. The influence of full and partial crowns on plaque accumulation, development of gingivitis and pocket formation. J Periodont Res 1970;5:219–24.

39. Silverman SI. Differential diagnosis. Fixed or removable prosthesis? Dent Clin North Am 1987;31:347–62.

40. Stein RS. Pontic-residual ridge relationship: a research report. J Prosthet Dent 1966;16:251–85.

41. Thompson VP, Del Castillo E, Livaditis GJ. Resin-bonded retainers. Part 1: resin bond to electrolytically etched non-precious alloys. J Prosthet Dent 1983;50:771–9.

42. van der Stelt PF. Improved diagnosis with digital radiography. Curr Opin Dent 1992;2:1–6.

43. Walton JN, Gardner FM, Agar JR. A survey of crown and fixed partial denture failures: length of service and reasons for replacement. J Prosthet Dent 1986;56:416–21.

44. Wanserski DJ, Sobczak KP, Monaco JG, McGivney GP. An analysis of margin adaptation of all-porcelain facial margin ceramometal crowns. J Prosthet Dent 1986;56:289–97.

Additional Resources

Garber DA, Adar P, Goldstein RE, Salama H. The quest for the all-ceramic restoration. Quint Dent Tech 2000;23:27–37.

Goldstein RE. Esthetics in dentistry. Philadelphia: JB Lippincott, 1976.

Goldstein RE. Diagnostic dilemma: to bond, laminate, or crown? Int J Periodont Restor Dent 1987;87(5):9–30.

Goldstein RE. Esthetic principles for ceramo-metal restorations. Dent Clin North Am 1988;21:803–22.

Goldstein RE. Change your smile. 3rd edn. Carol Stream, IL: Quintessence, 1997.

Goldstein RE, Adar P. Special effects and internal characterization. J Dent Technol 1989;17:11.

Goldstein RE, Feinman RA, Garber DA. Esthetic considerations in the selection and use of restorative materials. Dent Clin North Am 1983;27:723–31.

Goldstein RE, Garber DA, Goldstein CE, et al. The changing esthetic dental practice. J Am Dent Assoc 1994;125:1447–57.

Goldstein RE, Garber DA, Schwartz CG, Goldstein CE. Patient maintenance of esthetic restorations. J Am Dent Assoc 1992;123:61–6.

Gregory-Head B, Curtis DA. Erosion caused by gastroesophageal reflux: diagnostic considerations. J Prosthodont 1997;6:278–85.

Grippo JO. Abfractions: a new classification of hard tissue lesions of teeth. J Esthet Dent 1991;3:14–9.

Grippo JO. Noncarious cervical lesions: the decision to ignore or restore. J Esthet Dent 1992;4(Suppl):55–64.

Hacker CH, Wagner WC, Razzoog ME. An in vitro investigation of the wear of enamel on porcelain and gold in saliva. J Prosthet Dent 1996;75:14–7.

Harris EF, Butler ML. Patterns of incisor root resorption before and after orthodontic correction in cases with anterior open bites. Am J Orthod Dentofac Orthop 1992;101:112–9.

Hazelton LR, Faine MP. Diagnosis and dental management of eating disorder patients. Int J Prosthodont 1996;9:65–73.

Hertzberg J, Nakisbendi L, Needleman HL, Pober B. Williams syndrome—oral presentation of 45 cases. Pediatr Dent 1994;16:262–7.

Heymann HO, Sturdevant JR, Bayne S, et al. Examining tooth flexure effects on cervical restorations: a two year clinical study. J Am Dent Assoc 1991;122:41–7.

Hicks RA, Conti P. Nocturnal bruxism and self reports of stress-related symptoms. Percept Mot Skills 1991;72:1182.

Hicks RA, Lucero-Gorman K, Bautista J, Hicks GJ. Ethnicity and bruxism. Percept Mot Skills 1999;88:240–1.

Horsted-Bindslev P, Knudsen J, Baelum V. 3-year clinical evaluation of modified Gluma adhesive systems in cervical abrasion/erosion lesions. Am J Dent 1996;9:22–6.

Hsu LK. Epidemiology of the eating disorders. Psychiatr Clin North Am 1996;19:681–700.

Hudson JD, Goldstein GR, Georgescu M. Enamel wear caused by three different restorative materials. J Prosthet Dent 1995;74:647–54.

Hugoson A, Ekfeldt A, Koch G, Hallonsten AL. Incisal and occlusal tooth wear in children and adolescents in a Swedish population. Acta Odontol Scand 1996;54:263–70.

Ikeda T, Nishigawa K, Kondo K, et al. Criteria for the detection of sleep-associated bruxism in humans. J Orofac Pain 1996;10:270–82.

Imfeld T. Dental erosion. Definition, classification and links. Eur J Oral Sci 1996;104:151–4.

Imfeld T. Prevention of progression of dental erosion by professional and individual prophylactic measures. Eur J Oral Sci 1996;104:215–20.

Ingleby J, Mackie IC. Case report: an unusual cause of toothwear. Dent Update 1995;22:434–5.

Jagger DC, Harrison A. An in vitro investigation into the wear effects of selected restorative materials on enamel. J Oral Rehabil 1995;22:275–81.

Jagger DC, Harrison A. An in vitro investigation into the wear effects of selected restorative materials on dentine. J Oral Rehabil 1995;22:349–54.

Jarvinen VK, Rytomaa II, Heinonen OP. Risk factors in dental erosion. J Dent Res 1991;70:942–7.

Johansson A. A cross-cultural study of occlusal tooth wear. Swed Dent J Suppl 1992;86:1–59.

Josell SD. Habits affecting dental and maxillofacial growth and development. Dent Clin North Am 1995;39:851–60.

Josephson CA. Restoration of mandibular incisors with advanced wear. J Dent Assoc S Afr 1992;47:419–20.

Kaidonis JA, Richards LC, Townsend GC, Tansley GD. Wear of human enamel: a quantitative in vitro assessment. J Dent Res 1998;77:1983–90.

Kampe T, Hannerz H, Strom P. Ten-year follow-up study of signs and symptoms of craniomandibular disorders in adults with intact and restored dentitions. J Oral Rehabil 1996;23:416–23.

Kelleher M, Bishop K. The aetiology and clinical appearance of tooth wear. Eur J Prosthodont Restor Dent 1997;5:157–60.

Khan F, Young WG, Daley TJ. Dental erosion and bruxism. A tooth wear analysis from south east Queensland. Aust Dent J 1998;43:117–27.

Kidd EA, Smith BG. Toothwear histories: a sensitive issue. Dent Update 1993;20:174–8.

Kiliaridis S, Johansson A, Haraldson T, et al. Craniofacial morphology, occlusal traits, and bite force in persons with advanced occlusal tooth wear. Am J Orthodont Dentofac Orthop 1995;107:286–92.

Kleinberg I. Bruxism: aetiology, clinical signs and symptoms. Aust Prosthodont J 1994;8:9–17.

Knight DJ, Leroux BG, Zhu C, et al. A longitudinal study of tooth wear in orthodontically treated patients. Am J Orthod Dentofacial Orthop 1997;112:194–202.

Kokich VG. Esthetics and vertical tooth position: orthodontic possibilities. Compend Cont Educ Dent 1997; 18:1225–31.

Lambrechts P, van Meerbeek B, Perdigao J, et al. Restorative therapy for erosive lesions. Eur J Oral Sci 1996;104:229–40.

Lavigne GL, Rompre PH, Montplaisir JY. Sleep bruxism: validity of clinical research diagnostic criteria in a controlled polysomnographic study. J Dent Res 1996; 75:546–52.

Lee CL, Eakle WS. Possible role of tensile stress in the etiology of cervical erosive lesions of teeth. J Prosthet Dent 1984;52:374–80.

Lee CL, Eakle WS. Stress-induced cervical lesions: review of advances in the past 10 years. J Prosthet Dent 1996;75:487–94.

Leinfelder KF, Yarnell G. Occlusion and restorative materials. Dent Clin North Am 1995;39:355–61.

Leung AK, Robson WL. Thumb sucking. Am Fam Physician 1991;44:1724–8.

Levine RS. Briefing paper: oral aspects of dummy and digit sucking. Br Dent J 1999;186:108.

Lussi A. Dental erosion clinical diagnosis and case history taking. Eur J Oral Sci 1996;104:191–8.

Lussi A, Portmann P, Burhop B. Erosion on abraded dental hard tissues by acid lozenges: an in situ study. Clin Oral Investig 1997;1:191–4.

Mair LH, Stolarski TA, Vowles RW, Lloyd CH. Wear: mechanisms, manifestations and measurement. Report of a workshop. J Dent 1996;24:141–8.

Marchesan IQ, Krakauer LR. The importance of respiratory activity in myofunctional therapy. Int J Orofac Myol 1996;22:23–7.

Maron FS. Enamel erosion resulting from hydrochloride acid tablets. J Am Dent Assoc 1996;127:781–4.

Matis BA, Cochran M, Carlson T. Longevity of glass-ionomer restorative materials: results of a 10-year evaluation. Quintessence Int 1996;27:373–82.

McCoy G. The etiology of gingival erosion. J Oral Implantol 1982;10:361–2.

McCoy G. On the longevity of teeth. J Oral Implantol 1983;11:248–67.

McIntyre JM. Erosion. Aust Prosthodont J 1992;6:17–25.

Mehler PS, Gray MC, Schulte M. Medical complications of anorexia nervosa. J Womens Health 1997;6:533–41.

Menapace SE, Rinchuse DJ, Zullo T, et al. The dentofacial morphology of bruxers versus non-bruxers. Angle Orthod 1994;64:43–52.

Mercado MD. The prevalence and aetiology of craniomandibular disorders among completely edentulous patients. Aust Prosthodont J 1993;7:27–9.

Mercado MD, Faulkner KD. The prevalence of craniomandibular disorders in completely edentulous denture-wearing subjects. J Oral Rehabil 1991;18:231–42.

Metaxas A. Oral habits and malocclusion. A case report. Ont Dent 1996;73:27.

Millward A, Shaw L, Smith AJ. Dental erosion in four-year-old children from differing socioeconomic backgrounds. ASDC J Dent Child 1994;61:263–366.

Millward A, Shaw L, Smith AJ, et al. The distribution and severity of tooth wear and the relationship between erosion and dietary constituents in a group of children. Int J Paediatr Dent 1994;4:151–7.

Milosevic A. Tooth wear: an aetiological and diagnostic problem. Eur J Prosthodont Restor Dent 1993;1:173–8.

Milosevic A, Brodie DA, Slade PD. Dental erosion, oral hygiene, and nutrition in eating disorders. Int J Eat Disord 1997;21:195–9.

Milosevic A, Dawson LJ. Salivary factors in vomiting bulimics with and without pathological tooth wear. Caries Res 1996;30:361–6.

Milosevic A, Lennon MA, Fear SC. Risk factors associated with tooth wear in teenagers: a case control study. Community Dent Health 1997;14:143–7.

Morley J. The esthetics of anterior tooth aging. Curr Opin Cosmet Dent 1997;4:35–9.

Moses AJ. Thumb sucking or thumb propping? CDS Rev 1987;80:40–2.

Moss RA, Lombardo TW, Villarosa GA, et al. Oral habits and TMJ dysfunction in facial pain and non-pain subjects. J Oral Rehabil 1995;22:79–81.

Murray CG, Sanson GD. Thegosis—a critical review. Aust Dent J 1998;43:192–8.

Nel JC, Bester SP, Snyman WD. Bruxism threshold: an explanation for successful treatment of multifactorial aetiology of bruxism. Aust Prosthodont J 1995;9:33–7.

Nel JC, Marais JT, van Vuuren PA. Various methods of achieving restoration of tooth structure loss due to bruxism. J Esthet Dent 1996;8:183–8.

Nemcovsky CE, Artzi Z. Erosion-abrasion lesions revisited. Compend Cont Educ Dent 1996;17:416–8.

Neo J, Chew CL. Direct tooth-colored materials for noncarious lesions: a 3-year clinical report. Quintessence Int 1995;27:183–8.

Neo J, Chew CL, Yap A, Sidhu S. Clinical evaluation of tooth-colored materials in cervical lesions. Am J Dent 1996;9:15–8.

Nunn JH. Prevalence of dental erosion and the implications for oral health. Eur J Oral Sci 1996;104:156–61.

Nunn J, Shaw L, Smith A. Tooth wear—dental erosion. Br Dent J 1996;180:349–52.

Nystrom M, Kononen M, Alaluusua S, et al. Development of horizontal tooth wear in maxillary anterior teeth from five to 18 years of age. J Dent Res 1990;69:1765–70.

Okeson JP. Occlusion and functional disorders of the masticatory system. Dent Clin North Am 1995;39:285–300.

Osborne-Smith KL, Burke FJ, Farlane TM, Wilson NH. Effect of restored and unrestored non-carious cervical lesions on the fracture resistance of previously restored maxillary premolar teeth. J Dent 1998;26:427–33.

O'Sullivan EA, Curzon ME, Roberts GJ, et al. Gastroesophageal reflux in children and its relationship to erosion of primary and permanent teeth. Eur J Oral Sci 1998;106:765–9.

Owens BM, Gallien GS. Noncarious dental "abfraction" lesions in an aging population. Compend Cont Educ Dent 1995;16:552–62.

Paterson AJ, Watson IB. Case report: prolonged match chewing: an unusual case of tooth wear. Eur J Prosthodont Restor Dent 1995;3:131–4.

Pavone BW. Bruxism and its effect on the natural teeth. J Prosthet Dent 1985;53:692–6.

Pierce CJ, Chrisman K, Bennett ME, Close JM. Stress, anticipatory stress, and psychologic measures related to sleep bruxism. J Orofac Pain 1995;9:51–6.

Pintado MR, Anderson GC, DeLong R, Douglas WH. Variation in tooth wear in young adults over a two-year period. J Prosthet Dent 1997;77:313–20.

Powell LV, Johnson GH, Gordon GE. Factors associated with clinical success of cervical abrasion/erosion restorations. Oper Dent 1995;20:7–13.

Principato JJ. Upper airway obstruction and craniomandibular morphology. Otolaryngol Head Neck Surg 1991;104:881–90.

Ramp MH, Suzuki S, Cox CF, et al. Evaluation of wear: enamel opposing three ceramic materials and a gold alloy. J Prosthet Dent 1997;77:523–30.

Ribeiro RA, Romano AR, Birman EG, Mayer MP. Oral manifestations of Rett syndrome: a study of 17 cases. Pediatr Dent 1997;19:349–52.

Ritchard A, Welsh AH, Donnelly C. The association between occlusion and attrition. Aust Orthod J 1992;12:138–42.

Rivera-Morales WC, McCall WD Jr. Reliability of a portable electromyographic unit to measure bruxism. J Prosthet Dent 1995;73:184–9.

Robb ND, Cruwys E, Smith BG. Regurgitation erosion as a possible cause of tooth wear in ancient British populations. Arch Oral Biol 1991;36:595–602.

Rogers GM, Poore MH, Ferko BL, et al. In vitro effects of an acidic by-product feed on bovine teeth. Am J Vet Res 1997;58:498–503.

Schmidt U, Treasure J. Eating disorders and the dental practitioner. Eur J Prosthodont Restor Dent 1997;5:161–7.

Schneider PE. Oral habits—harmful and helpful. Update Pediatr Dent 1991;4:1–4, 6–8.

Schwartz JH, Brauer J, Gordon-Larsen P. Brief communication: Tigaran (Point Hope, Alaska) tooth drilling. Am J Phys Anthropol 1995;97:77–82.

Seligman DA, Pullinger AG. The degree to which dental attrition in modern society is a function of age and of canine contact. J Orofac Pain 1995;9:266–75.

Seow WK. Clinical diagnosis of enamel defects: pitfalls and practical guidelines. Int Dent J 1997;47:173–82.

Sherfudin H, Abdullah A, Shaik H, Johansson A. Some aspects of dental health in young adult Indian vegetarians. A pilot study. Acta Odontol Scand 1996; 54:44–8.

Silness J, Berge M, Johannessen G. A 2-year follow-up study of incisal tooth wear in dental students. Acta Odontol Scand 1995;53:331–3.

Silness J, Berge M, Johannessen G. Longitudinal study of incisal tooth wear in children and adolescents. Eur J Oral Sci 1995;103:90–4.

Silness J, Berge M, Johannessen G. Re-examination of incisal tooth wear in children and adolescents. J Oral Rehabil 1997;24:405–9.

Smith BG, Bartlett DW, Robb ND. The prevalence, etiology and management of tooth wear in the United Kingdom. J Prosthet Dent 1997;78:367–72.

Smith BG, Robb ND. The prevalence of toothwear in 1007 dental patients. J Oral Rehabil 1996;23:232–9.

Sognnaes RF, Wolcott RB, Xhonga FA. Dental erosion I. Erosion-like patterns occurring in association with other dental conditions. J Am Dent Assoc 1972;84:571–6.

Speer JA. Bulimia: full stomach, empty lives. Dent Assist 1991;60:28–30.

Spranger H. Investigation into the genesis of angular lesions at the cervical region of teeth. Quintessence Int 1995;26:183–8.

Steiner H, Lock J. Anorexia nervosa and bulimia nervosa in children and adolescents: a review of the past 10 years. J Am Acad Child Adolesc Psychiatry 1998;37:352–9.

Stewart B. Restoration of the severely worn dentition using a systematized approach for a predictable prognosis. Int J Periodont Restor Dent 1998;18:46–57.

Suzuki S, Suzuki SH, Cox CF. Evaluating the antagonistic wear of restorative materials when placed against human enamel. J Am Dent Assoc 1996;127:74–80.

Taylor G, Taylor S, Abrams R, Mueller W. Dental erosion associated with asymptomatic gastroesophageal reflux. ASDC J Dent Child 1992;59:182–5.

Teaford MF, Lytle JD. Brief communication: diet-induced changes in the rates of human tooth microwear: a case study involving stone-ground maize. Am J Phys Anthropol 1996;100:143–7.

Teo C, Young WG, Daley TJ, Sauer H. Prior fluoridation in childhood affects dental caries and tooth wear in a south east Queensland population. Aust Dent J 1997;42:92–102.

Thompson BA, Blount BW, Krumholz TS. Treatment approaches to bruxism. Am Fam Physician 1994;49: 1617–22.

Timms DJ, Trenouth MJ. A quantified comparison of craniofacial form with nasal respiratory function. Am J Orthod Dentofac Orthop 1988;94:216–21.

Touyz LZ. The acidity (pH) and buffering capacity of Canadian fruit juice and dental implications. J Can Dent Assoc 1994;60:448–54.

Turp JC, Gobetti JP. The cracked tooth syndrome: an elusive diagnosis. J Am Dent Assoc 1996;127:1502–7.

Tyas MJ. The Class V lesion—aetilogy and restoration. Aust Dent J 1995;40:167–70.

Ung N, Koenig J, Shapiro PA, et al. A quantitative assessment of respiratory patterns and their effects on dentofacial development. Am J Orthod Dentofac Orthop 1990;98:523–32.

Villa G, Giacobini G. Subvertical grooves of interproximal facets in Neandertal posterior teeth. Am J Phys Anthropol 1995;96:51–62.

Waterman ET, Koltai PJ, Downey JC, Cacace AT. Swallowing disorders in a population of children with cerebral palsy. Int J Pediatr Otorhinolaryngol 1992;24:63–71.

West NX, Maxwell A, Hughes JA, et al. A method to measure clinical erosion: the effect of orange juice consumption on erosion of enamel. J Dent 1998;26:329–35.

Westergaard J, Moe D, Pallesen U, Holmen L. Exaggerated abrasion/erosion of human dental enamel surfaces: a case report. Scand J Dent Res 1993;101:265–9.

Woodside DG, Linder-Aronson S, Lundstrom A, McWilliam J. Mandibular and maxillary growth after changed mode of breathing. Am J Orthod Dentofac Orthop 1991;100:1–18.

Yaacob HB, Park AW. Dental abrasion pattern in a selected group of Malaysians. J Nihon Univ Sch Dent 1990;32:175–80.

Yamaguchi H, Tanaka Y, Sueishi K, et al. Changes in oral functions and muscular behavior due to surgical orthodontic treatment. Bull Tokyo Dent Coll 1994;35:41–9.

Young DV, Rinchuse DJ, Pierce CJ, Zullo T. The craniofacial morphology of bruxers versus nonbruxers. Angle Orthod 1999;69:14–8.

CHAPTER 22

ESTHETIC REMOVABLE PARTIAL DENTURES

Roman M. Cibirka, DDS, MS, Carol Lefebvre, DDS, MS, Ronald E. Goldstein, DDS

The patient who has lost a number of teeth has several treatment alternatives. The patient may remain partially edentulous until esthetics or function is compromised, or treatment in the form of a fixed partial denture (FPD), removable partial denture (RPD), or implant(s) may be pursued. Orthodontics may be indicated for partially edentulous regions of limited size or to enhance the prognosis of the rehabilitation through other modalities.

The highly esthetic demands of contemporary dental patients compel dental practitioners to satisfy their requests. Removable partial dentures designed without prudence and skillfulness might result in functional or esthetic insufficiency. Esthetic deficiencies may be shrouded by functional criticisms. Patients may present with frequent functional complaints of unaccountable pain or inability to chew when, in fact, they are discontented with the appearance. Unesthetic RPDs can be avoided with appropriate diagnosis and design using conventional clasping or attachment-aided prostheses.

CLASSIFICATION OVERVIEW

Universal classification systems for the partially edentulous arch have been devised to enhance communication and aid in design. Although numerous classification systems exist, the most widely accepted is that proposed by Kennedy[21] and further modified by Applegate.[1] There are four classes in the Kennedy classification system (Figure 22–1). The Kennedy Class I consists of bilateral edentulous areas located posterior to the remaining natural teeth and is the most common of the partially edentulous situations.[12] The Kennedy Class II has a unilateral edentulous area located posterior to the remaining natural teeth. The Kennedy Class III consists of a unilateral edentulous area with natural teeth remaining both anterior and posterior to it. The rarest class of the Kennedy classification is the Kennedy Class IV, which is a single, bilateral (crossing the midline), edentulous area located anterior to the remaining natural teeth. Edentulous areas other than those determining the classification are termed modification spaces.

PRINCIPLES OF DESIGN

The prudent treatment plan embraces a comprehensive analysis of the patient's dentition and supportive soft tissues. The health and distribution of the teeth

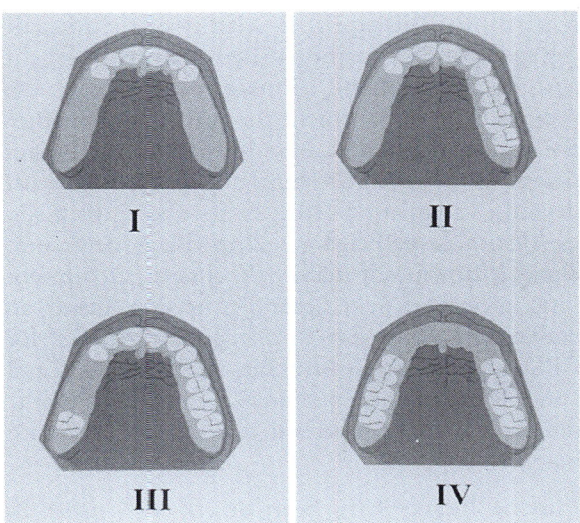

Figure 22–1: Kennedy classification. Kennedy Class I, bilateral distal extension; Kennedy Class II, unilateral distal extension; Kennedy Class III, unilateral edentulous area bounded by natural teeth; and Class IV, single bilateral (crossing the midline) area located anterior to the remaining natural teeth.

will influence partial denture component selection and the anticipated esthetics. Likewise, the quality of the supportive soft tissues dictates the measure of force transferred to the abutments and guides the component selection for the tooth-tissue–supported RPD. The greater the tissue support required, the more likely it is that the forces imparted to the abutment teeth will increase. The most destructive force is that of torque in the distal extension design. Minimization of torque should be considered of paramount importance in the design of the RPD.

Therefore, RPD design should be based on the available support. Kennedy Class I, II, and large IV RPDs are considered tooth tissue supported. In general, flexible direct retainer assemblies, mesio-occlusal rests on posterior distal extension abutments, and indirect retainers to limit rotation are indicated for tooth-tissue–supported RPDs.[4] Kennedy Class III and small IV are considered tooth-supported RPDs. In these situations, no additional support from the tissue is generally needed. For these designs, clasp assemblies may be more rigid, and indirect retainers are usually not indicated.

Examination of the patient requires clinical and radiographic diagnosis of the teeth and soft tissues for judgment of the support available for the partial denture. Radiographic interpretation should include (1) periodontal stature, (2) responses of the teeth to previous stress, (3) vitality of the remaining teeth, and (4) pathosis. The quantity or height and quality of bone support often predict the prognosis of an abutment tooth or may influence the design of a partial denture component. Proper diagnosis necessitates high-quality radiographs, devoid of angulation errors or processing blemishes. Vertical bone heights will provide a measure of clinical crown:root ratios. A clinical crown:root ratio greater than 1:1 should be considered an endangered abutment with a poor prognosis for RPD support. Stress-breaking direct retainers and contingency planning should be included in the design of partial dentures to use an abutment with marginal support.

Bone indices have been described;[32] however, they may be difficult to discern on certain radiographs. A 25% error in actual bone calcification levels may be found with normal radiographs. Optimum bone qualities are expressed as normal-sized interdental trabecular spaces that tend to decrease in size slightly near the coronal portion of the root. Normal bone responds favorably to stresses within clinical limits. Favorable reaction to stresses from an existing partial denture may be considered indicative of a future reaction to stress. Teeth that have experienced previous heavy stress from RPD support or in conjunction with abnormal occlusal forces and demonstrate normal to slightly condensed trabeculation, a dense lamina dura, and a heavy cortical layer are designated as having a positive bone index or factor. Abnormal stresses will be evidenced as a reduction in the size of the trabeculae being most pronounced adjacent to the lamina dura. The reduced trabeculae size may be termed bone condensation and should be indicative of aberrant forces that may lead to bone loss if the patient becomes less resistant. A compaction of trabecular spaces and significant alterations to the cortical layer or lamina dura may be considered a negative bone index or bone factor.

Lamina dura is considered a radiographic measure of abutment tooth health. The structure is hard cortical bone lining the sockets of the teeth with a primary function of withstanding mechanical strain. The lamina dura should be intact and cross interdental spaces to adjacent teeth as a fine, radiopaque white line.

The supportive elements will generally respond to build support where needed and predict the degree of future response. Mechanical insults from poorly designed RPDs may overload the remodeling capacity of the body, resulting in tissue destruction. Bone is approximately 30% organic and stores little protein; therefore, any alterations in body health will be reflected in the ability to maintain support. Systemic diseases that alter the reparative capacity of the body should be strongly considered with partial denture design. The patient's future health status and manifestations of aging should be considered in the selection of abutment teeth for loading.

USE OF A SURVEYOR

The dental surveyor is a fundamental instrument for RPD design and treatment planning. Additionally, the dental surveyor is indispensable for the laboratory technician to construct a partial denture and fabricate supportive elements such as surveyed, telescopic, or attachment restorations.

The surveyor may be used for diagnostic cast analysis, contouring abutment tooth restorations, placement of attachment retainers, milling internal rests, and reciprocal elements. Survey objectives include (1) determination of an acceptable path of insertion to eliminate interference with placement or removal, either hard or soft tissues; (2) identification of proximal tooth surfaces to be made parallel to act as guiding planes for placement and removal; (3) location and measurement areas of teeth for undercut and suitable esthetic clasp placement; (4) delineation of heights of contour; and (5) recording of cast position, or tripod, for future reference.[32,42]

An esthetic determinant of the survey is establishing one path of placement to minimize the retentive element and acrylic resin or denture base display. Retentive areas may influence the placement of retentive elements, so areas of retention should be selected to enhance the esthetic value of the RPD. When an anterior modification space is present, a path of placement should be selected to minimize excessive modification of adjacent abutment teeth and eliminate placement interferences. Anterior tissue undercuts may dictate a posteriorly directed path of placement to avoid excessive need for tissue blockout and inherent lip fullness from the overcontoured denture base flange. Restoration of highly esthetic anterior regions should be accomplished through fixed prosthodontics whenever possible or when the path of placement required for accomplishment of esthetics might limit the functional efficacy of the partial denture.

BIOMECHANICS

The design of an RPD must value the mechanics and the biologic considerations. Maxwell stated that "Common observation clearly indicates that the ability of things to tolerate force is largely dependent upon the magnitude or intensity of the force."[32] The structures supporting a partial denture, teeth, and residual ridges are "living things" subjected to forces. The attributes, frequency, and magnitude of the force will foretell the success or failure of the RPD and remaining dentition.

Forces applied to an RPD are generally classified into three cranial planes: vertical, sagittal, and coronal. However, it should be recognized that functional forces are a summation of individual vector forces in the three cranial planes. Hence, the actual force encountered by an abutment may be the result of two differing planar vector forces of varied intensity. Knowledge of the functional movements patients generate should be considered in the selection of abutment teeth, retainers, and partial denture design. Widely distributed abutment teeth with poor periodontal support in a patient with a parafunctional bruxism habit whose native diet includes nuts will obligate the dentist to develop a different design than for a patient with sound periodontal support and few other potentially damaging functional considerations.

A lever is a rigid rod supported somewhere between its two ends at a point, termed a fulcrum, which allows movement around that point.[32] The lever system allows magnification of force applied at one end of the rod proportional to the length of the rod from the fulcrum. Consequently, a small magnitude of force remote to the fulcrum will amplify to potentially destructive levels, depending on the design of the prosthesis. This is most apparent in distal extension designs where the length of the lever arm predicts the degree of force applied to the abutment teeth. Likewise, the dissimilar characteristics of support from the teeth and soft tissues yield rotation in three cranial planes.

The tooth:tissue dissimilarity of support is a preeminent concern in distal extension and Class I, II, or large IV partial denture designs. Class I, II, or large IV partial dentures derive a great deal of their support from the residual ridges and a limited amount from the abutment teeth. These types of RPDs generate the most potentially destructive lever forces. The fulcrum is generally established through a line connecting the most distal abutment teeth or the rests on those teeth. The Class III or small IV partial denture design is generally tooth supported with the fulcrum positioned between the abutment teeth bordering the edentulous space.

The residual ridge has a fibrous connective tissue covering the bone and underlying the mucosa. The thickness of subepithelial tissue will define the displaceability of the tissue overlying the residual bone. The displaceability and the amount of keratinized mucosa overlying the residual ridge will distinguish the amount of support anticipated from the edentulous regions. The periodontal ligament is comprised of collagenous fibers, blood vessels, and interstitial fluid to act as a shock absorber for the dentition. This ligament or membrane may vary in composition or thickness depending on the amount of force applied to the tooth. However, the compressibility of the residual ridge tissues and tooth ligament is not comparable. In fact, a tissue:tooth ratio of approximately 13:1 exists in healthy tissues.[32] This phenomenon requires careful deliberation when designing and constructing a distal extension partial denture.

Occlusion is of primary interest in the distal extension prosthesis. Accentuated occlusal forces or aberrant, parafunctional occlusal forces on the most remote portion of the distal extension base will impart a greater degree of leverage force to the supportive elements. Formation of a precise occlusal scheme will ensure harmonious function and enhance the prognosis of the abutment teeth.

Tooth morphology should be considered when evaluating potential abutment teeth. Clinical crown contours and occlusion will often direct retainer, major and minor connector selection, and rest seat placement.[18,35] Root anatomy is frequently overlooked as a critical component of the supportive element for a removable prosthesis. In general, single-rooted teeth are less favorable abutments than multirooted abutments. Divergent roots render more support than fused roots. Circular roots offer the least resistance to rotational forces than do oblong root contours. For this reason, premolars, particularly mandibular premolars, are poor choices to serve as solitary abutments for distal extension RPDs. Ideally, an FPD should be provided from the second premolar to the canine to avoid using the second premolar as a solitary abutment. Periodontally weakened roots provide disproportionately less surface area for anchorage owing to their conical shape.

PROBLEM SITUATIONS

Perhaps the most difficult situation is the distal extension RPD. This is complicated when the missing teeth are located unilaterally since functional requirements make it more difficult to esthetically mask the abutment attachments. However, if the entire arch is to be restored, then the situation becomes amenable to either an overdenture or precision attachment. If this is not the case, then the determination of the lower lip when smiling will help determine the type of attachment or clasp assembly to use.

SPECIFIC CLASP TYPES AND ESTHETIC CONSIDERATIONS

The use of conventional clasping in esthetic regions of the mouth can present difficulties with patient acceptance. Proper surveying and mouth preparation may circumvent complications. Clasps may approach undercuts from a suprabulge or infrabulge region. Proper abutment tooth selection for clasps and placement of the clasps far enough into the infrabulge or distal region will maximize the esthetic benefit. Ideally, suprabulge clasps should be placed in the middle one-third of the tooth in the region of the proximal plate. The retentive tip should be located in the gingival one-third but not encroach on the free gingival margin (Figures 22–2A and B). Placing the suprabulge clasp in this manner will improve the esthetic result and diminish the torquing forces applied to the tooth by the clasp. Infrabulge clasps will generally provide more enhanced esthetics, although they may have limitations to their use owing to anatomic considerations. The height of the vestibule, position of frena and soft tissue, or bony prominences may limit their application or necessitate preprosthetic surgery.

Circumferential Clasp

Owing to its rigidity, this suprabulge clasp is generally reserved for tooth-supported abutments in posterior regions of the mouth. It is a cast clasp of either a round or half-round configuration, both of which provide little flexibility. When serving as a retentive element, the clasp should only engage a 0.025-mm undercut to avoid excessive torquing of the tooth. This clasp may also serve as a bracing or reciprocal element and is positioned above the height of contour. Due to the relative size (thickness and diameter) of this clasp, use of the clasp above the height of contour for reciprocation should be limited in esthetic regions of the mouth. In situations where increased flexibility is necessary, but there is no place to remote solder a wrought wire clasp, such as the tooth-supported side of a Kennedy Class II arch, a cast round clasp may be used. A 20-gauge cast round clasp has been shown to have the same flexibility as a 19-gauge wrought wire clasp.[16]

I-, Y-, T-, or Modified T-Bar Clasp

The infrabulge approach of this clasp optimizes esthetics for patients with reasonably high lip lines or in situations where clasping of maxillary first or second premolars is indicated (Figure 22–3). It is

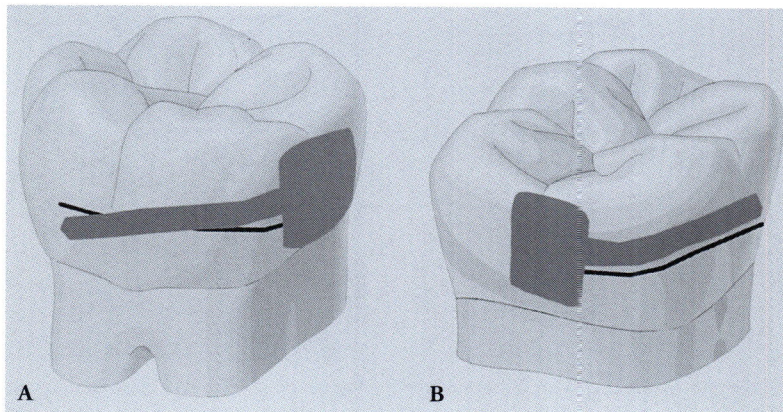

Figure 22–2A and B: Proper placement of the retentive and reciprocal arms. (A) The retentive arm exits the abutment tooth in the middle one-third and terminates in the gingival one-third; only the retentive tip (terminal one-third) is placed below the height of contour. (B) The reciprocal arm exits the abutment tooth in the middle one-third and remains completely above the height of contour.

generally cast as part of the framework and should exit the meshwork approximately one tooth distal to the abutment tooth. This allows for optimal tooth positioning without excessive grinding of the replacement tooth, which would reduce the cosmetic value of the denture tooth. In Figure 22–4, correct positioning of the approach arm of the I-bar allows the clasp to traverse from the framework through the interproximal embrasure region of the first and second replacement tooth. This will minimize the need to shorten the most anterior denture tooth to allow for the clasp to traverse from the framework more anteriorly.

The T- or Y-bar configuration achieves undercut engagement of 0.25 mm on either the mesial or distal surfaces of the tooth. A common error is to place both tips of the T- or Y-bar clasp into an undercut (Figures 22–5A and B). The esthetic value may be diminished if the anterior arm of the T- or Y- bar remains while using a distal undercut. Removal of the anterior arm should be considered, and a modified T-bar clasp should be selected (Figures 22–6A and B). A functional advantage of the modified T-bar is elimination of the mesial arm, limiting mesial undercut engagement of the clasp during a seating movement of the denture base toward the residual ridge. This will reduce the torque and distal tipping of the tooth. As a general rule, clasps should disengage during denture base movements toward the residual ridge and become active only on dislodging movements

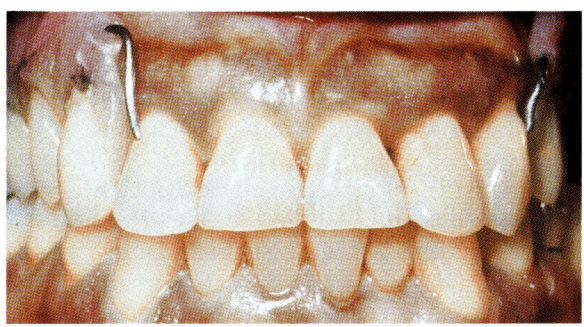

Figure 22–3: The use of the infrabulge bar (I-bar) clasp optimizes esthetics, particularly in the maxillary arch.

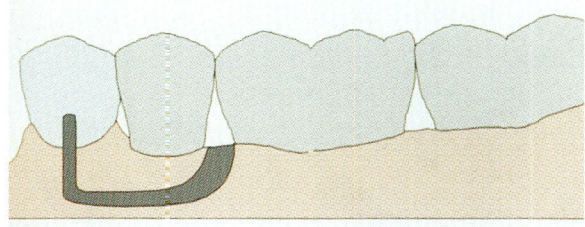

Figure 22–4: The approach arm of the I-bar is placed approximately one tooth distal to the abutment tooth. It exits the meshwork in the interdental area between the replacement teeth to minimize grinding of the replacement teeth.

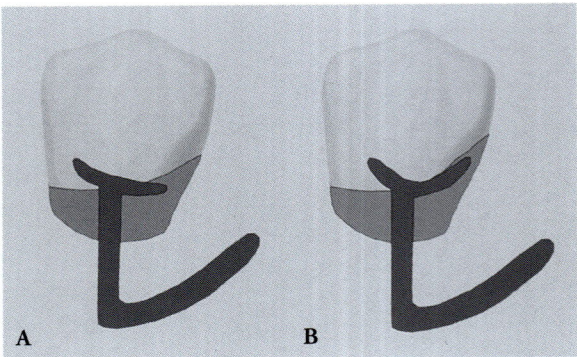

Figure 22–5A and B: Only one tip of the T- or Y-bar clasp should be placed in the retentive undercut. The other tip provides support only.

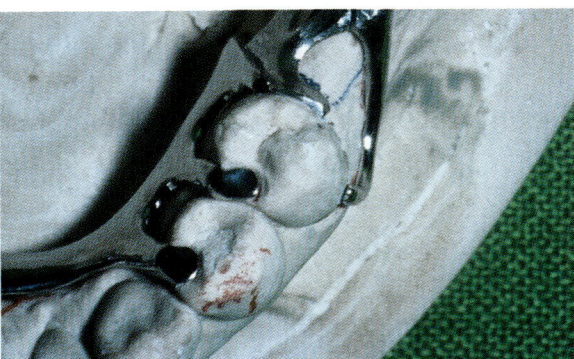

Figure 22–7: The RPI clasp design consists of a mesio-occlusal rest, proximal plate, and midfacial I-bar clasp (courtesy of Dr. John R. Ivanhoe).

away from the residual ridge. If the height of contour is located high on the tooth, this clasp design should not be used because of the space created under the approach arm.

Rest-Proximal Plate-I-Bar Clasp

The rest-proximal plate-I-bar (RPI) clasp, described by Kratochvil[24,25] and later modified by Krol,[26,29] consists of the following components: (1) mesio-occlusal rest, (2) proximal plate, and (3) I-bar clasp. The retentive tip of the I-bar should engage a 0.25-mm midfacial undercut (Figure 22–7). As for the T- or Y-bar clasps, the approach arm should traverse from the meshwork approximately one tooth distal from the abutment tooth. Esthetically, the RPI clasp fulfills all requirements of a conventional clasp yet demonstrates minimal tooth coverage, relatively limited metal display, and an infrabulge approach. The mesio-occlusal rest stabilizes the tooth and resists distal tipping. The design is indicated for distal extension situations and allows for disengagement of the clasp under occlusal force to the denture base. As with the T- or Y-bar, this infrabulge approach may not be desirable if adequate vestibular height is not present or anatomic structures, such as frena, are present. Infrabulge clasps may be more esthetically pleasing for patients with a low lip line.

Mesial Groove Reciprocation Clasp

The mesial groove reciprocation (MGR) clasp, described by McCartney,[31] is indicated for maxillary distal extension RPDs when canines serve as the abutment teeth (see Figure 22–3). Facial bracing is important because, unlike premolars, the mesiolingual contour of the canine does not usually present enough surface to resist distal movement. Adequate bracing is necessary to resist distal movement that would disengage the retentive portion of a distally placed clasp from the surface of the canine and result in a loss of retention.[20]

When necessary, the labial surface should be prepared so that its height of contour is at the same occlusogingival level as that of the lingual surface. A distal guide plane is not prepared. A 1-mm depression is prepared in the center of the distal half of the labial surface, gingival to its height of contour (Figures 22–8 to 22–10). Retention is attained with a 19-gauge cast or wrought wire I-bar engaging a 0.25-mm undercut on this surface. The MGR clasp incorporates a prepared mesial groove to provide reciprocation. A vertical mesial groove guiding plane 1 to 2 mm in length is prepared in

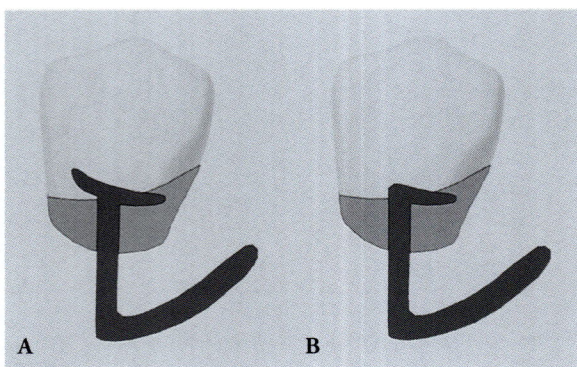

Figure 22–6A and B: The anterior tip of the T-bar clasp may be eliminated, producing the modified T-bar clasp.

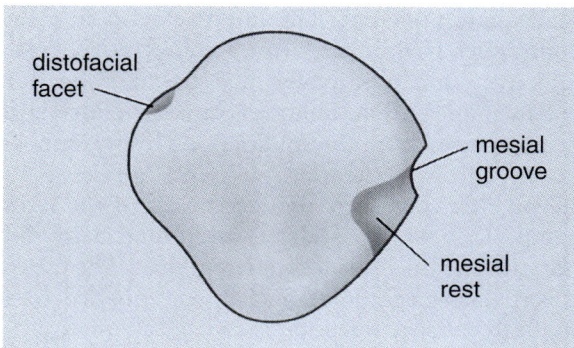

Figure 22–8: Mesial groove reciprocation clasp natural tooth preparation. A distal guide plane is not prepared. A 1-mm depression is prepared in the center of the distal half of the labial surface, gingival to the height of contour. A mesial groove that provides reciprocation extends over the mesial marginal ridge to a mesial rest seat.

the mesiolingual surface within the mesial marginal ridge enamel. To complete the abutment modification, the mesial reciprocation groove is extended over the mesial marginal ridge to terminate in a spoon-shaped mesial rest seat. Occasionally, a small amalgam restoration may be required when dentin is exposed while preparing sufficient depth for lateral force resistance.

Ring Clasp

This clasp is used for inclined maxillary or mandibular molars with natural undercuts on the mesiobuccal or mesiolingual surface, respectively. The ring clasp should never be used as an unsupported ring, known as a back-action clasp, as it cannot provide both reciprocation and stabilization.[32] It is usually designed with an additional bracing arm to prevent excessive flexing. An additional rest seat placed on the opposite side of the tooth enhances the rigidity of the clasp assembly and may aid in resisting further mesial migration of the tooth. All of the clasp assembly, except for the retentive tip, must lie above the height of contour. Consequently, it is not an esthetic clasp assembly and is reserved for molar abutments.

Embrasure Clasp

This clasp will be used in posterior regions of the mouth in the quadrant without an edentulous space, as in Class II situations. This clasp avoids excessive distal extension of the major connector. The embrasure clasp is a suprabulge clasp that should have an adequate sluiceway prepared through the embrasure of the abutment teeth to allow for proximal rests and emergence of the suprabulge clasp arm elements near the height of contour (Figures 22–11A and B). Adequate sluice-

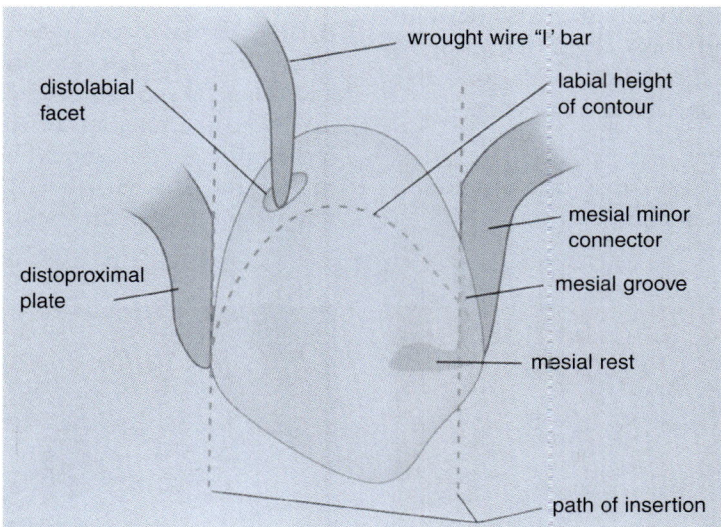

Figure 22–9: Mesial groove reciprocation clasp framework design. An I-bar engages a 0.25-mm undercut in the prepared depression on the distal surface. The mesial minor connector contacts the mesial groove and terminates in the mesial rest seat.

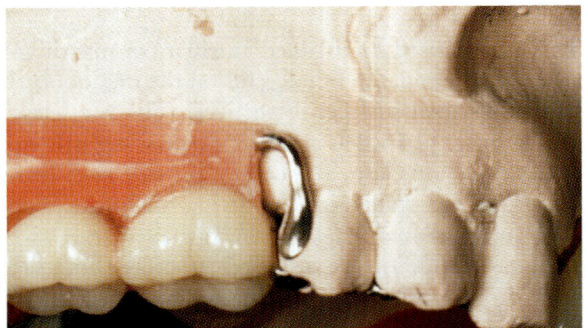

Figure 22–10: The mesial groove reciprocation clasp is indicated for maxillary teeth where esthetics is a concern.

way depth will also provide for proper metal thickness to ensure rigidity and avoid occlusal interference from the opposing dentition.

Combination Clasp

The combination clasp consists of a wrought wire clasp arm and cast reciprocal arm (Figure 22–12).[23] It is most frequently used adjacent to a distal extension base to promote stress-breaking characteristics to the abutment tooth. The wrought wire, being more flexible (less brittle), may be used in smaller diameter with less danger of fracture. Nineteen-gauge wrought wire in a 0.5-mm mesial undercut is generally indicated for canine and premolar distal extension abutments. Remote soldering of the clasp to the framework provides increased flexibility.[8] Due to its round form, light refraction is decreased, making the metal display less noticeable than with the broader surface of a cast clasp.

Retention Enhancement

Traditionally, enamelplasty or a cast restoration has been indicated for an abutment tooth with an inadequate undercut. The improvements in resin composites have made them a conservative, cost-effective, and minimally invasive method for enhancing retention. However, variable results have been reported from the studies using resin composite to enhance retention. In vitro studies have shown that cast I-bars produced wear of the resin composite,[43] whereas stainless steel round clasps did not cause a noticeable loss of retention.[13] The use of a partial-coverage porcelain laminate bonded to a tooth to enhance retention is a viable alternative.[14]

Rest Seats

In general, mesio-occlusal rest seats are indicated for posterior distal extension abutments when the occlusion permits.[24,49] For tooth-supported RPDs, rest seats are placed on either side of the modification space to prevent tissueward movement of the RPD and for ease of fabrication. Cingulum rest seats are indicated for anterior teeth. However, the lack of adequate enamel often precludes placement of a positive cingulum rest seat on the mandibular anterior teeth. Traditionally, incisal rests have been advocated for mandibular anterior teeth. Unfortunately, they are unesthetic, may interfere with the occlusion, and may increase torquing forces on the teeth. Bonded resin composite or metal rest seats have been shown to provide a satisfactory and esthetic alternative to the incisal rest (Figure 22–13).[44,48]

Flange Design

A labial flange in the anterior region is indicated when residual ridge resorption has occurred and additional lip support is needed. The flange should extend to the junction of the attached and unattached mucosa and should be contoured to blend in with the adjacent teeth. Also, the flange should not extend into an undercut apical to the adjacent

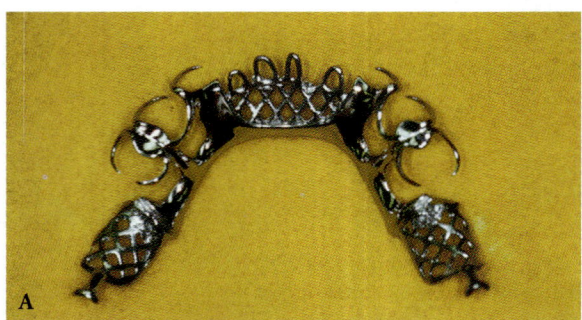 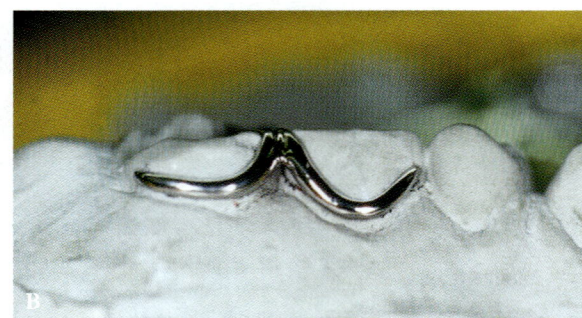

Figure 22–11A and B: The embrasure clasp is used on posterior teeth where no modification space is present.

Esthetic Removable Partial Dentures 677

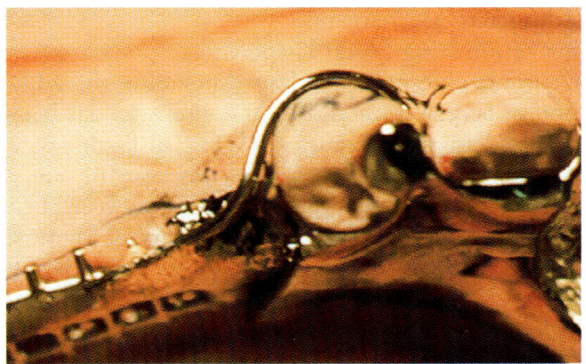

Figure 22–12: The combination clasp consists of a wrought wire retentive arm with a cast reciprocating arm or plated surface (courtesy of Dr. John R. Ivanhoe).

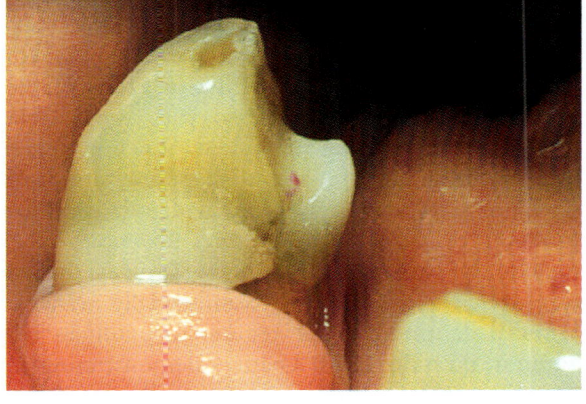

Figure 22–13: Bonded resin composite rest seat.

teeth.[38] Occasionally, tinting of the denture base to match the pigmentation of the patient may be indicated.[7,17,19]

Replacement Teeth

Teeth should be selected to match the size, shape, shade, and contour of the adjacent teeth. In some instances, it will be necessary to contour the tooth, and, occasionally, it may be necessary to stain the artificial tooth or place a restoration in the tooth to match adjacent teeth. A technique to modify the shade, contour, and occlusal contacting surfaces of denture teeth with light-polymerized resin composite has been described.[46] Microfilled resins for veneering facial surfaces are advocated because these are more easily polished and provide an improved esthetic appearance. These changes are most easily accomplished when the artificial tooth is fabricated from acrylic resin. The acrylic denture base resin should be contoured to match the size and contour of those of the adjacent teeth. The artificial teeth should be positioned to simulate the position of the natural teeth. If natural teeth remain, they may be used as a guide for placing the artificial teeth in a harmonious arrangement.

Other Esthetic Considerations

The patient should be assessed in totality rather than as an aggregate of singular entities. The potential consequence that one treatment has on another region of the mouth and the overall result requires careful appraisal. Although it is the intent of most practitioners to maximize the esthetic value of treatment for the patient, the esthetic awareness and desire of the patient merit consideration. The implementation of complex components, potentially increasing cost, maintenance, or difficulties with hygiene for a patient unconcerned with esthetics, is not prudent. However, the assessment of patient awareness needs to be bona fide. The apathetic patient can create postinsertion obstacles if a genuine esthetic concern is not detected. This type of patient will frequently respond to queries of esthetics with "Do whatever you think would look good, Doctor," or "I don't care about the appearance, as long as I can chew." Great caution should be exercised when managing the prosthetic care of these patients.

Skeletal anomalies that may effect esthetics should be brought to the patient's attention prior to treatment. Any discussion following the completion of care may often be interpreted as an excuse. Particular examples would include patients who believe that the RPD will correct skeletal discrepancies, overt facial wrinkling, or other cosmetic concerns normally requiring surgical intervention. A skeletal Class II patient or a patient with vertical maxillary excess will be particularly aware of a maxillary anterior modification space for the RPD. The excessive resin display or lip displacement justifies consultation prior to RPD construction, allowing the patient the opportunity to consider alternative treatment options to meet his or her esthetic needs.

Tooth morphology and anticipated placement require evaluation of presurgical diagnostic casts.

Most patients will request replacement of the missing dentition to maintain their previous esthetic situation. This should be readily accomplished, although if a suitable replacement is not feasible, the limitations should be discussed with the patient prior to commencing treatment. Encumbrances may be owing to tooth size or shape limitations or positioning difficulties, which may detract from the function of the partial denture. Examples may include the patient with natural anterior teeth that were much larger than the commercially available artificial dentition or the request to maintain the anterior tooth display in a patient demonstrating an excessive vertical overlap of the maxillary incisors. Clearly, esthetic and functional concerns may create the need for investigation of alternative treatment options or acceptance of the limitations by compromising either the esthetics or functional design. Any of these situations should remain well documented and explained to the patient completely.

ALTERNATIVE TREATMENT MODALITIES

In situations demanding maximal esthetics, alternatives to conventional RPD design must be in the practitioner's armamentarium. Alternative treatment modalities will often produce a result in prudent design with function and esthetics. The use of dental attachments is discussed in this chapter; however, finances, as well as dexterity or the ability to complete or maintain complex care, often dictate the need for conventional alternatives.

Adjunctive Mechanisms for Minimizing Metal Display

Camouflaging of RPD clasps, including the addition of acrylic resin and resin composite, has been reported in the literature.[33,39] The difficulty with the use of acrylic resins or resin composite to veneer to RPD metals lies in the differences between their abilities to flex and their coefficients of thermal expansion. Non-noble metals possess strength and resist significant flexure. However, resins are subjected to greater deformation from physical and thermal conditions. The resin composite matrix also tends to be brittle beyond its elastic limit. As a result, the abilities of the metals and resins to deform plastically are incompatible. Other concerns include the effect of the intraoral forces of mastication, the adjustability of veneered clasps, and the additional bulk of the clasp created by the addition of the veneering material. Excessive shortening and thinning of the clasp should be avoided to ensure rigidity and minimize the breakage potential of the clasp.[34]

Rotational Path Removable Partial Dentures

The rotational path RPD is a relatively uncomplicated method that eliminates the use of esthetically objectionable clasping in the anterior region of the mouth (Figures 22–14A and B).[22,27,28,50] It uses an anterior rigid portion of the framework and a conventional flexible posterior retentive clasp as the retentive components. The main advantage of this design is the minimal use of clasps. The esthetic result is enhanced, and the tendency toward plaque

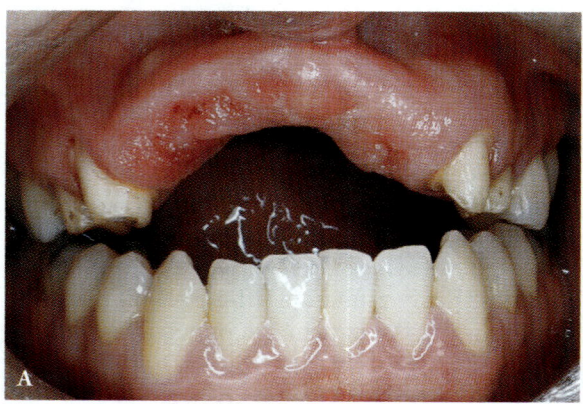
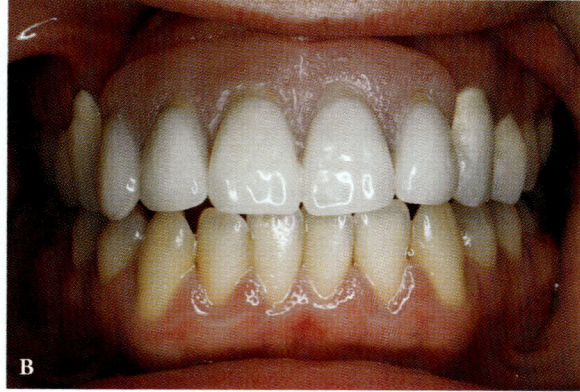

Figure 22–14A and B: *(A)* The maxillary anterior teeth were lost as a result of a traumatic injury. The bone loss in the anterior maxilla is significant. *(B)* The rotational path removable partial denture allows the elimination of anterior clasp arms to improve esthetics.

accumulation is reduced. However, both the clinical and laboratory procedures required for the rotational path RPD are technique sensitive.

The rotational path RPD should be limited to tooth-supported situations to prevent torquing of abutment teeth. This design also requires that positive rest seats be used. Cingulum and extended occlusal rest seats are indicated for canine and premolar abutments, respectively (Figures 22–15A and B and 22–16). For premolars, the rest seats should be extended to 1.5 to 2.0 mm deep occlusogingivally with nearly parallel facial and lingual walls. A restoration may be indicated to adequately contour the rest seat.

The cast is first surveyed at a 0-degree tilt to determine the adequacy of undercuts on the mesial surfaces of the anterior abutments and the distofacial

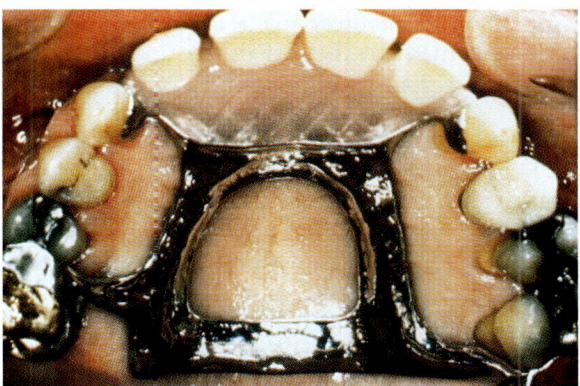

Figure 22–16: The rotational path design uses extended rests on the anterior abutments.

surfaces of the posterior abutments (Figure 22–17). The amount of undercut needed for the anterior teeth is 0.25 to 0.5 mm. This position is registered using tripod marks. The cast is then tilted until the undercuts of the anterior abutments are eliminated. The analyzing rod is then used to determine whether access exists for the rests to be seated. There must be no interferences for the anterior segment to go to place (Figure 22–18). If it is satisfactory, the second cast tilt should be registered on the cast with a second set of tripod marks (Figures 22–19A and B). Major connectors with minimal palatal or lingual tooth contact are indicated to avoid interferences to seating of the framework. It is important that during the framework try-in appointment, there is minimal adjustment of the anterior proximal plate; otherwise, the anterior retentive component may be lost. The rotational path RPD is not indicated for distal extension RPDs, arches with lingually inclined teeth, severely tapered arches, and arches with multiple edentulous areas.

ATTACHMENTS FOR REMOVABLE PARTIAL DENTURES

Diagnosis and Treatment Planning

The demands for highly esthetic dental restorations provide the catalyst for the attachment RPD. The esthetic expectations of a patient should be the primary directive for attachment use. The psychological component of treatment planning of the RPD remains crucial to the success or failure of the rehabilitation. Meeting the patient's esthetic and functional expectations while not exceeding the biomechanical attributes of the supportive structures will

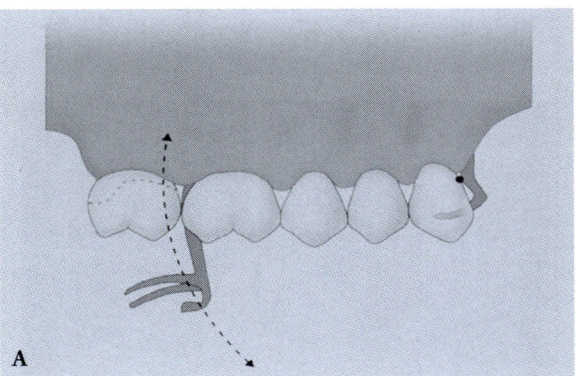

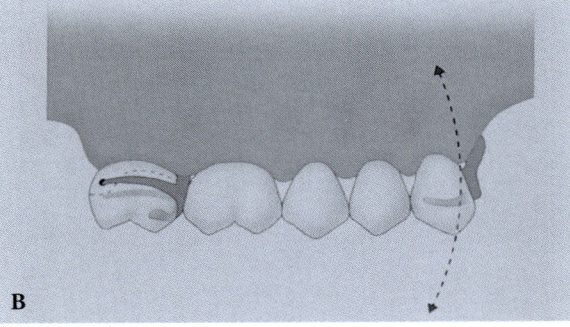

Figure 22–15A and B: (A) The rotational path removable partial denture uses an anterior rigid portion of the framework that engages an undercut and a conventional flexible posterior retentive clasp. After engaging the anterior undercut, the prosthesis is rotated into the fully seated position along an arc. (B) This arc demonstrates the arc along which the anterior rigid retainer would have to move for the prosthesis to be dislodged.

result in successful therapy. The anticipated function of the prostheses by the patient must not exceed the physiologic capacity of the teeth and tissues.

Proper treatment planning of the attachment RPD encompasses similar concepts to the conventional RPD. Fundamental biologic tenets must be adhered to for successful treatment. The components of guiding planes, rigid major and minor connectors, and indirect retention remain important in the philosophy of design. Suitable tissue preparation, accurate border extension, and tissue coverage without impingement are important adjuncts. Correct prosthetic planning will reduce the possibility of tissue abuse and enhance the prognosis for success.

Definition. An attachment is a connector consisting of two or more parts.[40] One part is connected to a root, tooth, or implant and the other part to a prosthesis. Attachment RPDs have been empirically termed "precision attachments" for years. The terminology of precision attachment partial dentures is frequently misused. Attachment partial dentures should be classified by the nature of the attachment fabrication, location, and biomechanical properties. Attachments used in RPDs are most commonly classified in the following manner: (1) precision, (2) semiprecision, (3) intracoronal: nonresilient and resilient, and (4) extracoronal: nonresilient and resilient.[3,36,40]

Attachments are subdivided into two general categories: precision and nonprecision.[9,40] Precision attachments consist of machined components of special alloys under precise tolerances within 0.01 mm. The metallurgic properties of the alloys are controlled to minimize the intra-attachment wear and are designed in a manner that affords most wear to occur on interchangeable elements. The intra-abutment portion of the attachment will generally evidence little to no wear, allowing accurate replacement while maintaining the specific tolerances designed. These systems allow ease of replacement interchangeability of the standard components.

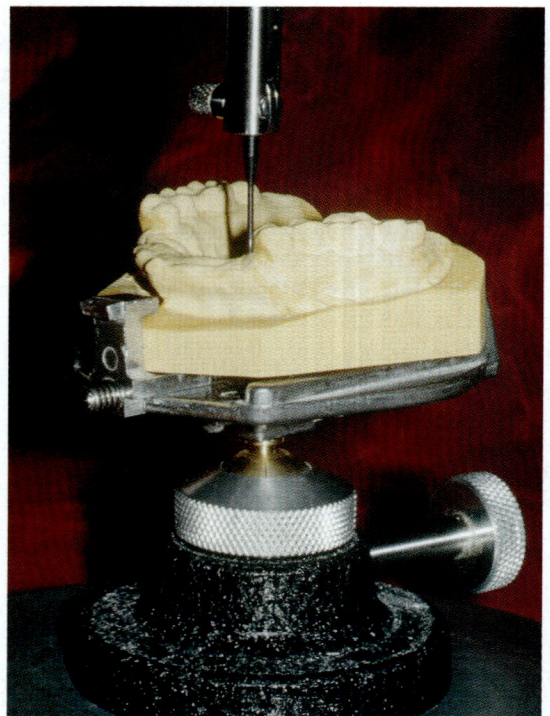

Figure 22–17: The cast is first surveyed with a 0-degree tilt to determine the adequacy of undercuts on the mesial surfaces of the anterior abutments and on the distal facial surfaces of the posterior abutments. This position is registered using tripod marks.

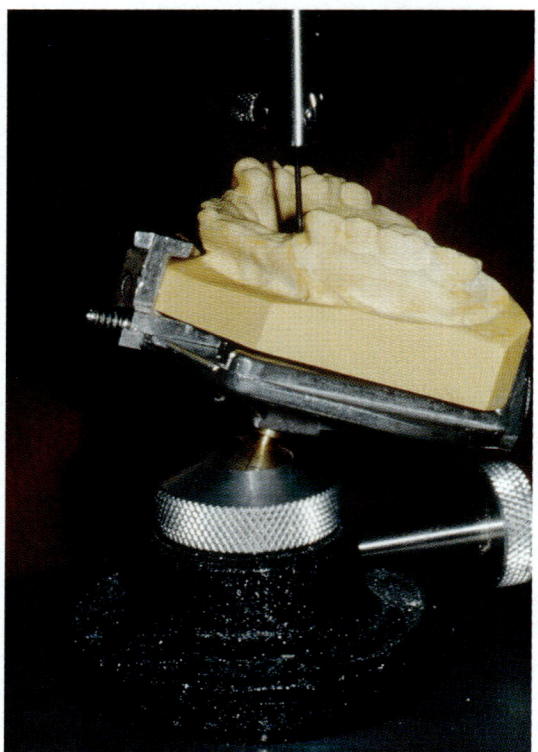

Figure 22–18: The cast is then tilted to eliminate the undercuts of the anterior abutments. This tilt is registered with a second set of tripod marks.

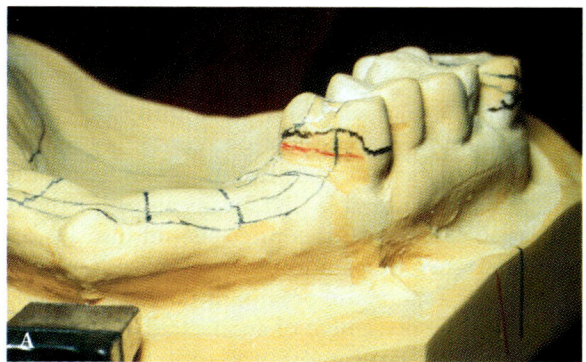
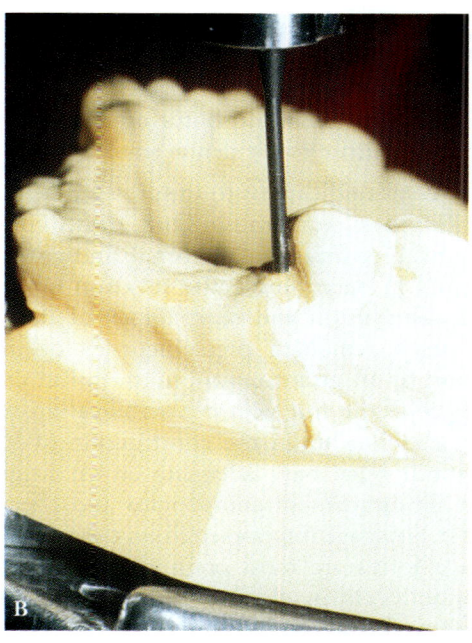

Figure 22–19A and B: The heights of contour made at the two paths of insertion. The superior height of contour is made at the 0-degree tilt. The inferior height of contour represents the path of insertion whereby the undercuts of the anterior abutments are eliminated. The area between the two lines represents the undercut into which the anterior rigid section of the framework is seated. Care must be taken during finishing and fitting of the framework in this area; otherwise, retention may be lost.

Semiprecision attachments require the direct casting of plastic, wax, or refractory patterns. They are considered semiprecision because they are subject to inconsistent water:powder ratios, burnout temperatures, and other variables. The resulting components may dimensionally change and reduce the preciseness of their accuracy of fit. The primary advantages of the semiprecision attachments are economy, ease of fabrication, and ability to be cast in a wide variety of alloys without the problem of coefficiency differences between the casting alloy and the attachment alloy.[9,40]

General Considerations for Attachments

The variability in the circumstances for use of attachments and the variety of attachments available preclude the establishment of a standard model. Selection should be based on the functional and physiologic requirements of the restoration. Consideration of the laboratory expertise in using particular attachments must be contemplated. Selection of an attachment with specific biomechanical and functional attributes may be finalized by the technician's ability to use the attachment and fabricate the prosthesis.

Attachment Use. A significant consideration in the selection of an attachment should be the long-term maintenance. Retrievability should be regarded with equality to function in the design and selection of an attachment for the esthetic RPD. Repeated use of similar attachments increases the knowledge of the practitioner and technician alike. This repetition will prove beneficial for efficacious delivery of care, management of difficult situations, and postoperative maintenance. The dental team should limit the application of dental attachments to a selection that meets the functional and esthetic requirements of the majority of patients and the level of expertise of the team. Other attachments may be considered periodically; however, use of other attachments may prove to be the rarity rather than the norm. This self-imposed limitation will ensure correct fabrication of the partial denture, untroubled delivery of care, and unrestricted maintenance of the prosthesis. Periodic planned or unplanned maintenance of the attachment prosthesis will be required. Consistent use of an attachment selection may safeguard adequate supply of replacement parts in the event of accidental breakage.[37]

Indications and Contraindications. The overwhelming indication for the attachment RPD is esthetics. Numerous skillfully designed conventional RPDs are not worn simply because the patient does not like the appearance. Elimination of the buccal or labial direct retainer or clasp arm is a key factor in establishing an esthetically acceptable design. Once the need for an attachment-assisted RPD is established, the selection of the attachment type should be based on the biomechanical, physiologic, and functional attributes of the patient or technical expertise of the dental team.[9,10]

The contraindications to the use of attachments in RPDs are numerous. One must consider anatomic, biomechanical, personal, and physiologic factors in determining the selection of attachments. The health and morphology of the abutment teeth remain a preeminent factor in the selection of an attachment. Short clinical crowns prove to be the foremost contraindication to the use of attachments in the construction of RPDs. The tooth must have adequate crown height to house the attachment components and effectively offset the leverage forces exerted on the crown. The leverage forces are most often observed in distal extension RPDs. In addition, adequate height must be present for the corresponding attachment components to be housed within the RPD framework or supportive acrylic resin while allowing proper artificial tooth placement.[3,9,10,36,37,40]

Adjunctive Procedures. Gingivectomy, or crown-lengthening procedures, may overcome the clinical disadvantage of short clinical crown height. This preprosthetic procedure will generally improve fixed prosthesis retention and resistance form and may increase the effective undercut, thereby enhancing the retention for a conventional clasping mechanism. This may avoid the need for placement of a surveyed crown when attachments are not a feasible treatment modality. Gingival crown-lengthening procedures may be required to provide adequate occlusal cervical space for attachment positioning while maintaining the functional attributes of the selected attachment to be used.

Orthodontic therapy should be considered with the presence of tipped or malpositioned teeth. The orthodontic correction of malpositioned teeth will avoid excessive tooth preparation, enhance vertical loading, avert the need for endodontics, and provide easier development of a common path of placement for the attachment partial denture. A particular degree of parallelism is required of all attachments. Orthodontic correction of malpositioning will allow proper attachment orientation. A nonresilient precision attachment requires the higher degree of parallelism.

Teeth with large pulps will not allow for incorporation of an internal box within the crown preparation to accommodate certain attachments.[3,9,10] The result of improper preparation would be an excessively overcontoured tooth leading to a periodontal liability. Endodontic therapy may be required in certain instances for the use of attachments. Endodontics should also be considered when preparation of a tooth with a large core restoration might provide little resistance to fracture. The placement of an intraradicular core might offer enhanced resistance to fracture under the functional loading of an attachment RPD.

The placement of attachments in pontics is an option that can avoid possible violations of biologic principles during tooth preparation or the need for adjunctive procedures (Figures 22–20A and B). The use of attachments lingually positioned in a traditional pontic or distally located in a cantilevered pontic has been described.[30]

Dexterity. Poor patient dexterity remains a strong contraindication for the placement of an attachment RPD. Patients lacking adequate hand coordination may encounter significant difficulty manipulating the prosthesis in the mouth. For some, it may be a virtual impossibility. While the average life expectancy of the population increases, more patients become potential candidates for RPD treatment. Debilitating diseases affecting neuromuscular control and joint mobility are likely to correspondingly increase. Arthritis, Parkinson's disease, cerebrovascular accidents, and other situations that influence fine motor skills might preclude efficacious attachment partial denture use or, at least, direct the attachment selection. Consequently, dexterity should remain a strong diagnostic consideration with all potential attachment RPD patients. Patients demonstrating average dexterity will generally be able to manipulate placement and removal with relative ease over time. A resilient attachment will generally be more easily accommodated rather than a rigid intracoronal attachment with a precise path of placement.

Cost. The design and construction of the complex attachment RPD treatment are costly. Cost in terms of time, effort, and resource commitment can be anticipated. The economic factors may predict the feasibility of using attachments. The prudent practitioner should anticipate an increased amount of diagnostic effort, laboratory expense, chair time, and maintenance in this form of therapy. These factors should be explained to the patient. The patient should anticipate charges for periodic attachment maintenance or replacement. Subsequently, these considerations support the use of a limited number of different attachments for efficacious delivery of care and reduced chair time.[37]

Oral Hygiene Maintenance. A final factor to be considered in the possible exclusion of attachment use for patients is the long-term maintenance of the prosthesis. It must be anticipated that periodic evaluation, adjustment, or replacement of attachment components will be required. The inability of patients to travel or return on a regular or periodic basis should be considered contraindications to the use of attachments. Oral hygiene may also be considered a parameter of attachment selection. Attachments will accumulate plaque and calculus, limiting the effectiveness or intended function of the attachment. Additionally, attachment use implicates the fabrication of full- or partial-coverage castings. Patients with high caries rates may experience a diminished prognosis with rehabilitations consisting of multiple fixed restorations.

Biomechanics and Support

Once a decision has been made to restore a region with an attachment prosthesis, the manner in which the vertical and horizontal forces are to be supported requires consideration. A partial prosthesis may be toothborne or tooth-tissueborne. The forces imparted to the prosthesis and its supportive elements should be as widely distributed as possible.

The periodontal health and support of the natural teeth should be considered in the selection of an attachment design. The forces should be equitably distributed over as many teeth as possible within the biologic and physiologic capacity of the supportive dentition. The denture bases should offer the broadest support possible for mucosal coverage.

Distal extension situations raise the dilemma of load distribution between the teeth and mucosa. The amount of soft-tissue compressibility over the distal extension residual ridge remains disproportionate to the abutment teeth. This phenomenon will create unharmonious movement of the partial denture, imparting leverage forces to the abutment teeth, possibly resulting in harm to the abutment teeth, mucosa, and residual ridge, if not considered in the selection of an attachment. Only teeth with suitable clinical crown height and periodontal stature should be considered for attachment use. The presence of excessive tissue compressibility or unsupported tissue might prescribe the need for preprosthetic surgical intervention.[3,9,10,36]

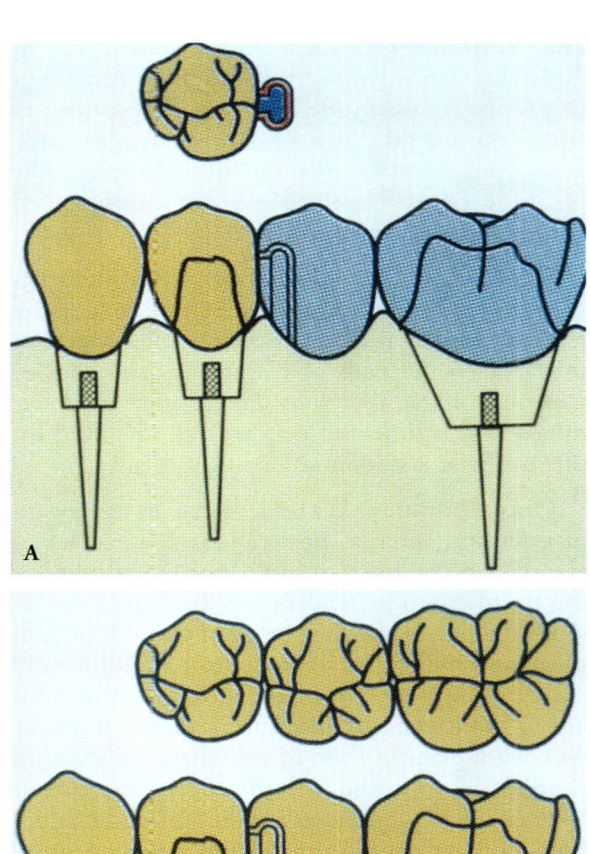

Figure 22–20A and B: Intracoronal attachment types such as the Score-BR, PDC, Omega-M, Beyeler, etc. (Attachments International, San Mateo, CA). *(A)* The female is placed upside down and cast to the anterior abutment. The male is waxed over the female, and the wax-up of the bridge is completed. *(B)* The bridge is invested, cast, and finished. (Reproduced with permission from Staubli P. Attachments and implants: reference manual. 6th edn. San Mateo, CA: Attachments International, 1996:13.)

Path of Insertion

With the aid of a surveyor, the anticipated path of insertion must be considered to develop appropriate guiding planes and attachment placement within the confines of the natural dentition. A less resilient attachment will generally dictate a smaller degree of tolerance or more parallelism relative to the path of insertion. Rigid and intracoronal attachments must closely accommodate nonsurgically correctable tissue/anatomic limitations or undercuts. For example, distal extension situations may require a distally inclined path of placement to accommodate extension into the retromylohyoid fossa, whereas an anterior modification space may require a labially inclined path of insertion and attachment orientation.[3,36]

Knowledge of the anticipated path of insertion may guide the attachment selection to a more resilient, universal design that can offer a greater tolerance to the path of placement. The path of insertion of the abutment crowns may be determined at this time and may indicate the need for preprosthetic endodontics or surgery.

Once a prosthesis has been placed along its path of insertion, anterior, posterior, and lateral forces alone or in combination influence the stability of the prosthesis. The tendency of the forces to dislodge the prosthesis must be counteracted through direct and indirect retainers. Direct retention may occur through friction of the attachment components, framework components with the teeth, or mucosal coverage of the denture bases. The forces of adhesion, cohesion, and surface tension between the base, saliva, and mucosa cause a pressure reduction on compression and further inhibit denture base movement.

Indirect Retention

Resistance to lateral displacing forces must be provided through rigid bracing components and the vertical height of the residual ridges. Bilateral distal extension bases use the mucosa and teeth of both sides of the dental arches for resistance to lateral forces. A force on one side of the arch is resisted by the components or tissue/base integrity of the contralateral side. This supports the increased stability usually found in bilateral distal extension bases as compared with unilateral designs. The design of certain attachments will provide indirect retention; however, the effectiveness of the indirect retention will vary. In attachment systems that offer little or no indirect retention, it must be incorporated in the framework design. In general, the more precise or rigid the attachment design is, the greater is the degree of indirect retention inherent in the design. Additionally, the more widely spaced the retainers are, the greater the support and stability are when compared with a design with retainers placed closely together.[3,9,10,36,37,40,41]

As attachment designs increase in the degree of indirect retention, generally, a greater amount of force to the supportive elements will be generated. Because of this increase in leverage forces transferred to the abutment teeth by the prosthesis, many teeth treated with castings incorporating attachments must be splinted to adjacent teeth. This concept safeguards the functional and biomechanical overloading of the supportive elements.[5,6,11,15]

Tooth Preparation

Preparation design should anticipate an increased degree of the forces to be applied to the teeth by the attachment mechanism. Avoidance of excessive taper, replacement of suspicious or weakened core restorations, and adequate axial wall height will reduce the risk of tooth fracture or decementation of the restoration. Therefore, most teeth will require full crown coverage for adequate retention and resistance form.

The preparations should consider the morphology of the tooth as related to the attachment selection. Adequate tooth structure must be present in all dimensions to allow incorporation of the attachment pattern yet retain the emergence profile and clinical crown contours of the tooth. Buccolingual, incisocervical, and mesiodistal space must be considered before a bur is placed to the tooth tissue. Alternative attachment selection or adjunctive procedures should be planned prior to preparation to allow for completion of the intended restoration and to enhance the functional and periodontal success of the restoration.

Attachment Selection Considerations

Proper attachment selection requires evaluation of five factors: location, function, retention, available space, and cost. Location can be subdivided into intracoronal, extracoronal, radicular, and bar type of attachments.[40]

Location. Intracoronal attachments are incorporated entirely within the contours of the cast crown for the tooth. It is imperative that adequate space exists in all three dimensions for both incorporation of the attachment and the maintenance of natural tooth contours to ensure proper use of the attachment and a positive prognosis of the restoration and the tooth. If it is not possible to place a box in the preparation to accommodate the matrix component of the attachment, an alternative attachment selection should be made. The advantage of the intracoronal attachment is that the forces exerted by the prosthesis are applied more closely to the long axis of the tooth. All intracoronal attachments are nonresilient and may require double abutting or splinting of the adjacent teeth. This form of attachment offers indirect retention and a more precise path of placement. Most wear will occur on placement and removal. In situations with diminished attachment length as a result of reduced interocclusal height, milled lingual bracing arms should be considered (Figures 22–21A to C). Careful consideration should be given to the amount of reduction in attachment length that will also allow for maintenance of the functional aspects of the attachment. Most manufacturers will state the optimal and minimal lengths of the attachment.

Extracoronal attachments are situated external to the developed contours of the crown. Normal emergence profile and tooth contours may be maintained while minimizing the amount of tooth structure preparation. The more conservative preparation reduces the risk of or need for devitalization.

The majority of extracoronal attachments have resilient attributes. This will improve the ability of patients demonstrating dexterity problems when inserting the prosthesis. However, the extracoronal positioning will increase the likelihood of hygiene difficulties. Patients will require fastidious hygiene instruction using floss and adjunctive periodontal aids to prevent food entrapment and calculus accumulation. Inadequate hygiene will generally result in hyperplastic tissue inflammation subjacent to the attachment apparatus.

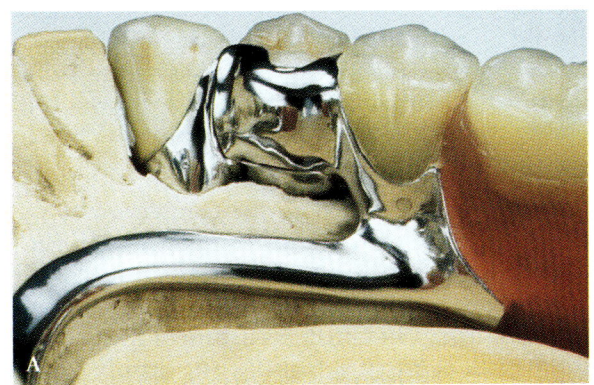

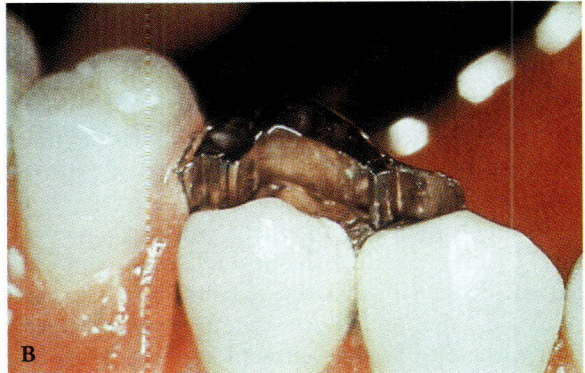

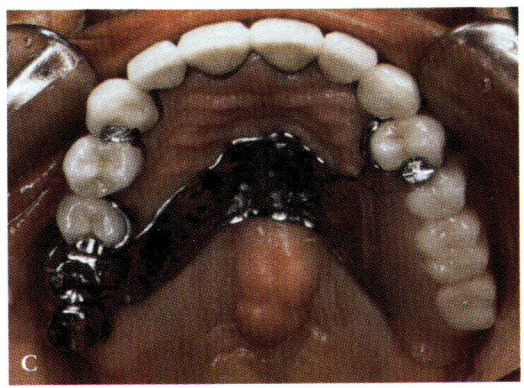

Figure 22–21A to C: *(A)* Milled lingual bracing arm on an RPD framework. The design allows development of normal crown contours with placement of the RPD. *(B)* The Biloc and Plasta attachment (Attachments International) allows the bracing arm to be incorporated into the crown contours. *(C)* A traditional lingual bracing or reciprocal arm may create bulk or result in tongue irritation.

Function. The functional attributes of an attachment require differentiation between the intention of the prosthesis as being solid or resilient. Kennedy Class III and small to moderate-size (replacement of less than seven teeth) Class IV tooth-supported prostheses should be considered solid, whereas large Class IV and distal extension I or II prostheses are increasingly tissue supported and should be considered resilient.

Rigid attachment mechanisms may include locking pins. Locking and nonlocking attachments allow for virtually no movement between the prosthesis and the abutment tooth. Resilient attachments allow for a spectrum of movement ranging from limited uniplanar to universal. Staubli has categorized rigid and resilient attachments into six classifications, from rigid to universal resiliency.[40] The higher classification number correlates with a greater degree of resiliency and suggests less torque transfer to the root or implant abutment. The classifications are shown in Table 22–1.

Retention. Retention of the attachment components may be based on frictional, mechanical, frictional-mechanical, magnetic, and suction characteristics. Frictional retention is developed by the resistance to the relative motion of two or more surfaces in contact. Greater intimate surface contact will usually correlate with an increase in the amount of retention. Mechanical retention implies the resistance to relative motion by means of a physical undercut. The degree of undercut and the ability to adjust the physical component will predict retention. Frictional and mechanical retention combines parameters previously discussed and should be considered in situations necessitating increased retention with appropriate abutment support. Magnetic retention is created by attraction of certain materials to a surrounding field of force produced by the motion of electrons and atomic alignment. This type of retention is not largely used and may be diminished by corrosion of the elements. Suction is created by a negative pressure similar to the intaglio surface of a denture to the supportive residual ridge.

Space. Space is a principal consideration for the selection of an attachment. Vertical space is measured from free gingival margin to the marginal ridge of the abutment. Avoidance of tissue impingement and maintenance of a proper emergence profile is paramount at the cervical region. Cautious placement of the superior aspect of the attachment will circumvent occlusal interferences. The length of attachments that rely on frictional retention should be maximized to maintain resistance to dislodgment. Placement of the attachment should be as low on the tooth as possible to reduce the tipping or leverage forces applied. Buccolingual space is equally important to avoid overcontouring the crown. Additional bulk will be required buccal and lingual to the attachment for the casting alloy. Proper analysis of mesiodistal measurement ensures proper proximal contour and will provide an indication of a need for boxes in the development of the preparation. The largest attachment possible should be selected. This requires careful preperparation analysis that includes the arrangement of denture teeth in a diagnostic wax-up. This will help ensure the highest functional and esthetic value to the reconstruction.

Cost. Cost is related to the complexity of the attachment and the material components. In general, precision attachments are precision machined from known, possibly noble alloys. The accuracy, manufacturing, and precious nature of the composition will demand a higher cost. Semiprecision attachments are made of plastic or other refractory materials subject to variables in the casting procedure, possibly leading to inaccuracies in the preciseness of fit. The greater simplicity in the manufacturing techniques significantly reduces the cost of using these attachments.

Intracoronal Attachments

Advantages. Intracoronal attachments, if used correctly, are incorporated entirely within the contours of the crown. This is advantageous for maintenance of tooth dimension and morphology. The positioning of the attachment near the long axis of the tooth allows force direction to be located along the

TABLE 22–1. Classification of Attachments

Class 1a	Solid, rigid, nonresilient
Class 1b	Solid, rigid, lockable with U-pin or screw
Class 2	Vertical resilient
Class 3	Hinge resilient
Class 4	Vertical and hinge resilient
Class 5	Rotational and vertical resilient
Class 6	Universal, omniplanar

Reprinted with permission from Staubli P. Attachments and implants. 6th edn. San Mateo, CA: Attachments International, 1996:5.

long axis of the tooth. This creates a more advantageous biomechanical loading and force transfer to the tooth with a reduction in adverse leverage forces. Maintenance of natural tooth contours and the ability to properly place an adjacent replacement tooth without excessive recontouring or alteration for adaptation around an external attachment generally make intracoronal attachments more esthetic. Less possibility of food entrapment near the gingival tissues will enhance long-term prognosis and comfort.[3,9,10,36,40,41]

Disadvantages. A disadvantage of intracoronal attachments is the more excessive tooth reduction required for proper positioning of the attachment. Teeth with large pulps or young patients often contraindicate the use of intracoronal attachments or necessitate endodontic therapy for attachment use. The three-dimensional size of the tooth will predict the functional or biomechanical success with this attachment. Large clinical crowns (at least 4 mm) are usually required for intracoronal attachments. Decreasing the length by one half reduces the retention by a factor of eight. This may be overcome by using a mechanical type of retentive element. The cost and precision of intracoronal attachments may be a limiting factor. Patient dexterity, maintenance, and repair are disadvantages or possible contraindications to the use of this type of attachment. Attachment alignment is critical due to the limited resilience and finite path of placement possible. This creates a limited path of placement for the prosthesis.[3,9,10,36,40,41]

It is our intention to present commonly used attachments that meet the considerations previously described. However, we recognize that other attachments similar in design and meeting the functional and biomechanical criteria for use may be prescribed. The intracoronal attachment obligates a sound abutment tooth and demand for high esthetic value. A clinical crown of greater than 4 mm is generally required with a similar faciolingual width. A preparation depth of the internal box will be approximately 2 mm. The frictional retention attachments must maximize clinical length to offer the greatest degree of retention. Generally, in situations where the clinical crown will be 3.5 mm or less, a mechanical retention attachment type should be considered.

Types of Intracoronal Attachments
Stern G/A, Stern G/L, and Stern Type 7 (Sterngold, Attleboro, MA). The Stern G/A, Stern G/L, and Stern Type 7 are intracoronal precision attachments providing frictional retention and allowing for some degree of adjunctive mechanical retention.[41] The Stern G/A attachment may be considered for segmenting an FPD, which may require modification to an RPD in the future. The gold alloy patrix offers an expansion slot on the gingival edge for enhancement of frictional retention. The Stern Type 7 does not offer conversion from an FPD to an RPD, although it has similar adjustment of the frictional retention through the use of expansion slots. The Stern G/A expansion slot design (Figure 22–22) allows for the patrix faceplate to remain flat against the matrix wall, thereby reducing wear. The Stern G/L employs a gingival latch mechanism to provide mechanical retention in addition to the frictional retention of the similar Stern G/A and Type 7 (Figure 22–23). The Stern G/L patrix is produced in two designs, the flat-back and ESI, and in two faciolingual widths, 0.70 and 0.96 inches. The width characteristics are axiomatic, although the shape characteristics predict the method of attachment to the RPD framework. The

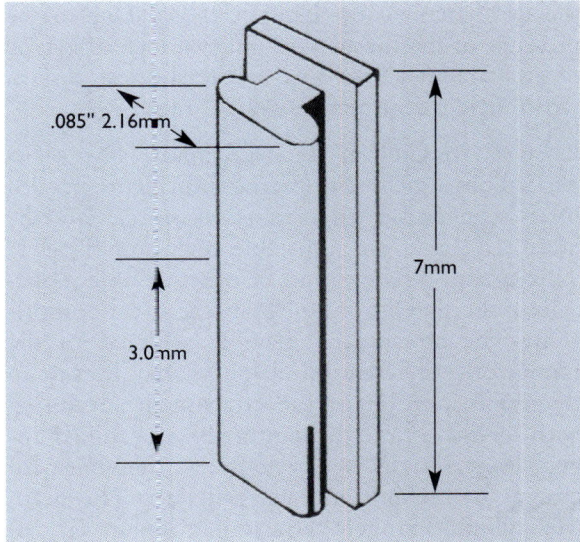

Figure 22–22: Stern G/A dimensions and illustration of expansion slot to allow for frictional retention adjustment. (Reproduced with permission from Sterngold, International. Advanced restorative products catalog. Attleboro, MA: Sterngold, 1998:14.)

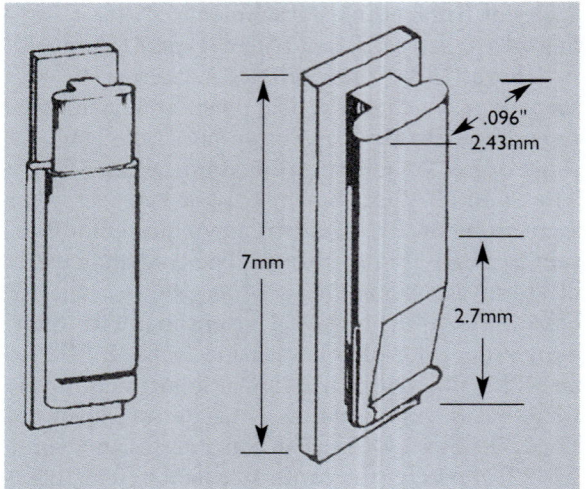

Figure 22–23: Stern G/L dimensions and illustration of an expansion slot to allow for frictional retention adjustment and gingival latch component. (Reproduced with permission from Sterngold, International. Advanced restorative products catalog. Attleboro, MA: Sterngold, 1998:15.)

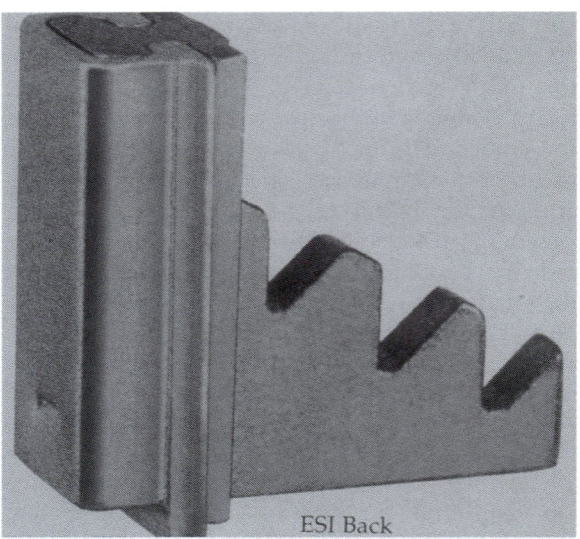

Figure 22–24: Stern G/L ESI back allows for resin retention to the RPD framework during attachment relation. Resin retention allows for retrievability of the attachment for ease of maintenance. (Reproduced with permission from Sterngold, International. Advanced restorative products catalog. Attleboro, MA: Sterngold, 1998:15.)

flat-back design requires soldering to the framework or casting a retentive arm to the attachment for resin retention within the denture base. The ESI offers greater versatility, allowing soldering, electrosoldering, and acrylic resin attachment to the RPD framework (Figure 22–24). Due to the presence of the mechanical gingival lock, this type of attachment allows one of the shortest clinical crown height requirements of 2.7 mm.

Swiss McCollum and Crismani. The Swiss McCollum attachment (Sterngold) (Figure 22–25) offers conversion characteristics similar to the Stern G/A and an adjustable retention flange.[40] This retention flange must be oriented to face buccally and ordered from the manufacturer appropriately. The attachment may be soldered to the framework, or retention elements may be cast to the patrix portion of the attachment for luting with acrylic resin to the denture base. A milled lingual ledge should be developed in the abutment crown for bracing arm construction. The Stern McCollum (Sterngold) attachment (Figure 22–26) offers an adjustment slot on the face of the patrix that allows access when the slot is situated lingually for cross-arch stabilization.[41] The Crismani attachment (Sterngold) has a similar adjustment slot design, although in cross-section resembles an

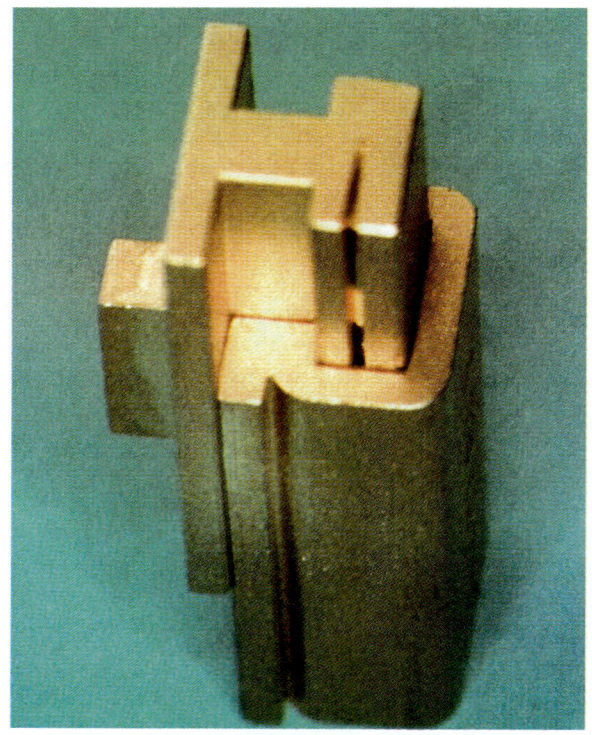

Figure 22–25: Swiss McCollum attachment (Sterngold). Note that the expansion slot must be positioned to face buccally.

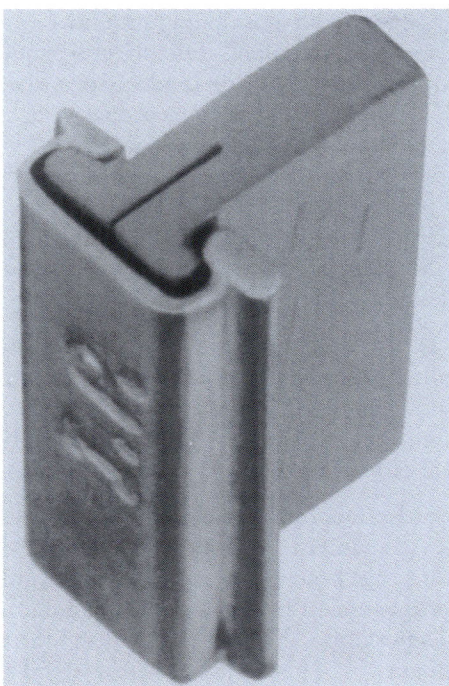

Figure 22–26: Stern McCollum (Sterngold) attachment. Note that the expansion slot is positioned on the face of the attachment oriented along the ridge crest. (Reproduced with permission from Sterngold, International. Advanced restorative products catalog. Attleboro, MA: Sterngold, 1998:16.)

inverted triangular shape rather than the T-shape of the Stern McCollum attachment.[40]

Schatzmann, Biloc and Plasta, and Score. The Schatzmann, Biloc and Plasta, and Score attachments (Attachments International, San Mateo, CA) offer conversion possibilities from FPDs to RPDs.[40] The Schatzmann attachment is an adjustable slide attachment providing frictional and mechanical retention. The mechanical plunger element is easily replaced chairside at minimal cost in time or expense. The Biloc and Plasta attachment, an intracoronal semiprecision attachment, offers a machined patrix in two alloy possibilities and a castable plastic matrix. A lingual bracing arm is highly recommended and is indicated in fixed, Kennedy Class I or II situations (Figure 22–27). The Score system offers multiple application options interchanging three semiprecision castable plastic patrix configurations with one castable matrix: the Score-PD, Score-BR, and Score-UP. The PD version combines frictional and mechanical retention, whereas the UP version incorporates a U-pin to lock the patrix and matrix segments together. This version (UP) allows for interchangeability to extracoronal resilient restorations using Dalbo (Cendres & Métaux SA, Biel, Switzerland), ASC 52 (Attachments), or Ceka-type attachments.

The patrix portion of the attachment types described are either similar in metallurgic properties or possess characteristics allowing a greater degree of wear when compared with the matrix. Consequently, the frictional wear of the patrix reduces retention and supports the adjustment capacity of the components. When the amount of wear or loss of retention exceeds the adjustment capacity, replacement of the patrix component is necessary. This clarifies the advantage of a precision-milled component. For replacement, a new patrix is purchased and replaced into the RPD without concern for casting inaccuracies or difficulties retrofitting the patrix portion to the abutment matrix, as might be experienced with semiprecision attachments.

Attachment connection to the RPD may be accomplished in a variety of ways, as previously described. Soldering to the framework remains the most permanent and possibly the most common method. However, acrylic attachment of the patrix or patrix portion of the attachment to the RPD provides the highest degree of retrievability. In acrylic attachment patrices, the worn patrix component is retrieved from the RPD, and the new patrix is luted into place with autopolymerizing acrylic resin, often without disturbing the artificial teeth (Figure 22–28). The disadvantages of this

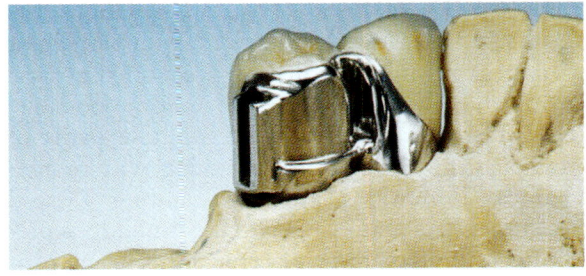

Figure 22–27: Biloc and Plasta attachment (Attachments International) allows for construction of an intracoronal attachment with a milled bracing arm. This design offers incorporation of the RPD bracing arm into the proper clinical crown contours. The mesial portion of the bracing arm is similar in orientation and function to the intracoronal portion of the attachment on the distal of the crown.

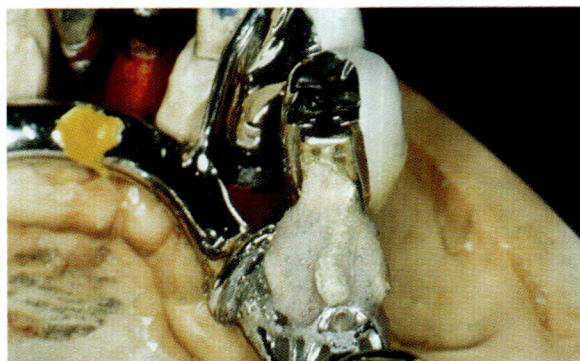

Figure 22–28: Patrix attachment with autopolymerizing resin to the RPD framework allows for easy retrievability and attachment replacement. This type of patrix placement increases the accuracy of the framework relation to the tissues and the abutment teeth.

technique are the discoloration and potential weakness of the resin. However, this technique remains more time and resource efficient than rebasing the RPD to retrieve a soldered-to attachment. A soldered technique requires artificial tooth removal and replacement owing to the excessive heat generated from the retrieval and resoldering of the patrix to the framework.

Extracoronal Attachments

Advantages. The advantages of extracoronal attachments include resiliency in certain designs and less abutment tooth preparation. The conservative nature of the preparation required would suggest less harm to the pulp and reduced risk of potential endodontic intervention. The resiliency in design provides advantageous stress-breaking characteristics in distal extension situations (ie, Class I or II arches). Attachment alignment is not as critical in highly resilient extracoronal attachments due to the omniplanar motion possible. This creates the advantage of multiple paths of placement for the prosthesis. Patients with biomechanical limitations not withstanding a rigid attachment apparatus or anatomic limitations precluding a finite path of placement are strong candidates for resilient attachments.[3,9,10,36,40,41]

Disadvantages. The adverse aspects of extracoronal classification include the potential for torque imparted by the attachment to the tooth and hygiene maintenance. Careful recall evaluation is necessary to ensure proper base–tissue relationships and fastidious oral hygiene. Tooth positioning around the attachment apparatus is often difficult and diminishes functional or esthetic value if adequate space is not available. Some resilient extracoronal attachments do not allow for "locking" to a rigid state. This may create difficulties with relining and rebasing procedures. Indirect retention and bracing are not incorporated into most extracoronal attachment designs and will necessitate the addition of components to provide these functions.[3,9,10,36,40,41]

As with intracoronal attachments, it was our intention to present commonly used attachments while understanding that other attachments similar in design and meeting the functional and biomechanical criteria for use may be prescribed.

Types of Extracoronal Attachments

Dalbo Attachment System (Cendres & Métaux SA). This attachment is one of the oldest and most successful extracoronal attachments and is classified as an adjustable, directed-hinge distal extension attachment.[40,41] This system features lateral stability, vertical resiliency, and hinge movement (Figures 22–29A to D). The advantages of the Dalbo system are the intrinsic direct retainer and excellent stability owing to the vertical beam. The attachment may be used in unilateral or bilateral applications (Figures 22–29E to J). The unilateral configuration provides a larger vertical bar for enhanced lateral stability. The attachment is offered in two sizes, although the mini version lacks vertical resiliency (see Figure 22–29D). The vertical resiliency is rendered through the presence of a spring and found only in the standard unilateral and bilateral designs. The difference between the standard and the mini is approximately 2 mm in clinical crown height requirement, 1.7 to 2.0 mm in preparation depth, and 1 mm in faciolingual width requirement. As in all extracoronal attachments, the amount of space required in the denture base is approximately 5.5 to 6.0 mm. This often creates difficulty with tooth placement and inadequate strength for the resin. The minimum amount of resin recommended should be strictly adhered to so as not to compromise the strength of the denture base in the region of the attachment. This extracoronal retainer offers a mechanism to "lock" the attachment for reline procedures.

Octolink. The Octolink System (Attachments International), an extracoronal precision/semiprecision attachment, furnishes a large degree of movement and is classified as a universal hinge with vertical resiliency (Figures 22–30A to D).[41] The patrix button is adjustable and is screwed into a metal keeper, or retention nut, which is retained in the acrylic denture resin or may be spot-welded to the RPD framework. The matrix becomes incorporated into the crown through either a cast-to technique or a castable plastic technique (Figures 22–30E to I). A minimum of 4.0 mm of vertical abutment tooth height is necessary, although a minimum of 6.0 mm of space is mandatory for the retentive keeper and patrix component in the denture base.

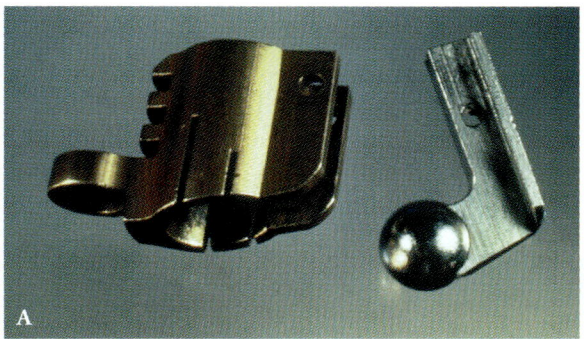
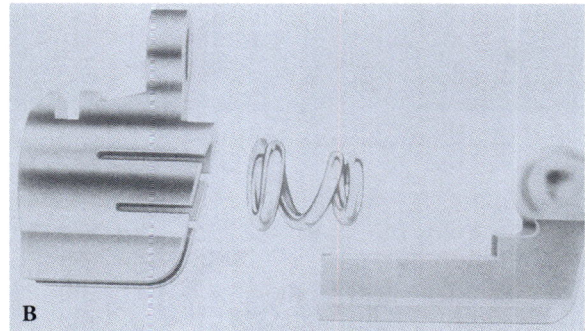
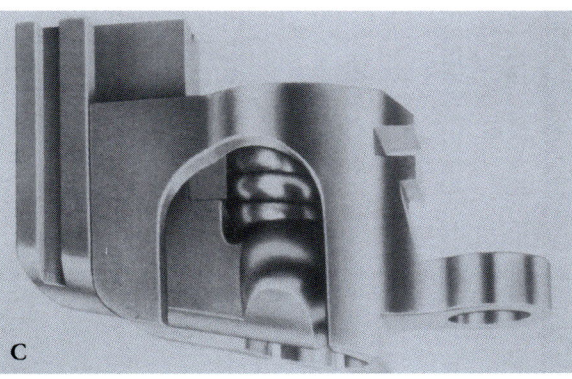
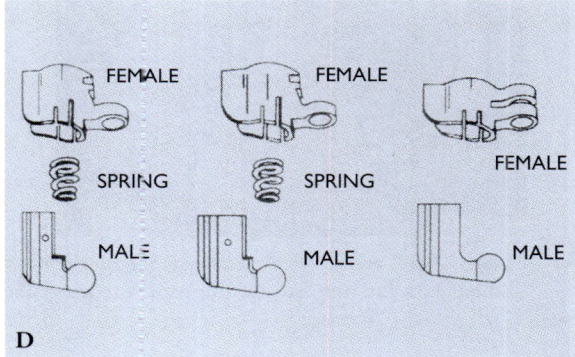

Figure 22–29A to D: (A) Dalbo attachment (Cendres & Métaux). (B) A spring allows for vertical resiliency, and a ball allows for horizontal rotation. (C) A compressed spring allowing for vertical resiliency. (D) Bilateral application, unilateral application, and mini (left to right).

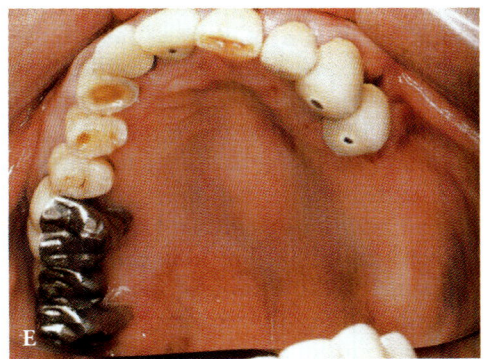
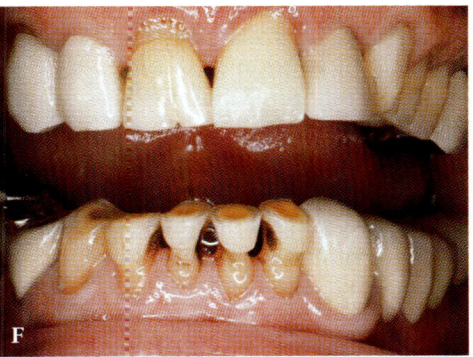

Figure 22–29E and F: This 75-year-old man wanted to improve both function and esthetics. Note the considerable wear in both the maxillary and mandibular dentitions.

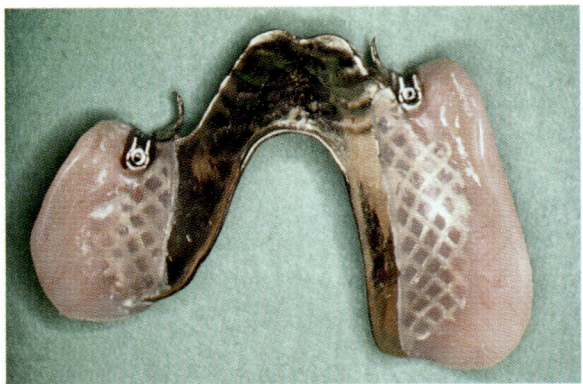

Figure 22–29G: A removable prosthesis with Dalbo attachments in place.

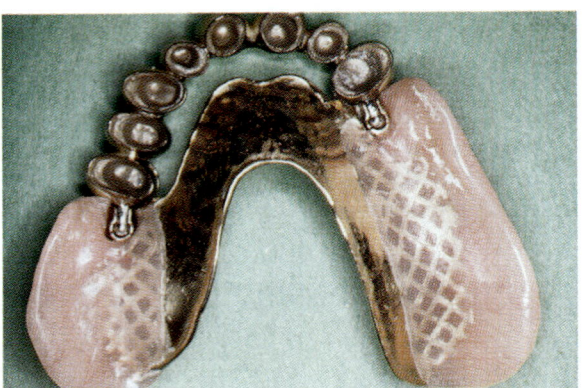

Figure 22–29H: The metal-ceramic framework is easily fixed to the Dalbo attachments.

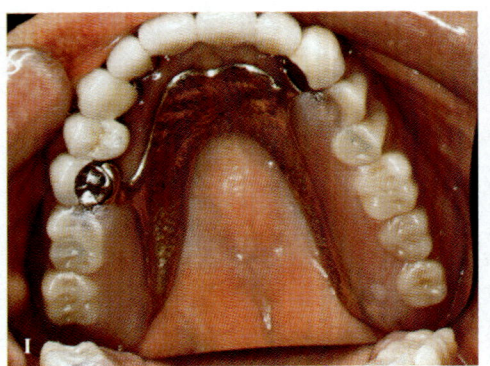
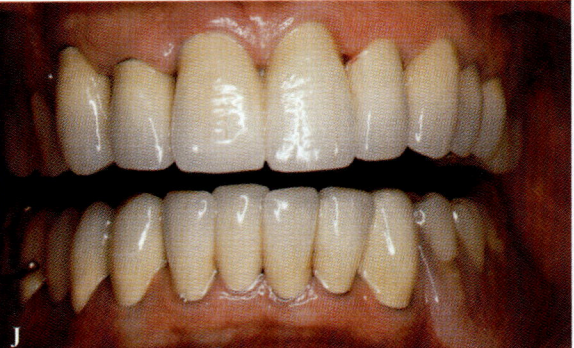

Figure 22–29I and J: Fixed metal-ceramic prostheses combined with Dalbo attachments provided maximum function and esthetics and were easy for this patient to insert and remove.

SA SwissAnchor. The SA SwissAnchor (Attachments International) is a semiprecision castable pattern providing either rigid or simultaneous vertical and hinge resiliency, depending on the design selected. A spacer will provide vertical resiliency. This system requires a vertical abutment tooth height of 3.5 mm. The patrix is screw retained in a keeper that is retained in the denture acrylic resin. This system is interchangeable with the regular Ceka.[40,41]

Stern ERA and Stern-RV. The Stern ERA and Stern-RV (Sterngold) are commonly used semiprecision attachment providing universal hinge and vertical resiliency (Figures 22–31A to E).[41] Retention may be varied through use of four color-coded nylon patrices indicating four levels of retention (Figures 22–31F and G). An optional metal jacket serves as a keeper for the patrix retentive element, which may be alternatively retained within the acrylic resin (Figure 22–31H). However, this is more difficult to change once retention is diminished. Patrices may be easily changed without the use of acrylic resin. The Stern ERA requires a minimum of 4 mm of vertical height, whereas the Stern-RV requires 3.5 mm of vertical space (Figure 22–32). No additional preparation depth is required for matrix incorporation to the crown restoration. A large space of 6.5 mm is required within the denture base for the patrix component and an additional 0.3 to 0.5 mm for the optional ERA Metal Jacket. The manufacturer recommends an additional 1.0 mm of denture base resin for patients demonstrating parafunction or "habitually strong occlusions." The patrix component is the variable between the Stern ERA and the Stern-RV. Both patrices fit with the selected matrix.[41,47]

Esthetic Removable Partial Dentures 693

Hader Vertical. This extracoronal semiprecision attachment (Attachments International) is compatible with conventional clasping on the contralateral side.[41] The resilience of the attachment allows slight hinging movement, although it will load abutment teeth more strongly than other resilient attachments. This attachment requires a 4.5-mm vertical tooth height without internal preparation limitations.

ASC 52 (Attachments International). The ASC 52 ball attachment functions well in limited space.[40] It is a universal attachment offering rotational and vertical movement. A spring-loaded

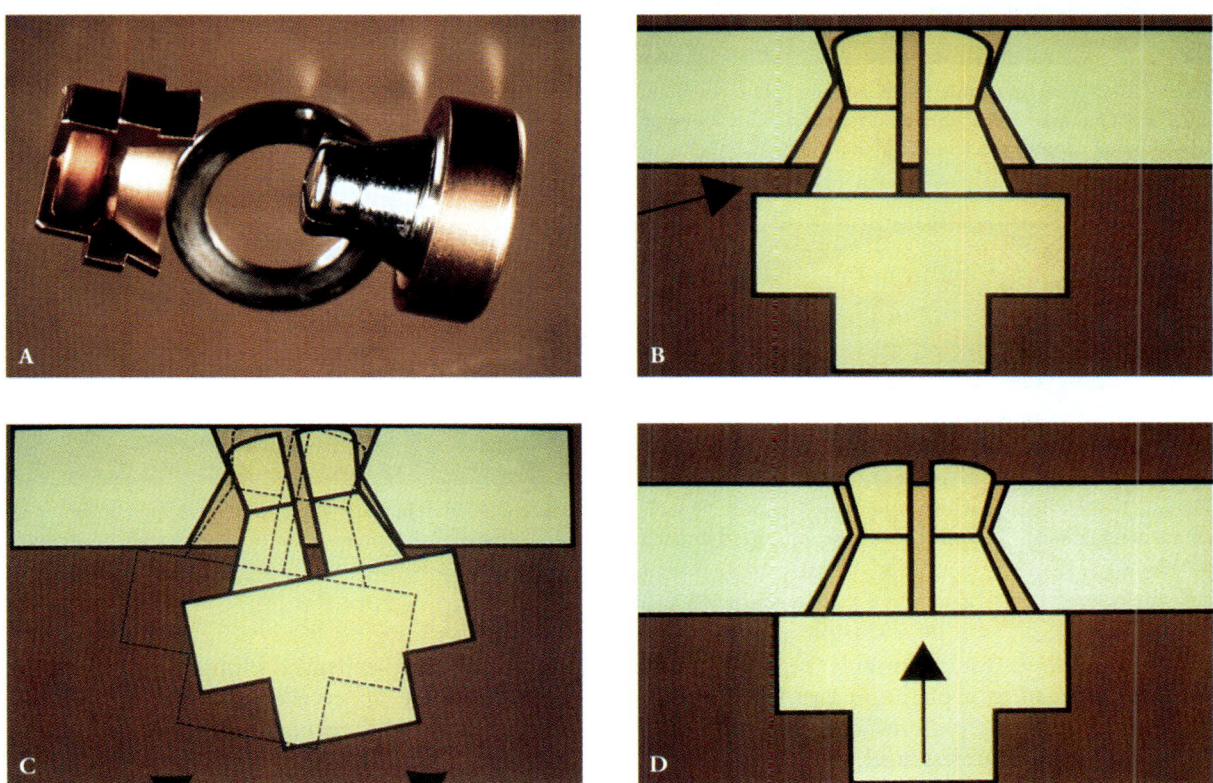

Figure 22–30A to D: *(A)* Octolink attachment (Attachments International). *(B)* Spacer used to allow for vertical resiliency. *(C)* and *(D)* Note the vertical and omniplanar resiliency of the attachment.

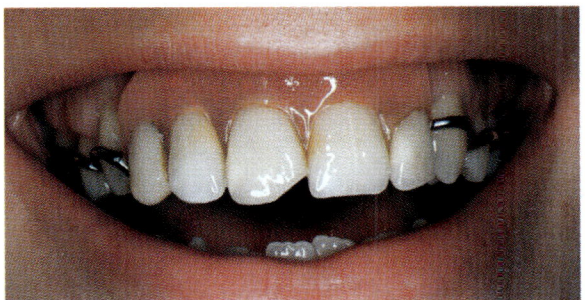

Figure 22–30E: This 30-year-old man was embarrassed because the clasps of his removable prosthesis showed when he smiled.

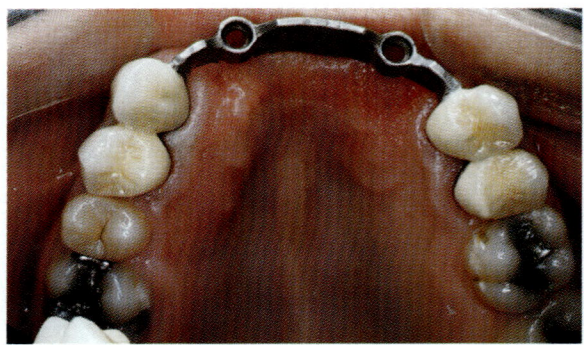

Figure 22–30F: A four-unit metal-ceramic splint combined with an Octolink (Attachments International) framework would better support the removable prosthesis.

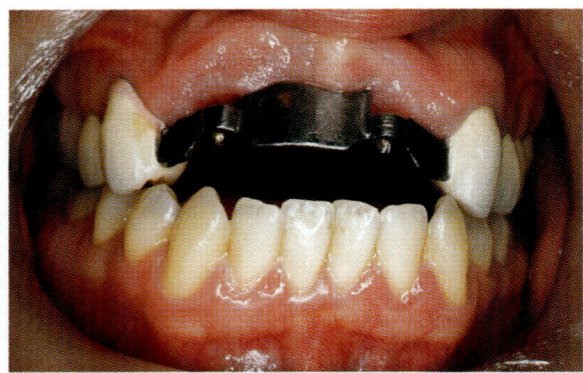

Figure 22–30G: This frontal view shows the adaptation of the metal framework to the alveolar ridge.

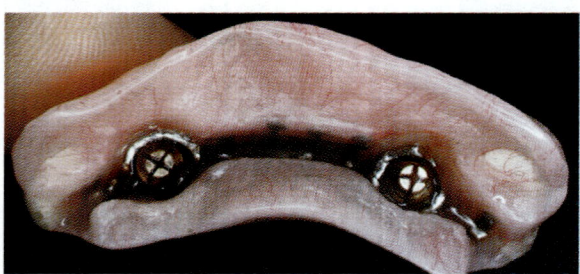

Figure 22–30H: This view shows how the Octolink (Attachments International) attachments will fit into the removable prosthesis.

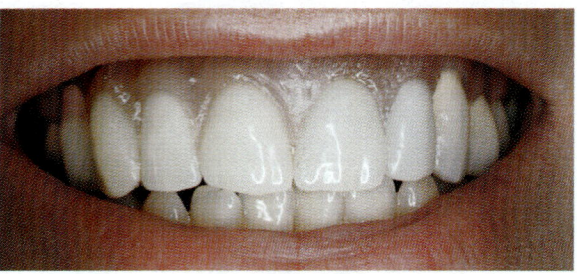

Figure 22–30I: The final smile shows the esthetic improvement offered by the combination of a secure attachment and a natural-looking acrylic flange.

connector allows for adjustable retention. The matrix is offered as a platinum cast-to alloy or a semiprecision plastic pattern. The precision patrix is constructed of stainless steel.

ORS-DE (Attachments). Superior stress-breaking characterizes this attachment.[40] This semiprecision castable plastic patrix pattern requires a minimum of 4.0-mm vertical height or nearly 6.0 mm of tooth height. The matrix will require a nearly identical amount of space within the denture base. A matrix O-ring may be retained in a metal retainer ring and provides easy retrieval and maintenance (Figures 22–33A and B).

Special Use Attachments

Special use attachments should be considered for limited use based on the esthetic, functional, or anatomic needs of the patient. These types of attachments augment the armamentarium of the practitioner, although they may often increase the complexity and expense. Plunger-type or pawl attachments are an excellent adjunct for esthetic anterior teeth with required function as retentive abutments.[2] Classified as an intracoronal attachment, the spring-loaded plunger allows for a full range of motion, mimicking a universal-type extracoronal design. This attachment may be used with conventional or attachment partial dentures. A reciprocal lingual arm should encompass 180 degrees and terminate in a rest seat. Matrix components or concavities are incorporated into the natural tooth or crown dependent on the situation or attachment, whereas patrix components are luted with acrylic to the framework and not soldered. Examples of plunger attachments are the Hannes anchor, the IC attachment, and the SwissTac/Tach E-Z (Attachments International) (Figures 22–34A to C).[40,41]

Splint bar designs incorporate Hader/EDS, Dolder, CM Bar & Rider or Ackermann clips, ABS, CBS, or PPM Bar Systems.[40,41] Selection is based on the

Esthetic Removable Partial Dentures 695

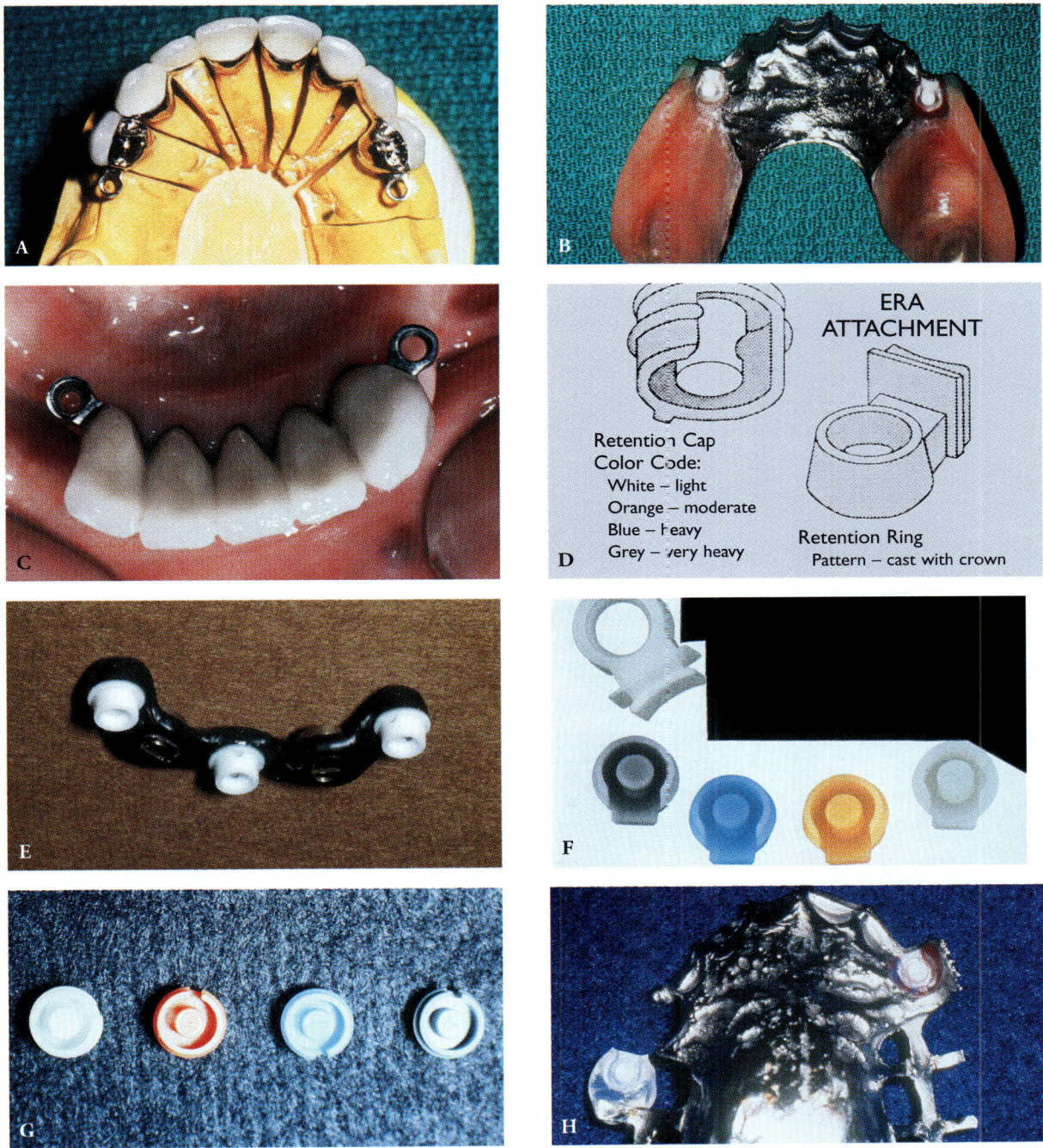

Figure 22–31A to H: *(A)* Maxillary bilateral distal extension application of Stern ERA attachments. *(B)* Male placement within an RPD framework (courtesy of Dr. Steven K. Nelson). *(C)* The need for parallelism with each other in the sagittal plane is not required. Note the splinting of fewer than six remaining anterior teeth. *(D)* Diagram of matrix and patrix components. The color-coded retentive cap has four different levels of retention. (Reproduced with permission from Sterngold, International. Advanced restorative products catalog. Attleboro, MA: Sterngold, 1998:21.) *(E)* An ERA attachment can be used with bar overdentures on implants or natural teeth. *(F)* Color-coded retentive caps and plastic pattern cast to abutment. (Reproduced with permission from Sterngold, International. Advanced restorative products catalog. Attleboro, MA: Sterngold, 1998:21.) *(G)* Color-coded retentive caps. *(H)* Retentive caps incorporated into the framework design and retained with autopolymerizing resin.

696 Esthetics in Dentistry

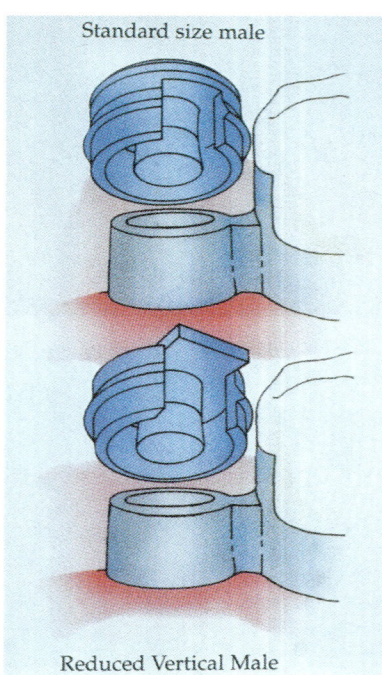

Figure 22–32: Comparison of the Stern ERA and the ERA-RV. The retentive cap varies in vertical height. (Reproduced with permission from Sterngold, International. Advanced restorative products catalog. Attleboro, MA: Sterngold, 1998:26.)

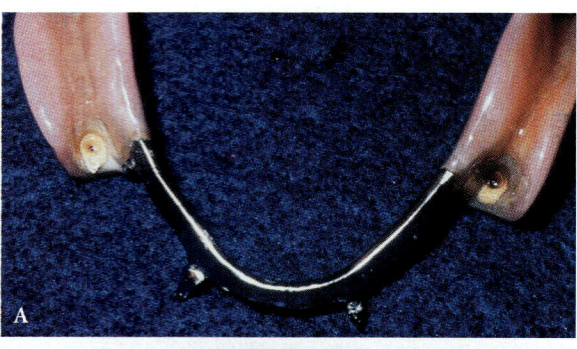

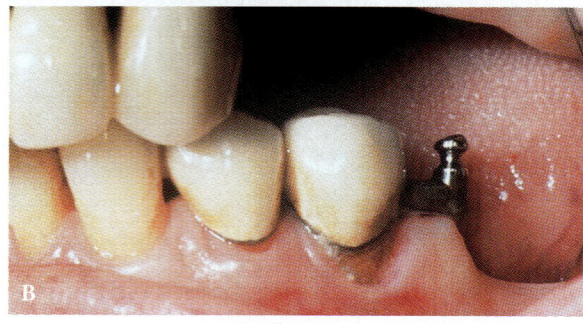

Figure 22–33A and B: *(A)* An ORS-DE matrix O-ring in an RPD framework. *(B)* An ORS-DE attachment in a distal extension application. Note that adequate vertical space is necessary for interocclusal clearance (courtesy of Dr. Steven K. Nelson).

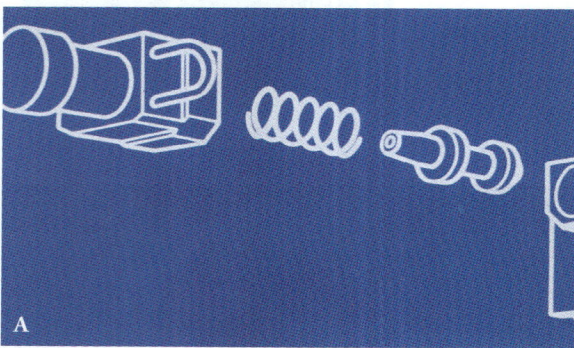

Figure 22–34A to C: *(A)* Diagram of an IC plunger attachment. *(B)* Female cast into abutment restoration. *(C)* Plunger and spring apparatus incorporated into resin or RPD.

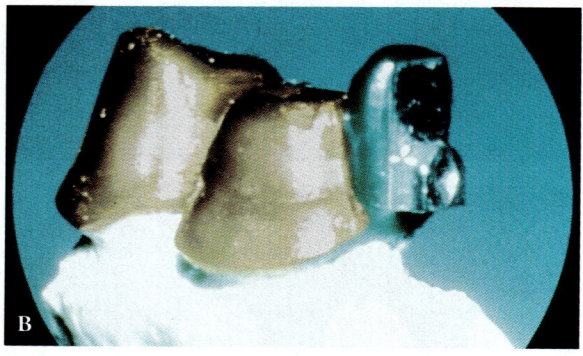

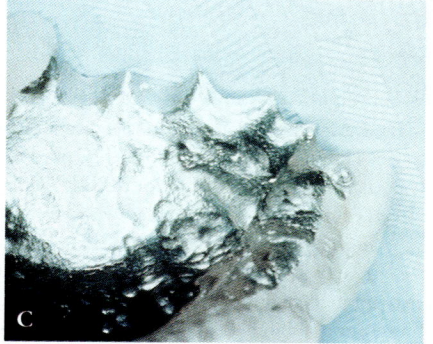

Esthetic Removable Partial Dentures

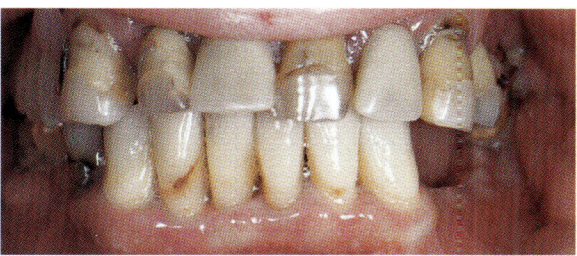

Figure 22–35A: This well-known 60-year-old attorney complained about his appearance. Examination revealed posterior bite collapse, extreme breakdown of his remaining teeth, and periodontal disease.

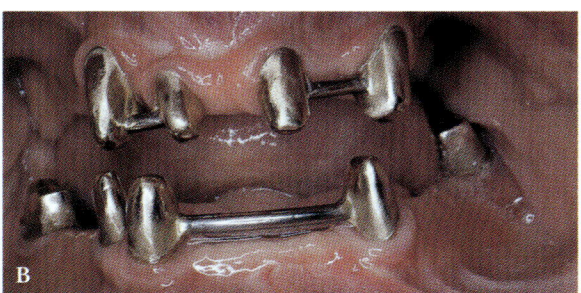 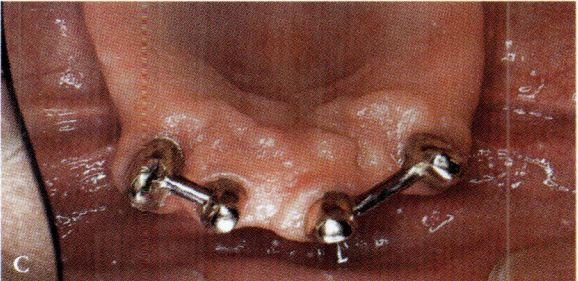

Figure 22–35B and C: Following periodontal surgery, maxillary and mandibular overdentures were constructed using Dolder bar attachments. Note the access that provides the patient with the ability for proper hygiene.

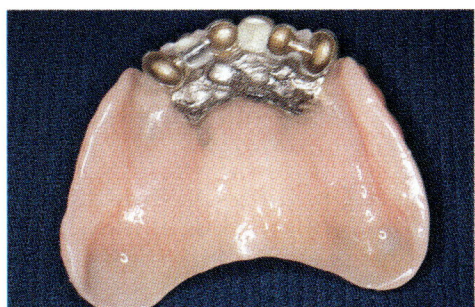 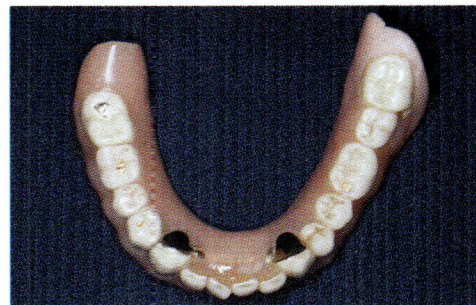

Figure 22–35D: This removable bridge provides excellent ridge adaptation plus Dolder bar secure retention for an ideal overdenture.

Figure 22–35E: This man wanted some exposed gold and a somewhat crowded anterior tooth arrangement for what he considered a "natural look."

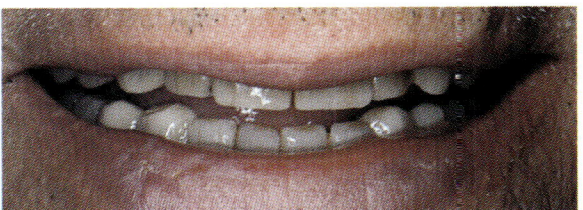

Figure 22–35F: A custom tooth staining and natural tooth arrangement gave him the appearance he thought appropriate.

degree of resilience, anatomic limitations, or convenience. The primary indication would be the splinting of abutment teeth while providing retention for the RPD. Careful consideration for the degree of resilience and interocclusal space for tooth arrangement must be provided (Figures 22–35A to F).

Dental implant placement offers a highly predictable treatment approach for overpartial dentures. Long tooth-bounded modification spaces requiring a significant amount of tissue support for the partial denture bases can benefit from application of overdenture abutment attachments on endosseous dental implants. Class I and II RPD classifications may have significant improvement in retention and stability by dental implant placement in the distal region of the edentulous residual ridge. The support offered by the overdenture concept using a dental implant would dramatically reduce the tipping and leverage forces imparted to the distal abutment teeth. This treatment modality may offer support comparable to the Class III RPD.

Milled lingual ledges have been described as an adjunctive component that will accommodate placement of lingual bracing arms, generally providing compensation for short attachment length.[40,41] A technique of providing frictional retention of components through precision milling has been described. Spark erosion technology to create precision milled fit has proved to be successful.[45] Adjunctive elastoclips may offer additional retention. The intimacy of fit developed with spark erosion or precision milling provides frictional retention, nearly eliminating any resilience. This type of attachment technology must be considered nonresilient and should be applied to the appropriate supportive elements. Additionally, the cost of this treatment approach may be prohibitive. A preprosthetic laboratory analysis of the anticipated cost may be useful in establishing the degree of remuneration required for the success of the rehabilitation.

References

1. Applegate OC. The rationale of partial denture choice. J Prosthet Dent 1960;10:891–907.

2. Bagley D. Versatile uses for plunger attachments. Trends Tech Contemp Dent Lab 1993;10:33–5.

3. Baker JL, Goodkind RJ. Precision attachment removable partial dentures. San Mateo, CA: Mosby, 1981.

4. Becker CM, Kaiser DA, Goldfogel MH. Evolution of removable partial denture design. J Prosthodont 1994;3:158–66.

5. Berg T, Caputo A. Load transfer by a maxillary distal-extension removable partial denture with cap and ring extracoronal attachments. J Prosthet Dent 1992;68:784–9.

6. Berg T, Caputo A. Maxillary distal-extension removable partial denture abutments with reduced periodontal support. J Prosthet Dent 1993;70:245–50.

7. Berte JJ, Hansen CA. Custom tinting denture bases by visible light cure lamination. J Prosthodont 1995;4:129–32.

8. Brudvik JS, Wormley JH. Construction techniques for wrought wire retention arms as related to clasp flexibility. J Prosthet Dent 1973;30:769–74.

9. Burns DR, Ward JE. A review of attachments for removable partial denture design: part 1. Classification and selection. Int J Prosthodont 1990;3:98–102.

10. Burns DR, Ward JE. A review of attachments for removable partial denture design: part 2. Treatment planning and attachment selection. Int J Prosthodont 1990;3:169–74.

11. Chou TM, Eick JD, Moore DJ, Tira DE. Stereophotogrammetric analysis of abutment tooth movement in distal-extension removable partial dentures with intracoronal attachments and clasps. J Prosthet Dent 1991;66:343–9.

12. Curtis DA, Curtis TA, Wagnild GW, Finzen FC. Incidence of various classes of removable partial dentures. J Prosthet Dent 1992;67:664–7.

13. Davenport JC, Hawamdeh K, Harrington E, Wilson HJ. Clasp retention and composites: an abrasion study. J Dent 1990;18:198–202.

14. Dixon DL, Breeding LC, Swift EJ Jr. Use of a partial-coverage porcelain laminate to enhance clasp retention. J Prosthet Dent 1990;63:55–8.

15. El Charkawi HG, El Wakad MT. Effect of splinting on load distribution of extracoronal attachment with distal extension prosthesis in vitro. J Prosthet Dent 1996;76:315–20.

16. Frank RP, Brudvik JS, Nicholls JI. A comparison of the flexibility of wrought wire and cast circumferential clasps. J Prosthet Dent 1983;49:471–6.

17. Gerhard R, Sawyer N. Dentures to harmonize with heavily pigmented tissues. J Am Dent Assoc 1966;73:94–5.

18. Goodkind RJ. The effects of removable partial denture design on abutment tooth mobility: a clinical study. J Prosthet Dent 1973;30:139–46.

19. Haeberle CB, Khan Z. Construction of a custom-shaded interim denture using visible-light-cured resin. J Prosthodont 1997;6:153–6.

20. Hansen CA, Iverson GW. An esthetic removable partial denture retainer for the maxillary canine. J Prosthet Dent 1986;56:199–203.

21. Kennedy E. Partial denture construction. Dental Items of Interest. 1928:3–8.

22. King GE, Barco MT, Olson RJ. Inconspicuous retention for removable partial dentures. J Prosthet Dent 1978;39:505–7.

23. Kotowicz WE, Fisher RL, Reed RA, Jaslow C. The combination clasp and the distal extension removable partial denture. Dent Clin North Am 1973;17:651–60.

24. Kratochvil FJ. Influence of occlusal rest position and clasp design on movement of abutment teeth. J Prosthet Dent 1963;13:114–24.

25. Kratochvil FJ. Partial removable prosthodontics. Philadelphia: WB Saunders, 1988.

26. Krol AJ. Clasp design for extension base removable partial dentures. J Prosthet Dent 1973;29:408–15.

27. Krol AJ, Finzen FC. Rotational path removable partial dentures: part 1. Replacement of posterior teeth. Int J Prosthodont 1988;1:17–27.

28. Krol AJ, Finzen FC. Rotational path removable partial dentures: part 2. Replacement of anterior teeth. Int J Prosthodont 1988;1:135–42.

29. Krol AJ, Jacobson TE, Finzen FC. Removable partial denture design outline syllabus. 4th edn. San Rafael, CA: Indent, 1990.

30. Lepe X, Land MF. Use of an intra-pontic attachment as cosmetic support for a removable appliance. Ill Dent J 1990;59;280–3.

31. McCartney JW. The MGR clasp: an esthetic extracoronal retainer for maxillary canines. J Prosthet Dent 1982;46:490–3.

32. McGivney GP, Castleberry DJ. McCracken's removable partial prosthodontics. 9th edn. St Louis, MO: Mosby, 1995.

33. Moreno de Delgado M, Garcia LT, Rudd KD. Camouflaging partial denture clasps. J Prosthet Dent 1986;55:656–60.

34. Morris HF, Brudvik JS. Influence on polishing of cast clasp properties. J Prosthet Dent 1986;55:75–7.

35. Myers RE, Pfeifer DL, Mitchell DL, Pelleu GB. A photoelastic study of rests on solitary abutments for distal-extension removable partial dentures. J Prosthet Dent 1986;56:702–7.

36. Preiskel HW. Precision attachments in dentistry. St. Louis: Mosby, 1968.

37. Schuyler CH. An analysis of the use and relative value of the precision attachment and the clasp in partial denture planning. J Prosthet Dent 1953; 3:711–4.

38. Smith BJ. Esthetic factors in removable partial prosthodontics. Dent Clin North Am 1979;23:53–63.

39. Snyder HA, Duncanson MG Jr, Johnson DL, Bloom J. Effects of clasp flexure on a 4-META adhered light polymerized composite resin. Int J Prosthodont 1991;4:364–70.

40. Staubli PE. Attachments & implants: reference manual. 6th edn. San Mateo, CA: Attachments International, 1996.

41. Sterngold-ImplaMed, Int. Advanced restorative products catalog. Attleboro, MA: Sterngold-ImplaMed, 1998.

42. Stewart KL, Rudd KD, Kuebker WA. Clinical removable partial prosthodontics. 2nd edn. St. Louis: Ishiyaku EuroAmerica, 1992.

43. Tietge JD, Dixon DL, Breeding LC, et al. In vitro investigation of the wear of resin composite materials and cast direct retainers during removable partial denture placement and removal. Int J Prosthodont 1992; 5:145–53.

44. Toth RW, Fiebiger GE, Mackert JR, Goldman BM. Shear strength of lingual rests prepared in bonded composite. J Prosthet Dent 1986;56:99–104.

45. Weber H, Frank G. Spark erosion procedure: a method for extensive combined fixed and removable prosthodontic care. J Prosthet Dent 1993;69:222–7.

46. Weiner S, Krause AS, Nicholas W. Esthetic modification of removable partial denture teeth with light-cured composites. J Prosthet Dent 1987;57:381–4.

47. Williamson RT. Removable partial denture fabrication using extracoronal attachments: a clinical report. J Prosthet Dent 1993;70:285–7.

48. Wong R, Nicholls JI, Smith DE. Evaluation of prefabricated linqual rest seats for removable partial dentures. J Prosthet Dent 1982;48:521–6.

49. Zach GA. Advantages of mesial rests for removable partial dentures. J Prosthet Dent 1975;33:32–5.

50. Zarb GA, MacKay HF. Cosmetics and removable partial dentures—the Class IV partially edentulous patient. J Prosthet Dent 1981;46:360–8.

Additional Resource

Goldstein RE. Esthetics in dentistry. 1st edn. Philadelphia: JB Lippincott, 1976:110–35.

PART 5

ESTHETIC PROBLEMS OF MALOCCLUSION

CHAPTER 23

RESTORATIVE TREATMENT OF DIASTEMA

Mark D. Dlugokinski, DDS, Kevin B. Frazier, DMD, Ronald E. Goldstein, DDS

One of the most challenging tasks of modern restorative dentistry is resolving the dilemma of spaces between anterior teeth. The presence of a diastema can be a problem because the esthetic value of anterior spacing varies between cultures, and the best treatment options are often rejected. To some, an anterior diastema is desirable, whereas others attempt to hide it with habits such as lip or tongue posturing.[6] Some patients have even resorted to daily applications of wax or cotton to disguise a diastema (Figures 23–1A and B). Treatment planning to correct a diastema may include orthodontics, restorative dentistry, or a combination of several therapies. Like most esthetic problems, the treatment of a diastema requires careful analysis and occasional consultation with specialists. Diagnostic casts, radiographs, and photographs or digital imaging are necessary to thoroughly evaluate a diastema. Anterior spaces should not be closed without first recognizing and treating the underlying cause(s).[4]

ETIOLOGY OF DIASTEMA

The etiology of diastema may be attributed to hereditary and developmental factors (Table 23–1).[10,18] Although hereditary determinants play a major role in causing diastemas, there is nothing that can be done to prevent them. Most of the other causes of diastema formation are preventable.

Maxillary lateral incisors are the most frequent congenitally missing permanent teeth, along with mandibular second premolars and the third molars. A missing tooth creates an obvious space problem in the immediate area and may lead to undesirable spacing in adjacent regions as the position of several teeth in a quadrant can be affected by the absence of one tooth. Small teeth and large jaws can lead to generalized spacing, whereas unerupted supernumerary teeth can create a diastema by their position between the roots of other teeth.[28] Anatomic factors such as those seen in atypical frenum positions may also contribute to diastema

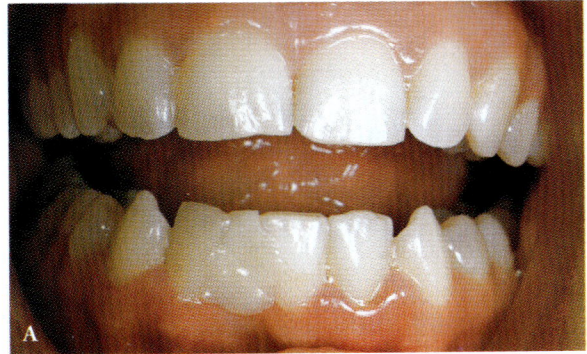 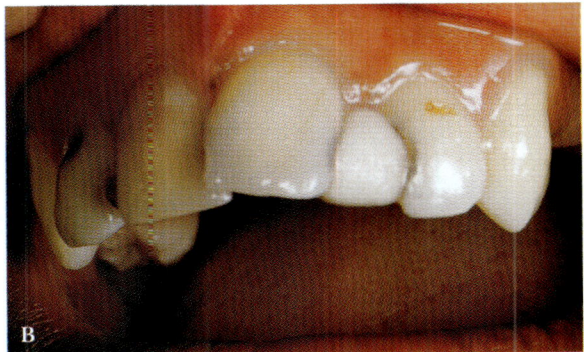

Figure 23–1A and B: Some patients resort to daily applications of materials such as wax (#25) or cotton (#10) to disguise a diastema.

TABLE 23–1. Factors Contributing to Diastema

HEREDITARY FACTORS	DEVELOPMENTAL FACTORS
Congenitally missing teeth	Habits
Tooth/jaw size discrepancy	Periodontal disease
Supernumerary teeth	Tooth loss
Frenum attachments	Posterior bite collapse

formation.[14] The presence of the frenum muscle fibers on the alveolar ridge influences the direction of tooth eruption and maintains separation of the adjacent teeth after eruption (Figures 23–2A to K). Although teeth can be moved together orthodontically in the presence of a frenum, once the active appliance is removed, the teeth tend to separate, reforming the diastema unless permanent retention is provided. An adequate border of attached gingiva is essential to successful orthodontic movement. Surgical removal or repositioning of the undesirable frenum attachment (and the creation of a stable area of attached gingiva in its place) prior to orthodontic repositioning reduces frenum-related diastema relapse.[7,16]

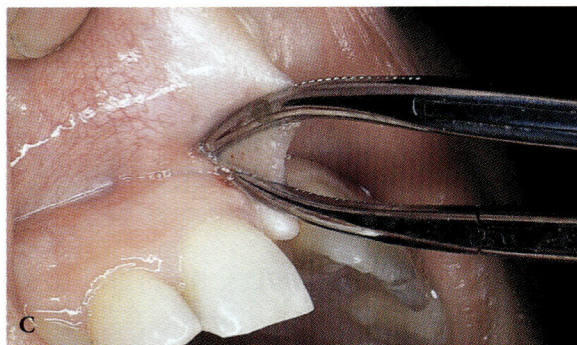

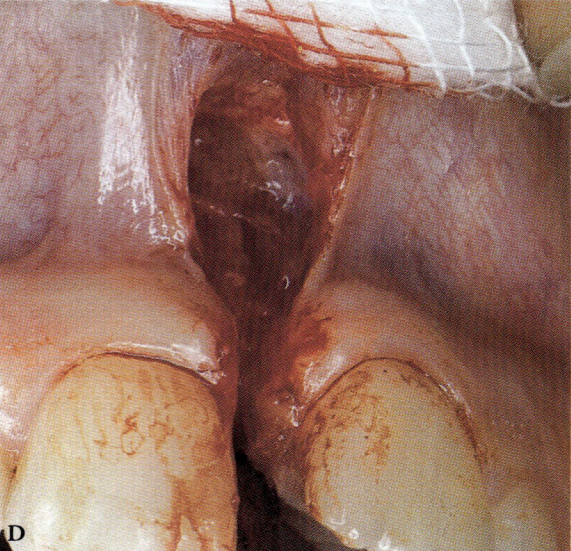

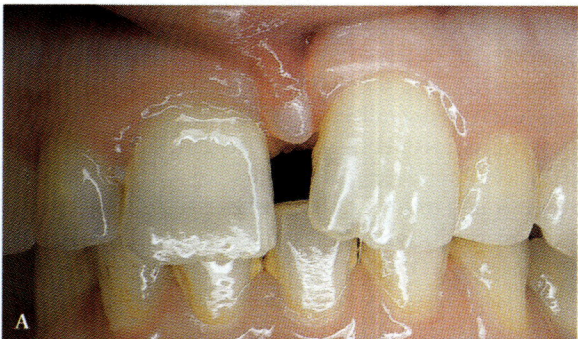

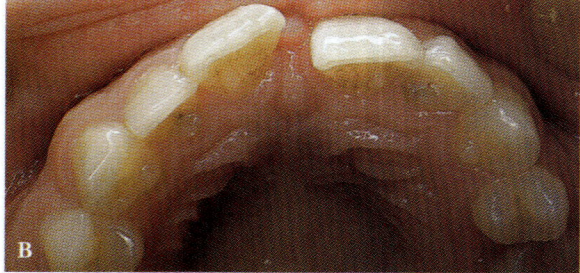

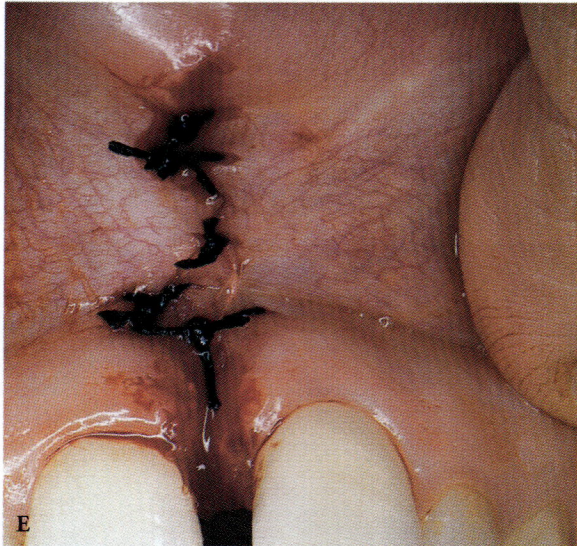

Figure 23–2A and B: This 23-year-old model was dissatisfied not only with the space between her teeth but also with the presence and form of the labial frenum.

Figure 23–2C to E: The labial frenum was surgically removed so that after her teeth were repositioned there would be no muscle interference.

Restorative Treatment of Diastema

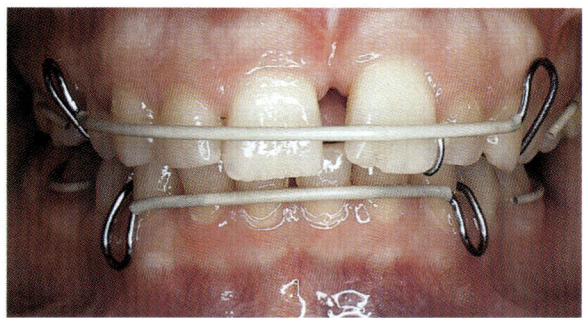

Figure 23–2F: After the tissue healed, removable Hawley appliances were placed. Note the tooth-colored Teflon tubing applied to the wire to mask the metal color.

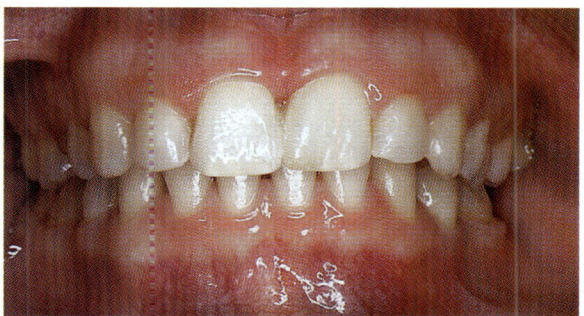

Figure 23–2H: Composite resin bonding was chosen to close the interdental space between the central incisors.

COMBINED THERAPY FOR FRENUM INVOLVEMENT

PROBLEM: A 23-year-old female presented with a large maxillary and a relatively small mandibular diastema (see Figures 23–2A, B, and K). The frenum protruded, and the left central incisor was rotated and in labioversion. Because the patient's profession was in fashion modeling, her chief complaint was that the presence of a space between her teeth was a liability to her.

TREATMENT: A frenectomy was performed (see Figures 23–2C to E). After healing, maxillary and mandibular Hawley retainers were designed for the patient (see Figure 23–2F). Note how a plastic coating that conceals the labial wires permitted the patient to wear the appliance while working. Therefore, she gained the advantage of wearing it more often. Figure 23–2F shows a maxillary appliance in position and the amount of space needed to close the diastema. Figure 23–2G illustrates the result of wearing the appliance for 18 hours per day for approximately 4 months. At this point, the central incisors were mechanically bonded with composite resin to mask the remaining interdental tissue space (see Figure 23–2H). Figures 23–2I and J show how

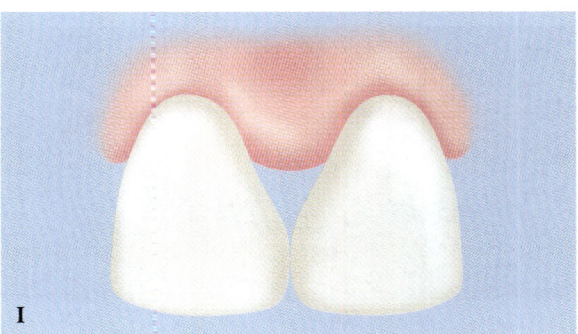

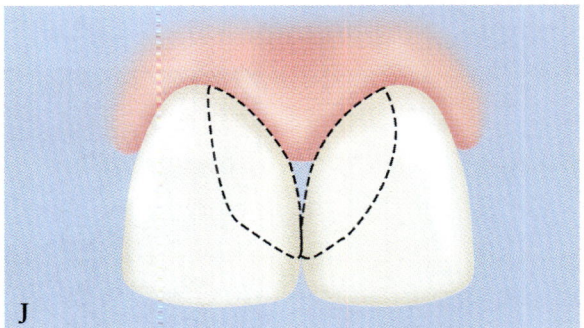

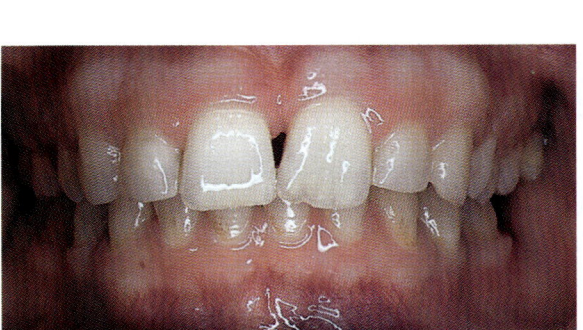

Figure 23–2G: After approximately 4 months of wearing the appliance 18 hours per day, the teeth were together.

Figure 23–2I and J: Composite resin bonding is the most conservative method to close an interdental space. (I) Before the restoration. (J) After the restoration outlining the surfaces involved with the restoration.

facial, mesial, and lingual surfaces were bonded to close the remaining interdental spaces.

It is sometimes possible to retain the interdental tissue if it is considered to be attractive. In this particular case, the protruding frenum looked like a small cyst, which the patient disliked, and was subsequently removed.

RESULT: Approximately 4 months of treatment were necessary to completely close and transform the patient's unattractive smile into an attractive one (see Figures 23–2K and L). The appliance was designed to be as unobtrusive as possible. Because of the patient's motivation and ability to tolerate the appliance, the movement was accomplished in less time than expected. Twenty-five years later, the patient wanted to update her smile. Following bleaching treatments, two porcelain laminates were fabricated for the central incisors (Figure 23–2M).

Among the most common developmental causes of diastemas are habits such as tongue thrust. Large tongues or abnormal swallowing patterns can cause tooth separation by forcing the tongue into lingual embrasures (Figures 23–3A and B). The habitual probing action of the tongue wedges the teeth apart. Chronic lip biting may also contribute to diastema formation due to the patient's habit of sucking the mangled lip mucosa against the teeth. Periodontal trauma with resultant spacing between the incisors can be caused by habits such as wedging a fingernail, toothpick, or other foreign object between the teeth (see Chapter 20, Figure 20–18). Other developmental causes of diastemas are obvious, such as the loss of a permanent tooth, or a more subtle cause, such as periodontal disease.[26] Tooth loss in the posterior region has been associated with anterior diastema formation as a result of posterior bite collapse.[15] In this case, the loss of posterior occlusal contacts alters the pattern of occlusal function, causing tooth migration and a decreased vertical dimension. The indirect result of this condition can be a flaring out of the maxillary incisors with space formation. The pressure from inflammatory exudate in an acutely involved periodontal pocket may

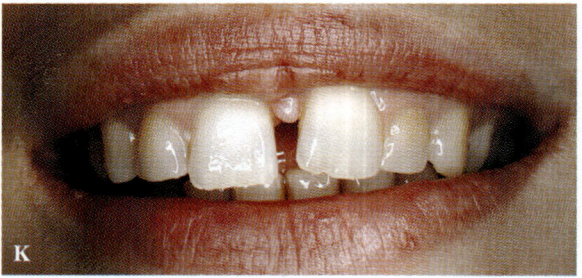
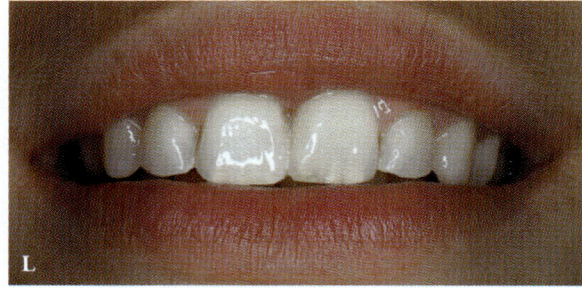

Figure 23–2K and L: A combination of minor orthodontic and restorative treatment helped to improve the smile in only 4 months.

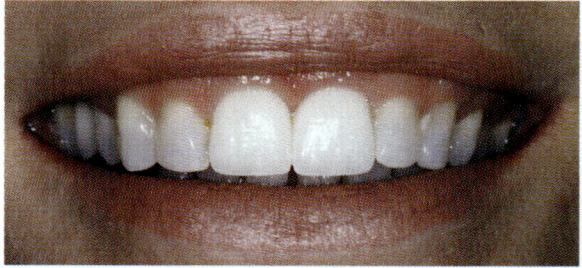

Figure 23–2M: Twenty-five years later, the patient wanted to update her smile. Bleaching treatments and two porcelain laminates were fabricated for the two central incisors to update the patient's smile to her satisfaction.

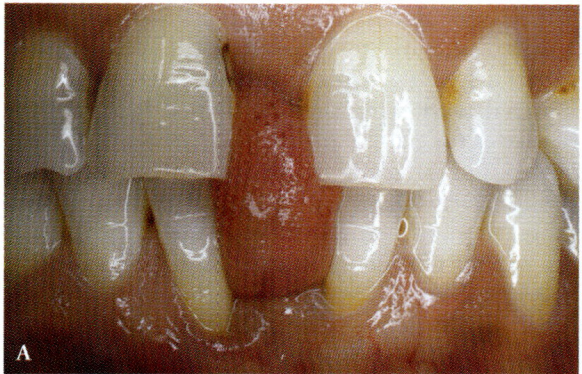 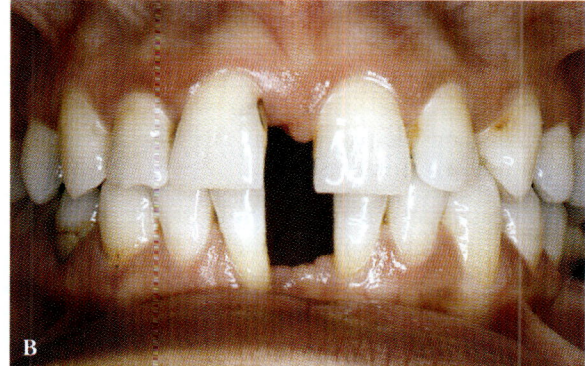

Figure 23–3A and B: This lady had a habit of forcing her tongue between both maxillary and mandibular anterior teeth, which caused her diastema to continue to enlarge.

facilitate localized tooth movement and the creation of a diastema. Prevention of tooth loss and maintenance of gingival health can prevent diastema formation that results from deterioration of the structure and function of the oral cavity.

DIAGNOSIS AND TREATMENT PLANNING

Although the presence of a diastema is self-evident, these spaces must not be closed without first addressing the underlying cause(s). As previously discussed, the etiology of diastema may be attributed to hereditary and developmental factors. On identifying these factors, the dentist should include the patient in the treatment planning process by presenting appropriate treatment alternatives, prognoses, and fees.

Identifying the cause(s) of a diastema will usually indicate the appropriate corrective treatment.[19] For example, diastema due to periodontal problems cannot be corrected predictably with restorations alone if alveolar bone has been lost and the teeth are mobile. Splinting or some other method of stabilization would have to be included in the treatment plan. When periodontal disease is causing the teeth to drift and separate, the acute pathology must be treated first. Final periodontal treatment can be postponed until after orthodontic therapy. Following orthodontic and periodontal therapy, any needed restorative treatment to achieve the final esthetic result may be performed.[1]

Although restorations are usually indicated to close multiple diastemas due to small teeth, other therapies may be needed to achieve an optimal esthetic result. Tooth repositioning may be necessary to even the spaces prior to restorations. Periodontal surgery may be required to provide additional clinical crown length to balance the increase in tooth width from restorations as spaces are closed. Additional teeth not directly affected by a diastema may need to be included in the restorative treatment plan to provide a proportional smile. Anytime a patient is considering extensive restorative treatment, he or she should first be given the opportunity to change the tooth color. Prerestorative bleaching can improve the esthetic result of any type of restorative therapy and should be considered when extensive dental treatment is planned. Tooth-whitening procedures allow thinner or more translucent restorations to be used when dark/stained tooth structure does not have to be masked. The preceding factors illustrate the importance of thorough diagnosis and comprehensive treatment planning for all types of diastema cases.

As patient acceptance of ideal treatment is the ultimate objective for the dentist in this phase, it is often necessary to allow the patient to visualize and judge the end result.[6] For simple diastema closures involving restorations, the chairside application of tooth-colored wax or unbonded composite resin to the patient's proximal tooth surfaces should provide a good indication of the result. For complex cases that involve several teeth or combination therapies (orthodontics and restorations), a diagnostic wax-up and computer imaging may be required to enable the patient to appreciate the anticipated result of extensive treatment (see Chapter 2, *Esthetics in Dentistry*, Volume 1, 2nd Edition).[17] When multiple disciplines are involved, such as orthodontics, surgery, and restorative dentistry, a case presentation conference (or teleconference) with all involved clinicians and the patient may facilitate acceptance of complex treatment plans.

Pre- and postoperative photographs or digital images can provide many benefits. Photographs of the results of treatment on other patients can be used to help current patients envision the possibilities associated with their own treatment and inspire confidence in the dentist's abilities. Photographs document the procedure and can be used to improve the chances for reimbursement from insurance carriers in certain cases. A duplicate set of pre- and post-treatment images given to a patient following treatment helps to prevent "buyer's remorse" and allows him or her to serve as a marketing advocate for the office when the dramatic before and after photos are displayed to family and friends. However, it is sound practice to use computer imaging of both close-up and full-face before and after images for best patient and doctor visualization.

TREATMENT TO CORRECT DIASTEMA

Orthodontic Repositioning

The traditional treatment modalities for diastema correction have included operative, surgical, periodontal, orthodontic, and/or prosthodontic procedures. In many cases of diastema, the treatment of choice is orthodontics (see Chapter 25). Too often, dentists compromise treatment with unnecessary restorations. This decision may result in sound tooth structure being sacrificed to correct a cosmetic problem, and, if so, it is an esthetic compromise in its truest sense. When a patient chooses to eliminate a diastema, the dentist is responsible for impressing on the patient the importance of choosing the best possible cosmetic treatment, namely, the one that best maintains the integrity of the oral cavity. An esthetic problem should be treated like any other dental condition. Just as the dentist is responsible for letting a patient know the best possible treatment to save a tooth, the clinician is obligated to inform the patient with an esthetic problem of the optimal method(s) of treatment.

When a diastema is best treated by orthodontics, the dentist should educate and motivate the patient to consider that type of therapy. No restorative material is equal to healthy tooth structure, and regardless of the time taken, skill employed, or material used, a restoration cannot duplicate the beauty of the natural dentition. In other words, the health and preservation of the natural dentition should always be foremost in our minds. Furthermore, there is a considerable monetary savings to the patient who chooses orthodontics over restorative dentistry due to the periodic repairs and/or remaking of the restoring dentition.

Localized spacing of the permanent teeth due to malalignment or resulting from an isolated habit is probably the optimal indication for treatment of a diastema with orthodontic repositioning. Any space-producing habit must be eliminated as part of the treatment, and it is essential that the patient understands that breaking the habit is ultimately his or her responsibility. The dentist's role in this situation is to identify the habit, educate the patient, and provide any habit-breaking appliances or techniques. Orthodontic treatment to close a diastema can be accomplished with the appropriate fixed or removable appliances followed by at least 6 months of stabilization with a fixed retainer. Permanent splinting is often necessary to prevent relapse when orthodontic treatment is the only therapy used to close spaces.[25]

A compromise can sometimes be found for the patient by electing to use a night guard that fits well. Even after postorthodontic stabilization, some space can continuously recur. The solution can be permanent splinting and tight-fitting fixed restorations. This works well if a patient resists using threaded floss, which is necessary for splinted teeth.

COMBINATION TECHNIQUE FOR CLOSURE OF A DIASTEMA

PROBLEM: This 39-year-old individual presented with diastemas between the maxillary central incisors and congenitally malformed lateral incisors. He had a marked overbite and fracture of a mandibular central incisor (Figure 23–4A).

TREATMENT: A removable maxillary appliance with finger springs was constructed to orthodontically reposition the central incisors together (Figure 23–4B). A mandibular lingual appliance was also

Restorative Treatment of Diastema

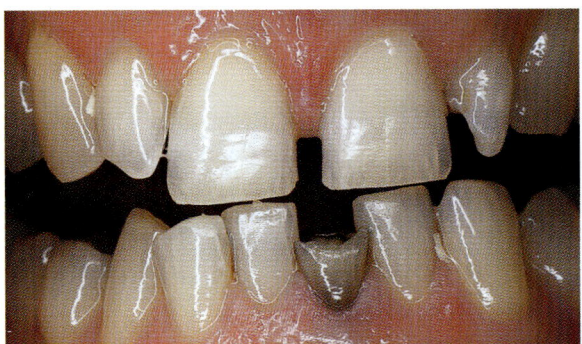

Figure 23–4A: This 39-year-old man was unhappy with his diastema, deformed laterals, and mandibular fractured incisor.

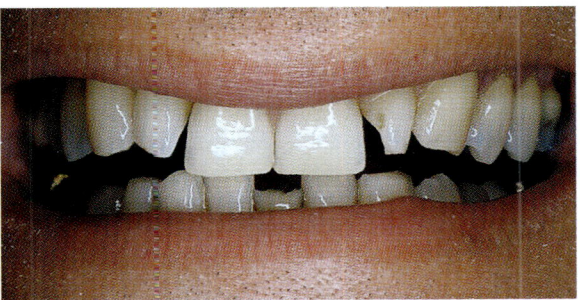

Figure 23–4B: A removable maxillary appliance with finger springs was used to bring the central incisors together.

used to upright the molars to regain lost vertical dimension and realign the crowded mandibular anterior teeth. After completion of orthodontic treatment, the maxillary central incisors were splinted together with composite resin to prevent future drifting and reformation of the diastema (Figures 23–4C and D). The adjacent maxillary lateral incisors were crowned to assist the stabilization of the central incisors and restore symmetry to the maxillary arch, eliminating their "peg-lateral" shape (Figure 23–4E). In addition, the mandibular left central incisor was crowned. The final smile achieved improved esthetics, health, and function (Figure 23–4F).

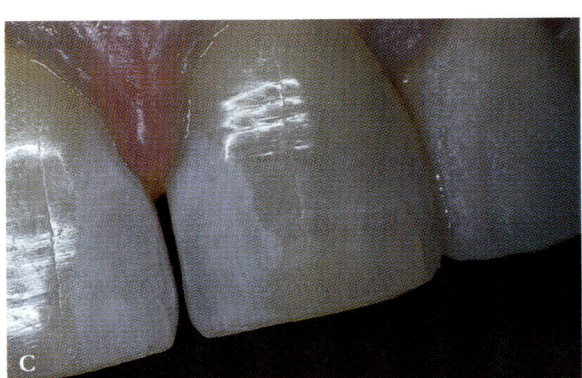

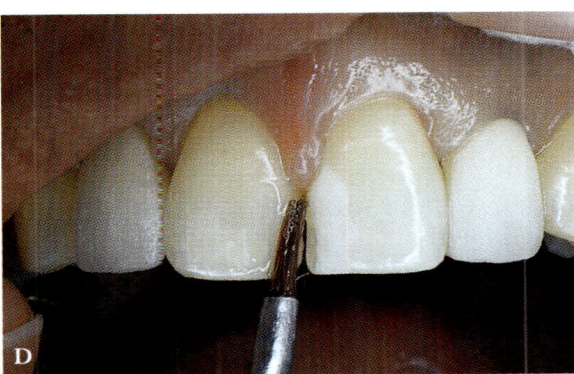

Figure 23–4C and D: The maxillary central incisors were bonded together with composite resin to help retain them in their new position.

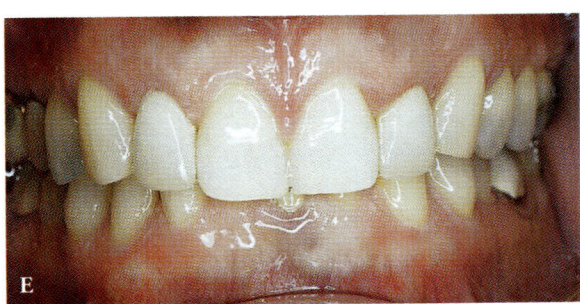

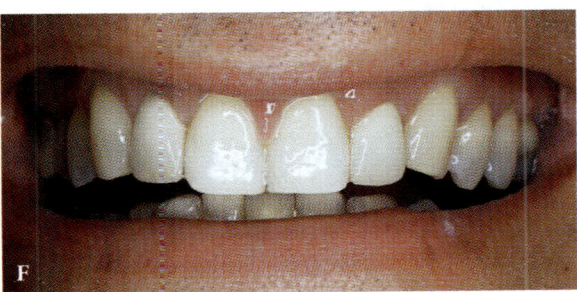

Figure 23–4E and F: The adjacent maxillary lateral incisors were crowned to help hold the central incisors in place and restore symmetry to the maxillary arch. The mandibular left central incisor also was crowned to complete the esthetic result.

RESULT: The success of this case is based on a close working relationship with the orthodontist to accomplish necessary repositioning before restorative procedures are begun. The final esthetic result could not have been achieved by crowning the four incisors alone. If orthodontics had not been employed, either the central or lateral incisors would have necessarily been overcontoured; in addition, the overbite would not have been corrected to any appreciable extent.

After orthodontic repositioning, it is sometimes necessary to splint teeth together to compensate for the resilient forces of the gingiva. Unless it is absolutely necessary, the central incisors should not be splinted together so the patient may readily maintain good oral hygiene with dental floss. An alternative to splinting central incisors together would be to bring the spaced central incisors together using either orthodontic wire or elastic ligature and then enlarge the mesial aspect of the adjacent lateral incisors with composite resin bonding. This technique is illustrated in the following case.

CLOSURE BY BONDING ADJACENT TEETH

PROBLEM: This 23-year-old man stated as his chief complaint that the space between his two front teeth had come back after they were restored several years ago with full porcelain crowns to correct the diastema (Figure 23–5A). It was believed that the teeth had drifted apart because of an existing periodontal condition that was further complicated by an occlusal problem.

TREATMENT: The mandibular incisors were adjusted to eliminate anterior interference and traumatic occlusion, followed by initiation of periodontal therapy. On completion of conservative periodontal therapy, an elastic ligature was placed around the maxillary central incisors to close the diastema. After wearing the elastic for several days, the patient returned with the space closed (Figure 23–5B).

To prevent future drifting of the central incisors and reformation of the diastema, the newly created space between the central and lateral incisors must be treated. Artus's shim-type articulating ribbon (Englewood, NJ) was used to protect the adjacent centrals from acid etching and bonding to the lateral incisors. This extremely thin material (5/10,000ths of an inch) is preferred over the much thicker Mylar or other materials to achieve the tightest contact possible. Figure 23–5C shows the ribbon in place with the lateral incisor etched and ready to be coated with composite bonding agent, followed by light cure for 20 seconds.

The addition of a single increment of composite resin is next adapted to the lateral incisor to close the diastema. This material is then polymerized (Figure 23–5D) labially and lingually. Lastly, the patient is instructed in the use of thin dental floss to properly cleanse the interdental spaces.

RESULT: Figure 23–5E shows the closed diastema, sufficiently stabilized by the lateral incisors. Regardless of whether the lateral incisors were

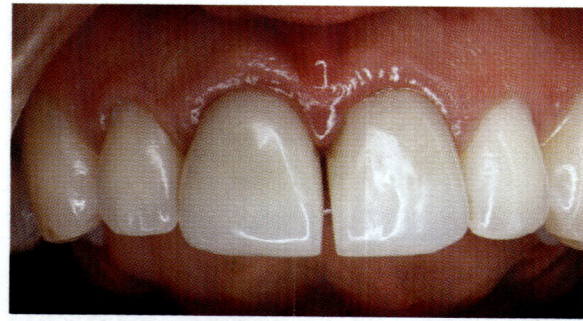

Figure 23–5A: This 23-year-old man presented with a new diastema formation between his previously crowned central incisors. The space had opened because of a periodontal condition complicated by traumatic occlusion.

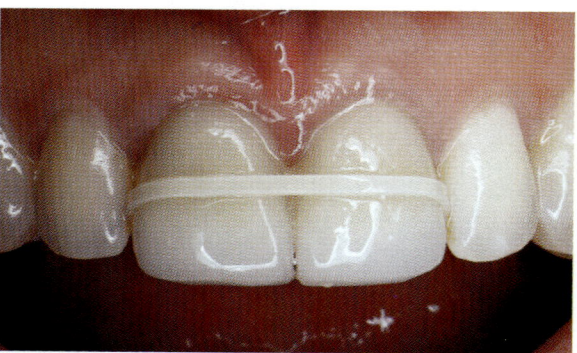

Figure 23–5B: After conservative periodontal therapy and occlusal equilibration, a rubber elastic was placed on the central incisors to close the diastema.

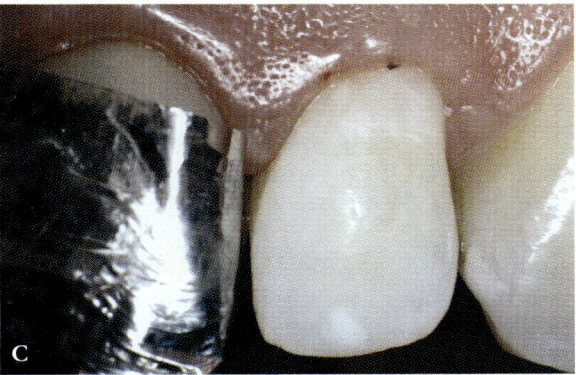 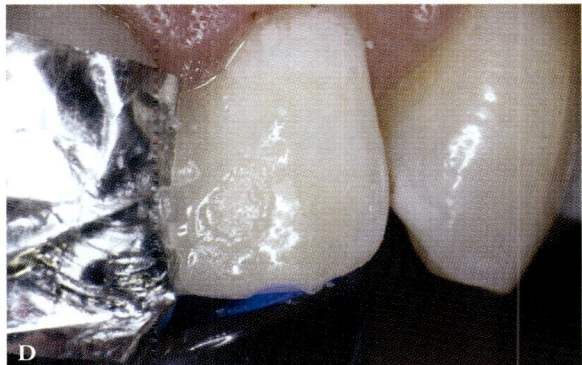

Figure 23–5C and D: The adjacent lateral incisors were tightly bonded using Artus shim stock (5/10,000th inch thick) to achieve the tightest closure possible.

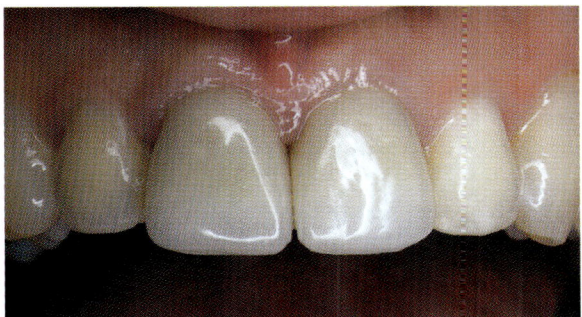

Figure 23–5E: After 24 months, the teeth continue to be held in position by the tightly bonded lateral incisors.

crowned, laminated, or bonded, it is essential that the contact area be broad so that the central incisors are held firmly in place. During closure, it is recommended to stabilize the central incisors with digital pressure while the composite resin is being applied and until it is polymerized.

Localized spacing due to missing teeth may require a combination of orthodontic and restorative treatment. Minor tooth movement to correct uneven, mesial distal drifting of spaced teeth can improve the esthetic result of corrective restorations by creating symmetric interdental spaces for individual restorations or through the formation of normal-sized edentulous spaces for a prosthetic replacement. Composite resin bonding can be used to do the final esthetic correction of remaining interdental spaces (Figures 23–6A and B).[22]

Orthognathic Surgery

Tooth repositioning cannot adequately eliminate generalized spacing of the anterior teeth resulting from tooth/jaw size discrepancies, skeletal malocclusions, or the single abnormally wide diastema. Restorative dentistry is often the best therapeutic option for correcting generalized spacing due to small teeth as they can be made artificially larger, thus filling the gaps (Figures 23–7A to D). Orthognathic surgery or an implant can treat the single, wide diastema that cannot be eliminated with restorations or a conventional prosthesis.[2,11,23,24] Diastema closure via surgical contracture of the arch can provide a stable and esthetic result if the patient is willing to assume the risks that are inherent with any surgical procedure and make the necessary financial commitment. However, restorative dentistry will sometimes be necessary to close any remaining diastemas following surgery.

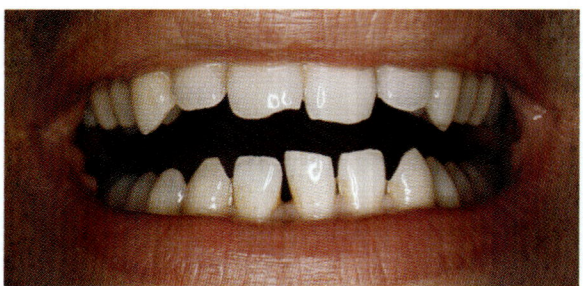

Figure 23–6A: This 29-year-old man had lost a mandibular tooth and the remaining teeth had shifted, exposing unattractive spaces when he talked or smiled.

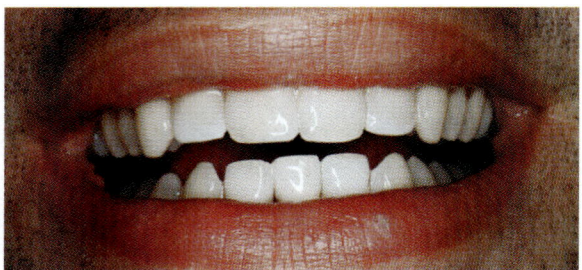

Figure 23–6B: After a one-appointment procedure with composite resin bonding and cosmetic contouring of both maxillary and mandibular incisors, the smile greatly improved. Note how much better the three remaining mandibular incisors appear when they are in balance with the rest of the mouth.

IMMEDIATE TEMPORARY CLOSURE OF A POSTERIOR DIASTEMA

PROBLEM: A 26-year-old female had undergone orthognathic surgery for her Class III protrusive malocclusion, which left a small diastema between the mandibular right cuspid and first bicuspid. The patient was very self-conscious of this space and adamantly declined other needed dental treatment until the space was closed (Figures 23–8A to C).

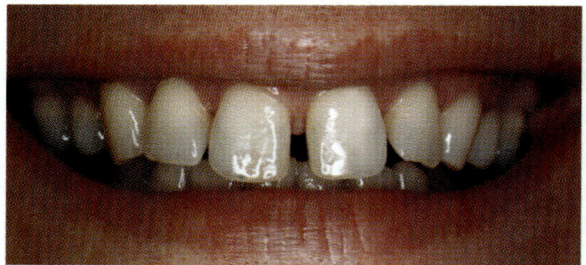

Figure 23–7A: This 24-year-old actress felt that she was being typecast because of her small and spaced anterior teeth.

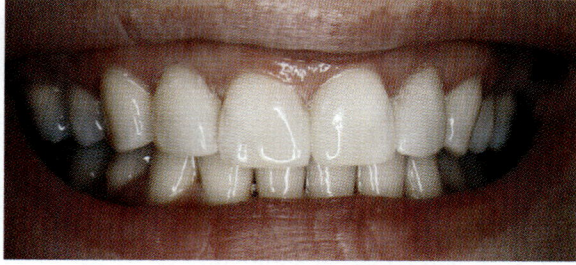

Figure 23–7B: Because the central and lateral incisors were too narrow for the patient's face, the teeth were bonded with composite resin to provide a more proportionate smile.

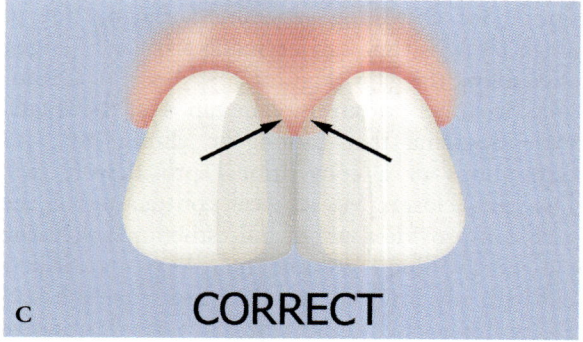

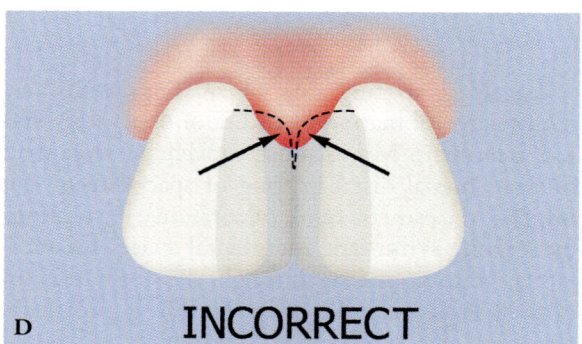

Figure 23–7C and D: (C) Illustrates the proper form in which the composite resin must be contoured to mask the interdental space while still allowing easy cleaning with dental floss. (D) Illustrates the improper form.

Restorative Treatment of Diastema 713

TREATMENT: Because a lack of sufficient space prevented the construction of a two- or three-unit fixed partial denture that would look symmetric and attractive, an alternative treatment was needed. The option of a second orthodontic treatment was deemed impractical as surgical orthodontics had already been employed as long-term treatment. The composite resin technique was chosen as both an immediate and economic solution. As previously stated in this chapter, if the diastema is large, both teeth must be treated. In this case, the distal surface of the cuspid and the mesial surface of the first bicuspid were etched and restored with composite resin to close the diastema (Figures 23–8D to F).

Because esthetics was the patient's chief concern, it was not imperative to completely close the space or obtain tight contact between these teeth. The patient was told that she would have to use dental floss to adequately clean the space. As each tooth was minimally bonded, neither appeared from a distance to be overly contoured or too large (see Figures 23–8E and F).

RESULT: The final result can be seen in Figures 23–8E and F. It is important to inform the patient

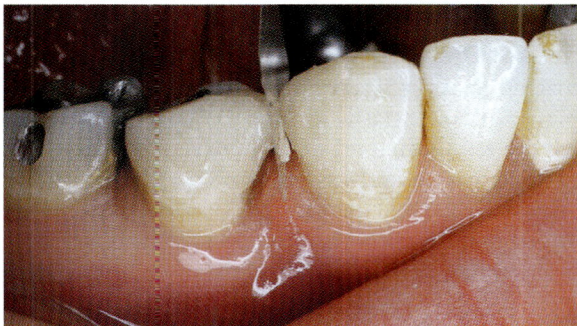

Figure 23–8D: Composite resin bonding was done on the adjacent proximating surfaces and separated by a Mylar strip.

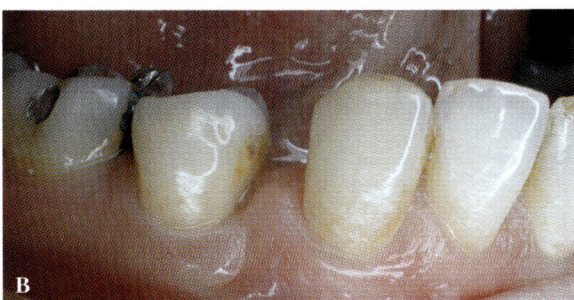

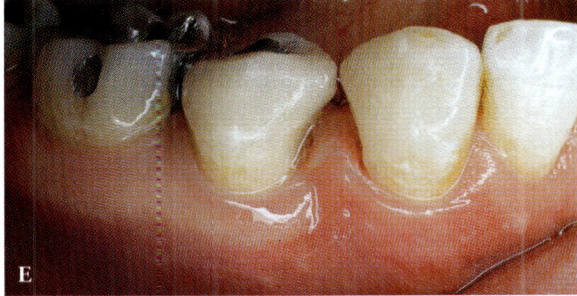

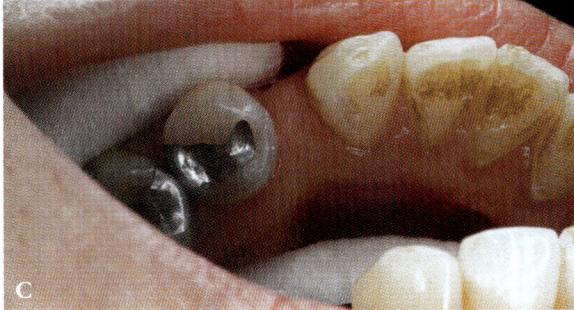

Figure 23–8A to C: This 26-year-old female was unhappy with the large diastema between the mandibular right cuspid and bicuspid following orthognathic surgery.

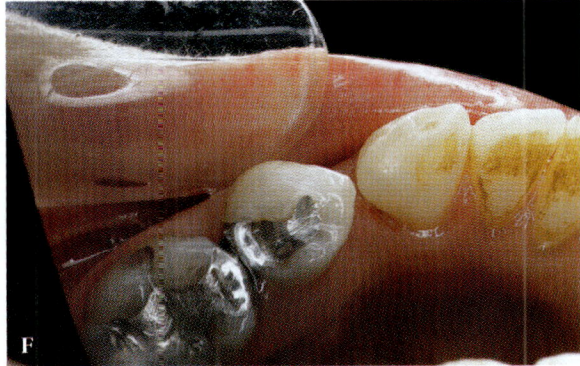

Figure 23–8E and F: The closure immediately after bonding.

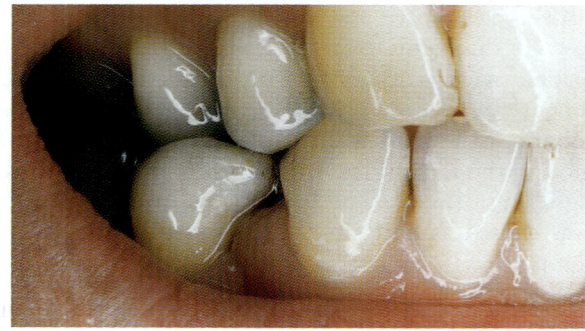

Figure 23–8G: The teeth remained acceptably closed after 5 years.

that no dental restoration is truly "permanent" and that composite resin closure of a diastema may require refinishing, repair, or remake every few years as discoloration and wear may occur. If longer life is achieved, the patient is satisfied (Figure 23–8G). It is hoped that, in time, the profession of dentistry may find a more "permanent" material or technique.

Esthetic Considerations for Restorative Options

When restorations are indicated for diastema closure, several esthetic factors must be considered. First and most obvious is the esthetic appearance of the individual teeth. The optimal proportions for a natural-looking maxillary incisor are an incisogingival length to mesiodistal width ratio of 1:0.6 (the tooth width should be approximately 60% of the length). When these proportions are violated, as often happens when large diastemas are closed with restorations, the restored teeth look "wrong" because they are out of proportion (see Chapter 9, *Esthetics in Dentistry*, Volume 1, 2nd Edition). The methods available to compensate for the extra width include lengthening the anatomic crown with a restoration, increasing the clinical crown length with periodontal surgery, or using restorative optical illusions to make a wide tooth appear narrow (see Chapter 8, *Esthetics in Dentistry*, Volume 1, 2nd Edition).

DIASTEMA CAUSED BY TEETH TOO SMALL

PROBLEM: This 28-year-old male store manager was so self-conscious about smiling that he adopted a more "serious" demeanor (Figure 23–9A) so that he would not have to smile.

TREATMENT: Esthetic analysis of the patient's smile, using a dental dial caliper, revealed teeth that were too small to be proportionate. Thus, even if orthodontics were chosen, the outcome would still

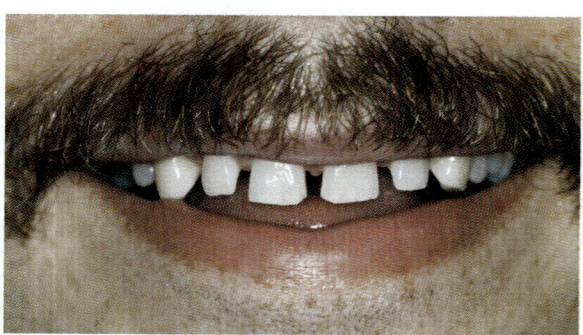

Figure 23–9A: This 28-year-old man presented with multiple diastemas and teeth too small for his facial structure.

result in a disproportionate smile. Therefore, the patient chose composite resin bonding as both an economic and immediate solution.

First, the shade selection was determined by testing different materials directly on the teeth. Once this was completed, a rubber dam was applied to maintain isolation during the procedures (Figure 23–9B). Next, the right central incisor was bonded to the predetermined mesiodistal width, measured again, and reduced slightly with a series of SoFlex discs (3M ESPE, St. Paul, MN) to exactly two of the spaces to be filled in (Figure 23–9C). Then the right central incisor was wrapped with a 5/10,000-inch thickness shim stock (Artus), held in place with an alligator clip, and the left central incisor was restored (Figure 23–9D).

Finishing procedures included the ET (Brasseler, Savannah, GA) series followed by SoFlex discs and strips. The final results of six bonded teeth can be seen in Figures 23–9E and F.

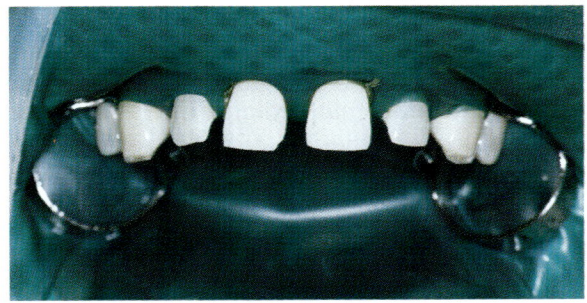

Figure 23–9B: A rubber dam was placed to maintain isolation during a multiple bonding procedure.

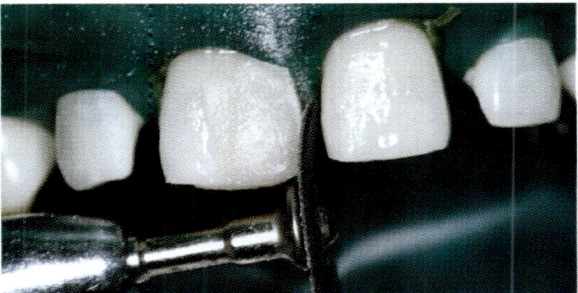

Figure 23–9C: The teeth were measured, sized, and proportionally bonded one by one.

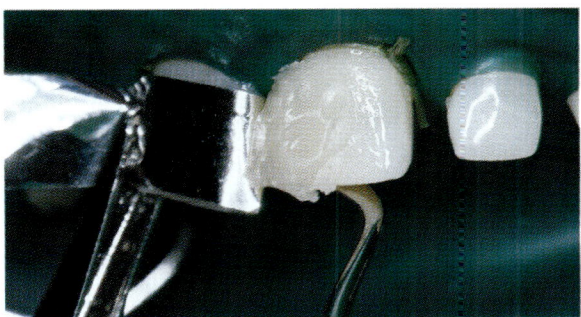

Figure 23–9D: After bonding the right central incisor, composite resin was placed on the left central incisor to close the space.

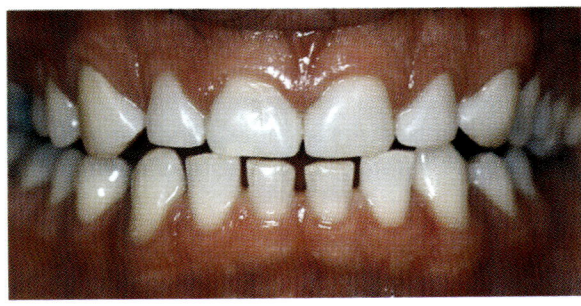

Figure 23–9E: The final results from bonding six anterior teeth.

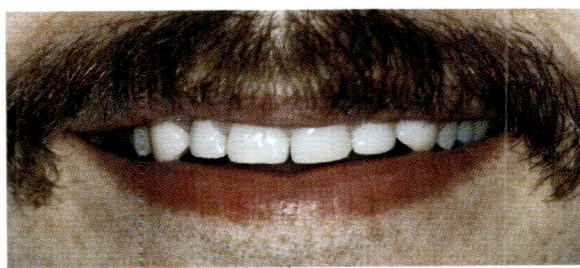

Figure 23–9F: One year later, the smile remained balanced and proportional for this patient.

RESULT: This balanced smile, shown 1 year later (see Figure 23–9F), is the product of reproportioning six teeth that were too small for the patient. Although orthodontics alone could have been used to close the spaces, the end result would not be as satisfying, both functionally and esthetically.

Lengthening the tooth by extending the incisal edge is the simplest method of maintaining proportionality of the individual tooth. However, the patient's occlusal scheme may not allow enough extra length to compensate for the added width because of the potential to create protrusive interferences. A complete examination and thorough analysis of the patient's occlusion would reveal this complication prior to starting the treatment phase. Lengthening the clinical crown by gingivectomy or an apically repositioned flap with osseous recontouring will provide the needed length to offset the extra width without creating potential occlusal interferences. Either of these options can enable you to close diastemas with natural-looking, proportional restorations, although the esthetic harmony of all of the anterior teeth must be considered as well.

The concept of the "golden proportion" as applied to a smile indicates that the apparent width (which is visible from a straight view of the patient from the midline) of each tooth on one side of the midline should be approximately 63% of the width of the tooth mesial to it. In other words, if the apparent width of the central incisor is assigned a value of 1, the apparent width of the lateral should be 63% of the central incisor's value (ratio of 1.6:1.0), and the visible portion of the facial surface of the canine should be 63% of the lateral incisor's value (see Chapter 9, *Esthetics in Dentistry*, Volume 1, 2nd Edition). Simply restoring two individual teeth in a proportional fashion of length to width to close a diastema does not mean that the final result will be esthetic if altering the golden proportion disrupts the symmetry of the entire smile (see Chapter 9, *Esthetics in Dentistry*, Volume 1, 2nd Edition).

There are esthetic considerations for periodontal surgery that are as important as those for teeth. Ideally, the position of the midfacial portion of the free gingival margin of the central incisors and the canines should be at the same height, whereas the free gingival margin of the lateral incisors is slightly coronal to the other two. Crown lengthening one tooth to achieve length to width proportionality may result in a decreased esthetic result because of the asymmetry of the gingival margins. Gingivectomies or apically positioned flap procedures should usually be carried out over several teeth, including all of the anterior teeth, to maintain esthetic harmony of the gingival contours. Occasionally, a single tooth may exhibit an improper gingival contour due to delayed passive eruption, and, in this case, a periodontal procedure for the individual tooth would be appropriate.

A wide tooth can be made to appear smaller than it is by altering its contours and using different color values in various parts of the tooth. The apparent face of the tooth is that portion of the facial surface that is isolated by the four facial line angles. The mesiofacial and distofacial line angles will influence what the eye perceives as the width of the facial surface of a tooth. A wide tooth can be made to look narrower by moving the mesio- and distofacial line angles toward each other, and a narrow tooth will look wider if these line angles are moved farther apart (see Chapter 8, *Esthetics in Dentistry*, Volume 1, 2nd Edition). Two adjacent teeth with different actual widths can look equally wide if the distance between the facial line angles is the same. Proximal contours, facial surface features, and color values can enhance the illusion provided by line angles as well. Wide and deep facial embrasures with lingually positioned contact areas give the illusion of narrow teeth, whereas constricted and shallow facial embrasures make teeth look wider. Horizontal or vertical "lines" added to the facial surfaces of teeth can make the tooth look artificially wider or longer as needed. Lighter color values on the facial surface of a tooth and darker values on the proximal surfaces will further contribute to the deception of tooth size. These illusions enable the dentist to make several teeth of different actual sizes look proportional in their widths by manipulating line angle location, proximal contours, surface texture, and color value. They are valuable adjuncts to treatment when compromises have to be made and ideal conditions are not available for closing diastemas and maintaining tooth proportionality or smile symmetry.

Direct Composite Resin Bonding

Although orthodontic repositioning may offer the most noninvasive or conservative method for diastema correction, this approach may be impractical, unaffordable, or unacceptable to the patient and may not even result in permanent closure of the diastema. In these situations, restorations are used as a means of closing a diastema rather than orthodontics, or as splints following tooth repositioning.[8] The size and number of the diastemas, functional and esthetic requirements of the patient, and pretreatment condition of the affected teeth influence the choice of restoration. The principles to be used in closing multiple spaces are illustrated in Figures 23–10A to F.

LARGE DIASTEMA CLOSED BY BONDING

PROBLEM: This 60-year-old airline travel agent presented with a large diastema of the maxillary central incisors (see Figures 23–10A and E). Advanced cervical erosion was also evident on her maxillary anterior teeth, especially on her right side.

TREATMENT: The teeth were slightly reproportioned by stripping and disking the distal surfaces of the central and lateral incisors (see Figure 23–10B). The key to successful restorative diastema closure is creating the illusion of a believable "natural" tooth width in the central and lateral incisors. Figure 23–10C shows a narrower width of the central incisors after the distal surfaces have been sufficiently reduced and ready for full-veneer bonding to close the central incisor diastema and restore the cervical defects. Final restoration is seen in Figure 23–10D.

RESULT: Figure 23–10F shows an entirely new smile with better proportioned teeth rather than two oversized teeth. Note that the cervical erosion on the maxillary right side has been simultaneously restored with composite resin bonding. The

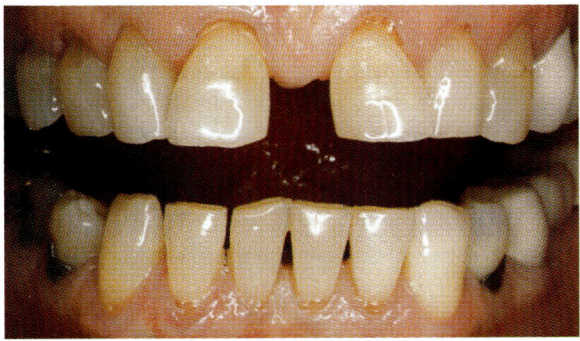

Figure 23–10A: This 60-year-old woman presented with a large diastema between her central incisors and cervical erosion on her maxillary anterior teeth.

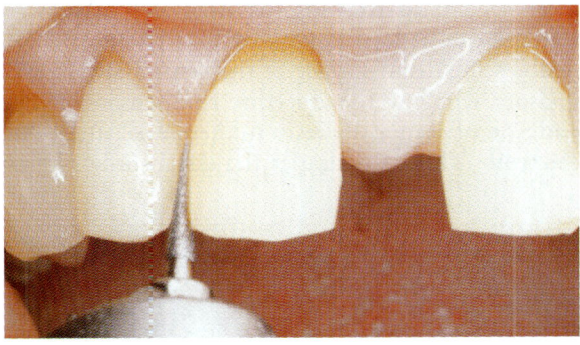

Figure 23–10B: Stripping and disking of the distal surfaces of the central and lateral incisors were done to slightly reproportion the teeth.

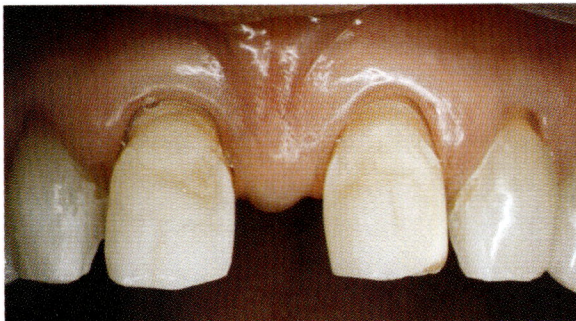

Figure 23–10C: The narrower width of the central incisors readies the diastema for closure.

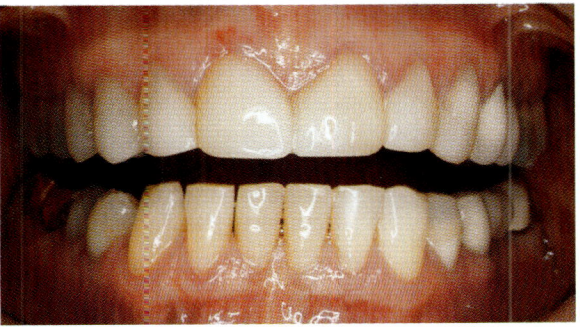

Figure 23–10D: The final full-veneer bonding closed the diastema and restored the cervical defects.

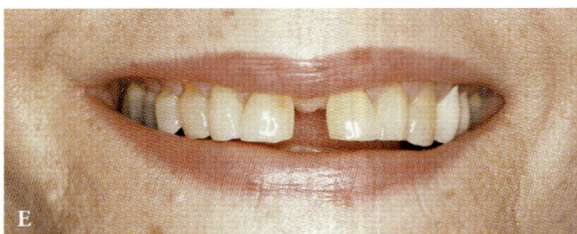 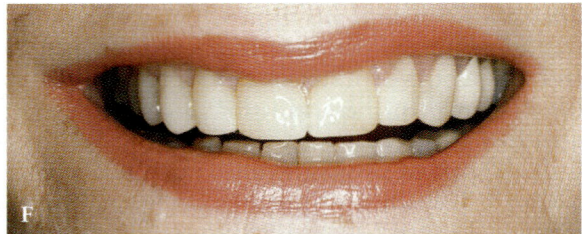

Figure 23–10E and F: Comparison of the before and after smiles shows an entirely new smile that is better proportioned by treating four anterior teeth. If only the two central incisors had been bonded, two oversized central incisors would have resulted.

mandibular anterior incisors were also cosmetically contoured to give them a level plane of occlusion. Comparing the before and after smiles (see Figures 23–10E and F) specifically illustrates how the patient's mid-upper lip naturally drops rather low, forming a "cupid's bow." This lowered lip line tends to mask the extra width of the central incisors, which also contributes to the illusion.

A schematic drawing of how this case was restored can be seen in Figures 23–11A and B. "X" denotes the distal surface of the central and lateral incisors, which were reduced to compensate for the addition of composite resin to the mesial surface of the teeth. This reduction of the distal surface helps to keep the mesially bonded aspects ("Y") of the central incisors in proper proportion. Any subgingival bonded areas must be meticulously contoured and finished so that the patient can maintain good dental hygiene and tissue health with the use of dental floss (Figure 23–11C).

The most practical restorative treatment to eliminate a small diastema between sound teeth is by direct bonding with composite resin (Figures 23–12A to H). Direct composite resin bonding is fast (one appointment) and reversible because mechanical tooth preparation is often unnecessary.[12] If an improved material or technique becomes available, it is relatively easy to remove the existing bonded composite and use the new method. Economics

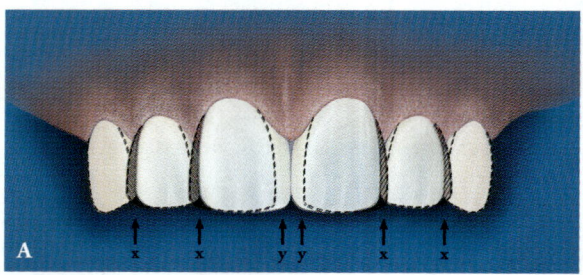 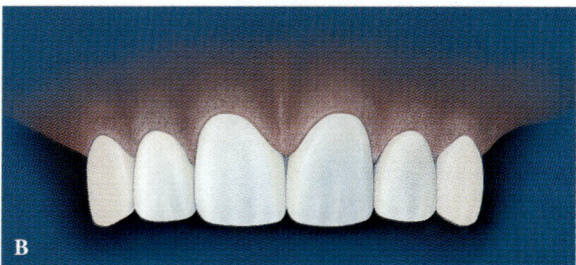

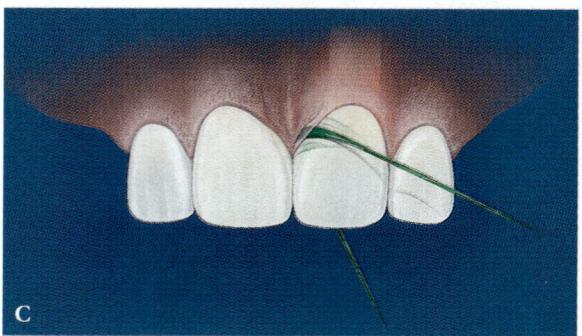

Figure 23–11A to C: (A) and (B) These drawings illustrate how the teeth of the patient in Figure 23–10 were restored to give a better proportioned smile (see text). (C) The shape of the bonding should be conducive to easy flossing.

Restorative Treatment of Diastema 719

is an additional advantage for the use of direct composite resin bonding as this technique is approximately one-third to one half the cost of porcelain laminates or crowns. The ability to save time, money, and tooth structure makes composite resin a popular choice with many dentists and patients.

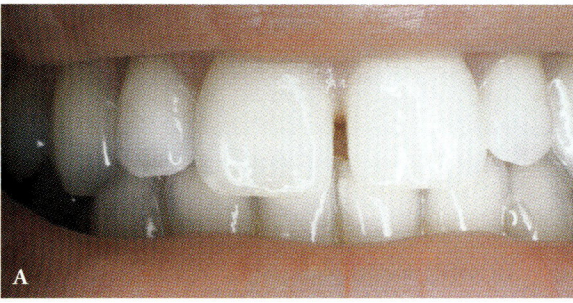

Figure 23–12A and B: The most practical method for closing a simple diastema is with composite resin bonding.

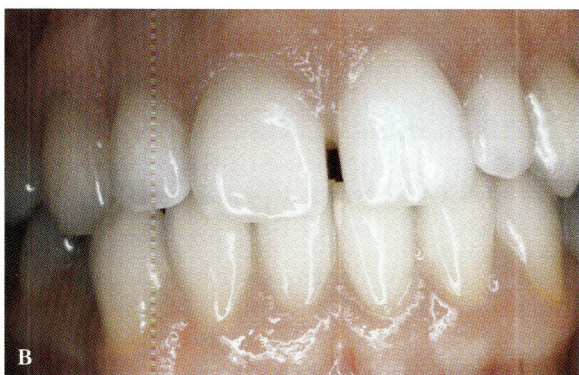

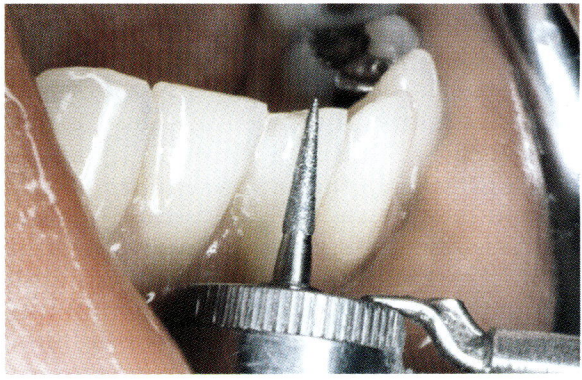

Figure 23–12C: Many times, it will be necessary to adjust the occlusion on the opposing arch to lessen the stress on the bonded incisors.

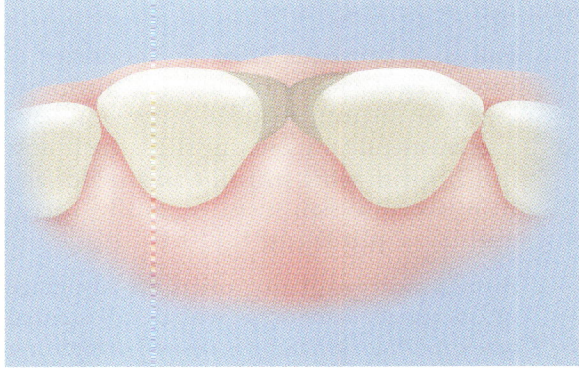

Figure 23–12D: This drawing illustrates that the composite resin will be bonded to labial, mesial, and lingual surfaces.

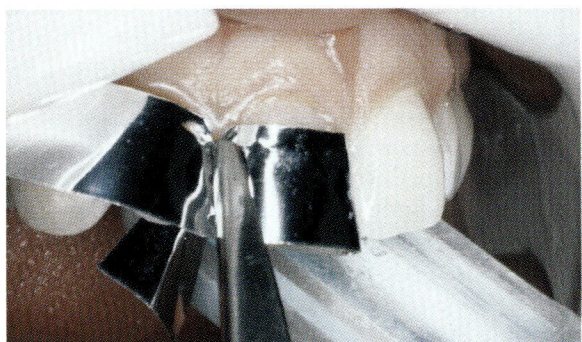

Figure 23–12E: It is important to measure the size of the space to be closed and bond each tooth separately using one half of the space for each tooth.

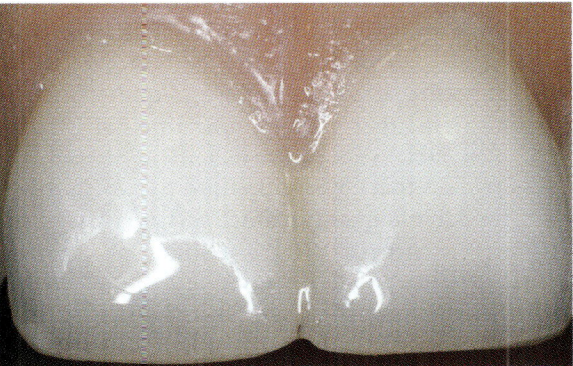

Figure 23–12F: The space is now closed. Note how invisible a self-contoured and polished margin can be.

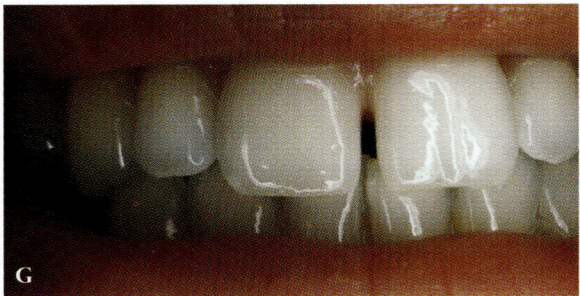 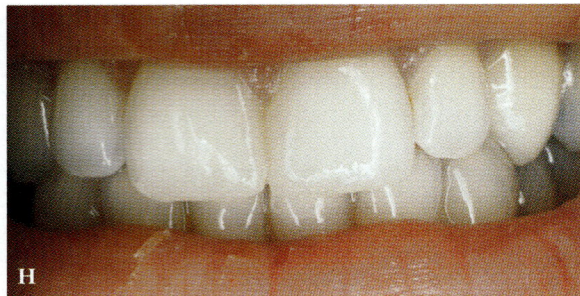

Figure 23–12G and H: The before and after comparison seems to confirm what this patient said: that even a small diastema can be distracting while observing the entire smile.

There are two design options possible with a composite resin restoration used to close a diastema: full labial veneer or proximal addition with labiolingual overlap. The decision to use a full-veneer technique rather than a proximal addition to close a diastema with composite resin is influenced by several factors:

1. Full labial veneering offers the advantage of concealing the restoration margins interproximally or lingually. Hidden restoration margins are useful for disguising slight shade mismatches with tooth structure and to hide any stain accumulation that eventually occurs after initial placement.

2. A full-veneer restoration offers the advantage of increased retention, which is essential when tooth lengthening is desired in addition to interproximal space closure. Tooth lengthening is needed to maintain an esthetic proportion of length to width for teeth when proximal additions are made to close spaces.

3. If only one diastema has to be closed, then three proximal surfaces (facial, mesial, and distal) per tooth need to be bonded. When only three proximal surfaces require composite resin, there is less indication for a complete labial veneer. An increment of composite resin that covers one-third to two-thirds of the labiolingual-proximal surface may be all that is necessary. This amount of coverage provides enough retention and allows a sufficient amount of material to be removed by polishing when future staining occurs.

4. Extremely translucent incisal edges on the teeth to be bonded may be a contraindication to using a complete labial veneer of composite. In this situation, confining the bonding material to the proximal surfaces will maintain the translucency of the incisal edges. As an alternative, choose a dark, medium, or light translucent shade of composite resin to blend in.[13]

In general, the choice of composite resin is influenced by the size of the space being closed in addition to the functional and esthetic requirements of the restoration.[20] If the space is small (1.5 mm or less), a microfilled composite material can be used alone to close the diastema. The occlusion should be evaluated for any aggressive contacts. Ideally, the lower incisors should have minimal occlusal function on the portion of the restorative material used to close the diastema. A deep overbite or heavy functional contacts may contribute to excessive wear or fracture of a microfilled composite. In these situations or in the case of a larger diastema (greater than 1.5 mm), a hybrid or microhybrid composite will offer greater wear and fracture resistance. A microfilled material can be veneered on the labial surface of a hybrid to provide a higher degree of luster and improved esthetics (Figures 23–13A to C).

Porcelain Veneers

The choice of porcelain laminates for diastema closure offers superb esthetics as the major indication for their use. Indirectly fabricated restorations are easier to contour, finish, and polish when compared with restorations that are created directly in the mouth. When several restorations will be required (multiple diastemas), laboratory-fabricated restorations allow the dentist to achieve perfection in proportioning multiple teeth (Figures 23–14A to K). Porcelain has excellent optical properties and can closely mimic enamel in appearance. Other advantages of porcelain veneers include resistance to surface staining and therefore less maintenance and increased wear resistance as compared with composite resin. Whereas composite resin restorations do not usually involve mechanical tooth preparation, porcelain laminates almost always require some enamel preparation and therefore should not be considered a reversible procedure.

The normal proximal finish line employed for porcelain veneers includes a chamfer labial to the interproximal contact when there are no interdental spaces present. The finish line for a porcelain veneer that is being used to close a diastema may approach a featheredge at the linguoproximal line angle, although a chamfer provides more edge strength.[21] The amount of extension toward the lingual surfaces can vary depending on the needs of the individual case. When incisal coverage is not needed, the amount of proximal extension toward the lingual can be minimal, approximately to the middle third or the middle of the tooth. When incisal edges are to be lengthened with veneers, or if translucency of the proximal segment of the restoration is not desired, more proximal extension, approaching the lingual-proximal line angle, is recommended. A lingually positioned proximal finish line on the diastema side of the tooth avoids preparation undercuts with the linguoincisal extension and also allows for a thicker interproximal increment of porcelain to reduce translucency.

FOUR PORCELAIN LAMINATES TO CLOSE DIASTEMAS

PROBLEM: This 21-year-old male model hesitated to smile because of his diastemas (see Figures 23–14A, G, and I). The patient was also concerned about the appearance of his inflamed gingiva adjacent to the left central incisor; subsequent exami-

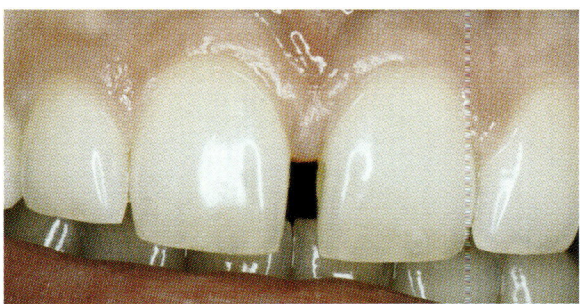

Figure 23–13A: When a diastema of this size is to be closed using composite resin bonding, a hybrid material should be chosen on the lingual surface for strength.

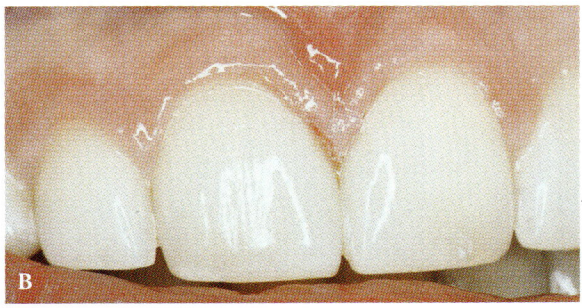

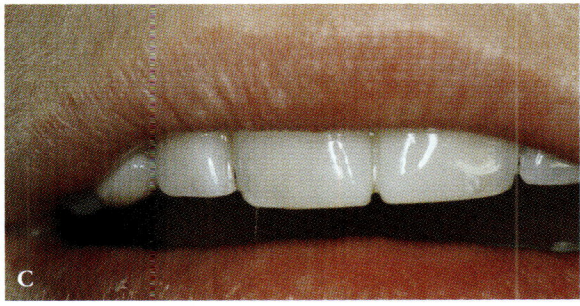

Figure 23–13B and C: To obtain a maximum "glaze" or polish to match existing enamel, a microfilled composite resin can be used on the labial surface. Note the glazed appearance of the labial microfilled polished composite resin.

nation showed an overextension of composite bonding. A main requirement of this patient was immediate esthetic treatment since he was leaving for Italy in 1 week. A second requirement was that no additional tooth be reduced, including the opposing teeth.

TREATMENT: To maximize longevity and esthetics, porcelain laminates were chosen as the most conservative treatment. Figure 23–14B shows the previously bonded left central incisor coated with dentin-disclosing solution to determine how much enamel was left. The tooth is washed, leaving red

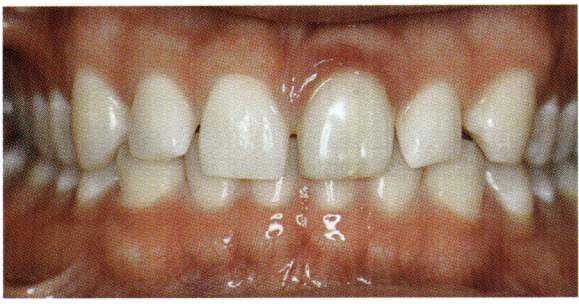

Figure 23–14A: This 21-year-old male model performed both runway and photography modeling without smiling because he disliked the spaces in his teeth.

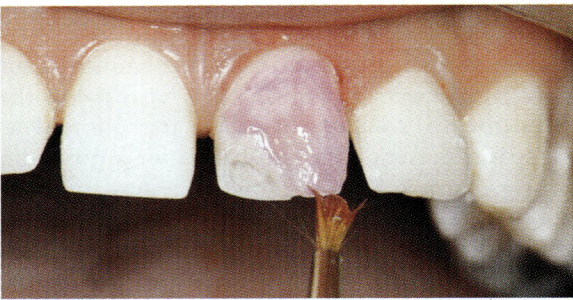

Figure 23–14B: Dentin disclosing solution is applied to determine how much enamel remained on this previously bonded left central incisor.

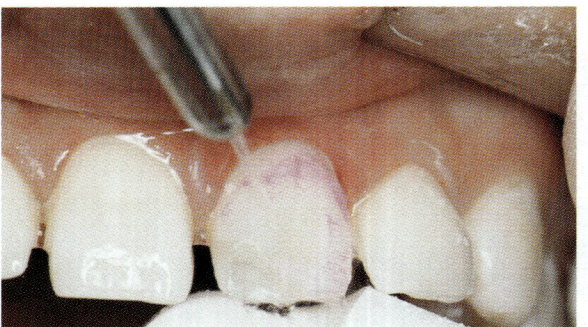

Figure 23–14C: Red dye indicates the areas of dentin.

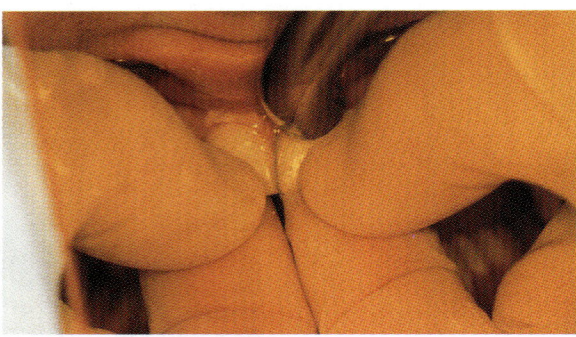

Figure 23–14D: A porcelain laminate is bonded to the left central incisor.

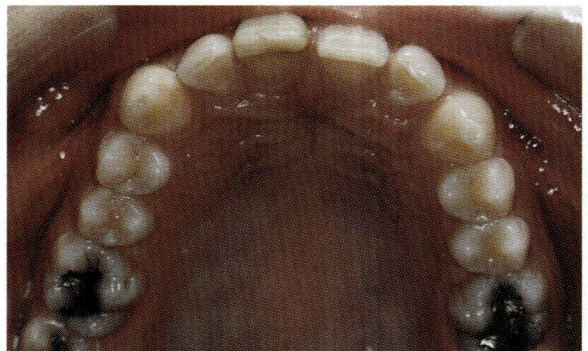

Figure 23–14E: This before occlusal view shows how much the left central incisor protruded prior to treatment.

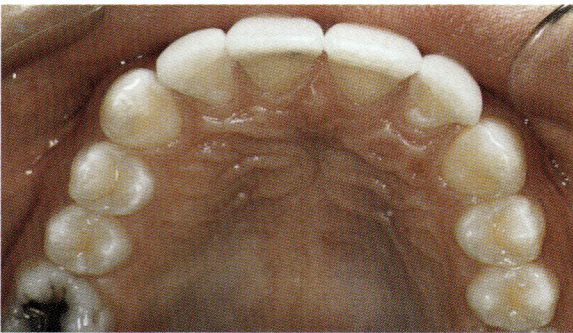

Figure 23–14F: Only four porcelain laminate veneers were necessary to eliminate the dark spaces between his teeth. Also note that the protrusion was eliminated.

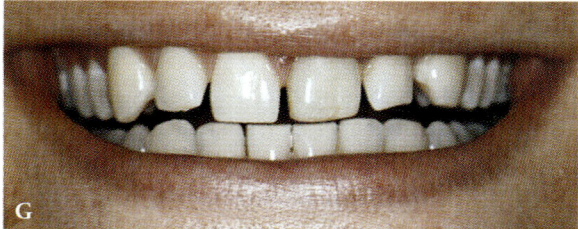 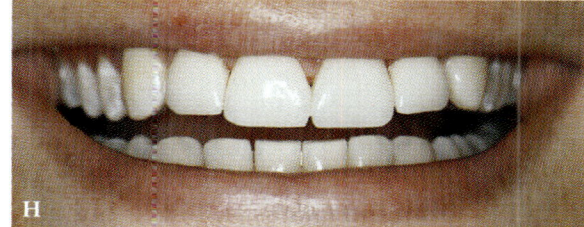

Figure 23–14G and H: Note the improvement in the smile by comparing the before and after pictures.

dye to indicate dentin areas (see Figure 23–14C). Figure 23–14D shows the left central incisor laminate being bonded into place. Figure 23–14E shows the occlusal view, indicating just how much the left central incisor protruded before restoration. Four porcelain laminates were used to create a symmetric arch with proper spacing (see Figure 23–14F). The improvement by the final result can be seen by comparing the before and after smiles (see Figures 23–14G and H). Note how the increased tooth size is well proportioned to the face (see Figure 23–14J). The conventional preparation for a porcelain laminate veneer when there is no diastema usually extends one-third to midway into the proximal surface (see Figure 23–14K). However, when closing diastemas, extend the proximal margins as far to the lingual surface as possible (Figure 23–14L). In addition, extending the preparation to the lingual surface allows for incorporating more translucent porcelain, which can keep the teeth from appearing too wide.

RESULT: Frequently, orthodontics is required to reposition teeth together to avoid the overly contoured appearance of restored teeth. Although this treatment could have been employed, the patient chose immediate esthetic correction over lengthy orthodontic treatment.

Full-Coverage Crowns

Prior to the introduction of laminates, direct composite resin bonding and full-coverage crowns were the only two restorative options available to treat a diastema. Crowns are indicated when the affected teeth are broken down and require additional support from a strong extracoronal restoration. Teeth that do not have a sufficient amount of enamel for bonding procedures can provide adequate retention when a full-coverage restoration design is used. When the teeth to be restored are in a poor pretreatment position, crowns can be used in place of orthodontics to "preposition" teeth without creat-

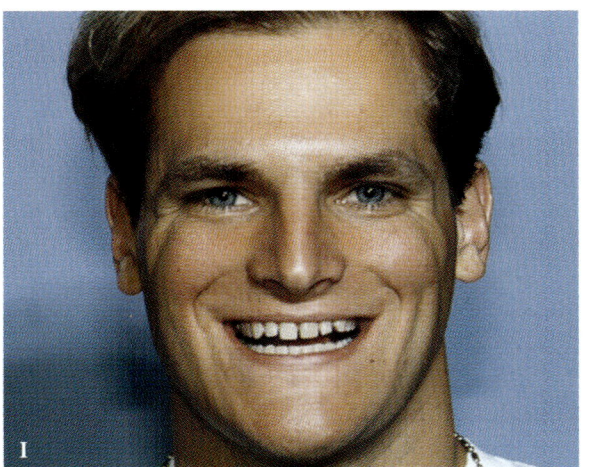 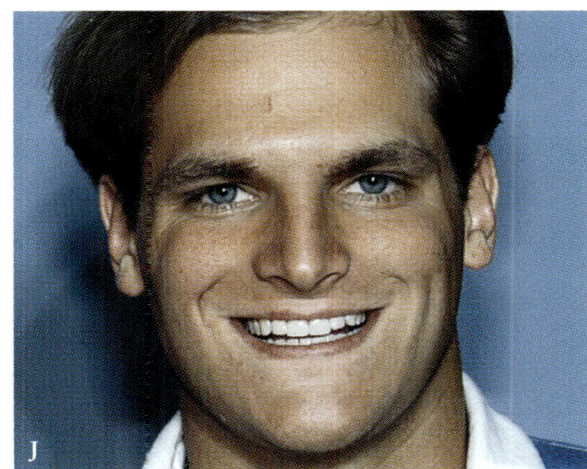

Figure 23–14I and J: These before and after pictures show how much better proportioned the larger teeth appear in full face. (Reproduced with permission from Goldstein RE. Change your smile. 3rd edn. Carol Stream, IL: Quintessence, 1997:122.)

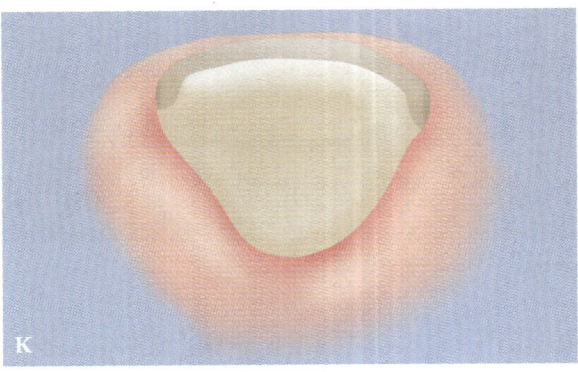
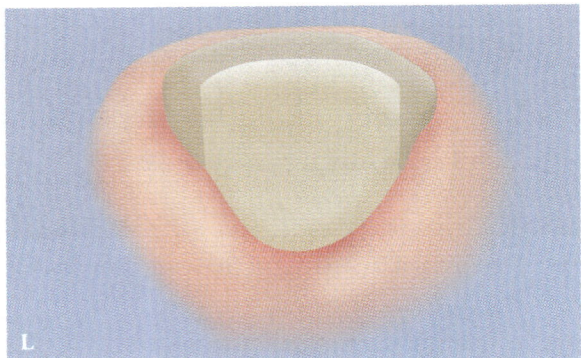

Figure 23–14K and L: (K) The conventional preparation for a porcelain laminate, when there is no space to close, usually extends one-third to midway into the proximating surface. (L) The revised preparation when increased opacity (or translucency) is desired; the proximal margins should be extended as far as possible to the lingual.

ing overcontoured restorations, which result when more conservative restorations are used.

When crowning, try to prepare as few teeth as possible that will still achieve an esthetic result. Although conservative dentistry is a worthy goal in itself, attempting to close a diastema by treating only one tooth will almost always result in esthetic failure, as in Figures 23–15A to D.

PROBLEM IN CROWNING ONE TOOTH TO CLOSE A CENTRAL DIASTEMA

PROBLEM: This 25-year-old actress and model presented with an oversized maxillary central incisor that had been crowned to close a central diastema (see Figure 23–15A). Note the extraordinary amount of space occupied by the left central incisor.

TREATMENT: The porcelain crown on the left central incisor was removed, margins were redefined, and the right central incisor was prepared for a full porcelain crown. However, if restored today, the right central incisor could have been more conservatively treated with a porcelain laminate or composite resin bonding. It was important, in this case, to construct temporary crowns that would esthetically balance the space and provide the dentist and technician with a guide for construction of the final restoration. It was felt that two central incisors were adequate to restore the anterior space. Note the tissue health around the temporary restorations, but stained acrylic, after 3 weeks of placement (see Figure 23–15B). Final restorations are shown in Figure 23–15C. Note that highlights, vertical lines, and texture are emphasized to give the illusion of a tooth appearing longer and narrower than it actually is. The effect can be appreciated by comparing

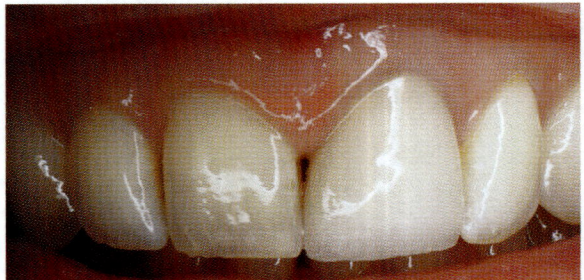

Figure 23–15A: This 25-year-old actress was unhappy with the result obtained with closing her wide diastema with a single central crown. Note the gingival inflammation caused by the overbuilt crown.

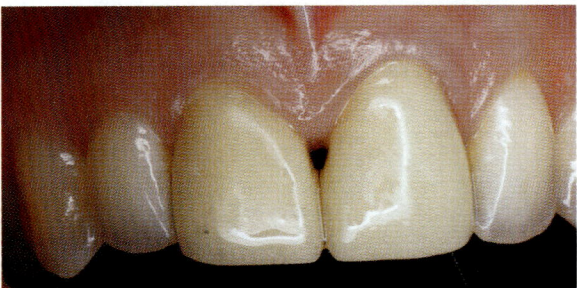

Figure 23–15B: Following conservative periodontal therapy, interim crowns were placed on both central incisors.

Restorative Treatment of Diastema 725

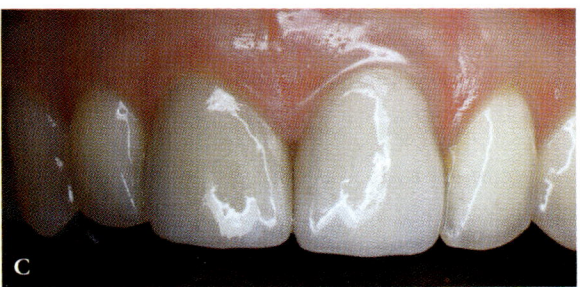
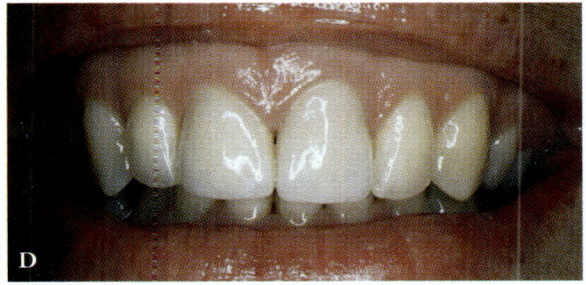

Figure 23–15C and D: Comparison of before and after treatment, which consisted of two all-ceramic crowns, shows a more esthetic result and acceptable tissue health. *(C)* Crown placement shows an esthetically pleasing result. *(D)* Nine years later, the esthetic result has been maintained.

before and after photographs (see Figures 25–15A and C). Note the horizontal highlights in the extra-wide crown on the left central incisor (see Figure 23–15A) and the vertical emphasis on the new central incisors (see Figure 23–15C). Figure 23–15D shows the lasting esthetic result 9 years later.

Result: The original mistake made in this case was to try to close a diastema between central incisors by altering only one. Unless both central incisors share restoration of the diastema, or if the single central incisor is not reduced on the distal to maintain an equal mesiodistal dimension with the adjacent central incisor, the result will be poor. The most realistic result in treating a diastema comes from a symmetric approach. This means bonding, laminating, or crowning two, four, or even several teeth to balance the existing space.

Normal-Sized Teeth

The previous cases discussed the occurrence of diastemas that are the result of small teeth. However, it is generally accepted that if a diastema coincides with normal-sized teeth, more teeth are used to close the space. This offers greater potential for shade matching and symmetry in size and shape. If there is a single diastema between the central incisors, and the teeth are in good occlusion, two, four, or several teeth may require crowns, bonding, or laminating, depending on the condition of the teeth.

SHAPING FOUR CROWNS TO CLOSE A DIASTEMA

Problem: A 20-year-old female presented with diastemas between her maxillary lateral and central incisors (Figure 23–16A). She had a poorly fitting crown on the maxillary right central incisor as well.

Treatment: In cases where diastemas are evenly distributed between the central and lateral incisors (Figure 23–16B), the best solution is laminating or crowning all four anterior teeth. If only the central incisors were laminated or crowned, the result would

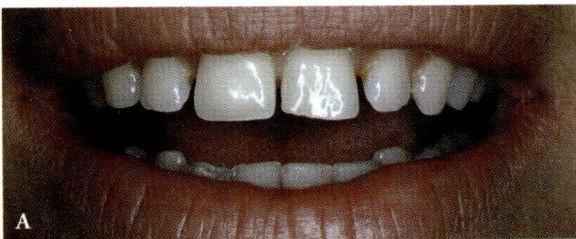

Figure 23–16A and B: This 20-year-old student was unhappy with the appearance of her smile. In addition to the multiple spaces, there was a labial flare to the teeth that made them look shorter than they actually were.

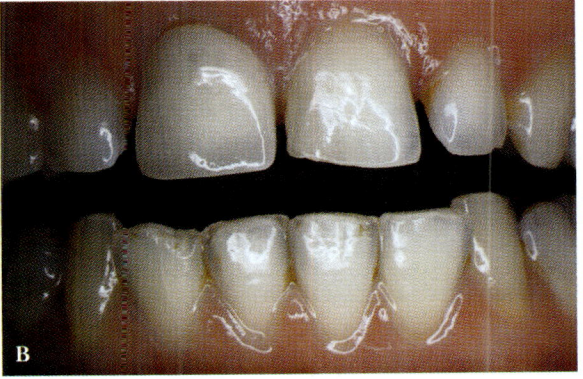

be less than ideal due to the overly contoured appearance of the centrals. Proportionally contoured and shaped crowns were constructed for the incisors and seated in place (Figures 23–16C and D).

RESULT: As previously stated, orthodontics is the preferred treatment of choice in closing diastemas involving normal-sized teeth. However, when correction by restoration is chosen, it is best to use an even number of teeth to close diastemas. Although the above case was successfully treated with four porcelain-fused-to-metal crowns, porcelain laminate veneering would probably be the treatment of choice today.

Principles in Shaping

In shaping crowns to close a space, several principles should be observed:[4]

1. Contacts should favor a lingual orientation. Figures 23–16E and F show the labial surface and how it is contoured ("S") toward that of the lingual surface. By controlling the reflection of light, the teeth can be made to appear thinner than they actually are. The distal and mesial line angles of the labial surfaces should be moved lingually and toward the midline of the tooth, leaving only a narrow surface width ("X") of the actual labial surface flat enough to pick up the light.[5]

2. Incisal embrasures should be more pronounced. Figure 23–16G shows widening and elongation of the incisal embrasures (ie, to help make the tooth appear narrower). The reshaping of the distal incisal angle should usually begin at point X or at the distolabial point of labial reduction.

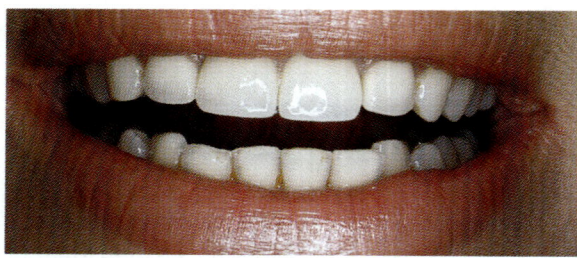

Figure 23–16C: Crowning the four maxillary incisors enabled the spaces to be closed and created better proportion between the central and lateral incisors.

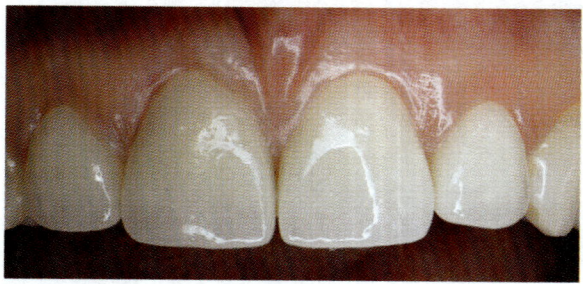

Figure 23–16D: This close-up view shows the improved interincisal distance achieved.

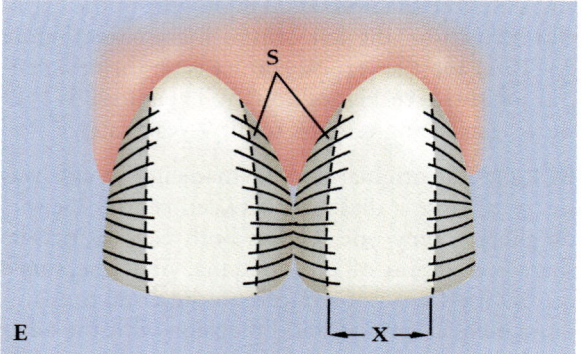

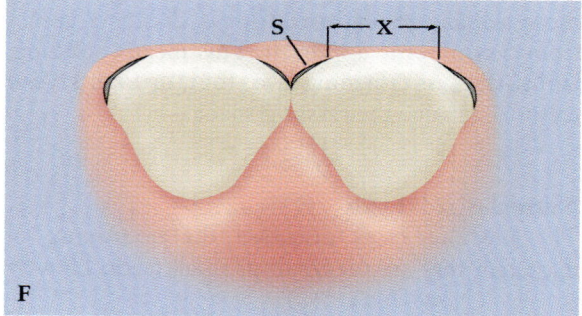

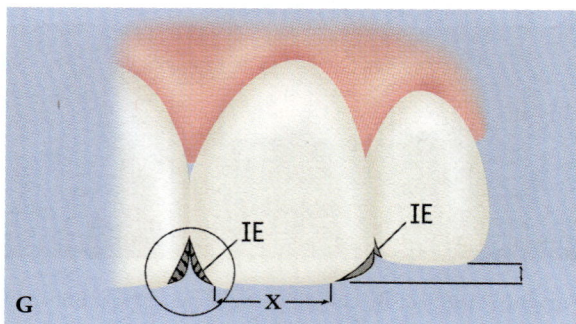

Figure 23–16E to G: These drawings illustrate the principles used in closing a diastema (see text). IE = incisal embrasures.

3. Vary the interincisal distances (see Figure 23–16G). Note the favorable illusion that this creates. The central incisors appear longer, enhancing the illusion of narrowness.[5]

Shaping tips: when closing teeth with either bonding or crowning, the primary objective is to create teeth that do not appear too wide:

1. Lengthen the central incisors slightly by decreasing the interincisal distance.

2. Move facial line angles toward the midline, thus giving the illusion of narrowness.

3. Consider crown lengthening if the patient has a high lip line.[4]

The two significant advantages of full-coverage crowns over other restorations at the present include increased fracture resistance to the forces of mastication (Figures 23–17A and B) and the ability to achieve maximum esthetics because the contours of the entire tooth can be easily controlled. When a restoration is indicated for diastema closure, the most conservative type should always be used as long as the result will provide a durable and esthetic result.

CROWNING SIX TEETH TO CLOSE MULTIPLE DIASTEMAS

PROBLEM: This 43-year-old male presented with multiple diastemas between the maxillary anterior teeth (see Figure 23–17A).

TREATMENT: Although porcelain laminates would be considered the preferred treatment of choice today, the option of full crowns was chosen when these teeth were restored. Therefore, six porcelain-fused-to-metal crowns were constructed to close the anterior diastemas because the natural teeth were too small for the space. Crowning with larger but proportionally sized teeth and using principles of illusion (see Chapter 8, Figures 8–32A and B, *Esthetics in Dentistry*, Volume 1, 2nd Edition) restored the man's appearance without overly contouring any of the crowns. Because the patient had a somewhat rugged look about him, anatomy was included in the restorations to give them natural-looking shape and texture. Some wear was simulated on the incisors, and a slight diastema was created between the central incisors to simulate the arrangement of the original teeth. The patient had objected more to the large spaces between the lateral incisors and cuspids than to the one between the central incisors as when he smiled it looked as if he were missing his teeth. The results can be seen in Figure 23–17B.

RESULT: Sometimes, it may take six crowns to close a diastema and create a symmetric result. There are times when a patient will want to retain natural characteristics and even duplicate a diastema on a smaller scale. If done well, this can effectively reproduce the realism and naturalness of the original dentition. If this case were to be restored using porcelain laminates, the esthetic principles illustrated here would be the same.

The main consideration in closing a central diastema is shown in Figures 23–18A to D. The central incisors are reduced more on the distal proximal surface than on the mesial as the majority of the diastema will be addressed by the mesial

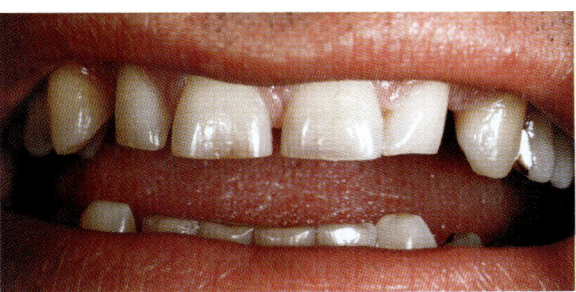

Figure 23–17A: This 43-year-old dentist was more concerned about the diastemas between his lateral incisors and cuspids than the space between the central incisors.

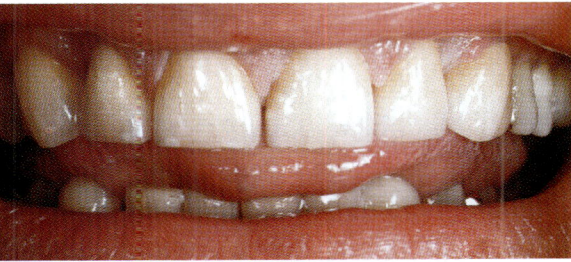

Figure 23–17B: Six aluminous porcelain crowns were placed to close the diastemas. However, the patient requested that a slight space be left between the central incisors to give him what he considered a more natural look.

728 Esthetics in Dentistry

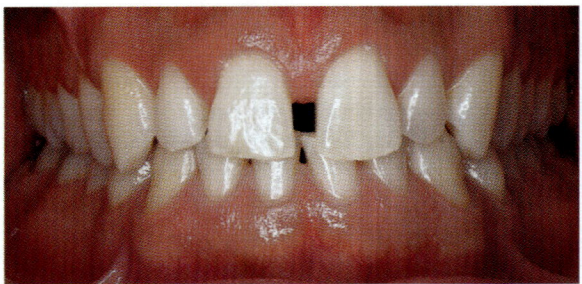

Figure 23–18A: This 27-year-old policeman wanted to close the space between his teeth without orthodontics.

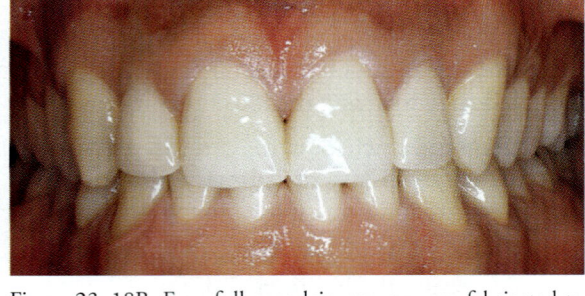

Figure 23–18B: Four full porcelain crowns were fabricated to proportionally close the space.

edges of the restored central incisors (indicated by "X," see Figure 23–18C). The lateral incisors will then assume a more mesial position. As much as possible, all of the teeth will have distally rounded incisal edges to reduce the amount of incisal edge that shows. The result is illustrated in Figure 23–18D. Note how directing the reflection of light gives the illusion of narrow teeth. The highlights are approximately in the center of the teeth (indicated by "X," see Figure 23–18D) rather than toward the distal surfaces ("Y").

Prosthodontic Replacement

When a missing permanent tooth (eg, maxillary lateral) is the cause of a diastema and the remaining teeth do not possess adequate mass to allow space closure by orthodontics, restorations are indicated.[27] The width of the diastema will determine the type of restoration that should be used because of the limitations imposed by tooth symmetry and esthetic proportioning of the teeth.

Small diastemas can be closed by individual restorations as long as the proximal extensions do not violate the optimal range of length to width ratios for the affected teeth. Large diastemas may be better restored by prosthetic replacements to preserve the proportions and symmetry of the anterior portion of the mouth. Prerestorative orthodontic treatment to equalize the space can usually improve the esthetic result and provide more options for restorative treatment. The options for prosthetic replacement of a missing anterior tooth include conventional porcelain-fused-to-metal bridge, resin-bonded bridge, fiber-reinforced resin bridge, and an implant-supported

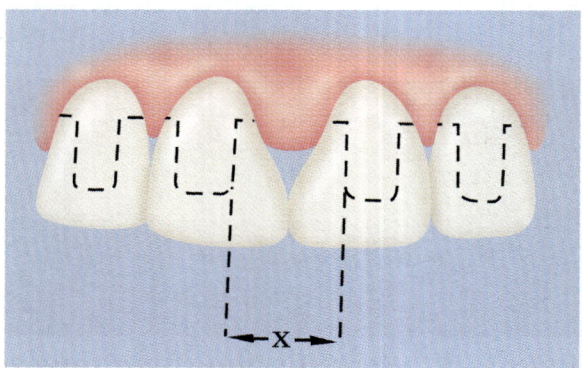

Figure 23–18C: This drawing illustrates the principle of reducing the tooth much more on the distal than the lingual surface, allowing more mesial placement of the lateral incisor crowns.

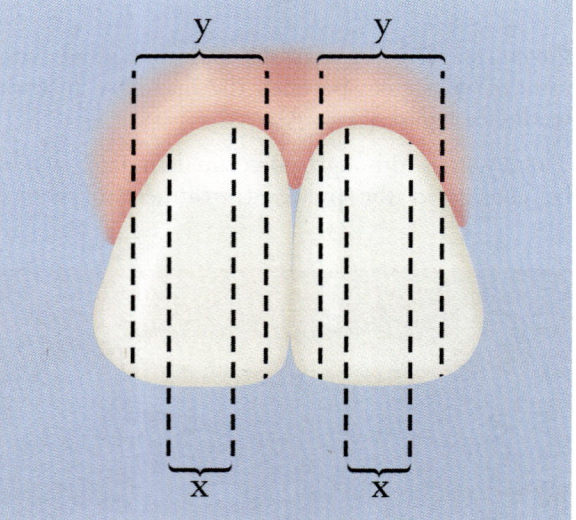

Figure 23–18D: When teeth are too wide, they should be contoured so that the labial surface does not appear too wide. Thus, the line angles should be more to the center of the tooth ("X" instead of "Y").

crown.[3,9] Esthetics, function, condition of the adjacent teeth, and patient finances influence the choices in this category.

Advanced Bone Loss

In instances where the patient has had posterior bite collapse and advanced bone loss, the anterior teeth tend to become splayed, resulting in large diastemas. Treatment of the resulting diastemas can consist of orthodontics combined with prosthodontics, extraction and implant therapy, and/or full-mouth rehabilitation. Such a case is illustrated in Figures 23–19 A to I using interim bonding followed by a telescopic fixed prosthesis.

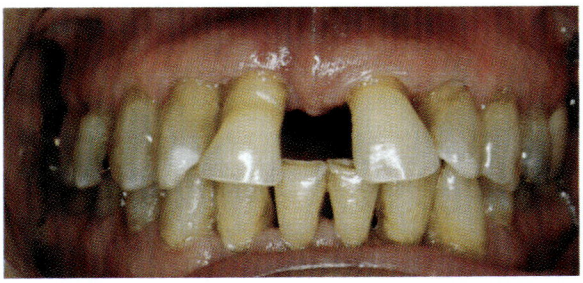

Figure 23–19A: This 65-year-old man was embarrassed by the appearance of his front teeth.

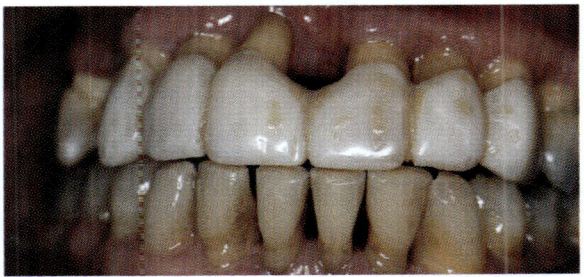

Figure 23–19B: Using the principles previously outlined in this chapter, composite resin bonding was done to immediately improve the patient's appearance and stabilize the dentition.

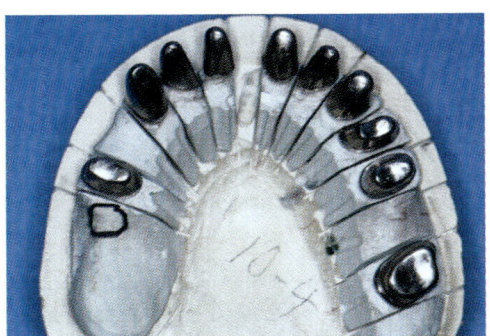

Figure 23–19C: Following periodontal therapy and interim stabilization for 3 months, a maxillary telescopic prosthesis was constructed. The gold copings are seen here on the model.

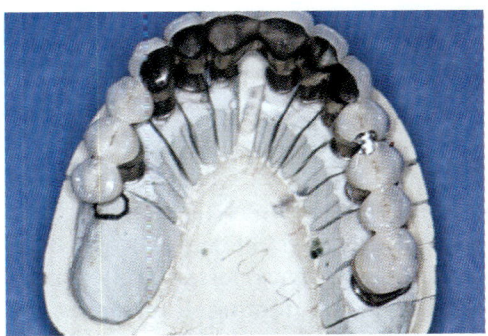

Figure 23–19D: The superstructure was constructed in two sections using a semiprecision attachment.

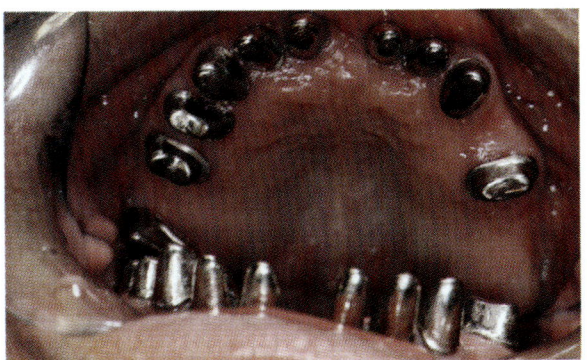

Figure 23–19E: The gold copings are seen here cemented in the mouth with final cement. This permits the superstructure to be cemented with soft cement so that it can be easily removed in the event that repairs are necessary. A further advantage in using "individual" telescopic copings is that the patient will require only minimal treatment if there is a superstructure cement washout.

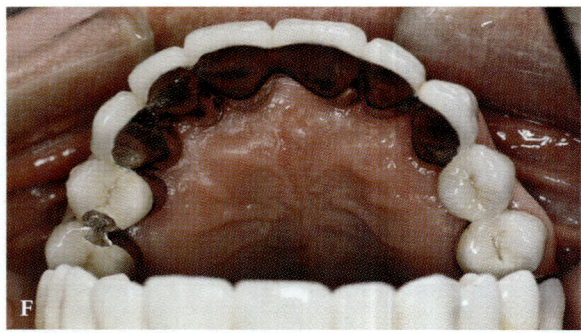 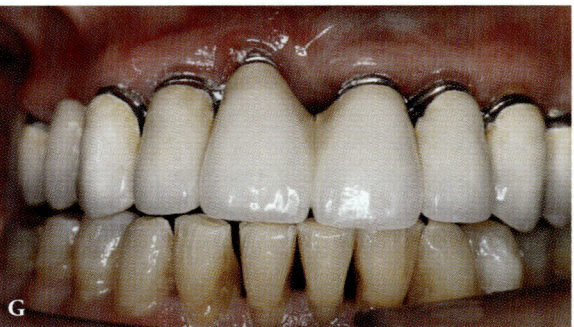

Figure 23–19F and G: The superstructure was first cemented with petrolatum and zinc oxide for 1 week to help fully seat the case.

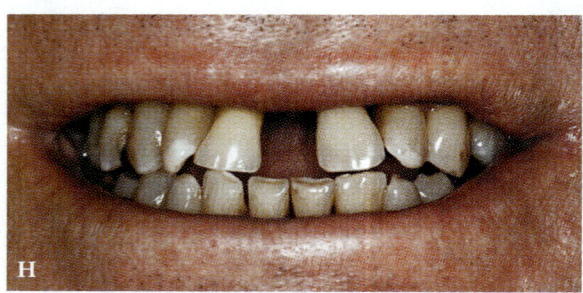 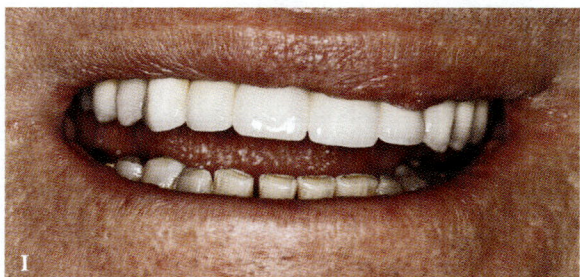

Figure 23–19H and I: Before and after treatment comparison show a greatly improved esthetic result. Note the patient's lower lip line. He felt comfortable that, because of his low lip line, none of the exposed metal margins would show.

SUMMARY

The esthetic significance of a diastema and the decision to close it is predominantly the choice of the patient. The dentist must possess a full appreciation of the factors contributing to diastemas and the various options available to treat them. Once the etiology of a diastema is identified, the patient should be informed of treatment alternatives, therapeutic time commitments, prognoses, and costs.

Regardless of treatment choice, the objective is to improve esthetics while preserving as much healthy tooth structure as possible. Good occlusion and maintenance of the supporting tissues are equally important to prevent diastema re-formation and failure of corrective therapies. The ability of the dentist to successfully manage diastemas is the mark of a clinician who practices esthetic dentistry according to sound, evidence-based principles.

References

1. Attia Y. Midline diastemas: closure and stability. Angle Orthod 1993;63:209–12.

2. Clark DC. Immediate closure of labial diastema by frenectomy and maxillary ostectomy. J Oral Surg 1968;26:273–6.

3. Davis RC. Prosthetically maintaining a dental diastema using single tooth implants. Implant Soc 1993;3(6):8–9.

4. Goldstein RE. Esthetics in dentistry. 1st edn. Philadelphia: JB Lippincott, 1976.

5. Goldstein RE. Esthetic principles for ceramo-metal restorations. Dent Clin North Am 1988;21:803–2.

6. Goldstein RE. Change you smile. 3rd edn. Chicago: Quintessence, 1997.

7. Goodman NR. Treatment of diastema: not always frenectomy. Dent Surv 1975;51(4):28–9, 32, 34.

8. Gribble AR. Multiple diastema management: an interdisciplinary approach. J Esthet Dent 1994;6:97–102.

9. Hagge MS, Clarke DA. Diastema preservation in resin-bonded fixed partial dentures. J Esthet Dent 1992;4:134–9.

10. Huang WJ, Creath CJ. The midline diastema: a review of its etiology and treatment [review]. Pediatr Dent 1995;17:171–9.

11. Kraut RA, Payne J. Osteotomy of intermaxillary suture for closure of median diastema. J Am Dent Assoc 1983;107:760–1.

12. Lacy AM. Application of composite resin for single-appointment anterior and posterior diastema closure. Pract Periodont Aesthet Dent 1998;10:279–86.

13. Larson TD. Techniques for achieving realistic color distribution in large composite resin restorations. J Am Dent Assoc 1986;112:669–72.

14. Leonard MS. The maxillary frenum and surgical treatment. Gen Dent 1998;46:614–7.

15. Martinez-Canut P, Carrasquer A, Magan R, Lorca A. A study on factors associated with pathologic tooth migration. J Clin Periodont 1997;24:492–7.

16. Miller PD Jr. The frenectomy combined with a laterally positioned pedical graft. Functional and esthetic considerations. J Periodont 1985;56:102–6.

17. Newitter DA. Predictable diastema reduction with filled resin: diagnostic wax-up. J Prosthet Dent 1986; 55:293–6.

18. Oesterle LJ, Shellhart WE. Maxillary diastemas: a look at the causes. J Am Dent Assoc 1999;130:85–94.

19. Popovich F, Thompson GW. Maxillary diastemas: a look at the causes. J Am Dent Assoc 1999;130:85–94.

20. Radz GM. Anterior esthetic bonded restorations using an improved hybrid composite. Compend Cont Educ Dent 1995;16:1204, 1206–7, 1210.

21. Rouse JS. Full veneer versus traditional veneer preparation: a discussion of interproximal extensions [review]. J Prosthet Dent 1997;78:545–9.

22. Sahafian AA. Bonding as permanent retention after closure of median diastema. J Clin Orthod 1978;12:568.

23. Sher MR. Surgical correction of the diastema. N Y State Dent J 1981;47:382–3.

24. Spilka CJ, Mathews PH. Surgical closure of diastema of central incisors. Am J Orthod 1979;76:443–7.

25. Sullivan TC, Turpin DL, Artun J. A postretention study of patients presenting with a maxillary median diastema. Angle Orthod 1996;66:131–8.

26. Towfighi PP, Brunsvold MA, Storey AT, et al. Pathologic migration of anterior teeth in patients with moderate to severe periodontitis. J Periodont 1997;68:967–72.

27. Wise RJ, Nevins M. Anterior tooth site analysis (Bolton Index): how to determine anterior diastema closure. Int J Periodont Restor Dent 1988;8:8–23.

28. Yamaoka M, Furusawa K, Yasuda K. Effects of maxillary anterior supernumerary impacted teeth on diastema [letter]. Oral Surg Oral Med Oral Pathol Oral Radiol Endod 1995;80:252.

Additional Resources

Goldstein RE. Diagnostic dilemma: to bond, laminate, or crown. Int J Periodont Restor Dent 1987;87(5): 9–30.

Goldstein RE. Esthetic principles for ceramo-metal restorations. Dent Clin North Am 1988;21:803–22.

Goldstein RE. Status report: dentistry in the 1980's. J Am Dent Assoc 1988;116:617–24.

Goldstein RE. Finishing of composites and laminates. Dent Clin North Am 1989;33:305–18.

Goldstein RE, Feinman RA, Garber DA. Esthetic considerations in the selection and use of restorative materials. Dent Clin North Am 1983;27:723–31.

Goldstein RE, Garber DA, Goldstein CE, et al. The changing esthetic dental practice. J Am Dent Assoc 1994;125:1447–57.

Goldstein RE, Garber DA, Schwartz CG, Goldstein CE. Patient maintenance of esthetic restorations. J Am Dent Assoc 1992;123:61–6.

Goldstein RE, Goldstein CE. Is your case really finished? J Clin Orthod 1988;22:702–13.

Goldstein RE, et al. Immediate conservative corrections of esthetic problems. J Dent Technol (Jpn) 1990;75: 50–9.

CHAPTER 24

RESTORATIVE TREATMENT OF CROWDED TEETH

Geoffrey W. Sheen, DDS, MS, Ronald E. Goldstein, DDS, Steven T. Hackman, DDS

Orthodontics is generally the first consideration when the patient presents with crowded teeth.[3,13,19,34] If a patient is unable to accept comprehensive orthodontic procedures, the general practitioner must determine whether the patient can be treated with minor tooth movement, restorations, extraction, or a combination of these procedures.

To analyze the treatment of crowded teeth, this chapter has been organized into the following sections: Treatment Considerations, Treatment Strategy, Treatment Options, and Unusual or Rare Clinical Presentations.

TREATMENT CONSIDERATIONS

Many patients have slightly crowded or overlapping anterior teeth that are not an esthetic problem. However, when an individual who finds this situation unesthetic seeks treatment, it may present a challenge for the dentist. Choosing the correct approach is the most important aspect of the treatment.[36]

Prior to properly developing a plan of treatment, the dentist should consider a number of preoperative conditions. A thorough evaluation of the patient will establish the basis for potential treatment options.[37] The areas to be evaluated include arch space, gingival architecture, influence of root proximity, smile line, emergence profile, and oral hygiene (Table 24–1).

Arch Space
The most significant factor in the treatment of crowded teeth is the available arch space, as well as how that space is occupied by the dentition. Locating space deficiencies and their degree will determine which teeth will require modification.

Berliner presented a classic formulation and clinical rule in his text that helps to make treatment of crowding more predictable. He stated:

> When the sum of the mesiodistal widths (at contact-point level from distal or right lateral to distal of left lateral) in any given segment measures more than the available arch space, when measured between the two points (obtained by dropping perpendicular lines from the mesial contact-point levels of the right and the left cuspids to the gingival line), the central and the lateral teeth will be buckled (displaced labially or lingually) or overlapped; conversely, when the sum of the combined mesiodistal widths of the central and the lateral teeth measure less than the available arch space (as indicated above), the involved teeth present diastemas.[2]

This formula can aid in the correction of crowded or spaced teeth by measuring the amount to be added or subtracted for the desired objective (Figures 24–1A to C).

Gingival Architecture
An often overlooked component of an esthetic smile is the gingival architecture. When there is crowding in the anterior region, certain teeth will be forced facially or lingually. In a Class II, Division 2 occlusion, for example, the maxillary lateral

TABLE 24–1. Treatment Considerations for the Correction of Crowded Teeth

Arch space
Gingival architecture
Influence of root proximity
Smile line
Emergence profile and oral hygiene

incisors may be positioned labially, and the gingival tissue will be forced more apically. This creates a discontinuity in the overall smile of the patient. Treatment considerations in this situation may require slight modification to the gingival architecture around the central incisors to create a more harmonious smile. If the patient's lip line hides the gingival discrepancy, then surgical intervention may not be necessary (Figures 24–2A to D).

Likewise, crowding in the mandibular anterior often results in the rotation or lingualization of the central or lateral incisors. The gingival tissue will therefore be positioned more incisally. It may be necessary to perform a crown-lengthening procedure prior to esthetic restoration of these teeth.[30,43]

Influence of Root Proximity

Root proximity may complicate the restoration of crowded mandibular anterior teeth. Root structures may be so close to one another that a separation is not possible. This creates gingival impingement that can be almost impossible to treat.

It may be necessary to extract one of the crowded teeth, leaving three incisors in place of four.[24] The decision should be based on radiographs and a study of the periodontium to determine the amount of bone present. If bone loss exists due to crowding, then extraction and repositioning are generally the treatment of choice. This can be successful when the teeth are properly proportioned. It is seldom noticeable to the patient. The tooth is extracted, and the remaining anterior teeth are repositioned, providing additional bone support. When small diastemas remain, the teeth can be bonded with composite resin or splinted to prevent further tooth movement.

In most cases, some form of retainer is advisable. The patient should be informed that he or she can

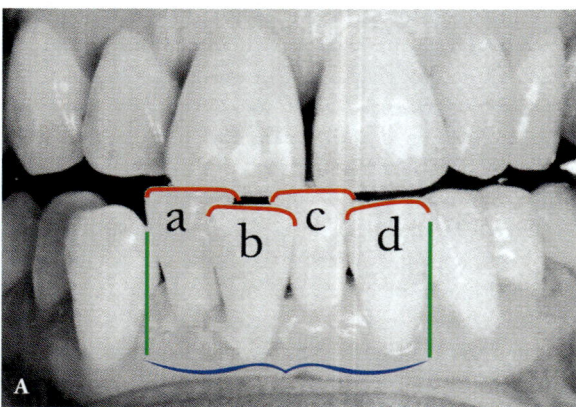
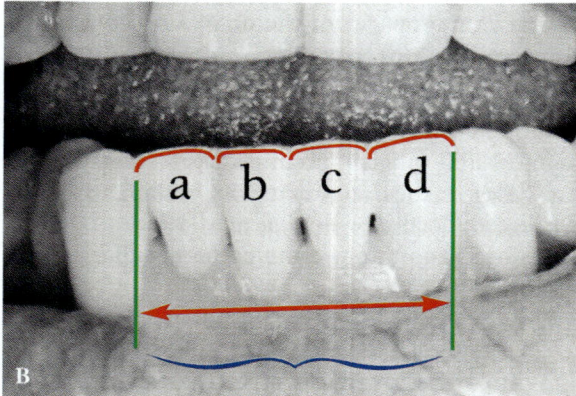
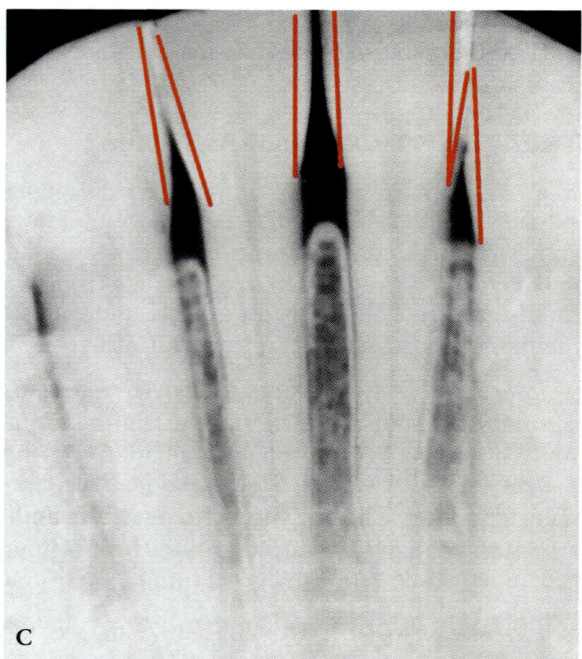

Figure 24–1A to C: *(A)* Preoperative view: note the relationship of the combined widths of the lower central and lateral teeth (A, B, C, D) to the extent of available arch space. Sum of combined tooth widths > available arch space, resulting in buckling. *(B)* Postoperative measurement, after remodeling of the lower central and lateral incisor teeth: the combined tooth widths equal the available arch space, and repositioning of the teeth became a feasible clinical procedure. *(C)* The proximal thickness of the enamel "caps" of the teeth on a lower anterior segment of the dental arch is indicated in outline. (Reproduced with permission from Berliner A. Ligatures, splints, bite planes and pyramids. Philadelphia: JB Lippincott, 1964:65.)

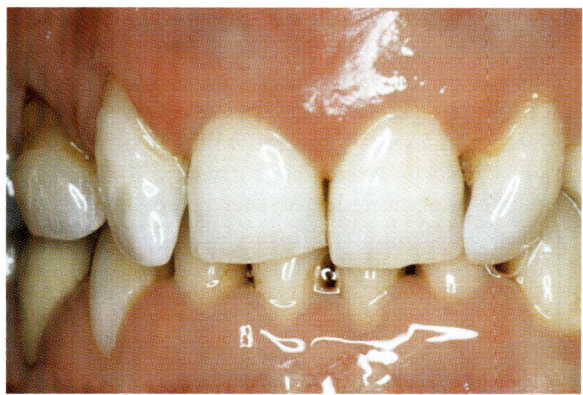

Figure 24–2A: This patient was dissatisfied with her crowded anterior teeth. Note how the gingival height differs between the central and lateral incisors.

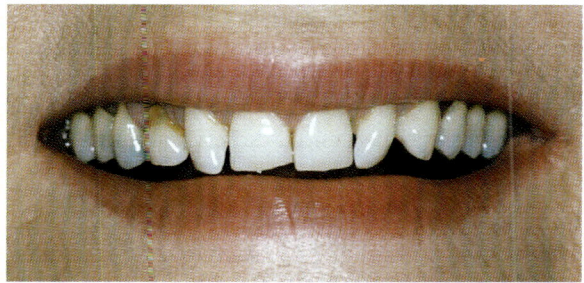

Figure 24–2B: The dissimilar gingival heights did not bother the patient because her natural smile line concealed these irregularities.

reduce the wearing time of the retainer provided that it does not fit too tightly each time it is placed. A tight fit might indicate some relapse. The patient should return for possible further treatment either to relax retentive gingival fibers or to adjust the occlusion to help equilibrate the stressful occlusal forces.

Smile Line

It is important to study the patient's smile line. The extent to which incisogingival tooth structure will show in the widest smile and in other expressions should be noted. If the patient will be embarrassed by a small metal collar or opaque margin of a porcelain-fused-to-metal crown, but there are occlusal demands for the strongest restoration possible, a porcelain butt margin on the labial surface of the crown is used. If occlusion is not a problem, an all-ceramic crown or other esthetic restoration, such as bonding or porcelain laminates, should be considered.[1]

Emergence Profile and Oral Hygiene

Many of the nonorthodontic treatment options discussed in this chapter are meant to "camouflage" malposed or malaligned teeth. Consideration must be given to the contours that will be created by the restorative process.[18,22,42] Often, these contours are unnatural and create areas around the teeth that the patient will find difficult to maintain with good oral hygiene. If these esthetic restorations are to survive, the dentist must consider the final contours being created, and the patient must be given the necessary instructions to maintain them.

TREATMENT STRATEGY

Development of an appropriate treatment plan for the correction of crowded teeth should follow a strategy. First, it is necessary to identify what type of correction and how much correction of tooth con-

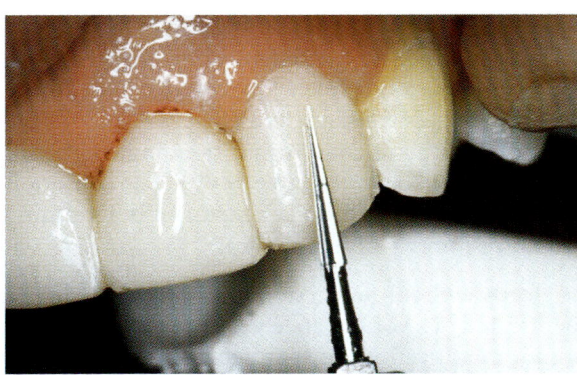

Figure 24–2C: After a slight reproportioning of the six anterior teeth, direct composite resin was placed and contoured (6-mm ET [Brasseler, Savannah, GA]). Note the maxillary cuspid, which was a retained deciduous tooth.

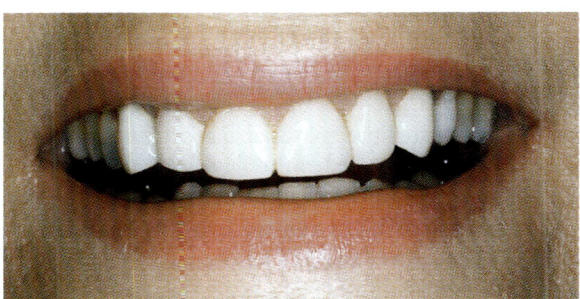

Figure 24–2D: The final result shows improved proportion in tooth size and form.

tours are required to achieve the desired esthetic results.[23,34] Then it becomes necessary to evaluate the dentition, identify clinical limitations to treatment, and select appropriate restorative options that will accomplish the desired esthetic outcome.

Identifying the Degree of Esthetic Correction Required
Following a process of evaluation and development of a problem list, the dentist may use this information to determine the degree of corrections required. Esthetic computer imaging can assist the dentist and the patient to visualize the proposed treatment.[5,17] The development of a diagnostic wax-up is a necessary procedure and may be used to confirm the viability of the proposed treatment developed by computer imaging.

Two sets of diagnostic casts should be made. One set will serve as a historical record of the patient's preoperative condition and should never be modified. The second set of casts should be used for the diagnostic wax-up.

Developing a diagnostic wax-up involves both the addition of wax to deficient areas of the dentition and the removal of stone as necessary to achieve the desired esthetic results. The diagnostic wax-up should be accomplished with attention to detail. Line angles, embrasure spaces, incisal lengths, and gingival contours must represent the desired results if this effort is to be an effective tool in the esthetic treatment of a patient.[25] Through this process, arch space deficiencies can be worked out, and specific modifications to each tooth involved can be identified.

Once completed, the diagnostic wax-up is used to develop additional clinical aids for the accurate and successful completion of the esthetic treatment plan. Polyvinylsiloxane interocclusal record material, such as Regisil 2x (DENTSPLY/Caulk, Milford, DE), is applied to the palate, lingual surface, and incisal edge of the wax-up to form a simple reduction guide. After the material has set, the matrix is carefully trimmed just to the facioincisal line angle. During preparation, the matrix is placed against the lingual surfaces of the teeth (the palatal coverage stabilizes the matrix). The desired incisal length and position of the facial surface (as developed in the diagnostic wax-up) can be identified, and adequate tooth reduction can be determined.

A provisional matrix can also be fabricated by using the same materials and technique. In addition to the palate, lingual surfaces, and incisal edges, the interocclusal record material also covers the facial surfaces and extends several millimeters onto the gingival tissue. The matrix formed will accurately duplicate the subtleties of the diagnostic wax-up. With proper embrasure form and gingival contours accurately duplicated in the provisional restorations, chairside adjustment will be significantly reduced.

A well-planned and executed diagnostic wax-up is an essential communications tool for both the patient and the laboratory.[8,21,41] Dental esthetics is truly in the eyes of the beholder. Everyone has a certain concept of how the teeth should look. Since provisional restorations are closely fabricated to the contours of the diagnostic wax-up,[10] the patient will have a chance to observe and identify any changes in contour and function he or she may desire. If necessary, changes can be made in the provisional restorations, and an impression of these newly contoured restorations can be made. The new cast will serve as a clinically evaluated diagnostic tool used to communicate this vital information to the laboratory.

In summary, a diagnostic wax-up will identify to what degree corrective contours must be made to idealize a crowded dentition. With knowledge of the specific modifications required for each tooth, the dentist can begin to select the proper treatment options.[35] This process should be undertaken whether the treatment is minor esthetic contouring or as comprehensive as a complete restoration of the anterior region with full-coverage crowns.

Identifying the Type of Restoration Required
There are many treatment options available to the dentist for correcting crowded teeth,[20,26,29,33] including esthetic contouring, bonding, porcelain laminates, and crowns (Table 24–2). The condition of the existing dentition is a factor in determining which restorative option is ideal.

Teeth without any restorations or caries should be treated as conservatively as possible. If only minor modifications to tooth contours are required to achieve the desired esthetic result, esthetic contouring and bonding provide the least invasive treatment options. Small existing restorations are easily incorporated into other restorative treatments.

TABLE 24–2. Treatment Options and Indications for the Correction of Crowded Teeth

PROCEDURE	INDICATIONS	CONTRAINDICATIONS	SEQUENCE	CRITERIA
Discing and orthodontics	Usually the first and best option for redistribution of significantly crowded teeth in the anterior region. Discing used to slightly modify width of specific teeth to reposition them into the dental arch	Inadequate supporting structures—bone, tooth roots, or gingival tissue. When immediate solutions are demanded by the patient	Cast analysis of available arch space and tooth size. Orthodontic consult. Cast surgery to reposition teeth into desired final position	
Esthetic contouring	Modification of line angles, incisal edges, or defects to create illusions of proper tooth size, shape, or position. Minimal alteration of tooth position	If contouring would expose dentin. If contouring would eliminate desirable occlusal or functional contacts	Following determination of the desired results by diagnostic wax-up	< 0.5 mm of facial reduction. < 1.0 mm of incisal reduction
Bonding	Addition of composite resin to modify apparent height and width of natural tooth by alteration of the shape and location of line angles. Diastema closure. Incisal edge modification of sound tooth structure. Minimal shade modification only	Inadequate enamel or supporting tooth structure. Severe occlusal loads placed on composite restoration. Modification of severe tooth discoloration	Following color modification (bleaching, etc.) of natural tooth structure. Following diagnostic wax-up to determine need for preoperative esthetic contouring	< 1.0-mm addition of composite resin
Porcelain laminate veneers	Indicated for esthetic rehabilitation of entire anterior segments. Individual teeth must be structurally sound. Changes can be additive, subtractive, or both. Shape/size, alignment, and color of the teeth may be modified	Weak supporting tooth structure. Multiple, large existing restorations. Minimal bondable tooth structure	Following diagnostic wax-up to determine need for preoperative esthetic contouring.	0.5 mm of reduction possible within enamel. < 25% exposed dentin. 2-mm maximum thickness of porcelain
All-ceramic crowns	Indicated for structurally weak teeth with large multiple restorations or when a more conservative restoration is contraindicated. All-ceramic crowns are indicated when esthetics is of primary importance. A favorable occlusal scheme should exist (canine guidance). Compatible opposing dentition or restorations	Unfavorable occlusal scheme. Bruxism. Significant vertical overlap with minimal occlusal clearance. When a more conservative restoration is indicated to achieve desired esthetic results	Following diagnostic wax-up to clearly define esthetic and functional objectives. Following proper build-up procedures	1.0-mm marginal reduction. Uniform, circumferential 90-degree shoulder margin. 2-mm incisal reduction

Caries in the teeth to be treated may require that more extensive restorations be considered, such as porcelain laminates or crowns. The size and location of the caries may dictate the design of these restorations.

The presence of a root canal-treated tooth,[14] with or without a post and core, may require a crown. In the crowded tooth scenario, this may be beneficial. The ability to reposition the crown into an ideal esthetic location can more easily be accomplished when the tooth has been treated with a root canal. Care must be taken, however, not to overextend or overcontour the final restoration, which would result in possible gingival irritation.

TREATMENT OPTIONS

Conservative treatments such as esthetic contouring,[11] discing combined with minor tooth movement, and bonding are available for minor corrections of crowded teeth. When corrections that are more substantial are required, porcelain laminates and crowns become the treatment of choice.[18]

Correction by Discing

If the evaluation of arch space, as previously described by Berliner,[2] shows that the combined addition of ABCD in the lower arch equals 21 mm (see Figure 24–1A) but the available space is 20 mm, the amount of crowding is 1 mm. Therefore, if minor movement or repositioning is attempted to realign the teeth, 1 mm of combined mesiodistal width can be sacrificed through discing. However, not all of the tooth surface will have to be lost from the central and lateral incisors. The mesial surfaces of the cuspids are also available and, under certain rare conditions, the distal surfaces of cuspids as well.

One limitation on reducing tooth structure through discing is the thickness of enamel on the teeth. Radiographs must be accurate enough to measure the available enamel. A measurement can be made of the proximal surfaces on each of the anterior teeth to predict the maximum reduction possible without perforating the dentin.

For example, if 0.25 mm is found to be the amount that can be reduced per proximal surface, then 0.5 mm can be reduced per tooth. Therefore, 3.0 mm could theoretically be reduced from the six anterior teeth by discing to increase the available arch space. In applying this to the earlier example of 1-mm crowding, there should be no repositioning problem.

The procedure for applying the above principle is as follows:

1. Measure the mesiodistal width of the individual teeth and the available arch space with a dental dial caliper.
2. Measure the enamel thickness by studying the radiographs of the involved anterior teeth (see Figure 24–1C). Peck and Peck caution that accessing enamel thickness from radiographs alone is subject to possible distortion.[32] Instead, they offer an arbitrary, but safe, guideline of 50% of the mesiodistal enamel thickness as the maximum limit of reproximation.
3. After determining that the amount of space necessary to realign the teeth is attainable without perforating dentin, disc the teeth accordingly. This can be done at one time, if the space is minimal, or over a period of time, depending on the conditions present. The patient can be instructed to return weekly or biweekly for stripping. Diamond separating strips (Compo-Strip, Premier Dental Products, King of Prussia, PA) should be used. If the teeth are extremely tight, use a Compo-Disc (Premier Dental Products) first for ease in initial discing. If considerable space is necessary, consider using an ET6 or ET9 30-micron diamond bur (Brasseler).
4. Repositioning can now be accomplished by any of several different methods shown in Chapter 25: Esthetics in Adult Orthodontics.

Correction by Bonding

The success of composite resin bonding has made immediate restorative correction of crowded teeth possible.[9,12] In most cases, it will be necessary to combine the treatments of composite resin bonding with esthetic contouring (see Chapter 11, *Esthetics in Dentistry*, Volume 1, 2nd Edition) to produce the greatest effect. As with all bonding techniques, the patient must be apprised of not only the esthetic life expectancy and limitations of the bonded restoration but also an estimate of how much maintenance may be required. The following example will show just how much can be accomplished through composite resin bonding.

Bonding and Esthetic Contouring to Eliminate Crowding

PROBLEM: This 30-year-old horse trainer had extremely large central incisors (Figure 24–3A). In addition, the mandibular centrals were crowded and rotated lingually (see Figures 24–3A and B).

TREATMENT: Although the patient was informed about the advantage of orthodontics as the ideal treatment, she nevertheless chose an immediate correction in the form of esthetic contouring and esthetic resin bonding. The central incisors were first contoured on the study cast to approximate the desired tooth size. Esthetic contouring was accomplished in both the maxillary (Figure 24–3C) and mandibular arches (Figure 24–3D). Next, the lateral incisors were bonded labially to round out a more symmetric arch (Figures 24–3E and F).

RESULT: By comparing occlusal views, one can see how effective the two procedures were in creating the illusion of straightness (see Figure 24–3F and Figure 24–3G). A more proportional smile can be seen by comparing Figures 24–3H and I.

Correction by Porcelain Laminates

The advantage in selecting porcelain laminates to correct crowded teeth is the ability for the labora-

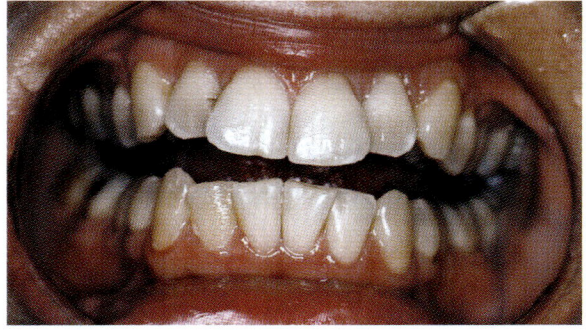

Figure 24–3A: This 30-year-old woman had extremely large central incisors with overlapping maxillary and mandibular teeth.

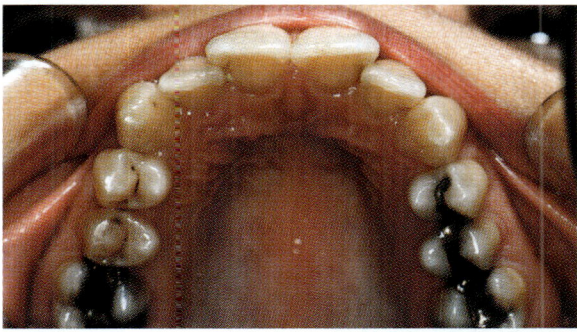

Figure 24–3B: An occlusal view showing the overlapping central incisors.

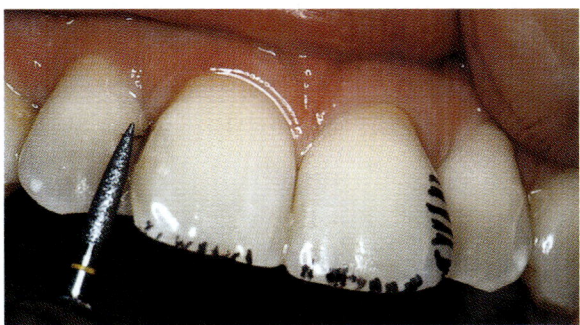

Figure 24–3C: Cosmetic contouring was first performed on the maxillary central incisors and mandibular anterior.

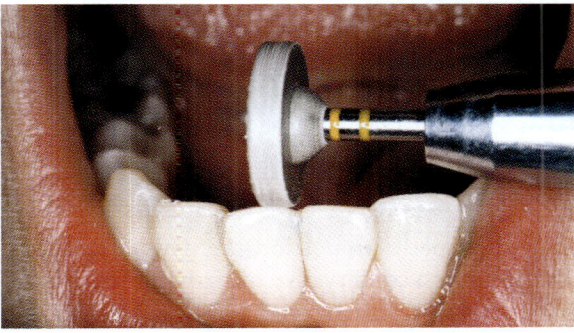

Figure 24–3D: After contouring the mandibular anterior teeth, they were polished with an impregnated aluminum oxide wheel (Cosmetic Contouring Kit, Shofu, Menlo Park, CA).

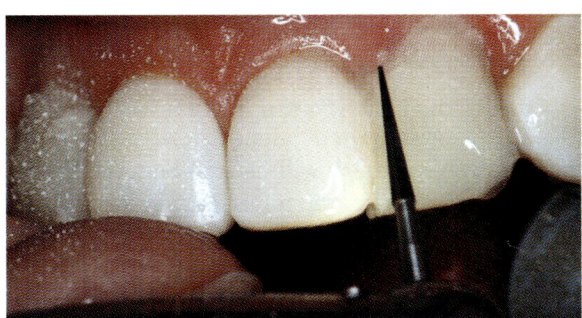

Figure 24–3E: Next, the maxillary laterals were bonded with composite resin and contoured and finished with ET carbide finishing burs (Brasseler).

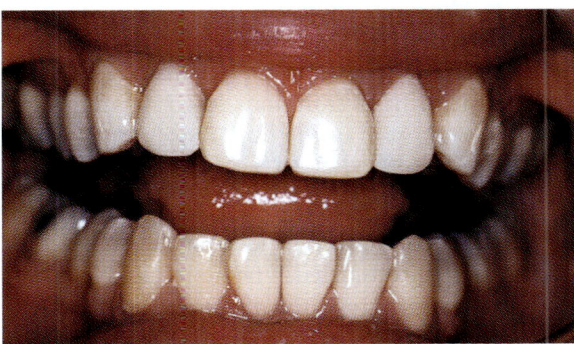

Figure 24–3F: Better tooth proportion and straighter-appearing teeth can be seen here before the final polishing.

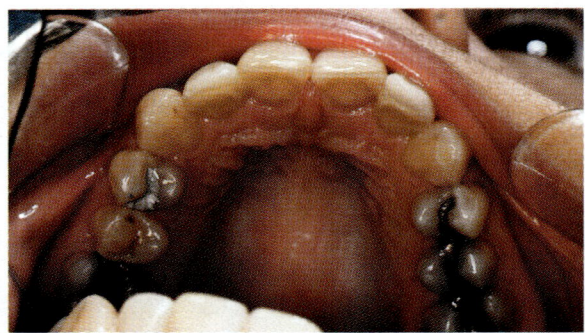

Figure 24–3G: Final result shows a straighter arc with more proportional teeth.

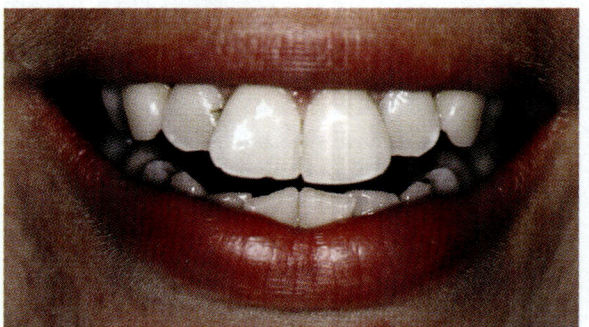

Figure 24–3H: Pretreatment view of the smile.

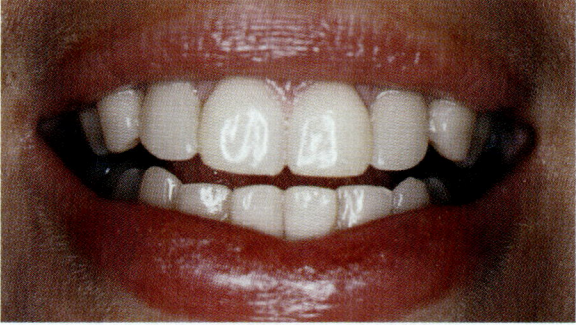

Figure 24–3I: Post-treatment view showing better harmony with the smile.

tory to properly proportion the new restorations. This permits a conservative solution to be used that will need less maintenance.[15,18]

When selecting porcelain laminates, determine arch space deficiencies on each side. Both lateral incisors may be rotated in a similar fashion, resulting in an equal amount of space on both sides of the arch. However, if one lateral is overlapped more than the other, the available space may be asymmetric. Correction may require shifting of line angles in the final restorations to create an illusion of equal dimension in the final restorations.

After reproportioning the anterior space, if the total space will result in teeth that would look much too narrow, building out the teeth in a slight labioversion should be considered. The more the buccal surface is positioned anteriorly, the wider the teeth will become. The added thickness will go unnoticed if it occurs throughout the restored teeth and results in an entire arc that is positioned labially from bicuspid to bicuspid. A curve that will look good from an occlusal and a labial view should be selected. It is usually possible to compromise by building out the other teeth slightly and lingualizing the most labially positioned teeth. How much and where the existing teeth will need reducing during the preparation of the teeth should be determined. This is easily accomplished by using a reduction matrix fabricated from a diagnostic wax-up. A good example of the above principles can be seen in Figures 24–4A to H.

Usually, the most severe reduction would resemble a similar amount of dentin loss, as in a full crown. Even if a tooth will have to be severely prepared for a laminate, the total loss would be much less with a laminate than for the crown. The worst scenario would be to require endodontic therapy by doing a vital extirpation of the pulp.

Following are several examples of the use of porcelain laminates to correct crowding in the anterior region.

Use of Diagnostic Wax-up and Matrices in the Correction of Crowding with Porcelain Laminates

PROBLEM: A 56-year-old businessman presented with a desire to straighten his anterior teeth. In addition, he was concerned about the wear and irregularity of the incisal edges of his teeth (see Figures 24–4A to C). Orthodontics was presented as a first option, but the patient declined this treatment option because of the lengthy treatment time that would be required.

TREATMENT: Because of uncertainty about the ability to achieve a satisfactory result using restorative treatment options to correct the significant rotation of the lateral incisors, diagnostic casts were made. A diagnostic wax-up was used to determine if appropriate modifications could be made that would correct this crowding.

Using a diagnostic cast, it was noted that the space available (see Figures 24–4D and E) for tooth #7 was 4.5 mm and for tooth #10 was 6 mm. The central incisors were evaluated, and tooth #8

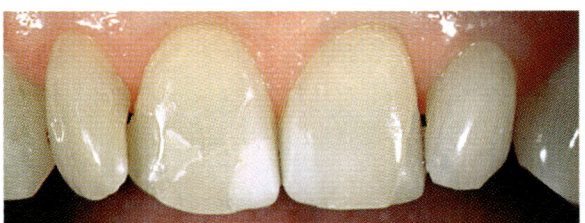

Figure 24–4A: Pretreatment—anterior view. Note the prominence of tooth #7 due to significant rotation and the slightly shortened appearance of tooth #10.

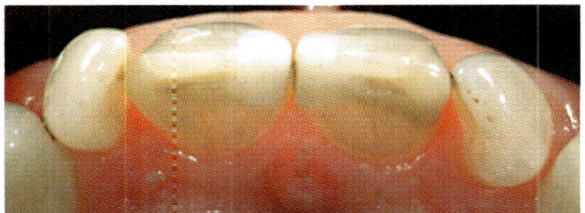

Figure 24–4B: Pretreatment—incisal view. Variations in available arch space for the lateral incisors are evident.

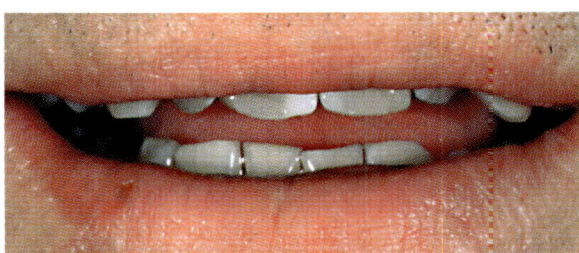

Figure 24–4C: Pretreatment—view of normal smile. Irregular incisal edges and incisal embrasures create an unbalanced esthetic appearance.

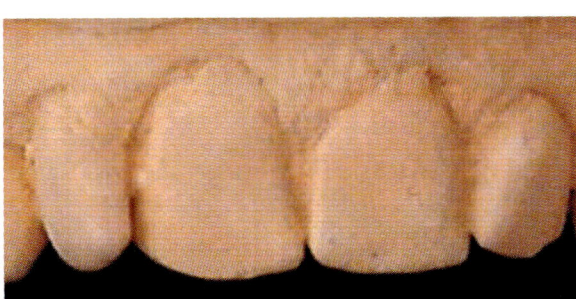

Figure 24–4D: Diagnostic cast—facial view.

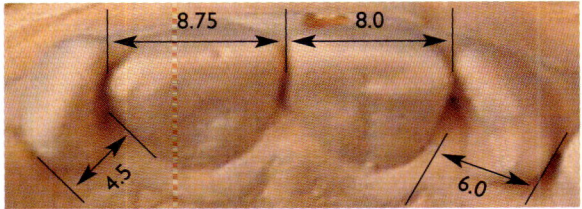

Figure 24–4E: Diagnostic cast—incisal view. By measuring the available arch space for each incisor, the source of the crowding problem was determined. The results of this analysis demonstrated a 1.5-mm deficiency in the area of tooth #7 and an excessive amount of arch space with tooth #8.

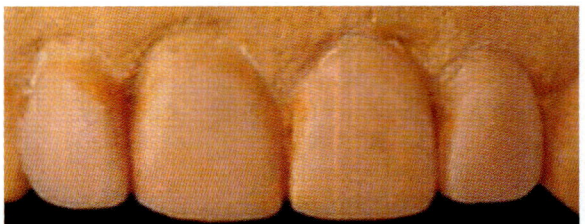

Figure 24–4F: Completed diagnostic wax-up—anterior view. Proposed reduction to the distal tooth #8 and additional width to the mesial of tooth #7 create a more harmonious distribution of tooth width in the arch.

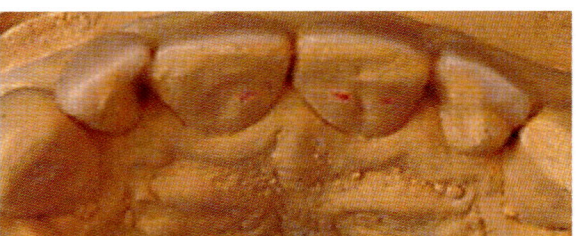

Figure 24–4G: Completed diagnostic wax-up—incisal view. The additional width required for tooth #7 was achieved by allowing the facial surface to remain slightly facial from the ideal arch form. This slight overlap was unnoticeable from an anterior view.

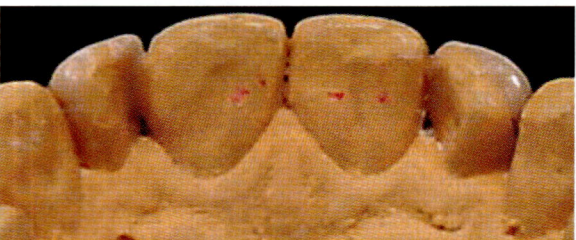

Figure 24–4H: Completed diagnostic wax-up—lingual view. The transition from the actual tooth position to the final tooth position created an unusual lingual embrasure on the mesial of both lateral incisors. Special instructions were given to the patient regarding oral hygiene in these areas.

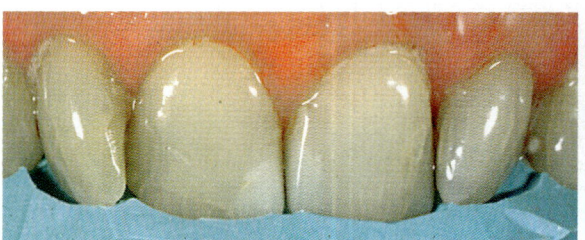

Figure 24–4I: Matrix of diagnostic wax-up used to identify areas of tooth structure beyond the desired final contours.

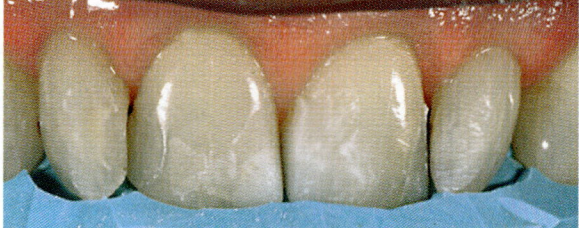

Figure 24–4J: Prior to final preparation of the teeth, only the excessive tooth structure was reduced using the diagnostic wax-up matrix as a guide.

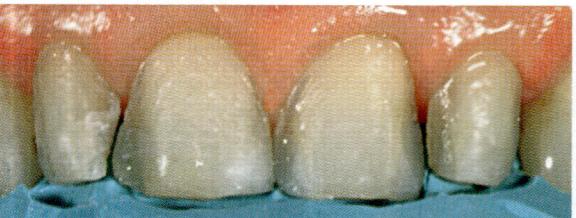

Figure 24–4K: Use of the diagnostic matrix to ensure proper incisal and facial reduction of the final preparations for porcelain laminate veneers.

was found to be 8.75 mm and tooth #9 was 8 mm. The crowding problem was then summarized as the deficiency in arch space of 1.5 mm for tooth #7 with an excessive width of 0.75 mm for tooth #8. If the distal of tooth #8 was reduced by 0.75 mm, then the space needed to be created for tooth #7 was 0.75 mm if both sides of the arch were to have a symmetric appearance.

Stone was removed from the prominent mesial line angles, and wax was added to the distal half of the lateral incisors to reduce the appearance of rotation (see Figures 25–4F to H). The central incisors were contoured to create a symmetric appearance and uniform width. Wax was added to the incisal edges to create a uniform length. Incisal embrasures were developed to define the width of each of the incisors. The facial surface and mesial edge of tooth #7 were allowed to remain slightly facial and overlapped with tooth #8. This facial positioning of the tooth (increasing the arch form in this area) provided the additional space needed to create an appropriately sized tooth.

Once it was determined that restorative treatment could adequately camouflage this patient's crowding, the decision was made to use porcelain laminates to accomplish this goal. The patient was then presented with this option, and he elected to proceed with treatment. A reduction matrix was fabricated over the diagnostic wax-up and trimmed to the facioincisal line angle. Figures 24–4I to K illustrate its use. Figure 24–4I shows the matrix in position prior to tooth reduction. This identified the amount of facial reduction necessary to bring the natural tooth back into the desired final contours. Figure 24–4J demonstrates the initial tooth reduction to achieve this. The teeth were then prepared for porcelain laminates, with the matrix being used to determine the proper incisal and facial reduction (see Figure 24–4K).

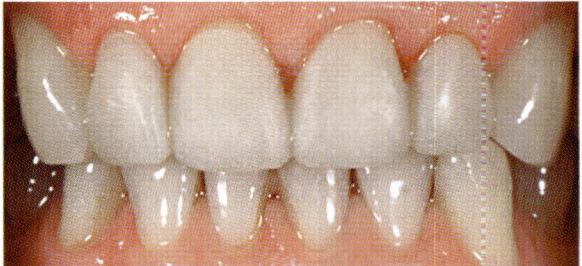

Figure 24–4L: Idealized provisional restorations fabricated using a second diagnostic wax-up matrix that remained untrimmed. From these restorations, the patient can accurately visualize the proposed results of the treatment.

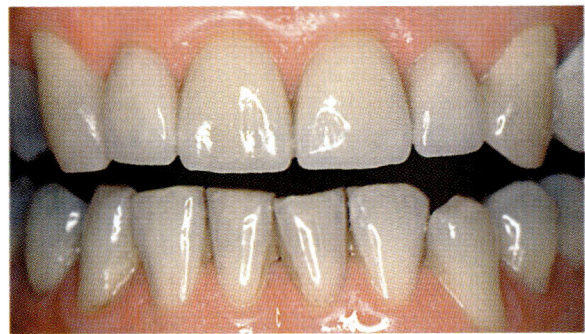

Figure 24–4M: Completed restorations—facial view. Note accurate reproduction of the diagnostic wax-up.

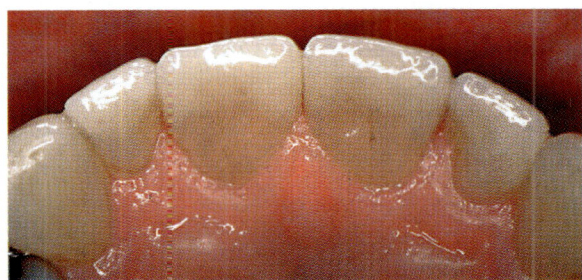

Figure 24–4N: Completed restorations—incisal view.

Provisional restorations were fabricated from a matrix formed over the diagnostic wax-up. The intended results of treatment were shown to the patient (Figure 24–4L). Following the patient's approval of esthetics, phonetics, and function, the laminates were completed (Figures 24–4M and N).

RESULTS: Porcelain laminates were used to correct significant crowding of four maxillary incisors with satisfactory results. The importance of the diagnostic casts, wax-up, and matrices in the overall planning, communication, and implementation of treatment was demonstrated.

Esthetic Contouring and Porcelain Laminates to Eliminate Crowding

PROBLEM: This 58-year-old housewife was concerned about her eroded, crowded, and stained front teeth (Figures 24–5A and B). Measurement with a dental dial caliper helped to accurately determine available space for reproportioning tooth size (Figure 25–5C). Although orthodontics was mentioned as a first step to an ideal solution, the patient preferred to accept a compromise treatment of porcelain laminates and cosmetic contouring. Although crowding was less of a concern to the patient (Figures 24–5D and E), she nevertheless decided to have straighter-looking teeth through a compromise treatment of porcelain laminates that would also esthetically correct the erosion and discoloration.

TREATMENT: Figure 24–5D shows the areas that will be esthetically contoured. Following contouring to reproportion spaces, Figure 24–5F demonstrates the gingival chamfer margin being placed with a two-grit LVS diamond bur (Brasseler). The occlusal view (Figure 24–5G) reveals just how much overlapping existed. Figure 24–5H shows the teeth

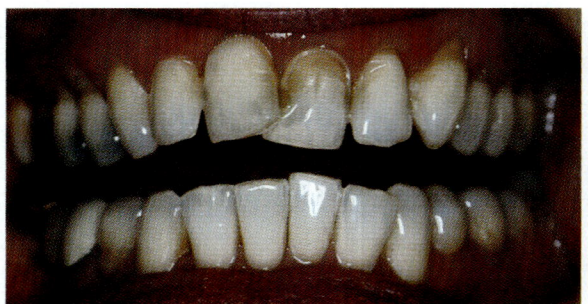

Figure 24–5A: This 58-year-old woman was dissatisfied with her crowded, eroded, and discolored teeth.

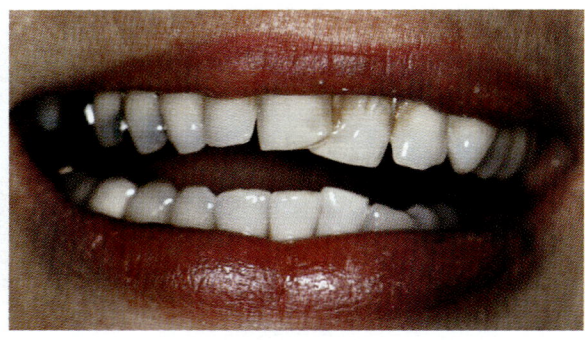

Figure 24–5B: Preoperative view.

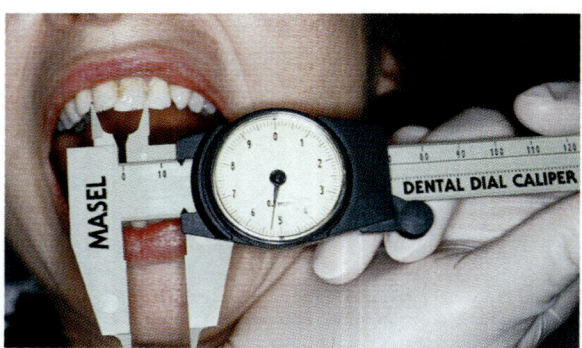

Figure 24–5C: Each tooth and the available space for the laminated teeth are measured with Dental Dial Calipers (Masel Enterprises, Bristol, PA).

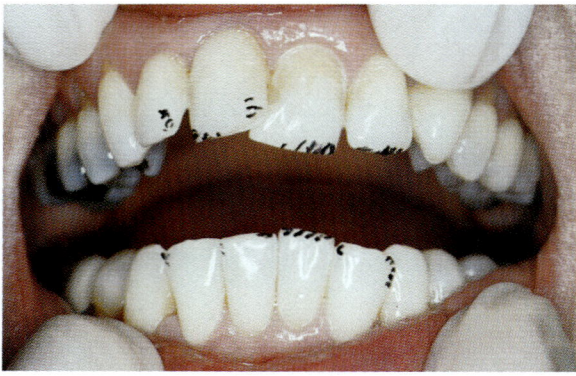

Figure 24–5D: The teeth are then esthetically contoured to begin creating the illusion of straighter teeth.

after esthetic contouring and tooth preparation have occurred, as well as how defective amalgam restorations were removed and glass ionomer bases were placed. Figure 24–5E shows finished laminates in place. Note the newly proportioned, straighter, and lighter-looking teeth. The final occlusal view also shows a new arch created by the laminates, building out teeth #9 and #10 and the new posterior laminate onlays on the upper right side.

RESULT: Before and after smiles can be seen by comparing Figures 24–5B and I. Esthetic contour-

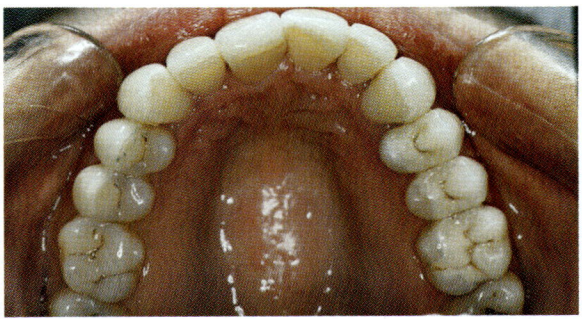

Figure 24–5E: Porcelain laminates were cemented from the right cuspid to the left second bicuspid; the laminate onlays were inserted on the maxillary right bicuspids and first molar.

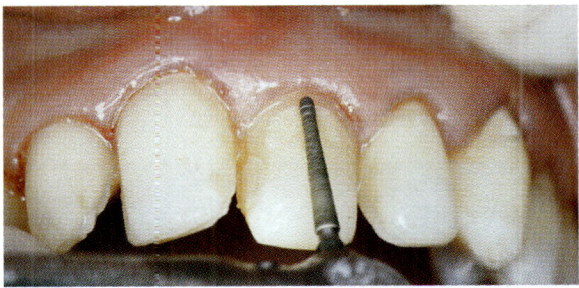

Figure 24–5F: The anterior teeth are prepared for porcelain laminates. A special two-grit diamond bur ([Brasseler]; see *Esthetics in Dentistry*, Volume 1, 2nd Edition, p. 346–7) helps prepare both the body and margin of the tooth.

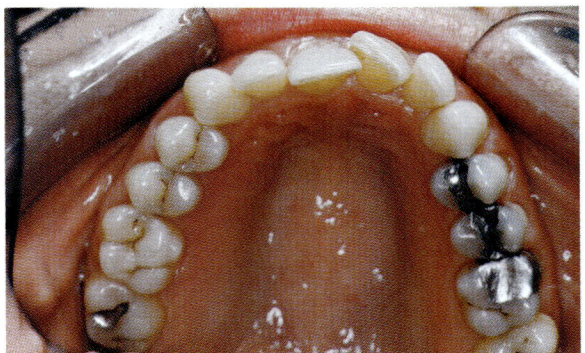

Figure 24–5G: The occlusal view shows the extent of overlapping in the central incisors.

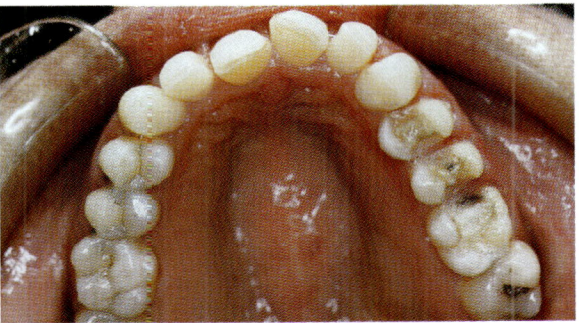

Figure 24–5H: This occlusal view shows the final tooth preparation. Note the patient's right posterior quadrant. The teeth were prepared for combination laminate/onlays.

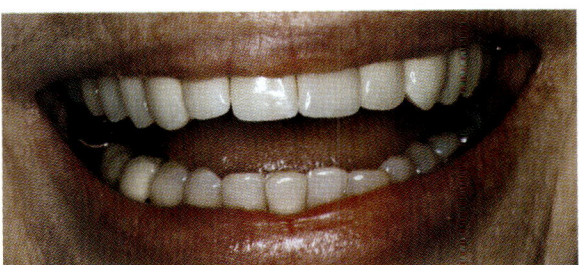

Figure 24–5I: Postoperative view of improved smile created by use of porcelain laminate veneers and esthetic contouring.

ing has also improved the alignment of the lower anteriors. Constructing the porcelain laminates indirectly allows the laboratory to better proportion tooth size.

Correction by Crowning

As in bonding, the first problem in restoring crowded teeth by crowning is tooth size. Each tooth needs to be or appear to be proportional. The more teeth that are crowned, the less distortion there is.[4,27,31] This means that if only one or two teeth are crowned, there may be a noticeable difference between the crowned teeth (which would be smaller) and the natural ones, depending on the space involved. However, it is possible to accomplish this by carefully shaping both the tooth to be crowned and the adjacent teeth to appear harmonious in size. Figures 24–6A to C provide an example of how one tooth can be crowned to relieve anterior crowding. After the adjacent central and lateral incisors were reshaped, a full porcelain crown was placed on the left central (see Figure 24–6B).

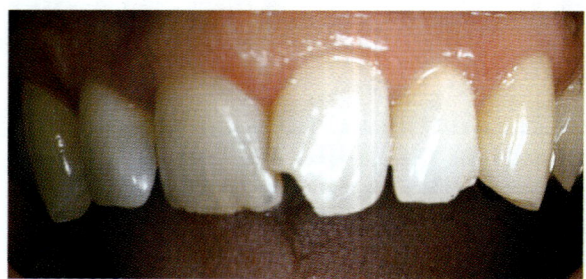

Figure 24–6A: This patient presented with chipped and crowded maxillary anterior teeth.

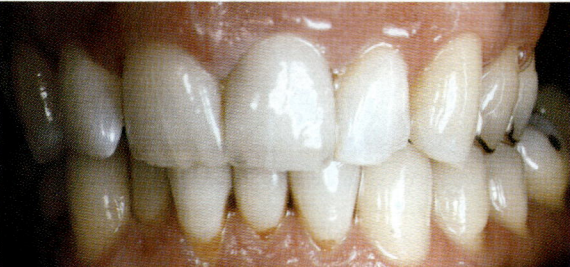

Figure 24–6B: A full porcelain crown was placed on the left central incisor; the right central and lateral incisors were esthetically contoured.

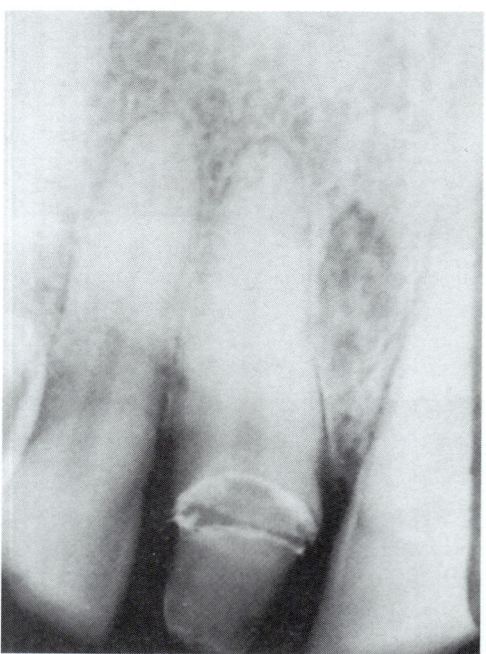

Figure 24–6C: The post-treatment radiograph shows the change in axial inclination for esthetic result.

An alternative solution is to reshape the existing teeth.[40] For example, in a maxillary anterior crowded condition, instead of merely crowning two central incisors, the lateral incisors can be reshaped by reducing the mesial surface slightly so that the adjacent central incisors can be enlarged. This same principle can be applied in other areas of the mouth. The teeth adjacent to crowns are always reduced to recover some of the space lost because of crowding. The more the adjacent teeth are reduced, the less noticeable is the distortion. An example of crowning six incisors to eliminate the crowding of anteriors follows.

Crowning to Eliminate Crowding

PROBLEM: This 38-year-old store owner presented with crowded and discolored maxillary and mandibular teeth (Figures 24–7A and B). Although orthodontic treatment was suggested as ideal treatment, he elected a compromise that consisted of bonding the mandibular and crowning the maxillary teeth.

TREATMENT: When teeth are as crowded as this, it is sometimes necessary to do a vital pulp extirpation to prepare the teeth for adequate porcelain thickness. Thus, tooth preparation and diagnostic wax-up were first completed on the study casts (Figures 24–7C and D). The patient was fully informed of the possibility of endodontic therapy. The actual tooth preparation can be seen in Figures 24–7E and F. Fortunately, the pulp had receded, so extirpation was not necessary. Electrosurgery was completed prior to impressions to improve access to the preparation margins. Six full porcelain crowns restored the esthetics of the maxillary arch (Figure 24–7G), whereas composite resin bonding helped restore mandibular esthetics. A maxillary occlusal night appliance was constructed for the patient to wear since the patient had a history of clenching while sleeping.

RESULT: The resulting smile with straighter and lighter teeth (Figures 24–7H and I) was most appreciated by the patient.

If crowded teeth are to be corrected with bonding, laminating, or full crowns, the central incisors must be proportioned correctly. This can be accomplished by either discing the mesial surfaces of adjacent uninvolved teeth or reducing the size of adjacent crowned teeth. For final esthetics, contouring of adjacent teeth should be considered.

The decision whether to laminate or crown should be made primarily on the position of the overlapping (protruding) teeth. To restore the arch on or near the labial-most position of the teeth, porcelain laminates can be used. However, if the choice is to use maximum position (including vital pulp extirpation), then crowns will probably be the best choice.

Crowning and Repositioning of Mandibular Anteriors. Although crowding can occur in both arches, it is more common in the mandibular anterior teeth. Treatment for these teeth is usually repositioning. There may be occasions when the orthodontist will choose not to reposition, and the patient may want these teeth bonded, laminated, or crowned. For teeth that are badly broken down or have significant gingival recession that has made them unattractive, bonding, laminating, or crowning can accomplish two things: it can restore and straighten each tooth to its proper form. How much correction can be achieved by repositioning is governed partially by root structure and crown inclination. If the axial alignments of the teeth are divergent, there is a limit to how much they can be straightened. If one of the teeth is in extreme labioversion, it is difficult to do much straightening without building the adjacent tooth somewhat thicker. This may create a gingival impingement on the tooth that is being overcontoured. Excessive labial reduction could cause pulp damage, so some compromise has to be reached. For this reason, repositioning is generally the better solution. Sometimes, a combination approach is the best solution. If the teeth are broken down and discolored and have unattractive, large restorations, partial repositioning can be attempted, and crowning may take care of the remainder of the problem. This way, the patient might not mind wearing an appliance for a short while. One of the main objections that patients have to orthodontic treatment is the length of time the appliances have to be worn.

748 Esthetics in Dentistry

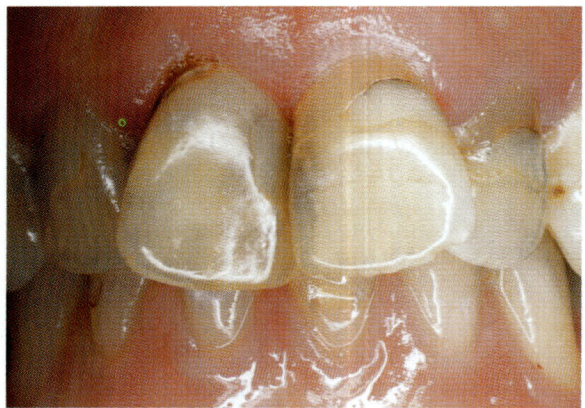

Figure 24–7A: This 38-year-old man wanted to improve his crowded maxillary and mandibular teeth.

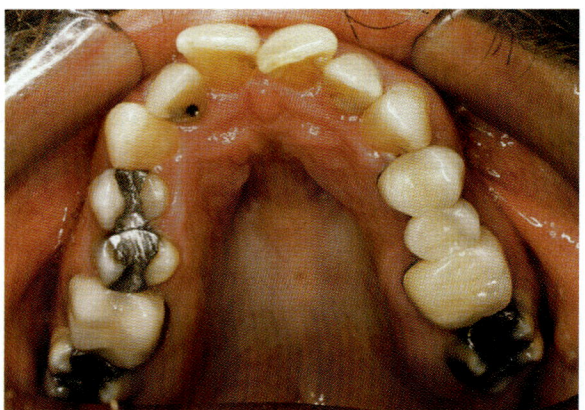

Figure 24–7B: This occlusal view shows why full orthodontic treatment was originally presented as the ideal treatment. The patient insisted on a "quick fix" solution.

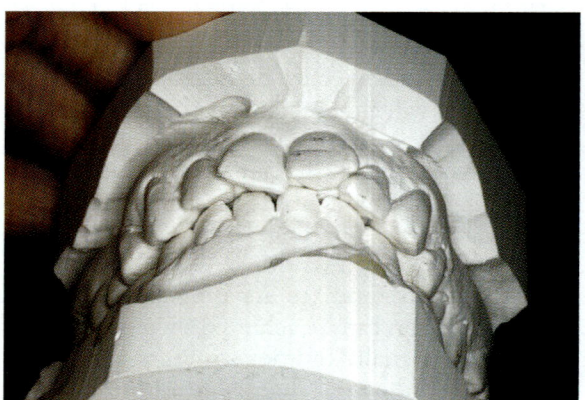

Figure 24–7C: Diagnostic casts show the extent of crowding in the maxillary anterior teeth.

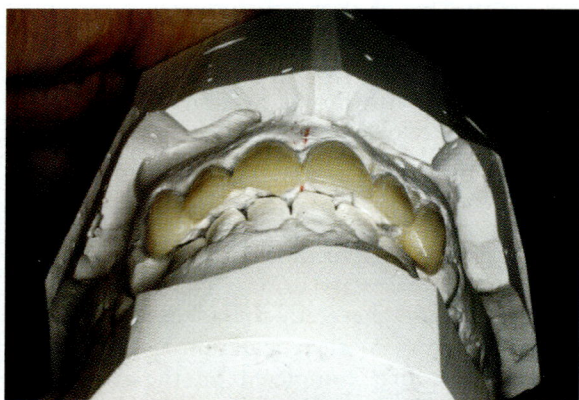

Figure 24–7D: A wax-up was completed to demonstrate to the patient and dental team how crowns could be used to accomplish the esthetic goal.

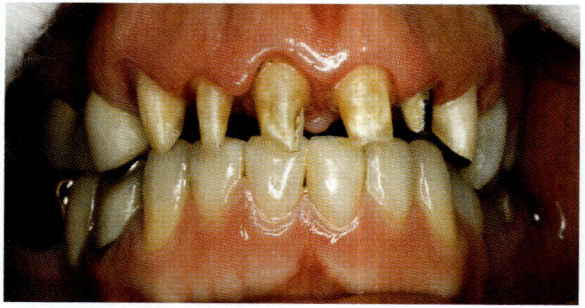

Figure 24–7E: Although the patient was warned that endodontic therapy might be necessary on the maxillary incisors, the teeth were prepared without pulpal exposures.

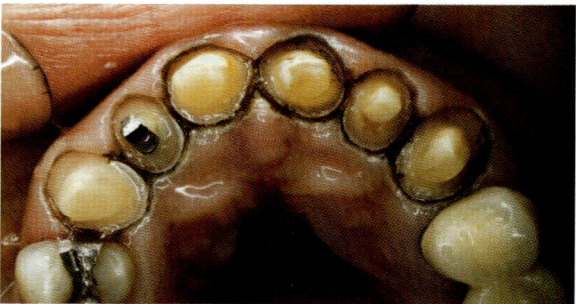

Figure 24–7F: The occlusal view shows the patient ready for impressions after electrosurgery for effective tissue displacement.

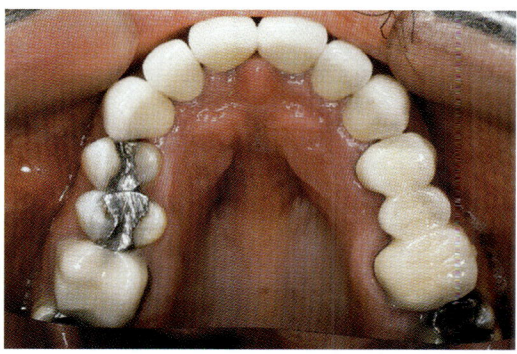

Figure 24–7G: The final six crowns show improved proportion and symmetry in the arch.

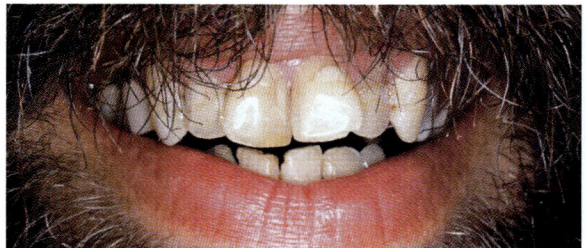

Figure 24–7H: Pretreatment smile.

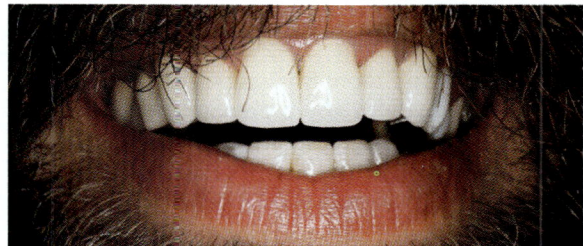

Figure 24–7I: Post-treatment smile with six maxillary full porcelain crowns and four mandibular incisors with bonded composite resins.

UNUSUAL OR RARE CLINICAL PRESENTATIONS

Occasionally, the dentist is presented with unusual dental problems associated with crowded dentitions. Some of these may include malposed and misaligned teeth, a protruding tooth, a retruded tooth, or the "lingually locked" tooth.[6,7,16,28,38,39]

Malposed and Misaligned Teeth

The method of choice for correcting malposition or misalignment of a tooth or teeth is orthodontia. For adults, consideration should be given to removable appliances, plastic or ceramic brackets, or lingual braces. However, it is sometimes possible to treat malposed or misaligned teeth without constructing special appliances. Provisional acrylic splints can be adapted to accomplish necessary repositioning.

An effective technique for repositioning crowded lower incisors is use of the provisional splint with small hooks. A composite resin stop that is mechanically bonded to the teeth helps keep the elastic from slipping. Some discing in the interproximal surfaces of the anterior teeth is necessary to create space for the incisors to move lingually. Finally, it is necessary to plan some sort of retention; either an A-splint or direct bonding with composite resin splint can be used.

Adult patients who come to the dentist for correction of malposed or misaligned teeth may think that they are too old for orthodontic therapy. The dentist will have to judge the importance of immediate facial esthetics to the patient. If repositioning is the best solution to the esthetic problem, then the patient should be advised and motivated to accept this therapy. When the patient will accept only those procedures that offer an immediate solution, then bonding, laminating, or crowning may be the only feasible compromises. Esthetic contouring should also be considered. Rather than no treatment, esthetic contouring may provide some compromise benefit.

The Protruding Tooth

In restoring a crowded labially positioned incisor, careful preparation can make the protruding tooth

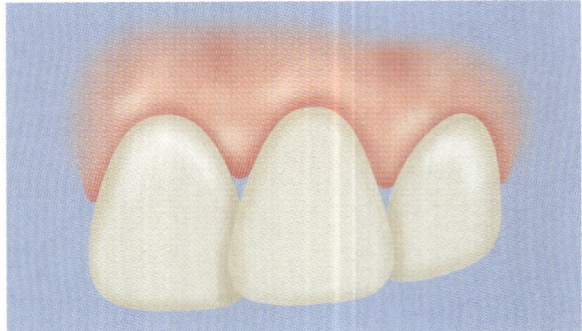

Figure 24–8A: The labial surface is reduced as far as possible without damaging the pulp. It is extremely important not to reduce the incisogingival height until the preparation is essentially complete.

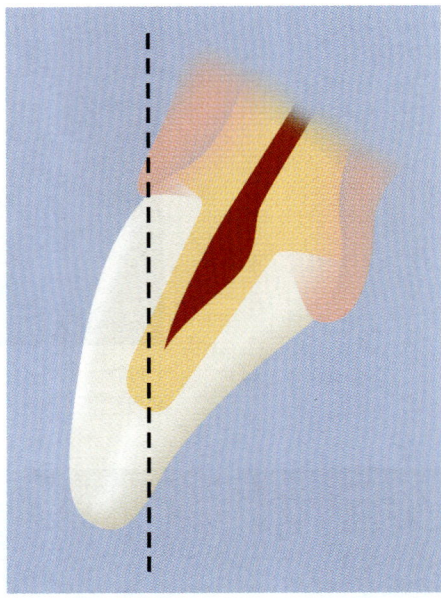

Figure 24–8B: The crowded labially positioned incisor requires a careful preparation to make it appear to be in a more lingual position.

appear to be in a more lingual position. Care must be taken to avoid a short preparation. The labial surface is reduced as far as possible without damaging the pulp; very little tooth structure is removed from the linguoincisal surface (Figures 24–8A and B). It is extremely important not to reduce the incisogingival height until the preparation is essentially complete. This will help avoid a short preparation. If the labial protrusion is so extreme that the pulp may become involved, the dentist may perform vital pulp extirpation.[2] Such radical procedures should be undertaken only when appearance is extremely important and the patient is completely aware of the possible consequences and has signed an informed consent for treatment.

The Retruded Tooth

This esthetic problem is similar to that of the protruded tooth. However, realignment of the tooth in linguoversion frequently necessitates reduction and recontouring of the opposing teeth to allow for clearance of the newly crowned, bonded, or laminated tooth. To achieve the desired result, a large bulk of the tooth structure may have to be removed from the linguoincisal surface of the opposing tooth. Esthetic results can then be achieved by crowning or laminating. If a porcelain-fused-to-metal restoration is desired, the lingual side can be covered with a thin layer of metal, and the labial porcelain may be built out to correct alignment. Laminating can be especially useful since virtually no enamel needs to be reduced on the labial surface, with only linguoincisal enamel being reshaped to mask the amount of retrusion present.

The Lingually Locked Tooth

If a lingually locked tooth is fully erupted, it can be restored to correct position by pulp extirpation and placement of an off-center endodontic post and porcelain crown. However, if the tooth is too short and in moderate linguoversion, this treatment may be impractical. A porcelain shoulder is prepared on the labial, and the porcelain is built up butted against the labial gingiva. The patient must be warned that oral hygiene must be scrupulous. It is far better to try to convince the patient of the advantages of repositioning the lingually locked tooth than to try to restore it in place. In severe situations, a third choice involving extraction and moving the remaining teeth together with elastic thread ligature or bonded brackets may be indicated.

TO BOND, LAMINATE, OR CROWN?

The following questions should be considered:

1. What is the size of the crowded tooth? Will bonding make the tooth too bulky? Bonded lower anteriors are more susceptible to this problem.
2. How much enamel is left for bonding? Are there very large restorations that, once

removed, will lessen the retention for a bonded restoration?

3. What is the appearance of the enamel? Is it badly stained or discolored so that a large amount of opaquer plus several layers of composite resin will be required to mask the defects? If so, then lamination and crowning are the better choices.

4. Does the patient have a bad habit that may stain a bonded restoration? Heavy smokers or coffee/tea drinkers may choose laminating or crowning to lessen the amount of postoperative discoloration.

5. Is there an economic problem? Frequently, patients may wish to have their teeth laminated or crowned, but finances enter into the decision since bonding is less expensive than either crowning or laminating.

6. How long does the patient expect the restoration to last? Chances are that both laminating and crowning can provide much longer life than direct bonding with composite resin.

References

1. Bello A, Jarvis RH. A review of esthetic alternatives for the restoration of anterior teeth. J Prosthet Dent 1997;78:437–40.

2. Berlinger A. Ligatures, splints, bite planes, and pyramids. Philadelphia: JB Lippincott, 1964.

3. Burstone CJ, Marcotte MR. Problem solving in orthodontics: goal-oriented treatment strategies. Chicago: Quintessence, 2000.

4. Chiche GJ, Pinault A. Esthetics of anterior fixed prosthodontics. Chicago: Quintessence, 1993.

5. Crispin B. Contemporary esthetic dentistry: practice fundamentals. Chicago: Quintessence, 1994.

6. Curry FT. Restorative alternative to orthodontic treatment: a clinical report. J Prosthet Dent 1999; 82:127–9.

7. Cutbirth ST. Treatment planning for porcelain veneer restoration of crowded teeth by modifying stone models. J Esthet Restor Dent 2001;13:29–39.

8. Derbabian K, Marzola R, Arcidiacono A. The science of communicating the art of dentistry. J Calif Dent Assoc 1998;26:101–6.

9. Dietschi D. Free-hand composite resin restorations: a key to anterior esthetics. Pract Periodont Aesthet Dent 1995;7(7):15–25.

10. Donovan TE, Cho C. Diagnostic provisional restorations in restorative dentistry: the blueprint for success. J Can Dent Assoc 1999;65:272–5.

11. Epstein MB, Mantzikos T, Shamus IL. Esthetic recontouring: a team approach. N Y State Dent J 1997;63(10):35–40.

12. Fahl N Jr, Denehy GE, Jackson RD. Protocol for predictable restoration of anterior teeth with composite resins. Pract Periodont Aesthet Dent 1995;7(8):13–21.

13. Foster TD. A textbook of orthodontics. 2nd edn. Oxford: Blackwell Scientific, 1982.

14. Fradeani M, Aquilino A, Barducci G. Aesthetic restoration of endodontically treated teeth. Pract Periodont Aesthet Dent 1999;11:761–8.

15. Garber DA, Goldstein RE, Feinman RA. Porcelain laminate veneers. Chicago: Quintessence, 1988.

16. Gleghorn TA. Use of bonded porcelain restorations for nonorthodontic realignment of the anterior maxilla. Pract Periodont Aesthet Dent 1998;10:563–5.

17. Goldstein CE, Goldstein RE, Garber DA. Imaging in esthetic dentistry. Chicago: Quintessence, 1998.

18. Goldstein RE. Esthetics in dentistry. Vol. 1. 2nd edn. Hamilton, ON: BC Decker, 1998.

19. Graber TM, Vanarsdall RL. Orthodontics: current principles and techniques. St. Louis: Mosby, 2000.

20. Heyman HO. Conservative concepts to achieving anterior esthetics. J Calif Dent Assoc 1997;25:437–43.

21. Jun S. Communication is vital to produce natural looking metal ceramic crowns. J Dent Technol 1997; 14(8):15–20.

22. Kokich VG. Esthetics: the orthodontic-periodontic restorative connection. Semin Orthodont 1996;2(1): 21–30.

23. Levine JB. Esthetic diagnosis. Curr Opin Cosmet Dent 1995;3:9–17.

24. Lieberman MA, Gazit E. Lower incisor extraction—a method of orthodontic treatment in selected cases in the adult dentition. Isr J Dent Med 1973;22:80.

25. Magne P, Magne M, Belsor V. The diagnostic template: a key element to the comprehensive esthetic treatment concept. Int J Periodont Restor Dent 1996;16:560–9.

26. Margolis MJ. Esthetic considerations in orthodontic treatment of adults. Dent Clin North Am 1997;41:29–48.

27. Narcisi EM, Culp L. Diagnosis and treatment planning for ceramic restorations. Dent Clin North Am 2001;45:117–42.

28. Narcisi EM, DiPerna JA. Multidisciplinary full-mouth restoration with porcelain veneers and laboratory-fabricated resin inlays. Pract Periodont Aesthet Dent 1999;11:721–8.

29. Okuda WH. Creating facial harmony with cosmetic dentistry. Curr Opin Cosmet Dent 1997;4:69–75.

30. Oringer RJ, Iacono VJ. Periodontal cosmetic surgery. J Int Acad Periodontol 1999;1:83–90.

31. Paul SJ, Pietrobon N. Aesthetic evolution of anterior maxillary crowns: a literature review. Pract Periodont Aesthet Dent 1998;10(1):87–94.

32. Peck H, Peck S. Reproximation (enamel stripping) as an essential orthodontic treatment ingredient. London: Transactions of the Third International Orthodontics Congress, 1975.

33. Portalier L. Composite smile designs: the key to dental artistry. Curr Opin Cosmet Dent 1997;4:81–5.

34. Proffit W, Fields HW. Contemporary orthodontics. 3rd edn. St. Louis: Mosby, 2000.

35. Rada RE. Interdisciplinary management of a common esthetic complaint. Gen Dent 1999;47:387–9.

36. Roblee RD. Interdisciplinary dentofacial therapy. Chicago: Quintessence, 1994.

37. Rufenacht CR. Principles of esthetic integration. Chicago: Quintessence, 2000.

38. Salama M. Orthodontics vs. restorative materials in treatment plans. Contemp Esthet Restor Pract 2001;5:20–30.

39. Shannon A. Reconstruction of the maxillary dentition utilizing a nonorthodontic technique. Pract Periodont Aesthet Dent 1999;11:973–8.

40. Singer BA. Esthetic dentistry: a clinical approach to techniques and materials. Philadelphia: Lea & Febiger, 1993.

41. Small BW. Laboratory communications for esthetic success. Gen Dent 1998;46:566–8, 572–4.

42. Studer S, Zellweger V, Scharer P. The aesthetic guidelines of the mucogingival complex for fixed prosthodontics. Pract Periodont Aesthet Dent 1996;8:333–41.

43. Wilson TG, Korman KS. Esthetic periodontics (periodontal plastic surgery). Chicago: Quintessence, 1996.

CHAPTER 25

ESTHETICS IN ADULT ORTHODONTICS

Paul Yurfest, DDS

In honor and memory of Dr. Marvin C. Goldstein, mentor and teacher.

It is the rare patient who understands that ideal orthodontic form and function are the foundation of esthetic treatment. When orthodontic remedies are prescribed as a first line of treatment but rejected by the patient, then all subsequent esthetic procedures become compromise treatments. This is not necessarily a negative; it is just a fact.

The quest to practice optimal esthetic dentistry requires an understanding of certain fundamental aspects of orthodontics and orthodontic therapies. This chapter does not address the radiographic analysis (cephalometrics) necessary to make a thorough evaluation in orthodontic complexities. However, it is imperative to master these analyses before undertaking a complex orthodontic plan. This discussion will focus on the treatment of limited problems requiring less complex types of orthodontic appliances and limited tooth movement to achieve a specific esthetic result. More difficult esthetic problems that are treated with complex orthodontic therapies will also be shown to demonstrate the scope of available treatments.

When a patient is asked what an orthodontist does, the likely response is usually something about "straightening teeth" or "fixing a smile." The typical patient's idea of orthodontic treatment remains based on the concept that he or she would have to wear "metal braces," that these braces are uncomfortable, and that they are unattractive. Therefore, if we are to motivate our patients to consider orthodontic treatment, we must also demonstrate the range of alternative esthetic orthodontic treatment options. The practice of esthetic dentistry requires an understanding of the techniques that are now available for orthodontic therapies that can assist the dentist in pursuing an acceptable esthetic result.

When dental and dentofacial esthetics are concerned, orthodontic therapy should be an integral consideration in any treatment plan. Modifying tooth position in anterior teeth prior to the fabrication of esthetic restorations such as porcelain laminate veneers, composite resin bonding, or crowns may greatly enhance the final esthetic and functional result. Factors such as restoration width and length are greatly affected when crowding, spacing, protrusion, or retrusion is present prior to initiating prosthetic restorative procedures. Sometimes, orthodontic treatment alone can be the definitive treatment of choice to satisfy the patient's esthetic issues. There is, of course, reluctance by many patients to undergo orthodontic treatment. Advances in the comfort, esthetics, and efficiency of orthodontic treatment and appliances (clear braces, lingual braces, Invisalign [Align Technology, Santa Clara, CA] [computer-assisted tray fabrication], removable braces, and heat-activated gentle-force wires) have done much to make orthodontic therapy more appealing, especially for adult patients.

PREVENTIVE TREATMENT

The concept of prevention in general health care has had a slow acceptance rate when compared specifically to the dental component. Dental professionals and patients alike have historically embraced preventive dental care. However, disregarding orthodontic preventive diagnostics is a disservice to patients that should be addressed. Too many adults who have had lifelong preventive dental care are suddenly diagnosed with a significant dental malocclusion. Severe overbite, where the upper front teeth cover the lower front teeth when the patient occludes, is a problem that the primary caregiver (dentist or dental hygienist) should easily recognize. Patients should be informed of the long-term destruction that such a condition can cause. The developing dentition (Figures 25–1A and B) requires attention from an orthodontic perspective prior to eruption of all of the permanent teeth. Severe crowding, midline shift, and developing crossbite are problems that will likely become worse and eventually cause needless wear to the anterior teeth if left untreated. Patients with these conditions should be diagnosed by the general dentist and, when appropriate, referred to an orthodontist.

ORTHODONTIC TOOTH MOVEMENT

When a tooth is repositioned, the entire tooth attachment, including bone and gingiva, migrates with it. This is particularly important where there is uneven gingival height at the maxillary central incisors. Figure 25–2A shows maxillary incisors that are unequal in length because of wear. After orthodontic extrusion of the left central incisor and incisal contouring, the teeth appear to be more equal in length (Figure 25–2B). The ability to reposition both bone and gingiva as the tooth moves is an attractive feature of orthodontic treatment.

RETENTION

The importance of postorthodontic stabilization (retention) cannot be overstated. Many adult patients seek treatment for esthetic problems that were orthodontically treated years earlier but not retained past a few years. Patients who seek re-treatment report that they simply stopped wearing retainers a few years after completing orthodontic treatment and have had a gradual regression in their tooth position. Patients must be motivated to wear retainers at least occasionally throughout their adult years to prevent significant tooth movement. The issue of patient compliance can be negated with fixed orthodontic retainers (Figures 25–3A to C). The major deficiency of fixed retainers is the difficulty they present to the patient when flossing between the teeth that hold the retainers. A patient who had difficulty with flossing in general would not be a good candidate for fixed retention. The bonded maxillary lingual retainer, in addition to causing flossing difficulties, could also come in contact with the incisal edges of the mandibular anterior teeth and may cause undesirable pressure on the anterior teeth of both arches.

CROWDED TEETH

Expansion Therapy: Nonextraction Treatment

A moderate crowding with a Class II cuspid (Figure 25–4A) can be treated with a conservative approach using the Crozat expansion appliance and bonded brackets (Figures 25–4B to F). An alternative treatment that could achieve esthetic results would be a restorative option such as porcelain laminate veneers. This would entail the removal of enamel and the challenge of creating esthetic anterior restorations. The patient should be informed that the additional benefit of orthodontic rather than restorative treatment in this situation is avoidance of maintaining and/or replacing the veneers because of chipping or gingival recession.

The patient in Figures 25–5A to C presented a more severely constricted and crowded problem and was opposed to extracting any teeth. The Crozat expansion appliance was placed for 18 months to create pressure against the inside base of the posterior teeth. The amount of expansion achieved (Figures 25–5D and E) was sufficient to

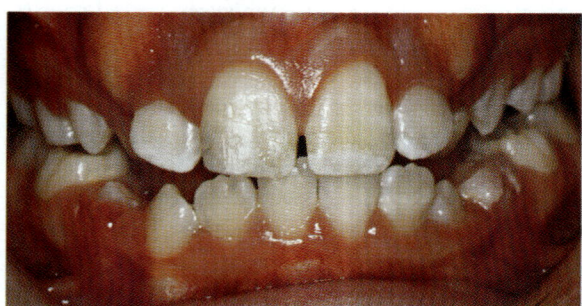

Figure 25–1A: Front view of a mixed dentition patient age 11. Notice the midlines that do not coincide, anterior open bite, and crossbite tendency of the upper premolars indicating a constricted maxillary arch.

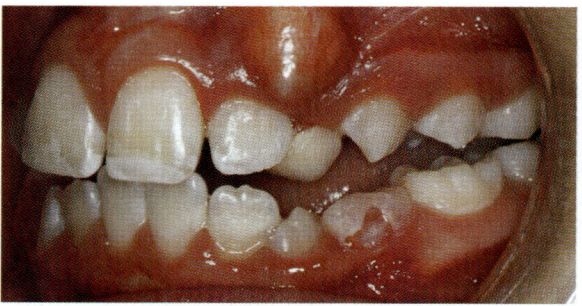

Figure 25–1B: Side view shows a large canine "bulge" that indicates significant trouble in the eruption process of the maxillary canines.

Esthetics in Adult Orthodontics 755

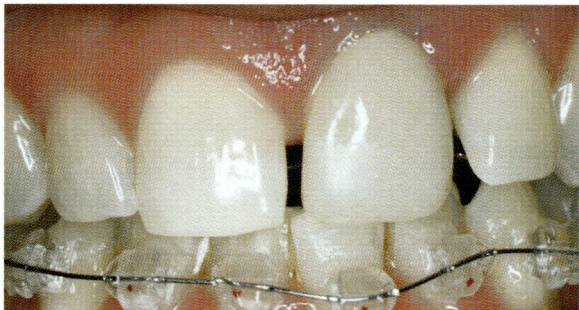

Figure 25–2A: Maxillary central incisors of equal length with lingual braces to extrude (bring down) the left central incisor, making the gingival margins the same height, and to close the spaces.

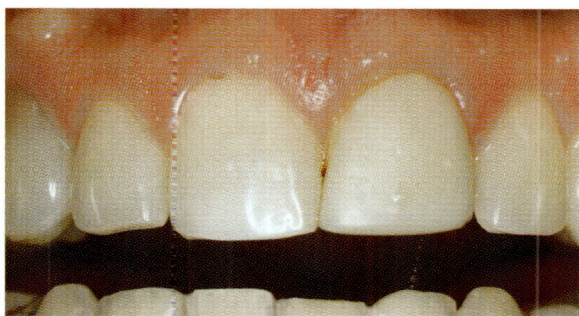

Figure 25–2B: After orthodontics. Note that the gingival margins of the central incisors are at the same level, and the incisal edges have been evened.

begin tooth alignment using direct bonded clear brackets (Figure 25–5F). The treatment was an esthetic success, with all of the teeth in good alignment and the dental arches nicely formed (Figures 25–5G to I).

Lower Crowding with Slight Underbite (Class III)

Figures 25–6A to D show a patient with more significant crowding complicated by anterior crossbite and anterior open bite. Lingual upper and clear lower braces were used to correct the problem.

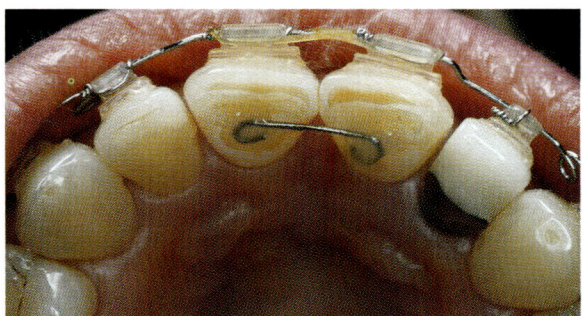

Figure 25–3A: Bonded fixed lingual retainer on the maxillary central incisors placed prior to removal of labial braces to maintain a closed midline space.

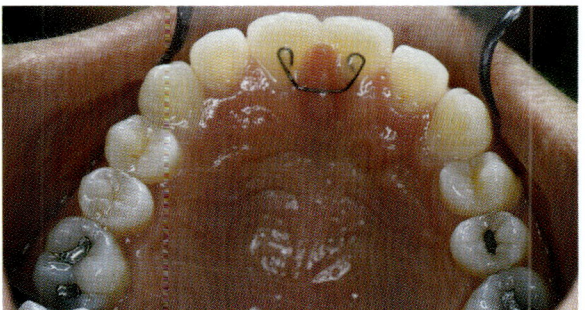

Figure 25–3B: Bonded retainer designed to avoid a swollen gingival papilla.

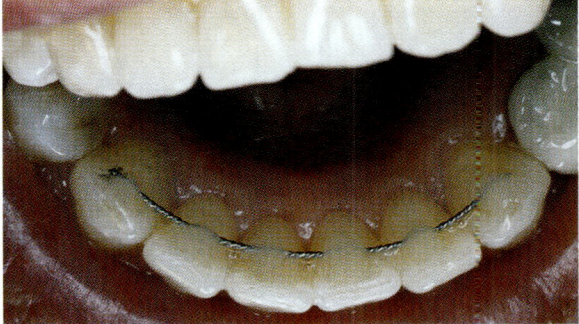

Figure 25–3C: Bonded fixed lingual retainer on the lower anterior teeth.

756   Esthetics in Dentistry

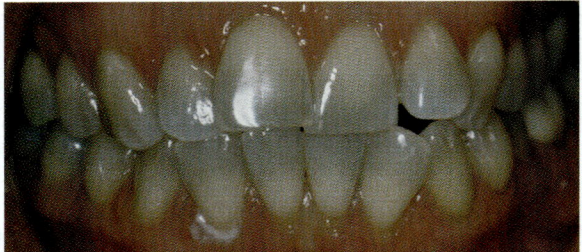

Figure 25–4A: Pretreatment view of a crowded constricted dentition. Note the constricted upper canines and the upper right canine directly on the lower canine (Class II).

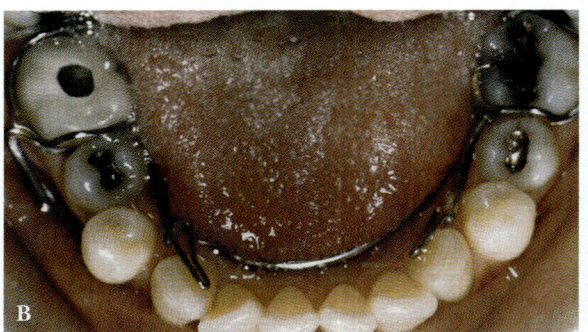 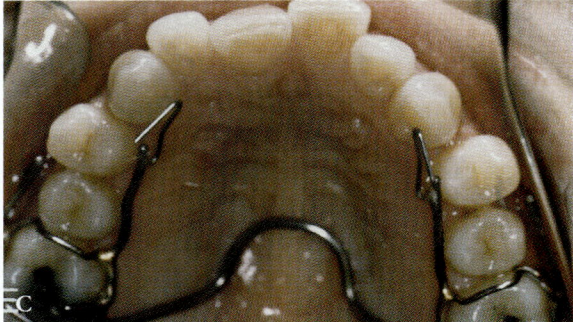

Figure 25–4B and C: Occlusal views during treatment with Crozat removable appliances. Note the spaces that were created in the bicuspid regions through gradual expansion of the dental arches.

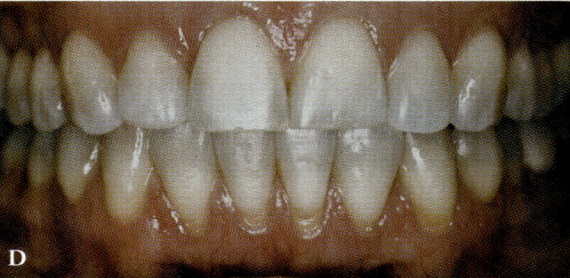

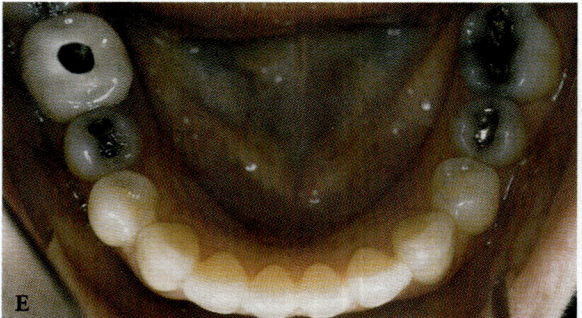 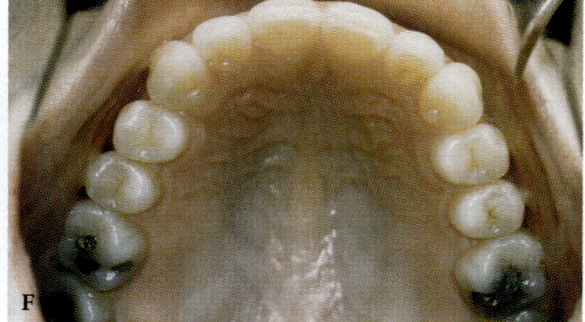

Figure 25–4D to F: Post-treatment views of the completed treatment. The dental midlines no longer meet, but tooth alignment and intercuspation of the posterior teeth have been improved.

Esthetics in Adult Orthodontics 757

The Crozat appliance can create generalized expansion and sufficient intra-arch space for tooth repositioning even in the severest cases (Figures 25–7A to F). The completed treatment is shown in Figures 25–7G to I.

When the width of the maxillary and mandibular arches is insufficient to allow the teeth to align without crowding (Figure 25–8) or there is a posterior crossbite (Figure 25–9), a course of orthodontic therapy should be undertaken to expand the

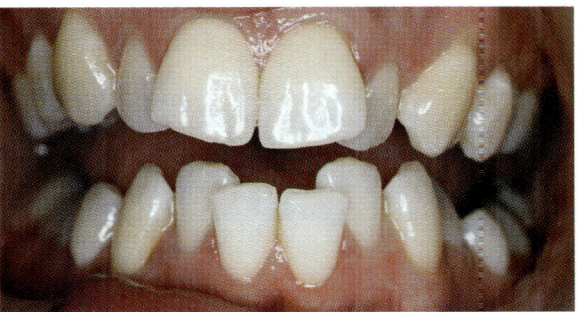

Figure 25–5A: Preoperative anterior view with teeth apart to show incisal irregularities.

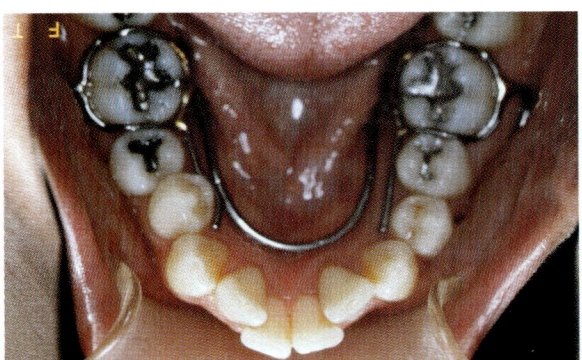

Figure 25–5B: Lower occlusal view showing extreme constriction and crowding and Crozat removable expander.

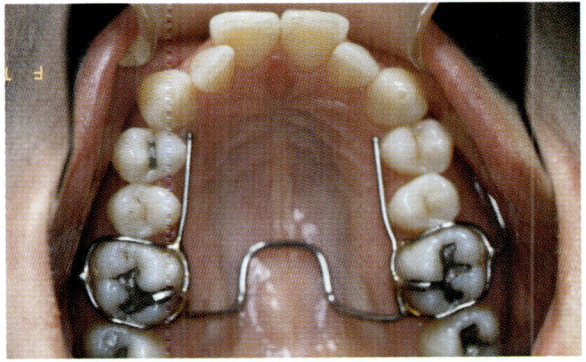

Figure 25–5C: Upper occlusal view with crowding and constriction.

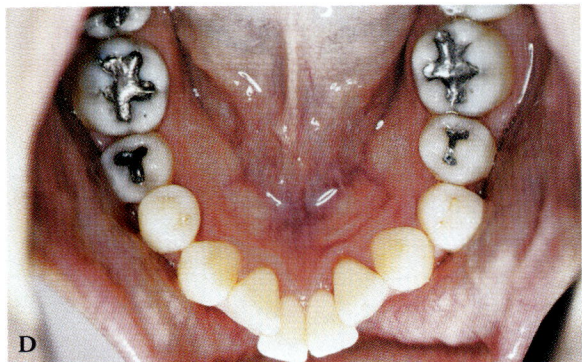

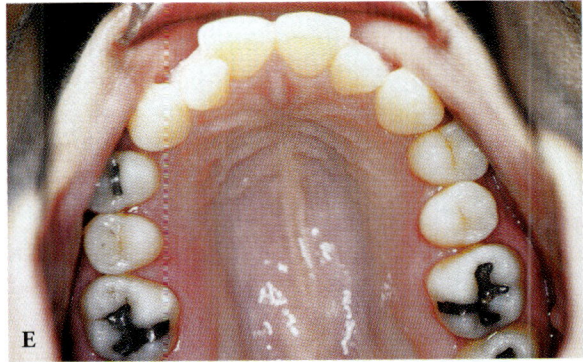

Figure 25–5D and E: Upper and lower occlusal views after the Crozat appliance has expanded the width of the dental arches and created space for incisor alignment.

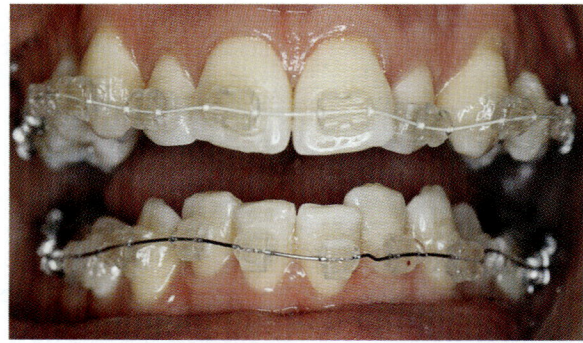

Figure 25–5F: Intraoral view of the teeth with direct bond brackets to align and detail the position of the teeth and refine the occlusion after Crozat expansion.

deficient arches. The expansion will diminish the negative smile space (dark spaces between the cheeks and the bicuspids and molars) and create a more favorable environment for tooth alignment and improved occlusion.

Class I Severe Crowding with Extractions

A routine procedure in orthodontic therapy was the extraction of permanent teeth. This was largely because the profession was guided by early research that considered a flat profile as the optimal esthetic

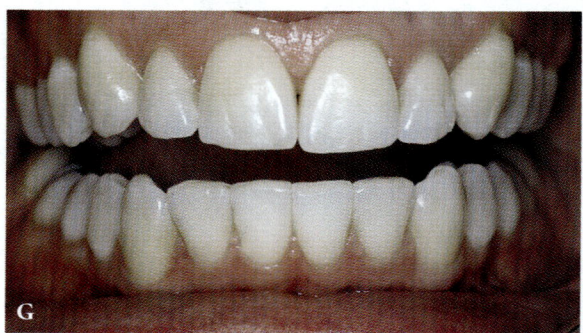

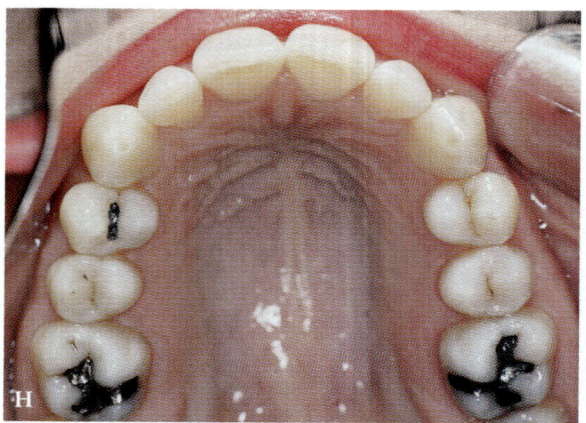

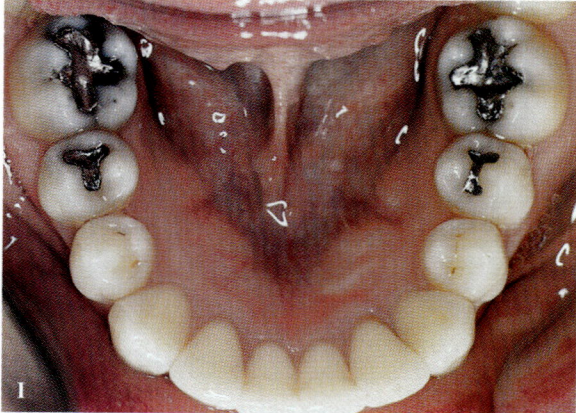

Figure 25–5G to I: Views of the completed treatment. Note the widened arch forms and reduced overjet.

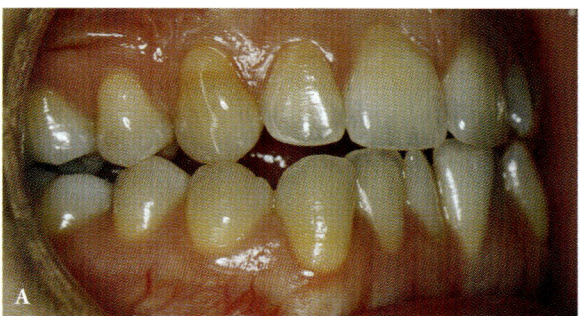 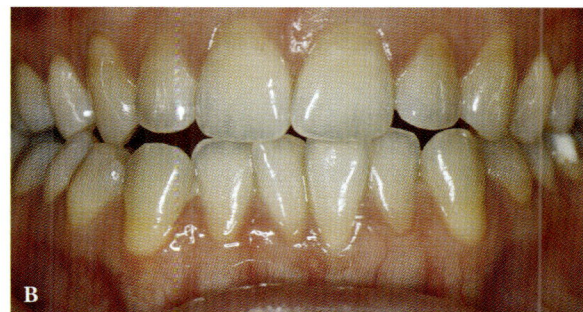

Figure 25–6A and B: Intraoral views of lower crowding. Note the forward position of the lower right canine relative to the upper canine and the lack of overjet.

result. This treatment concept has been replaced by a less stringent desire for a flat profile and a concern for possible negative side effects of bicuspid extractions. However, in some cases, severe crowding cannot be resolved without extractions. Bicuspid extractions were selected for the patient in Figure 25–10A to maintain the permanent mandibular cuspids in the occlusal scheme. The final result (Figure 25–10B) was obtained with some consequence to the gingiva of the mandibular cuspids. Note the labial gingival recession of the left mandibular cuspid in comparison with the gingiva of the mandibular right cuspid, which shows no change from the original height.

The unesthetic smile in Figures 25–11A and B is owing to the high position of the maxillary permanent cuspids. The natural eruption of the cuspids was inhibited by the lack of space in the maxillary arch. Extraction of the bicuspids was required to provide adequate space for the cuspids. Esthetic combination bracket therapy (Figure 25–11C) using a lingual orthodontic appliance on the anterior teeth and standard labial appliances on the posterior teeth achieved the excellent esthetic results seen in Figures 25–11D and E.

DIASTEMA

Early Treatment

Figure 25–12A shows a patient with a large maxillary midline diastema that is not only unesthetic but, more critically, is also preventing the eruption of the maxillary lateral incisors. The treatment consists of the bonding of orthodontic brackets to the maxillary central incisors, placing a contoured rectangular arch wire, and using chain elastics to draw the teeth together (Figures 25–12B and C). This should all be held in position until the maxillary lateral incisors are fully erupted (Figure 25–12D). After the maxillary lateral incisors are completely erupted (Figure

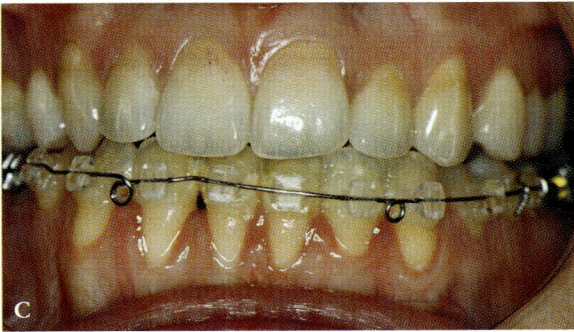 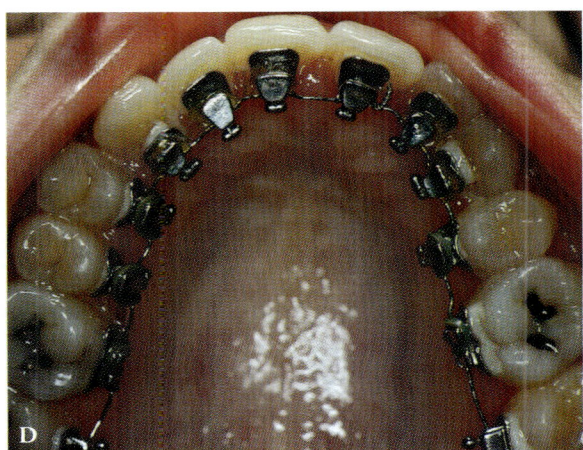

Figure 25–6C and D: Intraoral views of the corrected dentition with upper lingual and lower clear brackets. There is noticeable inflammation of the tissues near the lower incisors.

760 Esthetics in Dentistry

25–12E), the patient is ready for corrective orthodontics for the Class II right and midline correction.

Diastema Correction

The patient in Figure 25–13A has a large midline diastema and a severe overbite that would preclude retraction of the maxillary anterior teeth. Retraction of the maxillary anterior teeth to close the space would cause significant interference between the maxillary and mandibular incisors. Figure 25–13B shows the completed orthodontic treatment with the ideal overbite and overjet.

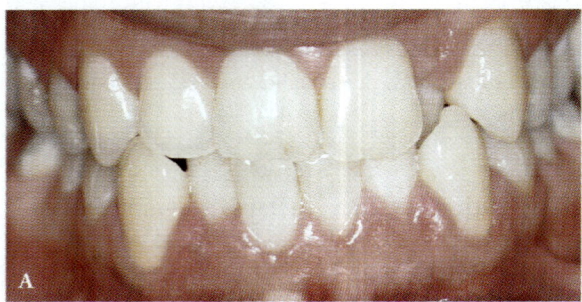 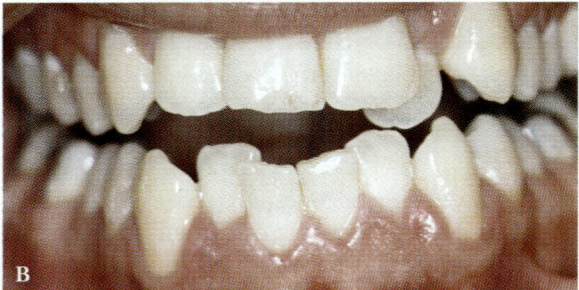

Figure 25–7A and B: Pretreatment intraoral photographs of severe crowding resulting in incisor crossbite and uneven lower incisal height.

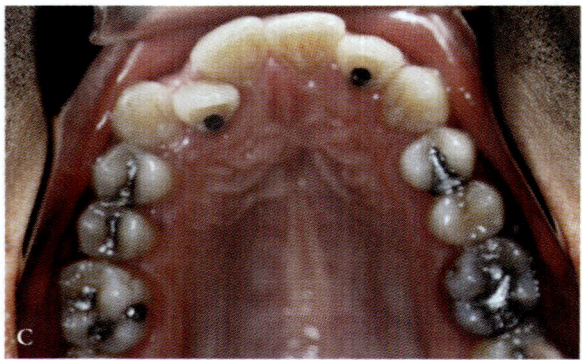 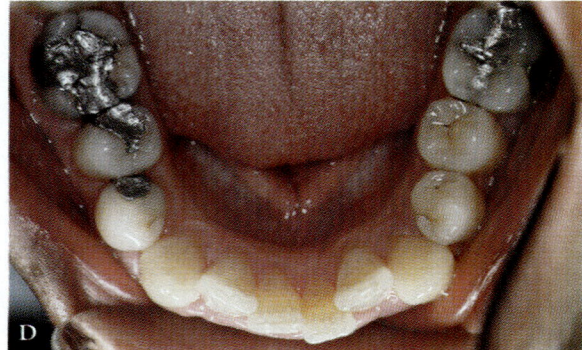

Figure 25–7C and D: Preoperative occlusal views of maxillary and mandibular arches.

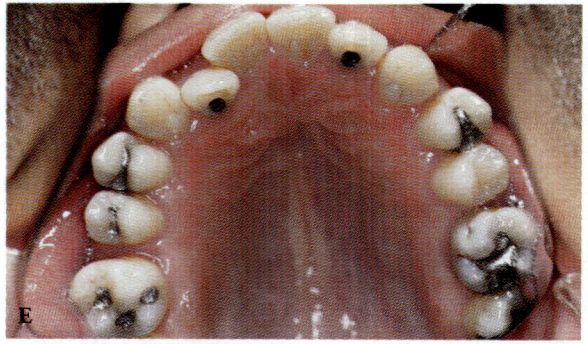 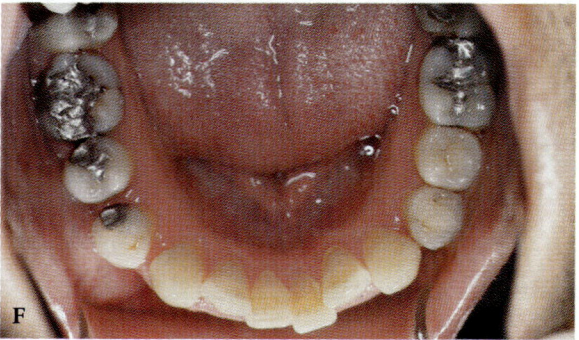

Figure 25–7E and F: Occlusal photographs after expansion with the Crozat expansion appliance. Note the spaces in the premolar region. The patient is now ready for bonded brackets.

Esthetics in Adult Orthodontics   761

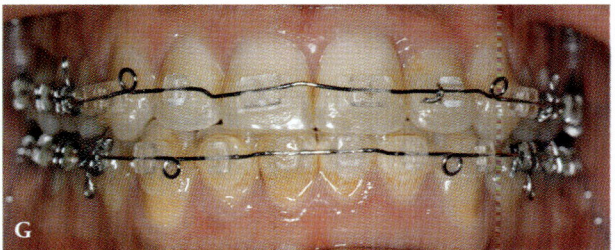

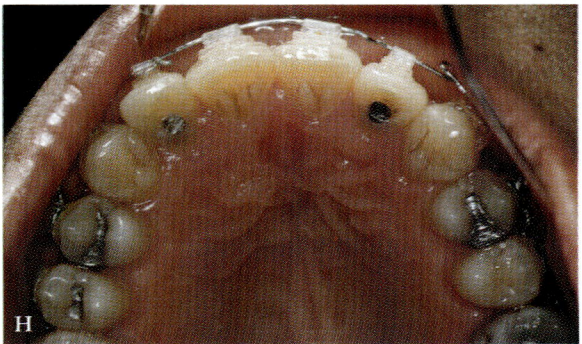

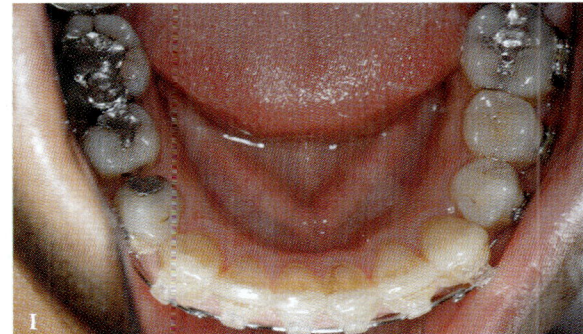

Figure 25–7G to I: Completed treatment prior to bracket removal.

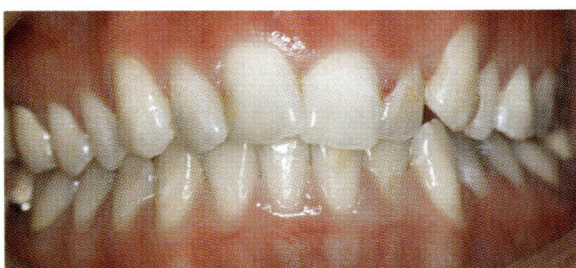

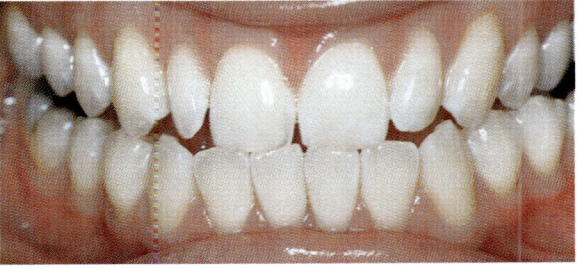

Figure 25–8: Severely constricted upper and lower dental arches causing crowding of the dentition and an inward tilt of the teeth and needing expansion.

Figure 25–9: Constricted upper dental arch causing posterior crossbite and posterior open bite and needing posterior upper expansion.

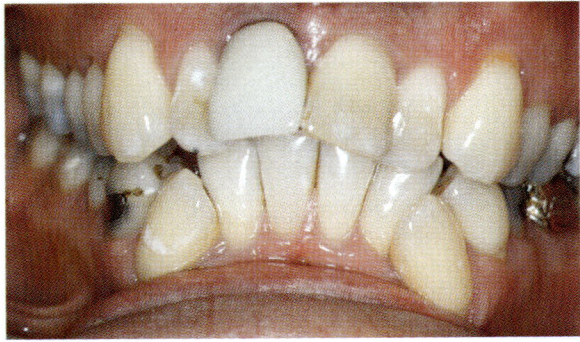

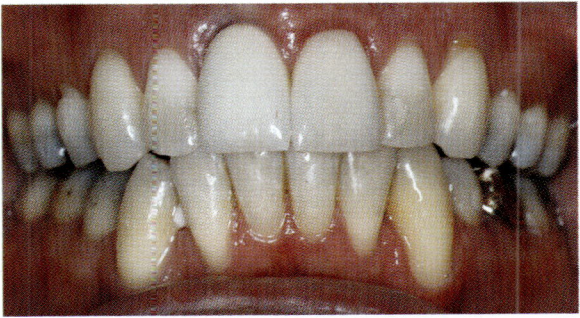

Figure 25–10A: Pretreatment intraoral photograph showing severe lower canine displacement and crowding.

Figure 25–10B: Post-treatment photograph after extraction of the four first bicuspids and treatment with clear orthodontic brackets. Note the gingival recession of the lower left canine.

762 Esthetics in Dentistry

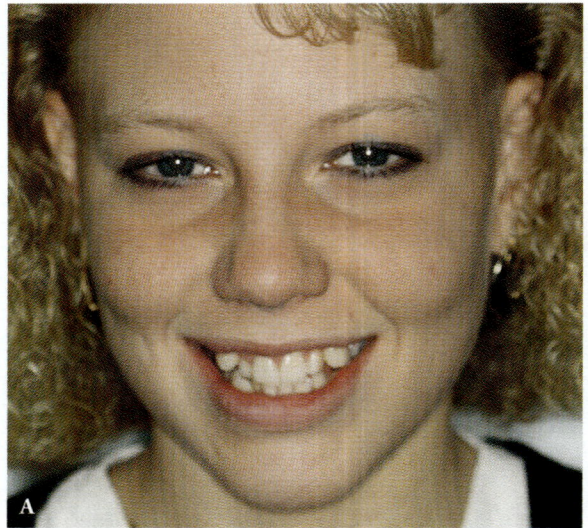

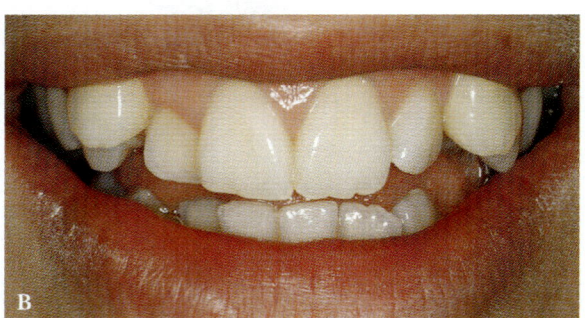

Figure 25–11A and B: Unesthetic smile caused by misplaced maxillary canines.

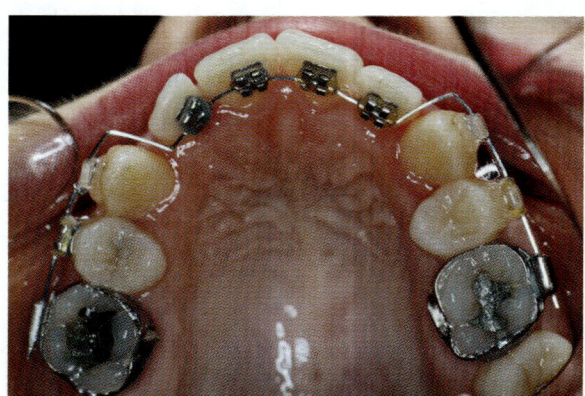

Figure 25–11C: This photograph shows the canines moved into the bicuspid spaces with the orthodontic brackets behind the anterior teeth and on the labial surfaces of the posterior teeth.

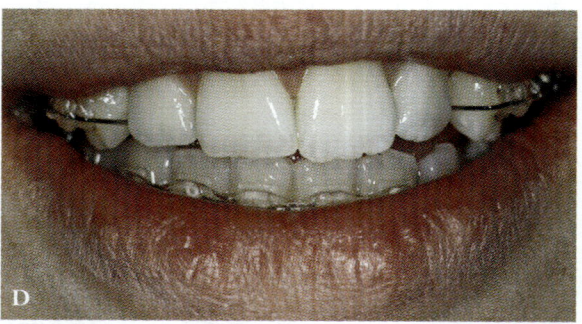

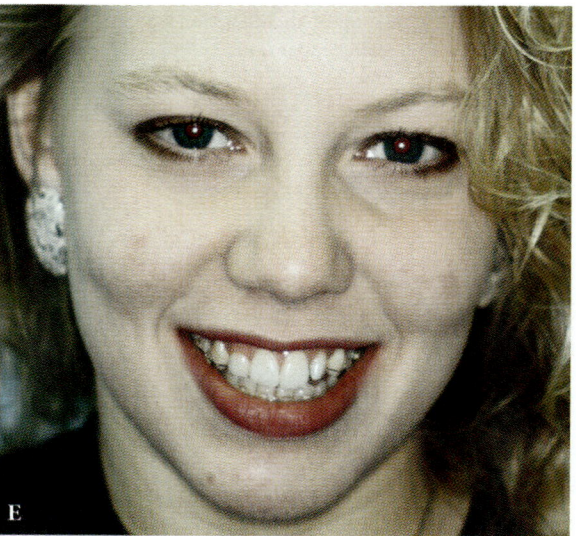

Figure 25–11D and E: Facial and smile photographs near the completion of treatment.

Esthetics in Adult Orthodontics 763

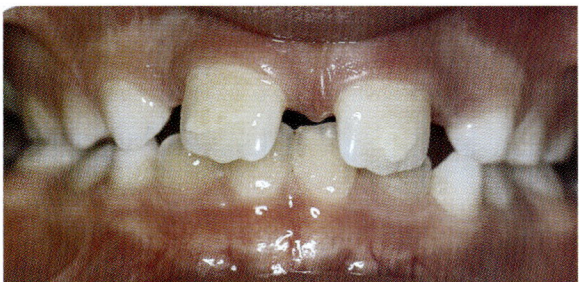

Figure 25–12A: Large midline diastema preventing eruption of the lateral incisors.

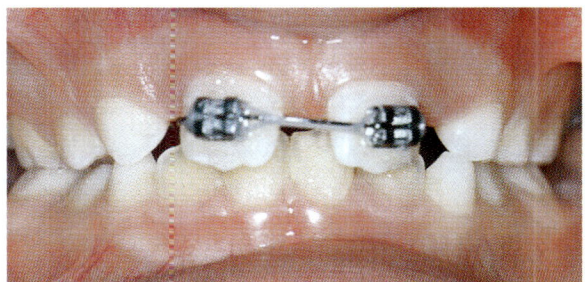

Figure 25–12B: Early treatment initiated to close the space.

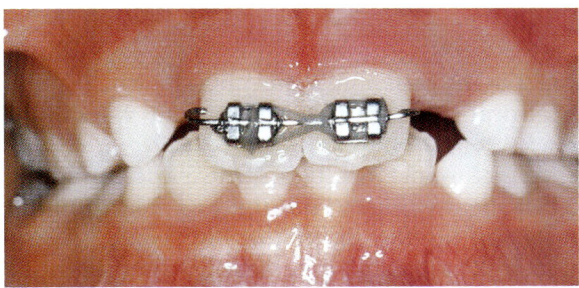

Figure 25–12C: Space closure completed.

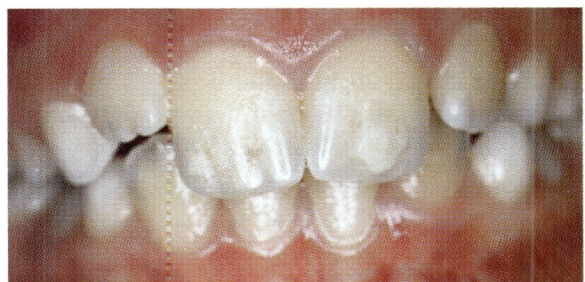

Figure 25–12D: Lateral incisors erupting.

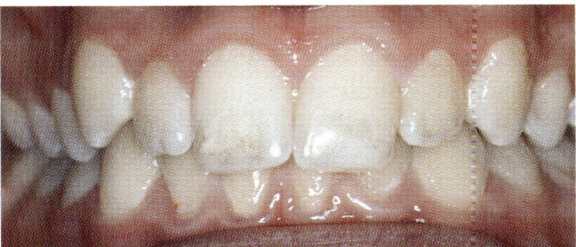

Figure 25–12E: After complete eruption of all permanent teeth and prior to initiation of orthodontic treatment to correct the overbite and Class II on the right side.

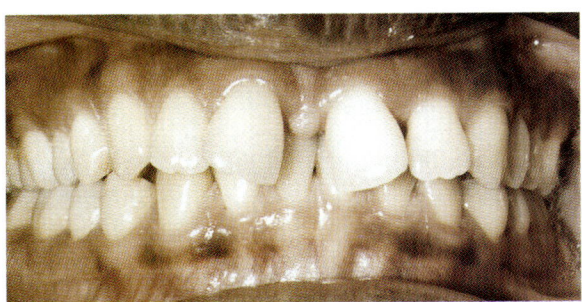

Figure 25–13A: Large midline diastema complicated by a very deep overbite.

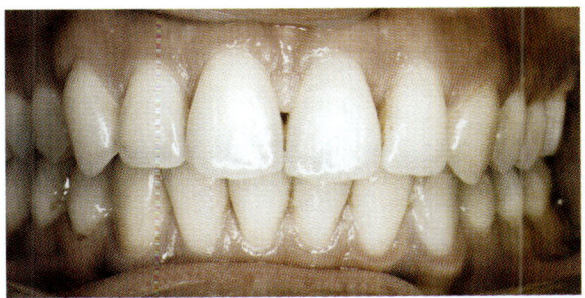

Figure 25–13B: Completed orthodontic treatment with corrected overbite.

Table 25–1. Maxillary Midline Diastema Diagnosis Chart*

Figure 25–14	Normal-sized teeth with spaces in the upper and lower anteriors Sufficient overjet owing to missing two lower incisors	Can be treated with any of the following methods: Invisalign, Hawley removables, or laminates
Figure 25–15	Extruded and protruded #8 and #9 that are in contact with the lower incisors	Improved esthetics with laminates; better with orthodontics to flatten, intrude, and close spaces
Figure 25–16	Greatly protruded and spaced #8 and #9 that are large and in contact with the lower incisors and a deep curve of Spee	Poor esthetic improvement with laminates Refer for complete orthodontic treatment

*Figures 25–14, 25–15, and 25–16 show a common problem that is likely to be encountered in clinical practice. The similarity is a midline diastema that the patient and the practitioner want closed. The differences between them is what will help to decide how treatment should progress.

Diastema Differential Diagnosis

Certain criteria must be evaluated when attempting to correct a maxillary diastema in an adult patient:

- Is there sufficient overjet to retract the incisors to close the diastema without interference from the mandibular incisors?
- Is the overbite sufficient to allow retraction of the anterior teeth without contacting the mandibular incisors?

Criteria are compared in Table 25–1. These criteria were sufficiently met in the patient in Figures 25–14A and B, who has a maxillary midline diastema and sufficient overjet with minimal overbite. The maxillary anterior teeth can be retracted using a Hawley appliance or maxillary braces alone without mandibular braces for bite opening.

Figure 25–15 shows a patient who has sufficient overjet but too much overbite, which causes the mandibular incisors to contact the lingual surface of the maxillary incisors. Retraction of the maxillary teeth causes excess interference with the incisal edges of the mandibular incisors. This case requires treatment with both maxillary and mandibular braces for orthodontic space closure; a Hawley appliance would not be sufficient for correction. The patient in Figures 25–16A and B has multiple maxillary anterior spaces that also require correction with conventional orthodontics rather than a Hawley appliance because of the severe overbite and overjet.

CROSSBITE

The decision to correct a dental crossbite rests on a number of factors:

- Is the crossbite anterior or posterior?
- Is it functional (ie, causes no problems) or harmful?
- If it is posterior unilateral, does it cause a mandibular shift to one side?
- Is it an esthetic problem?
- Is there a skeletal component, or is the problem limited to the teeth?

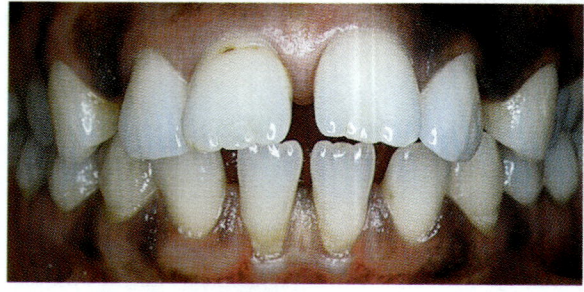 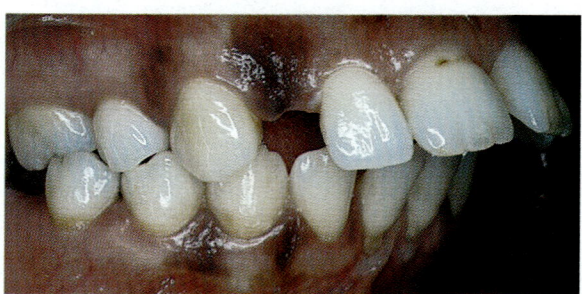

Figure 25–14A and B: Midline diastema with sufficient overjet and minimal overbite to allow space closure with an upper Hawley.

Esthetics in Adult Orthodontics

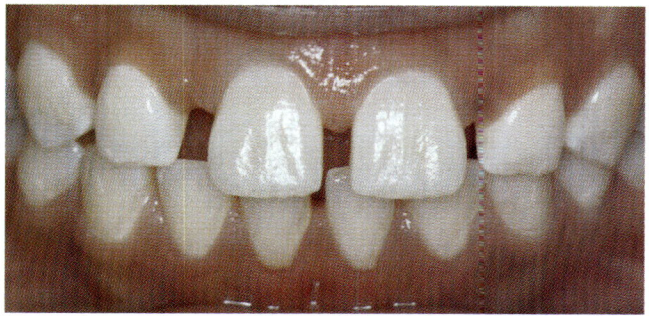

Figure 25–15: Maxillary midline diastema with sufficient overjet but upper incisal contact with the lower incisors preventing easy space closure.

Not all crossbites require correction. Some crossbites cause no functional or esthetic problems, such as an isolated first molar, and do not necessarily require correction.

Posterior Crossbite

The diagnosis of a unilateral posterior crossbite involving all of the posterior teeth on one side requires an analysis of the dental and facial midlines. The occlusion shown in Figure 25–17A is an excellent example of a mandibular shift caused by a constricted maxillary arch. Note how the mandibular dental midline and the entire mandible (Figure 25–17B) are deviated 3 mm to the side of the posterior crossbite. This patient deviates markedly to the left. This is a diagnostic feature of a maxillary constriction that requires bilateral maxillary expansion to correct. Once the maxilla is bilaterally expanded, the mandibular midline will usually not shift. When diagnosing this situation, it would have been easy to assume that the patient had only a unilateral crossbite.

Anterior Crossbite

Diagnosis of an anterior crossbite, as depicted in Figures 25–18A and B, is augmented by the use of a cephalometric film that examines the basic underlying skeletal pattern. In this case, a prognathic mandible (lower jaw more forward) was diagnosed. The decision was made to extract the mandibular left and right first bicuspids because the patient did not want orthognathic surgery to push back the mandible. Orthodontic therapy resulted in space closure for both the maxillary and mandibular arches and correction of the anterior crossbite (Figures 25–18C and D).

Short Lower Jaw (Class II, Division 2) with Extrusion of the Maxillary Anterior Teeth

The maxillary anterior component of this particular malocclusion gives rise to a number of esthetic factors in addition to the underlying Class II interdigitation of the cuspids and posterior teeth. Among these are, in particular, the lingual inclination of the maxillary central incisors and the extrusion of the

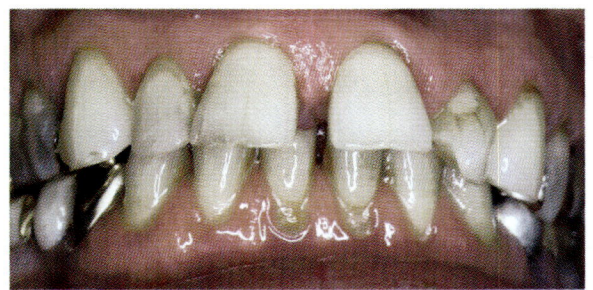 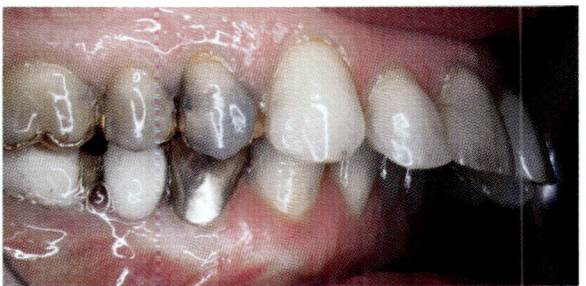

Figure 25–16A and B: Upper spacing with severe overbite and overjet requiring comprehensive orthodontic treatment for space closure.

maxillary anterior teeth beyond the plane of occlusion. The extrusion can produce a gummy smile (Figure 25–19A), which can be corrected through orthodontic torquing and intrusion of the maxillary anterior teeth. Correction requires the use of a full-bonded Edgewise orthodontic appliance with the addition of a torquing auxiliary (Figure 25–19B) that will push back the roots of the maxillary incisors and establish proper incisal inclination (torque). The final result (Figures 25–19C and D) shows the maxillary incisors intruded to the level of the occlusal plane and a Class I occlusion.

Severe Overbite

Untreated overbite (Figure 25–20) will, in time, lead to severe wear of the incisal edges of the mandibular and/or the maxillary teeth. This can easily be overlooked unless the practitioner carefully observes the mandibular anterior teeth in full centric occlusion. Once in this position, not more than 50% of the mandibular teeth should be covered by the maxillary incisors.

There are two distinct causes of excess anterior overbite that, when left untreated, will cause excessive incisal wear:

- *Extrusion of the maxillary incisors.* This can be a significant cause of a "gummy smile" because the gingival margins of the maxillary central and lateral incisors are more incisally (lower) positioned than the posterior buccal segments (see Figures 25–19A and 25–21A to B). Intrusion with full fixed orthodontic appliances is required to obtain better functional and esthetic tooth position.

- *Extrusion of the mandibular anterior quadrant (cuspid to cuspid).* The mandibular six anterior teeth are significantly higher than the posterior teeth. Typically, the mandibular arch appears normal except for the fact that there is a severe marginal ridge discrepancy between the cuspid and the first bicuspid (see Figures 25–20 and 25–22A). Although the severe deep overbite seems obvious, a dentist did not diagnose it until the patient was 35 years old. After orthodontic treatment prior to restorative treatment, the restorative dentist can create a more esthetic restorative result. Figure 25–22B shows the severity of the overbite. Figure 25–22C shows the correction.

Patients with these problems routinely state that they were never informed by their dentist that they had an overbite and were never advised to seek orthodontic treatment. Figure 25–23 shows a subtle overbite that can easily be overlooked by the general dentist. This should be treated with appropriate orthodontic therapy; otherwise, if left untreated, excessive incisal wear may result.

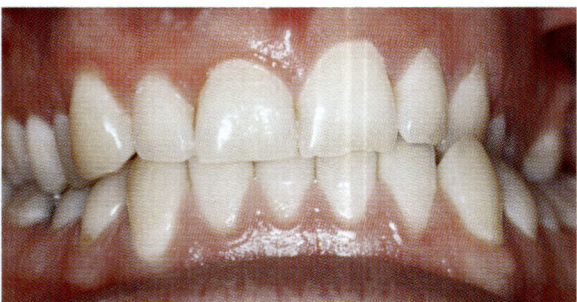

Figure 25–17A: Unilateral posterior crossbite with a marked midline discrepancy indicating there is a shift of the mandible. This means that the maxillary arch is most likely constricted on both sides.

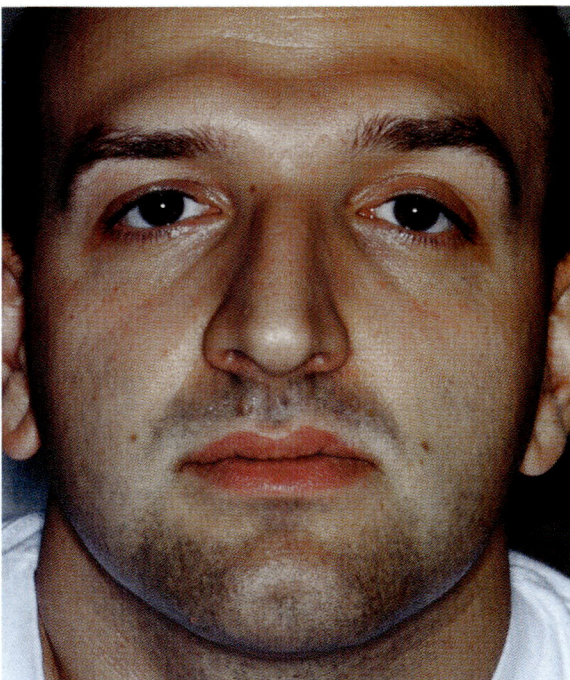

Figure 25–17B: Facial view showing the mandibular shift to the left.

Esthetics in Adult Orthodontics 767

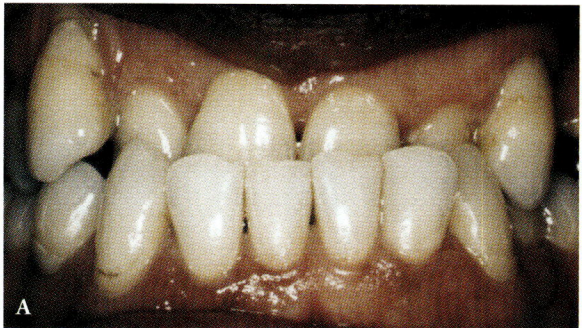 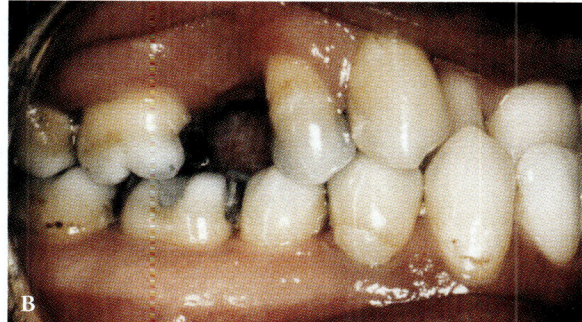

Figure 25–18A and B: Anterior crossbite and missing maxillary first bicuspids.

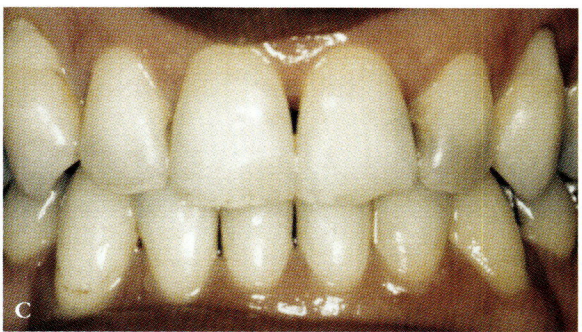 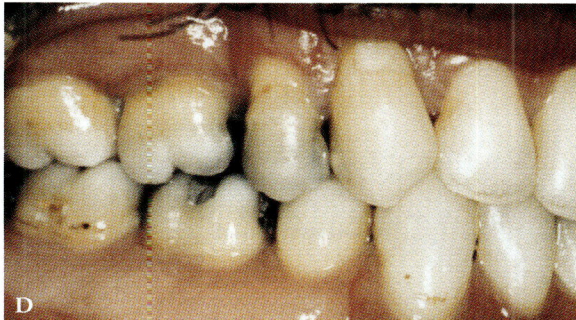

Figure 25–18C and D: Post-treatment results after extraction of the lower bicuspids and space closure of the missing teeth.

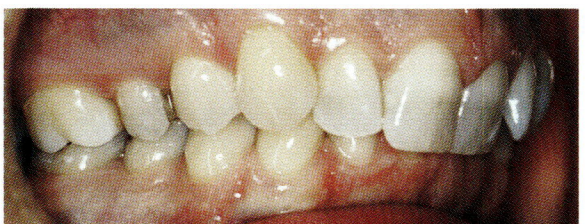 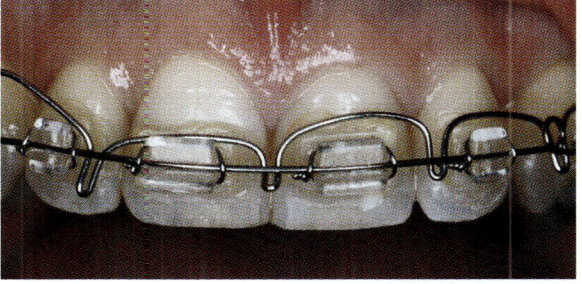

Figure 25–19A: Severe overbite and extrusion of the maxillary teeth combined with a Class II bite relationship. Note the backward angle (torque) of the upper anterior teeth and their position below the level of the occlusal plane.

Figure 25–19B Torquing auxiliary to push back the roots of the upper anterior teeth.

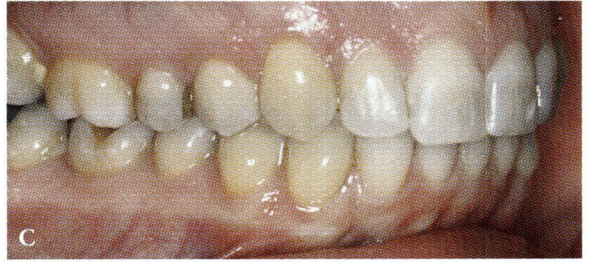 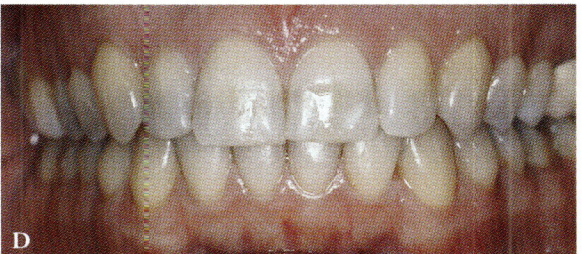

Figure 25–19C and D: Completed treatment after intruding the upper anterior teeth and widening the arch in the premolar area.

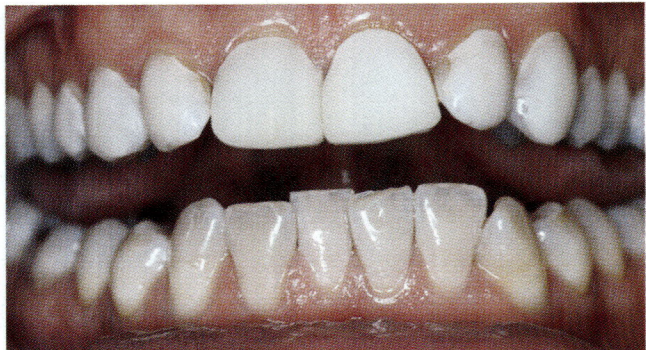

Figure 25–20: Severe wear on the upper and lower anterior teeth caused by untreated overbite and bruxism.

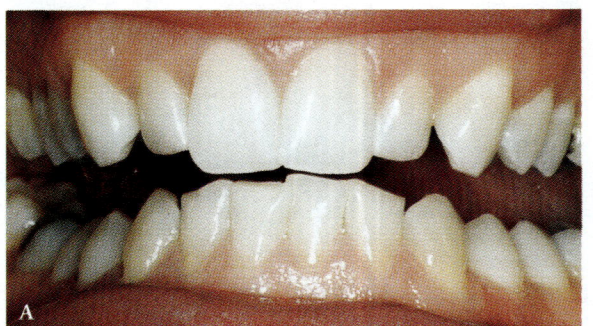 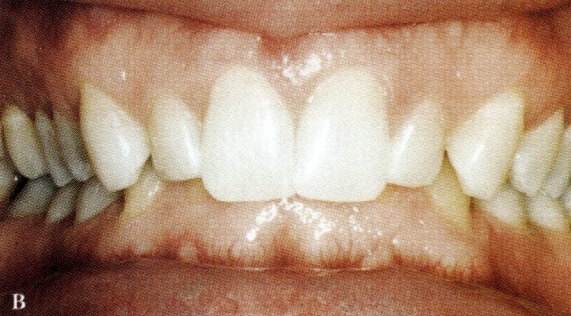

Figure 25–21A and B: Extrusion of the maxillary incisors below the level of the posterior teeth and the occlusal plane. Note the level of the upper incisal gingiva.

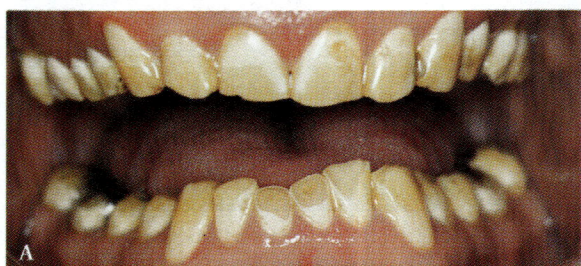 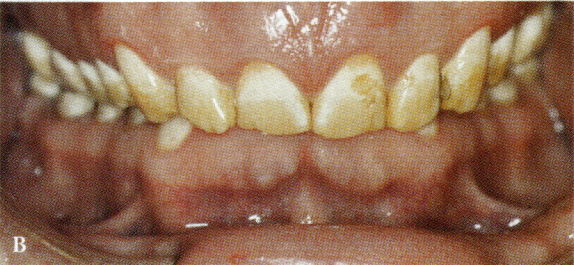

Figure 25–22A and B: Severe overbite with extrusion of the lower anterior teeth. Note extreme wear on lower incisors.

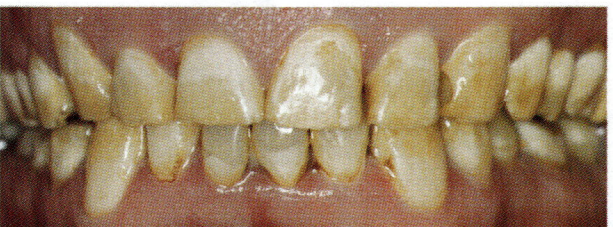

Figure 25–22C: Corrected overbite after orthodontic treatment.

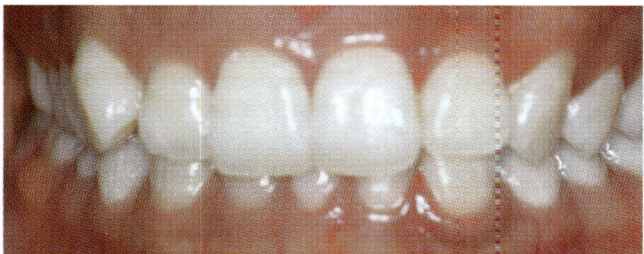

Figure 25–23: An easily overlooked overbite that needs correction.

INTERDISCIPLINARY TREATMENT

Many patients present with a variety of problems such as missing teeth, drifting, crowding, malocclusion, and extrusion that require the intervention of several dental disciplines. As dental professionals, we can never assume what the patient will accept or reject as the appropriate esthetic treatment or goal. The wise dentist develops a group of fellow practitioners of differing specialties who can review the diagnostic work-up of a patient whenever there is a question of potential issues that may compromise the final esthetic result. Not only is it the best service we can provide to our patients, it is also our responsibility to gather, analyze, and present all possible options for treatment so that they can make informed decisions. Only the patient can determine how much time, money, and effort that he or she is willing to invest, as well as what is a personally esthetic result. These issues are discussed more thoroughly in Chapter 2, "Esthetic Treatment Planning," *Esthetics in Dentistry*, Volume 1, 2nd Edition; however, the following generalized, comprehensive approach may be used as a sequence of interdisciplinary treatment:

- Restorative and periodontal evaluation
- Orthodontic referral and evaluation
- Determination of an initial plan between the restorative dentist and/or the periodontist (if necessary) and the orthodontist
- Removal of decay and infection
- Initiation of an orthodontic treatment plan
- Periodic consultations between the restorative dentist and the orthodontist to evaluate progress and possible alterations to the treatment plan necessitated by patient cooperation, infection, or difficulties in tooth movement (not all teeth move as planned) during orthodontic treatment. Increased periodontal monitoring is essential during adult orthodontic treatment.
- Removal of braces and initiation of restorative treatment plan
- Orthodontic retention

Figure 25–24A depicts a patient who requires interdisciplinary evaluation. Note the uneven spacing of the maxillary anterior teeth and the small maxillary left lateral incisor. Figure 25–24B was the result of efforts of the following specific dental disciplines:

- Soft-tissue management
- Orthodontics
- Implant prosthodontics (sometimes started during orthodontics)
- Fixed prosthodontics
- Removable prosthodontics

ESTHETIC FORMS OF ORTHODONTIC TREATMENT

Computer-Assisted Treatment Trays (Invisalign)
The search for an esthetic method of repositioning teeth has been ongoing. If patients can have an esthetically acceptable method of repositioning their teeth, they can more easily be motivated to accept an ideal treatment plan that includes orthodontics. An innovative orthodontic corrective procedure was introduced in 1999 that uses a series of clear, removable, hard acrylic trays similar to bleaching trays. A computer program designs the orthodontic correction in a series of stages similar to the numerous drawings of animated cartoons. For each of these

stages of tooth movement, a single acrylic tray is made. The patient wears this tray for 2 to 3 weeks to accomplish a small amount of tooth movement. There may be as few as 5 or as many as 60 stages, depending on the complexity of the problem. Careful and constant supervision is required, particularly because patient compliance is more of a factor for success than in most other orthodontic techniques. Figures 25–25A and B show a typical case that falls within the guidelines for successful treatment with computer-assisted tray therapy. Beyond the patient compliance factor, the several situations that are unsuitable for computer-assisted therapy include the following:

- When teeth are still erupting
- When extractions are required
- When a correction will be greater than 4 mm
- An overbite greater than 50%
- Crowding greater than 6 mm to be corrected to ideal
- Impacted teeth that need to erupt
- When severely tipped teeth must be uprighted
- When severely rotated cuspids and bicuspids require correction
- When tooth extrusion or intrusion greater than 3 mm is required
- When cuspids or molars require more than 3 mm to achieve a Class 1 occlusion
- Surgical-orthodontic cases
- Treatment of temporomandibular joint problems

Lingual Appliance Therapy

Lingual orthodontic therapy was introduced as an esthetic alternative to conventional braces. There are a few limitations for lingual appliance therapy, particularly concerning the technical demands on the orthodontist when bending the finishing wires. There is an increased amount of patient "chair time" and an associated increased cost factor that can limit the use of the appliances. Also, some cases must be completed with labial appliances. However, almost every type of malocclusion can be treated with lingual braces.

The patient in Figure 25–26A desired a flattening of her profile. She had four first bicuspids removed, lingual braces placed on the maxillary teeth (Figures 25–26B and C), and clear braces placed on her mandibular teeth to reduce treatment cost. Acrylic pontics were bonded onto the mesial surface of the maxillary second bicuspids to help mask the space from the missing bicuspids until the anterior teeth could be retracted. As the space closed, the pontics were trimmed to allow continued tooth movement.

Removable Appliance Therapy

Many perspective orthodontic patients are interested in correcting their problems with a "retainer." These patients are referring to the removable Hawley appliance that, for decades, has helped countless patients who would not wear fixed appliances. The patient in Figures 25–27A and B requires limited tooth repositioning, and a "retainer" with springs that tuck in the mesial surface of the lateral incisors was selected. A diamond disk removes sufficient enamel from both sides of the lateral incisor (Figure 25–27C) to allow the teeth to move in the desired

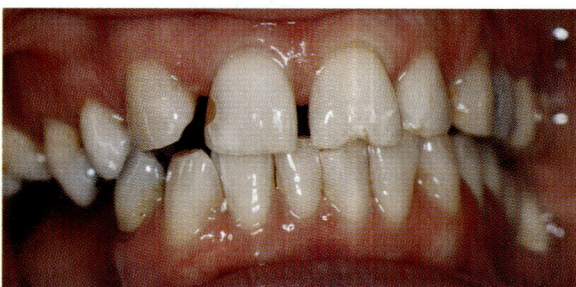

Figure 25–24A: A case that will require the talents of several dental disciplines to achieve an esthetic and functional result. Note the missing tooth #7, spacing missing posterior teeth.

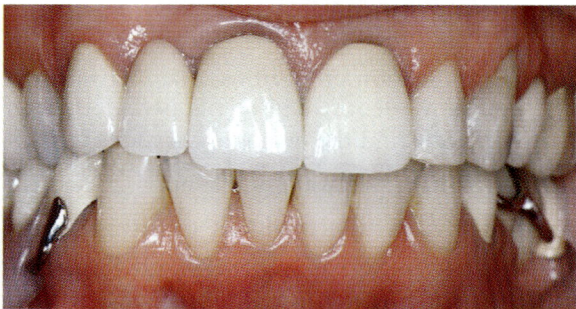

Figure 25–24B: After orthodontics and completed restorative treatment with crowns, implants, and a removable prosthesis.

Esthetics in Adult Orthodontics   771

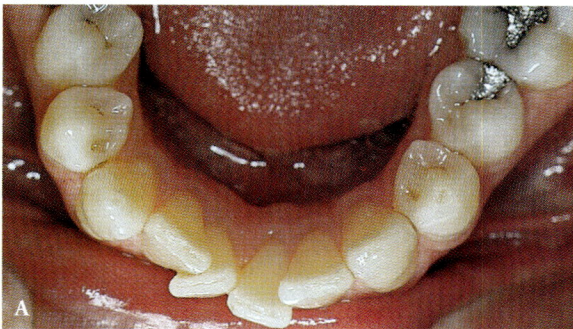 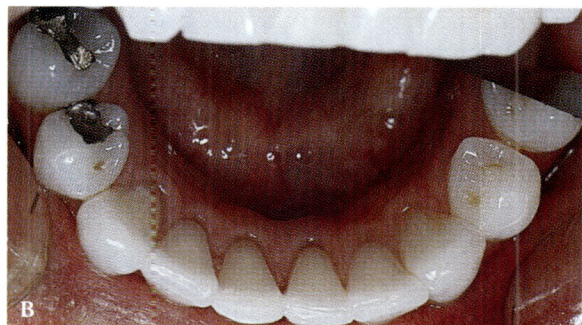

Figure 25–25A and B: Before and after treatment with removable tray therapy in which the lower incisors were aligned.

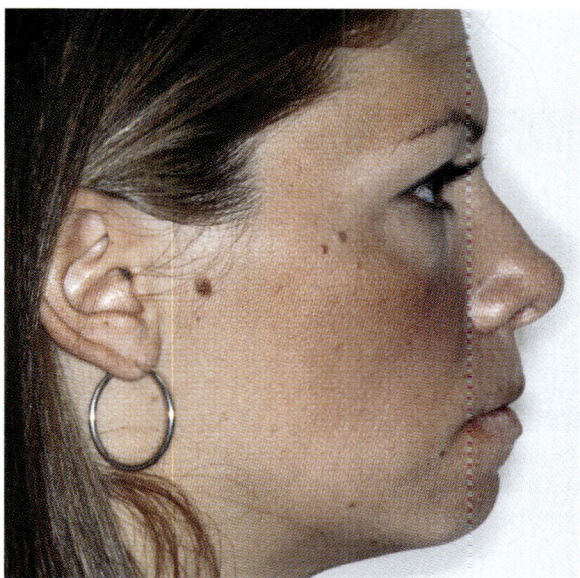

Figure 25–26A: Profile view of a patient wishing reduction of a protrusive profile.

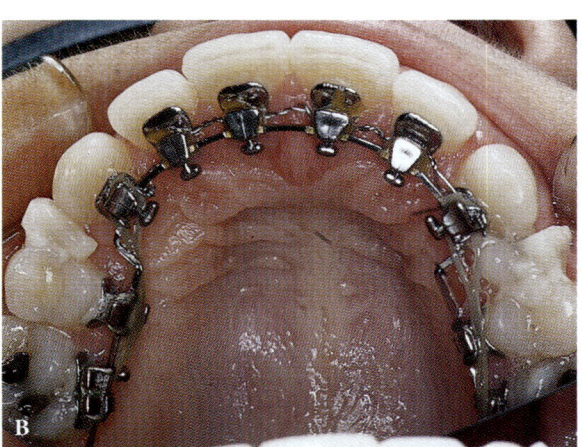 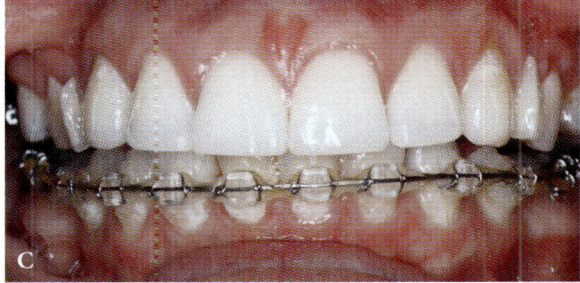

Figure 25–26B and C: Treatment photographs after removal of the first bicuspids and placement of pontics in the upper extraction spaces to minimize the visual impact of the extractions.

manner. The important issue here is to remove the enamel completely to the gingival margin so that the enamel is not touching the adjacent teeth, preventing the intended movement. The appliance was made with wax in the area of tooth movement (behind the mesial surface of the lateral incisors) so that tooth movement would not be prevented by any acrylic on the appliance (Figure 25–27D).

Another example of limited tooth movement is shown in Figures 25–28A and B. The lateral incisor has rotated outward and will be corrected with a Hawley appliance and a finger spring.

Indications for this appliance are small rotations of anterior teeth, anterior spaces, and limited tooth tipping. Limitations are rotated posterior teeth, posterior spaces, bite correction, and maxillary midline diastemata when the mandibular incisors contact the maxillary incisors.

CONCLUSION

When patients can consider two or more treatment options (that include different appliances, time frames, costs, and, possibly, outcomes), they are more likely to accept treatment. Surprisingly, it will sometimes even be full metal brackets for a rather long duration. In any event, both general or esthetic dentists and orthodontists are urged to incorporate flexibility and compromise in their treatment

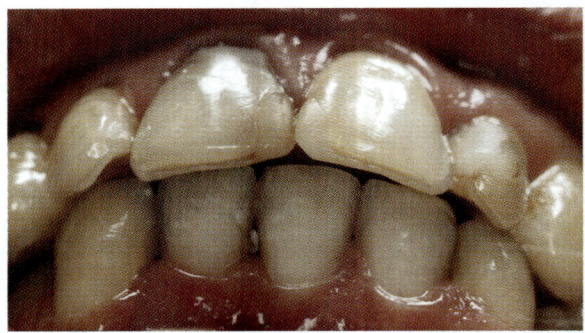

Figure 25–27A: A problem ideally suited for treatment with a Hawley appliance; rotated upper lateral incisors that have sufficient overjet to allow for tooth movement.

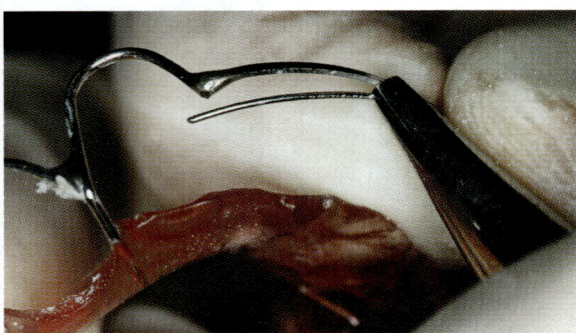

Figure 25–27B: Rotation springs are activated to apply pressure to the desired tooth surface when the appliance is in the mouth.

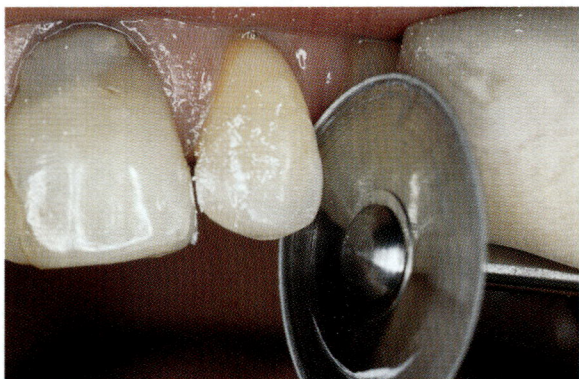

Figure 25–27C: Interproximal tooth reduction is accomplished on the mesial and distal surfaces down to the gingival margin to ensure that there is no enamel still in contact that would prevent tooth movement. A diamond stone (DET-GF, Brasseler, Savannah, GA) can also be used.

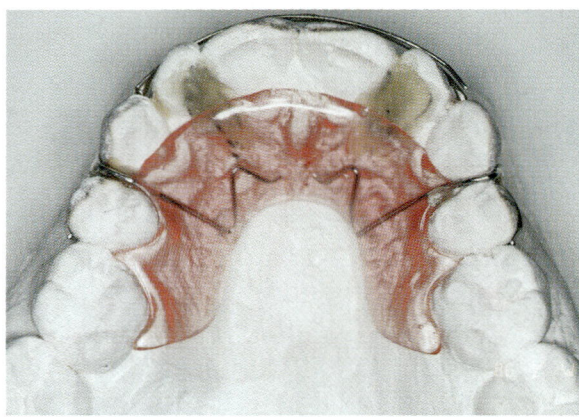

Figure 25–27D: Waxing the model to prevent acrylic from contacting the mesiolingual surface of the teeth to be moved.

Esthetics in Adult Orthodontics 773

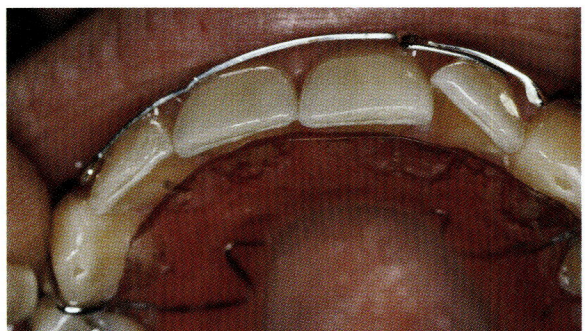

Figure 25–28A: Appliance in place to move in the mesial surface of the lateral incisor; note the large space between the mesial surface of the lateral and the appliance.

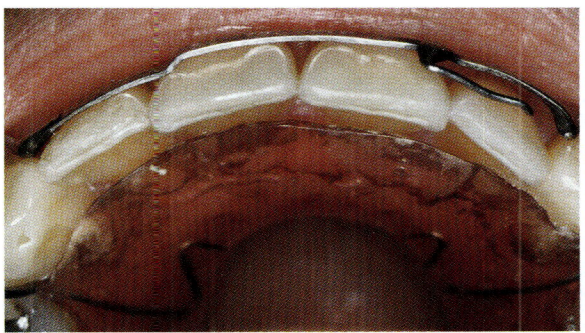

Figure 25–28B: Treatment almost completed. Sufficient enamel has been removed from the lateral incisor to allow it to fit into a smaller space.

Table 25–2. Common Esthetic Orthodontic Problems and Possible Solutions

PROBLEM	FACTORS	SOLUTIONS
Maxillary midline diastema	Large central incisors and space larger than 4 mm sufficient overjet Insufficient overjet Normal to small central incisors and large space	Hawley appliance to retract and close space Complete treatment with brackets or Invisalign Orthodontics and veneers
Narrow dental arches	Protrusion and crossbite Crowding	Orthodontic expansion Extraction if required with orthodontics
Mild crowding and spring	Good occlusion Poor occlusion	Interproximal tooth reduction aligner or Invisalign Complete orthodontics
Severe crowding	Good occlusion Poor occlusion	Consider removal of a lower incisor and use Invisalign Consider expansion, tooth narrowing, and orthodontics

plans. Contemporary dental patients expect esthetic appliance options, and, regardless of the final treatment choice, everyone benefits when patients are able to make informed decisions. The available treatment methods presented here all have a place in the esthetic orthodontic care of our patients. A summary of problems and solutions are presented in Table 25–2. Any dental problem that requires better tooth position for a better esthetic restorative result should have an orthodontic consultation.

Additional Resources

Azizi M, Shrout MK, Haas AJ, et al. A retrospective study of angle Class I malocclusions treated orthodontically without extraction using two palatal expansion methods. Am J Orthod Dentofacial Orthop, 1999;116:101–7.

Bishara SE, Ortho D, Jakobsen JR. Profile changes in patients treated with and without extractions: assessments by lay people. Am J Orthod Dentofacial Orthop 1997;112:639–43.

Brightman B, Hans MG, Wolf GR, Bernard H. Recognition of malocclusion: an education outcomes assessment. Am J Orthod Dentofacial Orthop 1999;116:444–51.

Cowan R Jr. Treatment of a patient with a Class II malocclusion, impacted canine, and severe malalignment. Am J Orthod Dentofacial Orthop 2000;118:693–8.

Derakhshan M, Sadowsky C. A relatively minor adult case becomes significantly complex: a lesson in humility. Am J Orthod Dentofacial Orthop 2001;119:546–53.

Fujuita K. New orthodontic treatment with lingual bracket mushroom arch wire appliance. Am J Orthod 1979;76:657.

Goldstein MC. Adult orthodontics. Am J Orthod 1958;39:400.

Goldstein MC. Adult orthodontics and the general practitioner. J Can Dent Assoc 1958;23:261.

Goldstein MC. Orthodontics in crown and bridge and periodontal therapy. Dent Clin North Am 1964; July:449–59.

Goldstein MC, Fritz ME. Treatment of periodontosis by combined orthodontic and periodontal approach. J Am Dent Assoc 1976;93:985.

Goldstein R. Dental esthetics. Philadelphia: JB Lippincott, 1977.

Hemmings KW, Darbar UR, Vaughan S. Tooth wear treated with direct composite restorations at an increased vertical dimension: results at 30 months. J Prosthet Dent 2000;83:287–93.

James RD. A comparative study of facial profiles in extraction and nonextraction treatment. Am J Orthod Dentofacial Orthop 1998;114:265–76.

Klontz HA. Facial balance and harmony: an attainable objective for the patient with a high mandibular plane angle. Am J Orthod Dentofacial Orthop 1998;114: 176–88.

Kurz C. The use of lingual appliances for correction of bimaxillary protrusion. Am J Orthod Dentofacial Orthop 1997;112:357–63.

Laino A, Melsen B. Orthodontic treatment of a patient with multidisciplinary problems. Am J Orthod Dentofacial Orthop 1997;111:141–8.

Miller RJ. Invisalign: current application and future direction. Presented at the 101st Annual Session of the AAO, Toronto, May 5, 2000.

Newman GV. Current status of bonding attachments. J Clin Orthod 1973;7:7.

Oliva de Cuebas J. Nonsurgical treatment of a skeletal vertical discrepancy with a significant open bite. Am J Orthod Dentofacial Orthop 1997;112:124–31.

Pearson L. Rapid maxillary expansion with incisor intrusion: a study of vertical control. Am J Orthod Dentofacial Orthop 1999;115:576–82.

Pintado M. Variation in tooth wear in young adults over a two-year period. J Prosthet Dent 1997;77:317–20.

Poling R. A method of finishing the occlusion. Am J Orthod Dentofacial Orthop 1999;115:476–87.

Rivera SM, Hatch JP, Dolce C, et al. Patients' own reasons and patient-perceived recommendations for orthognathic surgery. Am J Orthod Dentofacial Orthop 2000;118:134–40.

Sarver DM, Ackerman JL. Orthodontics about face: the re-emergence of the esthetic paradigm. Am J Orthod Dentofacial Orthop 2000;117:575–6.

Shue-Te Yeh M, Koochek A-R, Vlaskalic V, et al. The relationship of 2 professional occlusal indexes with patients' perceptions of aesthetics, function, speech, and orthodontic treatment need. Am J Orthod Dentofacial Orthop 2000;18:421–8.

Smith BG, Bartlett DW, Robb ND. The prevalence, etiology, and management of tooth wear in the United Kingdom. J Prosthet Dent 1997;78:367–72.

Smith SW, English JD. Orthodontic correction of a Class III malocclusion in an adolescent patient with a bonded RPE and protraction face mask. Am J Orthod Dentofacial Orthop 1999;116:177–83.

Spyropoulos MN, Halazonetis DJ. Significance of the soft tissue profile on facial esthetics. Am J Orthod Dentofacial Orthop 2001;119:464–71.

Tung AW, Kiyak A. Psychological influences on the timing of orthodontic treatment. Am J Orthod Dentofacial Orthop 1998;113:29–39.

Wilson JR. Treatment of a Class II, Division 2 malocclusion with one congenitally missing and one malformed lateral incisor and a palatally impacted maxillary canine. Am J Orthod Dentofacial Orthop 1998;114:55–9.

CHAPTER 26

SURGICAL ORTHODONTIC CORRECTION OF DENTOFACIAL DEFORMITY

John N. Kent, DDS, John D. Stover, DDS, MD, PhD

All of dentistry has become more aware of the relationship of the dentition to the facial bones and their impact on facial appearance. The precise, artistic work of the esthetic restorative dentist can be enhanced by orthodontic and surgical optimization and rejuvenation of the facial hard- and soft-tissue framework for the dentition. Such things as abnormal muscle function, lip incompetence, a variety of occlusal problems, and disturbances in facial bone growth contribute to facial disharmony. Today, the recognition and demand for correction of malocclusion and abnormal facial contour in adults are a significant topic in the practice of dentistry and in the specialties of orthodontics and oral and maxillofacial surgery. It is essential that all practitioners continually update their knowledge of the expanding treatment options provided by general dentists and specialists alike.

From the turn of the century through the 1950s, the treatment of dentofacial abnormalities was limited largely to correction of mandibular prognathism by osteotomies of the ramus or body of the mandible. During the following decade, owing to the pioneering efforts of Hugo Obwegesser and other European surgeons, surgical procedures were developed to correct mandibular retrognathism, chin deformities, and excessive maxillary growth. Dr. Obwegesser's appearance at the Walter Reed Army Medical Center in 1966 was the inspiration for the beginning of subsequent American contributions. Since that time, numerous procedures to treat the entire spectrum of dental, skeletal, and soft-tissue abnormalities have been developed. Optimal esthetic and functional results are now obtainable for all patients with a variety of occlusal and facial defects, as seen in textbooks by Hinds and Kent; Satorianos and Sassouni; Bell, Proffit, and White; Epker and Wolford; and Epker and Fish. Significant clinical and basic science research articles in the oral and maxillofacial surgery and orthodontic literature continue to provide outcome analyses of traditional orthodontic and orthognathic procedures and innovative progress in areas such as adjunctive soft-tissue procedures and evaluation of emerging biomaterials. The introduction of rigid fixation principles with bone plates and screws in the 1980s has eliminated intermaxillary fixation (jaws wired shut) in most patients. Recent applications in the 1990s of distraction osteogenesis are offering innovative solutions to difficult deformities. Applications include single jaw distraction, combined maxillomandibular distraction, and mandibular widening.

Unquestionably, some dental malocclusions do not need concomitant orthodontic and surgical procedures and will respond nicely to either modality alone. However, most skeletal malocclusions are too severe to be treated by either specialty alone. A successful outcome that remains stable for the long term often requires a multidisciplinary approach. After an appropriate diagnosis is made, the restorative dentist, orthodontist, and surgeon must evaluate the patient and then together formulate a comprehensive treatment plan, clearly communicating the proper sequence for the satisfactory completion of all dental, orthodontic, and surgical procedures. Communication among all parties involved must continue throughout treatment and long-term follow-up. This chapter presents the sequence of events the patient will encounter including the examination, case presentation, orthodontic treatment, surgical procedures, and follow-up management. Finally, a detailed description of common dentofacial abnormalities is presented in a problem-oriented fashion with illustration of treatment results.

FACIAL ESTHETICS

The planning of corrective surgery for dentofacial deformities is surely one of the best examples of the interaction of art and science in the field of dentistry. Although beauty may be skin deep, understanding facial esthetics requires an in-depth knowledge of how subcutaneous fat, muscle tone, and particularly the underlying supporting skeleton combine and interact to produce the facial appearance.

Modern concepts of facial esthetics, especially in America, are influenced by classical ideals. As professionals, we must strive to be objective in our analysis and planning but must also be aware of cultural biases, physical and racial characteristics, and, most importantly, the patient's desires. The evaluation of the face must be critical of form as it relates to function. Treatment should never alter one to the detriment of the other. In an attempt to evaluate facial form, there are five significant factors that should be considered objectively: age, body type, race, symmetry, and proportion.

The age of a patient is an important determinant of facial form. Underlying skeletal structures are not fully expressed until late adolescence. In adults, there is relative stability of the facial skeletal structure; however, during the aging process, generalized demineralization of bone occurs, which can have subtle effects on form. The distribution of subcutaneous tissue shifts with age, particularly with changes in fat deposits that may result in ocular, temporal, and buccal fat loss and accentuation of the underlying skeletal structures. The skin loses elasticity and begins to wrinkle and sag. Hair may recede, thin, and gray. Dimensional changes can also occur with the loss of teeth and associated alveolar bone.

Body type relates to age and sex and is generally reflected in facial form. Basic body types include endomorph (asthenic) types who are thin and angular, mesomorph (sthenic) types who are well proportioned and square, and endomorph (pyknic) types who are heavy set and rounded. Proper relation of facial form to body type is essential for desirable balance.

Racial characteristics are increasingly important in today's society. These qualities should be appreciated and should not limit the achievement of esthetic improvement in facial reconstructions. Asians will tend to have rounded faces, and their profile will be straight or slightly concave without defined anterior projection of the zygomas, nasal dorsum, or chin. Those of African origin will tend toward a convex profile with a flat forehead and nasal dorsum juxtaposed with bimaxillary dental alveolar protrusion, prominent lips, and a less defined chin. Northern Europeans, after whom most cephalometric norms were developed, tend to exhibit a straight or slightly convex profile with a defined anterior projection of the nose, zygomas, and chin.

The last two factors, symmetry and proportion, are most easily discussed together and of the five factors listed lend themselves to quantification most readily. Soft- and hard-tissue measurements are recorded in the frontal and profile views, and treatment can be designed to maximize the esthetic end result.

On frontal view, the face can be divided vertically into thirds (Figure 26–1): the upper third is

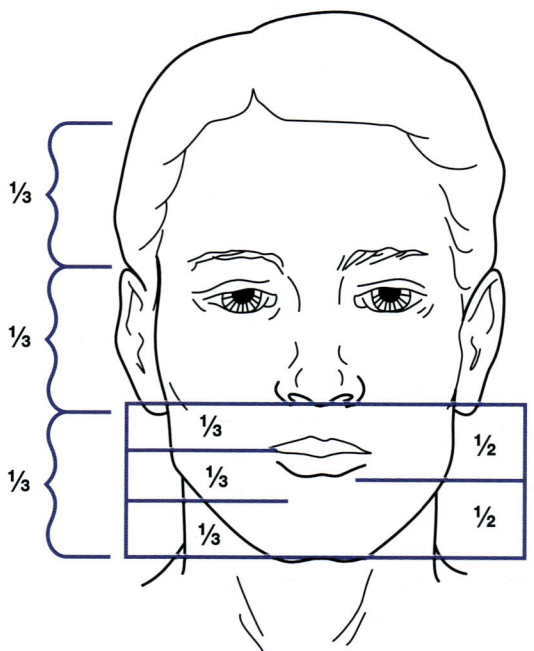

Figure 26–1: Frontal view of the face. Upper, middle, and lower thirds are delineated. Lower third is further divided into halves and thirds.

from the upper hairline to the glabella, the middle third is from the glabella to the subnasale, and the lower third is from the subnasale to the menton. A one-to-one ratio indicates ideal esthetic proportions. The lower third can further be divided in half, with the division at the vermilion border of the lower lip, or in thirds, with the upper third ending at the oral commissure (see Figure 26–1).

Symmetry and proportion can be judged on frontal examination by dividing the face into fifths, with each fifth being equal to the eye width (Figure 26–2). Midline points should lie on an axis, dividing the face in half, and all paired facial structures should be nearly equidistant from this axis. The intercanthal distance should be one eye width and should correspond to the width of the alar cartilages. The oral commissures should lie on vertical axes tangent to the medial limbus of each eye, and the distance between each axis should be one and one half times the width of the eye (see Figure 26–2).

Additional proportion evaluations are evident on profile examination. Nasal projection can be judged by the nasofrontal angle (115–130 degrees), the nasofacial angle (30–40 degrees), and a nasomental angle (120–132 degrees). Using a vertical line from the glabella to the menton, a perpendicular line drawn to the nasal tip should be 55 to 60% of the distance from the point of intersection to the nasion. The distance from the nasal tip to the subnasale should equal the distance from the subnasale to the vermilion border of the upper lip (Figure 26–3). Also, on profile examination, the interplay between the lip, chin, and neck can be evaluated (Figure 26–4). The mentocervical angle should be 80 to 95 degrees. The depth of the labiomental sulcus, measured using a line from the lower lip to the soft-tissue menton, should be approximately 4 mm.

The "ideals" described above should not be used to establish definitive treatment objectives in all patients. These are only guidelines by which facial harmony may be defined and from which ideas regarding treatment planning may be derived. There are numerous other measures, angles, and analyses that may be employed to aid in the diagnosis of a dentofacial deformity. Regardless of what data are collected and which analysis is used, final treatment decisions must be tailored to the individual patient. It is probable that the most important treatment planning information obtained will come from listening to the patient's own treatment goals.

WHO ARE THE CANDIDATES?

Combined surgical-orthodontic management is a complex and lengthy process with significant risks, costs, and inconvenience. The prospective patient must understand what is involved without "glossing over" the facts. It is especially important to listen to the patients' perception of the problem and then determine what they want to achieve as a result of treatment. If their expectations are inconsistent with their overall behavior, mode of dress, and level of health awareness, questions about their motives should be forthright. If they have a significant deformity and want to be "perfectly normal" or are suffering psychologically, they may be desperately hoping that treatment will enhance their image and success in life. The best possible result of treatment may not satisfy them.

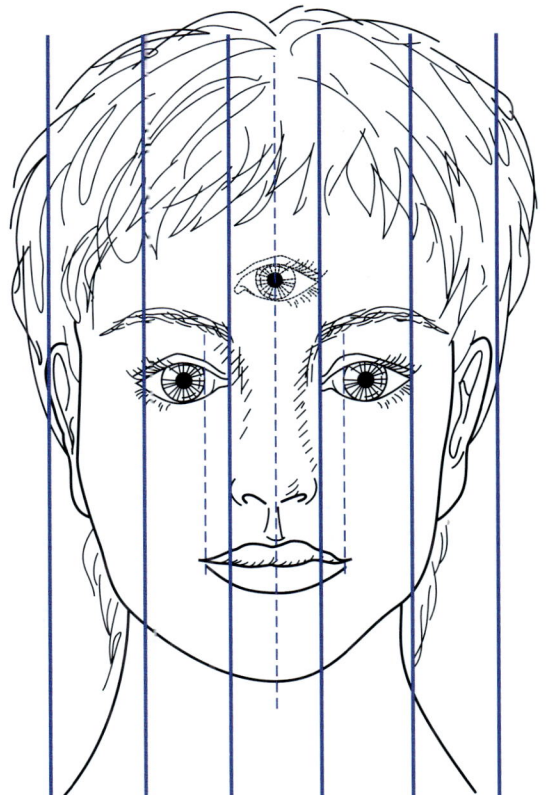

Figure 26–2: Frontal view of the face. Sagittal division of the face into fifths with each fifth equal to one eye width.

778 Esthetics in Dentistry

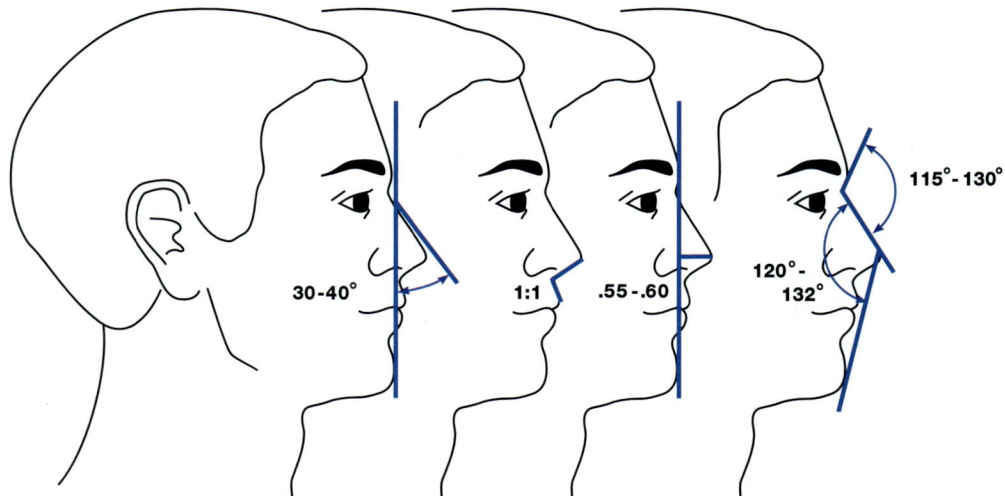

Figure 26–3: Profile views of the face relating the nose to the forehead, lips, and chin. Nasofrontal, nasofacial, and nasomental angles are described, as well as linear measurements of nasal tip projection.

In growing individuals, combined surgical-orthodontic treatment is generally avoided. Although most juvenile deformities can be rectified by influencing the growth process, psychological embarrassment or significant impairment of speech and masticatory function may warrant surgical procedures before facial growth is complete. In such cases, it is clearly explained to the patient and parents that further treatment may be necessary. Typically, the surgical phase of treatment is deferred until late adolescence, when growth is complete. Serial hand radiographs are compared to ensure maturation of epiphyseal plates. Distraction osteogenesis is increasingly being used to correct defor-

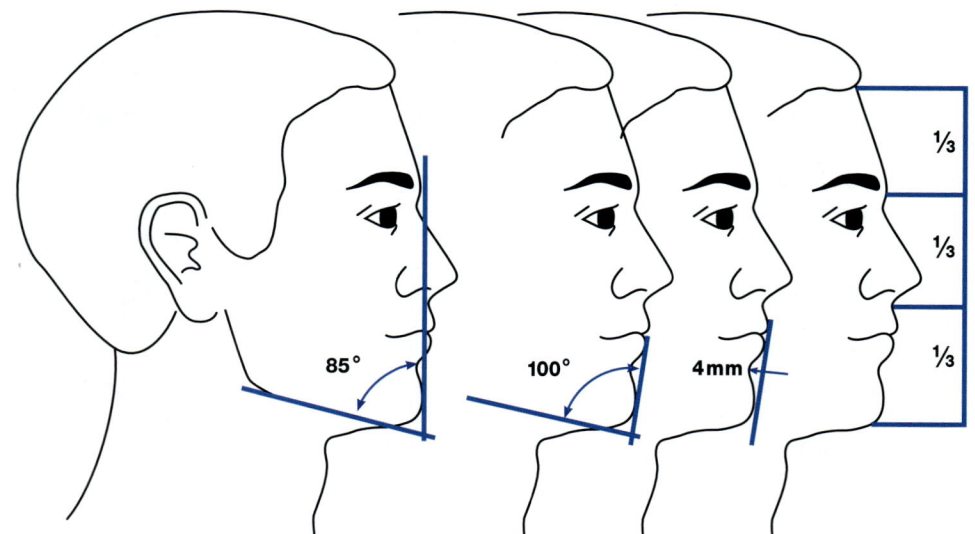

Figure 26–4: Profile views of the face relating the chin to the lips and neck and the labial mental sulcus to the lower lip and chin. The mental cervical angle is described.

mities in growing patients. Exciting research in this area is progressing rapidly as innovative applications of distraction are being applied not only to growing patients but also to adults.

There are many adults with malocclusions who exhibit little or no facial disharmony and who can be properly treated with orthodontics alone. However, if a true skeletal imbalance exists, orthodontic treatment cannot achieve proper gnathologic relationships, esthetics, and tooth position over basal bone simultaneously. In cases of severe skeletal disharmony, orthodontic treatment alone usually will not satisfactorily improve the facial profile. In fact, the occlusion may be improved at the expense of the esthetic relationships. The orthodontist should determine prior to initiating treatment whether and to what degree there is a skeletal component to the deformity. In the case of a significant skeletal deformity, the oral and maxillofacial surgeon should be consulted to discuss surgical options.

Adult Class II malocclusions corrected orthodontically are classically treated by extractions in the upper arch only and maximum retraction of the upper anterior segment. This may result in a flat upper lip, excessive uprighting of the upper incisor, which affects the posterior occlusion, causes spacing in the upper arch, and creates shallow incisal coupling. This type of treatment imposes a requirement of extensive headgear use or Class II elastic traction. If extensive Class II elastics are used, lower second bicuspids are often extracted to prevent flaring of the lower incisors.

Orthodontic treatment of Class III malocclusion usually results in severe lingual inclination of the lower incisors and does not correct excess chin prominence. There is little opportunity to bodily retract the lower incisors owing to the very narrow alveolus. Often, extractions are performed in both arches since Class III posterior occlusal relationships are notoriously unsatisfactory. One of the most difficult factors to overcome is the bilateral posterior crossbites often found with this type. If the midpalatal raphe is patent, it is possible to orthopedically expand the maxilla using "jackscrew"-type devices. Since this raphe will fuse in the late teens or early twenties, many adults cannot be treated with palatal expansion. Compromises will need to be accepted if orthodontics alone is the only alternative.

Since extraction therapy will average a minimum of 18 to 24 months, many adults will not accept treatment because of the time factor. Some will balk at using headgear or rubber bands. Others will insist on wearing plastic or lingual brackets, making incisor retraction even more difficult.

In these days of increased consumer awareness, the orthodontist and surgeon must be scrupulously truthful about all details and risks of proposed treatments even if they cause the patient to decline treatment. When the patient needs and receives guarantees and when the team members are overly enthusiastic, the situation is ripe for mishap. It is common practice to write out in detail a complete diagnostic report citing the treatment modalities and risks and mail signed copies to the patient and other team members. A report such as this, when accompanied by a signed consent form and signed prediction tracings, will substantiate a claim that the patient was fully informed and consented to the treatment.

FIRST VISIT

The first and most important step for the patient is the recognition that a dentofacial abnormality exists. The patient may have abnormalities in both the maxillary and mandibular regions requiring eventual orthodontic and surgical treatment of both jaws. At this point, the patient should be instructed that additional examination and tests are necessary to accurately locate the deformity and describe treatment possibilities. Each member of the team (general dentist, orthodontist, oral and maxillofacial surgeon) examines the patient, formulates a diagnosis, and prepares a treatment sequence. The length of orthodontic treatment, types of surgical procedures, cost, and complications cannot be discussed until the diagnostic records are taken and a treatment plan is formulated.

Diagnostic Records

To identify the dentofacial deformity and formulate treatment recommendations, diagnostic records usually include a panoramic radiograph, a lateral cephalogram, study casts, and facial, profile, and intraoral photographs. The panoramic radiograph is preferred by the orthodontist and surgeon for assessment of bone size, shape, pathology, and determination of osteotomy sites. The standardized lateral cephalogram is used for performing cephalometric analyses and subsequently making cephalometric prediction tracings. Additional records such as temporomandibular joint (TMJ) films, frontal cephalograms, and mounted casts are also used in selected cases.

Cephalometric Analysis. There are over 300 cephalometric measurements or analyses described in the literature for facial soft-tissue and bony architecture. Even though they provide language by which we communicate, they have limitations. Unavoidable error exists in taking and analyzing the cephalogram, partly because they are susceptible to geometric distortions. The "normal" data to which comparisons are made are derived from "ideal" individuals, and comparisons become less reliable as extremes in skeletal deformity are approached. Neither the cephalogram or the particular analysis to which the derived data are compared is most important from the diagnostic standpoint—rather, it is how these data correlate with the overall examination and treatment goals. Cephalometrics is more useful for documenting progress and change as the treatment unfolds than for the actual diagnostic process itself. The cephalometric tracing is created on acetate paper overlaid on the cephalogram (Figure 26–5A). Changes over time can be compared by superimposing tracings on each other.

Cephalometric Prediction Tracings. The cephalometric prediction tracing predicts the changes that should occur as a result of orthodontic or surgical treatment. For example, the work-up of a patient with a Class II malocclusion with vertical maxillary excess, mandibular retrognathism, and chin deficiency requires several tracings. Tracing 1 is the patient's existing dentofacial deformity (see Figure 26–5A). An overlay of tracing 2 (Figure 26–5B) on tracing 1 demonstrates maxillary orthodontic tooth movement, superior repositioning of the maxilla by Le Fort I osteotomy, and autorotation of the mandible. Tracing 3 demonstrates the advancement of the mandible by sagittal split osteotomy performed simultaneously with the maxillary surgery (Figure 26–5C). If necessary, a horizontal osteotomy of the chin or a chin implant is placed for augmentation as shown in tracing 4 (Figure 26–5D). Tracing 5 demonstrates a superimposition of all predicted hard- and soft-tissue changes on tracing 1 (Figure 26–5E). It is important to use the tracings without cephalometric lines, angles, and measurements, which are necessary for diagnostic purposes, as they may be confusing to the patient.

Prints of the patient's profile and frontal appearance can be enlarged to a full-size head image using the patient's cephalometric radiographs for sizing. Careful cutting and pasting of the prints using cephalometric overlays provide dramatic realization of post-treatment results (Figures 26–6A and B). Most orthodontic-orthognathic work-ups today are done with any one of several sophisticated computerized software programs. Digital cephalograms are superimposed on digital lateral facial photographs and captured into the prediction software application. Proposed orthodontic and orthognathic movements are made with the mouse, and the predicted facial form is displayed. Although these visual representations have great value in showing patients what changes can be made, it must be made clear that these are ideal treatment goals. One cannot guarantee that the end result will always be as predicted ideally.

Facial and Intraoral Photographs. All facial portraits should be of the head in an erect, natural, unstrained posture against a neutral-colored background. Teeth should be in occlusion, with the lips relaxed. For patients with lip incompetence, a second portrait should be taken with the lips closed to depict the amount of lip strain present. Frontal and profile portraits are taken. In Class II deformities, it is helpful for diagnostic purposes to take a second profile view with the mandible postured forward. In Class III deformities secondary to horizontal maxillary deficiency, it is demonstrative to take an additional profile portrait with a layer of gauze under the upper lip. Facial photographs also include smiling and maximum opening views if hypomobility exists. Finally, photographs of the patient's anterior and posterior occlusion in centric relationship and centric occlusion are taken, as well as occlusal views of the maxilla and mandible denoting arch form.

Study Casts. Full-arch casts should be trimmed in centric relation according to the methods described in undergraduate orthodontic textbooks. This trimming is necessary since many of the deformities are "nonocclusions," which cannot be accurately articulated when the models are held by hand. In severe cases, as well as cases that will undergo significant vertical changes as a result of

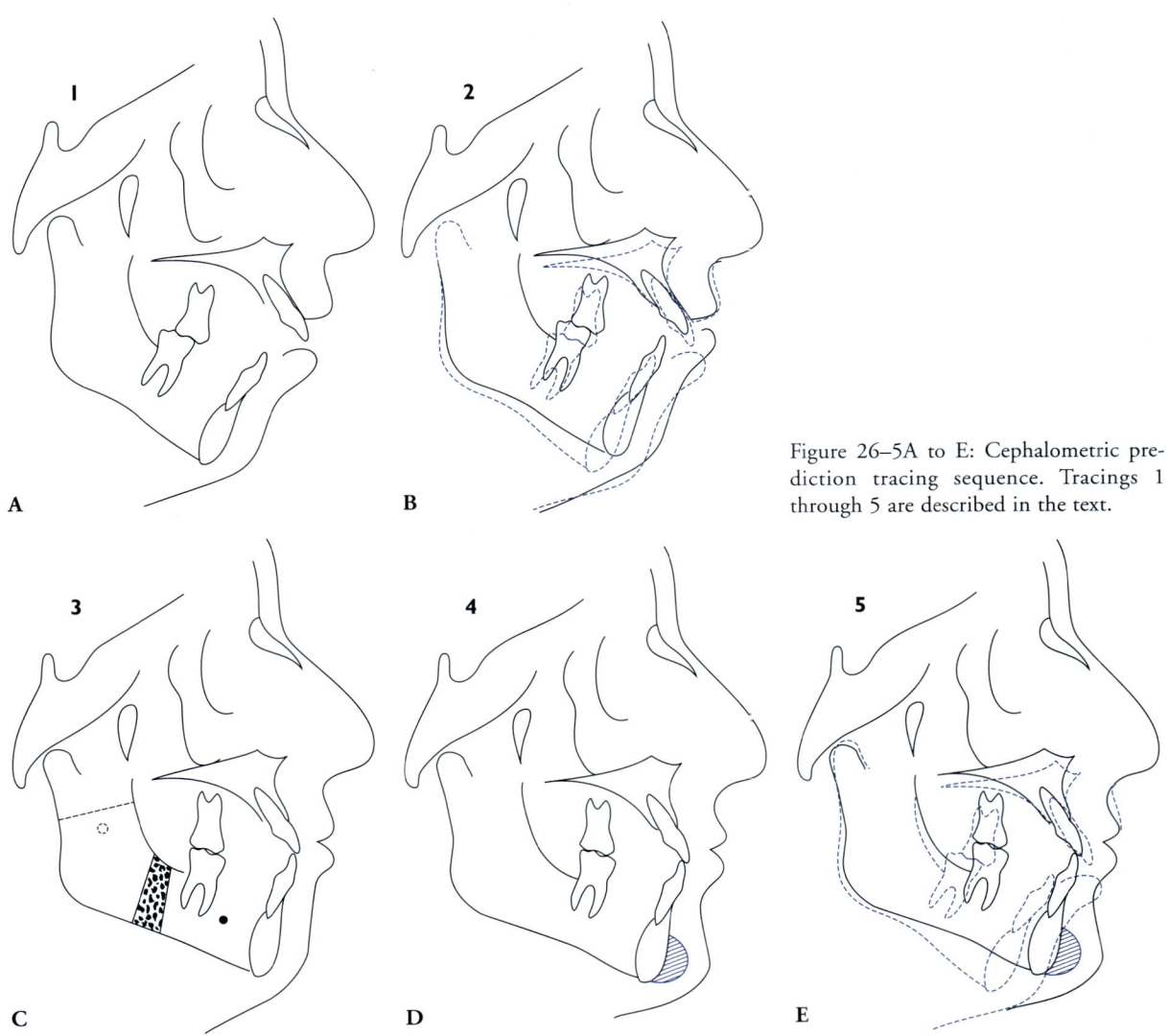

Figure 26–5A to E: Cephalometric prediction tracing sequence. Tracings 1 through 5 are described in the text.

treatment, mounting of the casts on an articulator with hinge-axis records will be necessary. The decision of precision hinge-axis versus the arbitrary hinge-axis determination is dictated by individual circumstances such as TMJ deterioration or dysfunction, degree of mandibular autorotation, and obvious asymmetry, among others.

CASE PRESENTATION VISIT

Once the diagnosis and general treatment plans have been formulated, the team, consisting of the patient's dentist, orthodontist, and oral and maxillofacial surgeon, renders a final integrated treatment plan. The most effective manner in which to coordinate and present all of this information would be at a conjoint conference among all of the parties involved.

The role of the primary dentist is to coordinate the efforts of the specialists through the diagnostic process and treatment period since maintenance of the final result will be relegated to him or her. The general dentist should restore the dentition only to prevent dental emergencies during the surgical and orthodontic treatment. Defective restorations, caries, infection, and periodontal disease must be controlled, and oral hygiene must be monitored.

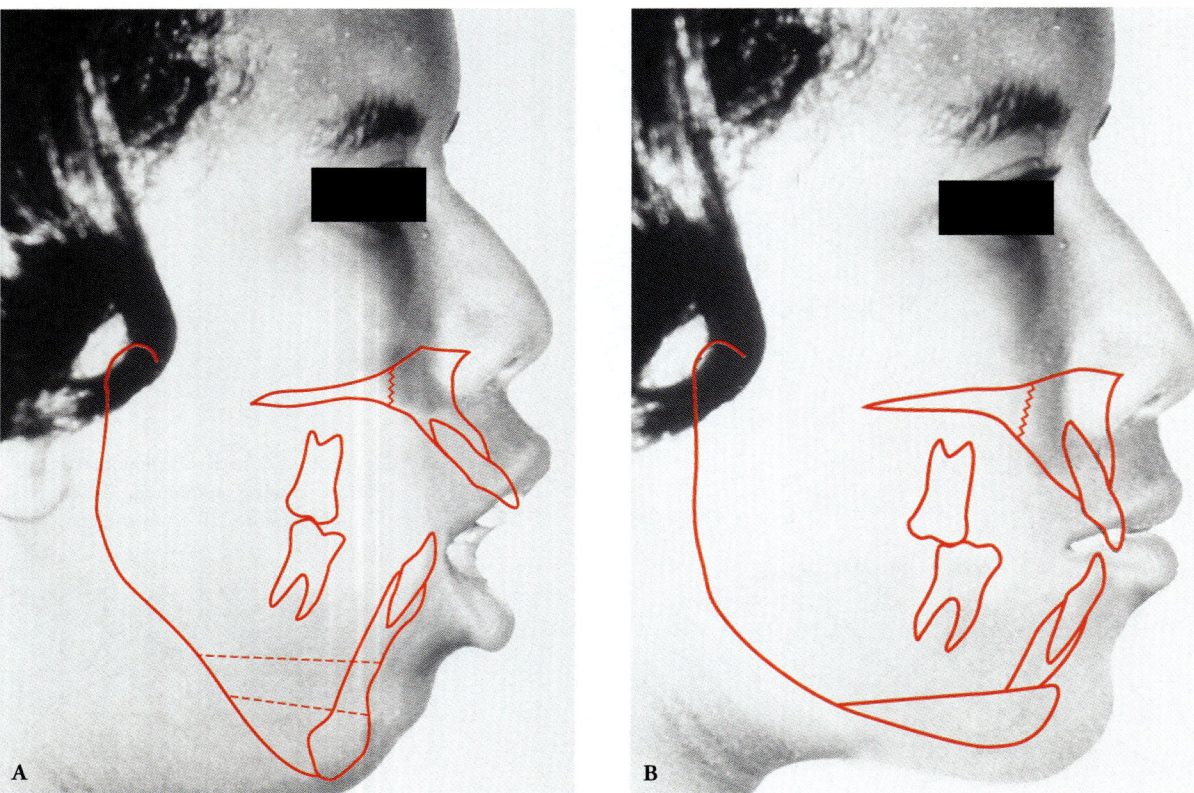

Figure 26–6A and B: Cutting and pasting of preoperative cephalogram and photograph to predict postoperative outcome.

Since the periodontal structures will be challenged during orthodontic and surgical treatment, optimal control and management of periodontal disease should be corrected immediately and monitored throughout the treatment.

It is beneficial to decide at the outset whether conventional orthodontics or a combined surgical-orthodontic treatment plan will be followed. Because of existing skeletal imbalance and facial disharmony, the axial relationships of the teeth are often compromised. For example, lingually inclined lower incisors in mandibular prognathism or labially inclined lower incisors in mandibular retrognathism are naturally occurring dental "compensations" that must be corrected before any surgery is performed. This idealization of the tooth-to-bone relationship will not only enhance the final skeletal–dental balance but will also provide the surgeon with a greater opportunity to reorient the skeletal framework sufficiently to render a substantial improvement in the facial appearance.

Therefore, it is essential that the orthodontist explain to the patient that the presurgical "decompensation" of the dentition accentuates the deformity and can make the malocclusion, facial profile, and speech temporarily worse (Figures 26–7A to F). The patient must understand that this ultimately improves the bony support for the teeth and maximizes the esthetic changes resulting from upcoming surgical procedures.

In most instances, considerable effort is extended in the presurgical phase to arrange the dental arches so that a nearly ideal occlusion is achieved by the surgical procedure. This will leave only short-term orthodontic detailing or perfection of the final occlusal schemata postsurgically. This approach offers several important advantages. Once surgery is completed, the patient is usually anxious to be finished. Second, and most importantly, if the immediate postoperative occlusion is stable, then the occlusion is more likely to remain stable for the long term.

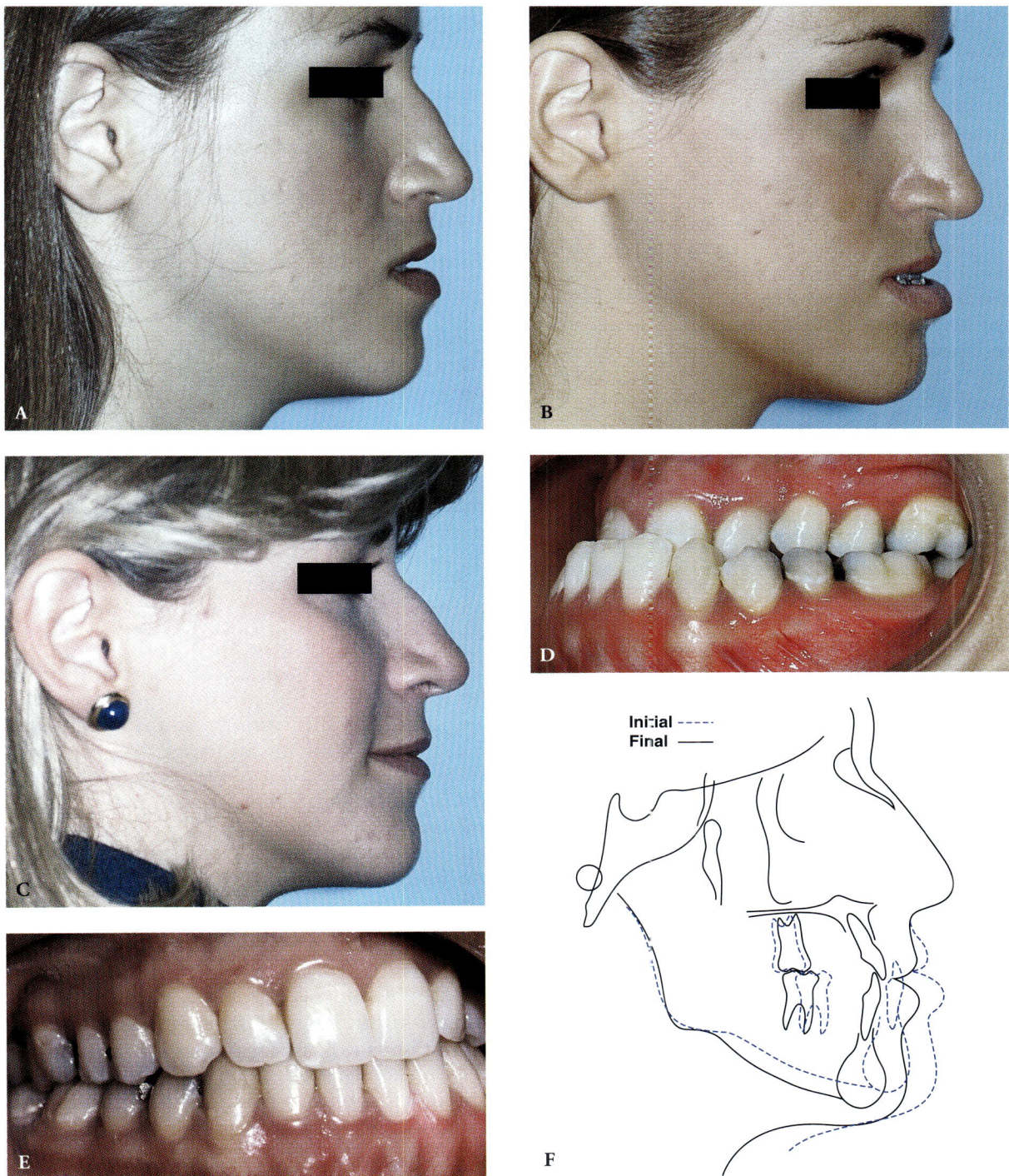

Figure 26–7A to F: Correction of mandibular prognathism and Class III malocclusion. (A) Preorthodontic profile of a patient with mandibular prognathism and flat cheekbones. (B) Postorthodontic, preoperative profile with lower incisors flared to remove dental compensations. Patient intentionally looks worse from orthodontic treatment. (C) Four-year postoperative profile. Surgery included augmentation with cheekbone implants and vertical subcondylar osteotomy of the mandible. (D) Initial pretreatment Class III malocclusion. (E) Final Class I occlusion. (F) Pretreatment and final tracing 4 years after surgery.

PRESURGICAL VISIT

When it is felt that the presurgical goals of arch alignment have been achieved, a set of progress records consisting of models, a cephalogram, and a panoramic radiograph will be obtained to verify that the patient is ready for surgery. Additional orthodontic treatment may be necessary to satisfy surgical goals.

A week or two before surgery, the patient should visit his or her general dentist for a thorough prophylaxis and fluoride treatment. The orthodontist will solder brass surgical lugs to a full-sized passive rectangular arch wire for application of intermaxillary fixation (IMF) wires that will be placed during surgery. Even though the surgeon will be primarily responsible for the care of the patient during the postsurgical healing phase, the general dentist and orthodontist should be available.

POSTSURGICAL TREATMENT

At the conclusion of a 6- to 8-week period, whether or not IMF is used, the surgeon will notify the orthodontist that he or she may begin definitive orthodontic treatment if clinical and radiographic examination indicates satisfactory healing. If bone segments begin to relapse, the orthodontist, working in concert with the surgeon, can nonsurgically re-establish the correct maxillomandibular relationship with elastics.

When occlusal splints are removed, the surgeon instructs the patient in the use of "training" elastics to preserve the skeletal alignment. Orthodontic follow-up as soon as possible is recommended. The orthodontist will inspect the mouth for loose or damaged brackets, wires, etc. Patients will typically continue the training elastics on a tapering basis for 1 to 2 months. The surgery wires are removed as soon as the patient is opening comfortably and are replaced with light passive round wires. The objective during and immediately after the surgery is to not produce orthodontic movement and possible surgical relapse. The patient should also be instructed in mobilization exercises to regain the full range of condylar motion. Occasionally, a physical therapy referral will be indicated.

Ideally, the final phase of orthodontic treatment should be straightforward, with most patients completing treatment 4 to 8 months after surgery. Tooth positioners may be used for a short period after the braces are removed, except in openbite cases. They are usually followed by more traditional retentive devices such as Hawley appliances and bonded lingual wires. Occasionally, a chin-cup is worn at night if relapse or additional growth is anticipated.

SURGICAL COMPLICATIONS AND RISKS

Fortunately, severe complications are rare. Certain surgical procedures carry a higher risk and are discussed in their respective sections. Patients must be adequately informed of these risks, particularly if there is no alternative in the selection of a surgical procedure.

Complications, particularly infections, from orthognathic surgery were not uncommon in the past. Today, however, proper selection of surgical procedures, refinement of surgical techniques, improved methods of postoperative fixation with bone plates, control of edema, use of antibiotics, and increased knowledge of the treatment of postoperative infections have resulted in a low incidence of complications.

Most common surgical procedures last 2 to 5 hours. The intraoral approach is most common and provides wide exposure of the maxilla and mandible while minimizing facial scars. An exceptional case may require an extraoral approach, particularly when mandibular bone grafts are used. Injuries to the teeth can occur with segmental alveolar osteotomies. With preoperative widening of the interdental space by orthodontics and careful technique, the injury to teeth can be avoided.

Blood loss can be significant during these procedures but is reduced with the increased use of hypotensive anesthesia. Transfusions of blood may be necessary in "double jaw" or more lengthy cases. The technique of autologous transfusion, in which the patient predonates blood 2 to 3 weeks preoperatively, has significantly decreased the incidence of complications associated with transfusions.

Stabilization of the operated segments is tantamount to proper healing, prevention of infection, and predictability of long-term stability. Bone segments are stabilized with bone plates and screws. Intermaxillary fixation, routinely required in the past, is now used primarily for cases involving significant mandibular setbacks or if bone plates and screws fail to immobilize jaw segments or are not possible. Early mobilization promotes faster functional bone healing, more rapid return of masticatory function, and facilitation of nutritional maintenance during the early postoperative period.

Postoperative discomfort is generally mild and can be handled with the conservative use of analgesics. Since there is a potential for significant postoperative edema, it is imperative to have informed the family that the patient may look much worse than he or she feels. Surgical dietary counseling and the availability of commercially prepared high-calorie, high-protein supplements can minimize weight loss postoperatively and maintain the nutritional balance required for normal wound healing.

DIAGNOSIS AND TREATMENT

Common dentofacial deformities are described in terms of their facial, skeletal, and dental characteristics. Treatment sequencing, orthodontic principles, and surgical procedures are now presented as a guide to the most frequently occurring deformities.

Mandibular Excess

The facial soft-tissue characteristics of classic mandibular skeletal prognathism or excess are primarily manifested in the profile view (see Figure 26–7A). There is a prominence of the lower lip and chin, a flat mentolabial fold, a normal to slight increase in the lower anterior facial height, a normal to obtuse gonial angle, and an appearance of sallow or deficient zygomas. From the frontal view, an increase in the lower anterior facial height and a flatness or lack of contour in the area of the zygomas and chin is usually evident. Cephalometrically, the point A-nasion-point B (ANB) angle is decreased, whereas the facial angle, sella-nasion-point B (SNB) angle and the lower anterior facial height are increased. The maxillary incisors are flared, and the lower incisors are lingually inclined. A negative overjet, Class III cuspid and molar relationships, and bilateral crossbites are common. In addition, these cases are generally characterized by severe arch length discrepancies in both arches.

Orthodontically, upper first bicuspids may be removed to correct crowding and flaring of the upper incisors. The lower arch is often treated without extractions since arch length is gained by tipping the incisal edges forward. This produces proper axial inclination of the incisors and fullness in the lower lip (see Figure 26–7B). The resulting worsening of the facial appearance will maximize the facial esthetic result when the mandible is set back by surgery (see Figures 26–7C to F). If mandibular extractions are required, the second bicuspids are usually removed to minimize retraction of the lower incisors. Class II mechanics, or reverse orthodontics, which accentuate the deformity, are often used to achieve these presurgical orthodontic goals. The increase in negative overjet allows for a normal incisor relationship postsurgically and will re-establish a normal mentolabial soft-tissue contour. Bilateral posterior crossbites evident presurgically are usually resolved with the surgical mandibular setback.

At least three variations of prognathism exist. Dentoalveolar prognathism is a horizontal prominence of the lower lip and dentition only. Since the chin is relatively normal in its relation to the upper face, profile prediction tracing of the surgical setback makes the patient appear "chin deficient." Orthodontics alone or alveolar osteotomies are therefore indicated rather than ramus surgery. A transfer of the inferior border may be necessary in bimaxillary prognathism with open bite for graft source and shortening of the facial height (Figures 26–8A and B). Alveolar osteotomies are usually stabilized using splints without IMF. Pseudo or false prognathism is a relative expression of mandibular horizontal excess secondary to a horizontal or vertically deficient maxilla. Correction of the maxillary midfacial deficiency will often obviate the need for mandibular surgery. The diagnosis and treatment are discussed in the section on maxillary deficiency. Prognathism may also be unexpressed in patients with vertical maxillary excess (VME). The features of true prognathism become evident when the maxilla is moved superiorly to a normalized position and the mandible autorotates upward and forward.

Surgery for correction of most prognathic cases consists of intraoral osteotomies in the ramus, either vertical subcondylar, inverted "L," or sagittal split type. Occasionally, a body ostectomy is indicated. The intraoral vertical subcondylar osteotomy (VSO) or vertical ramus osteotomy (VRO) is performed through a mucosal incision lateral to the midpoint of the anterior border of the ramus extending down to the vestibule opposite the first

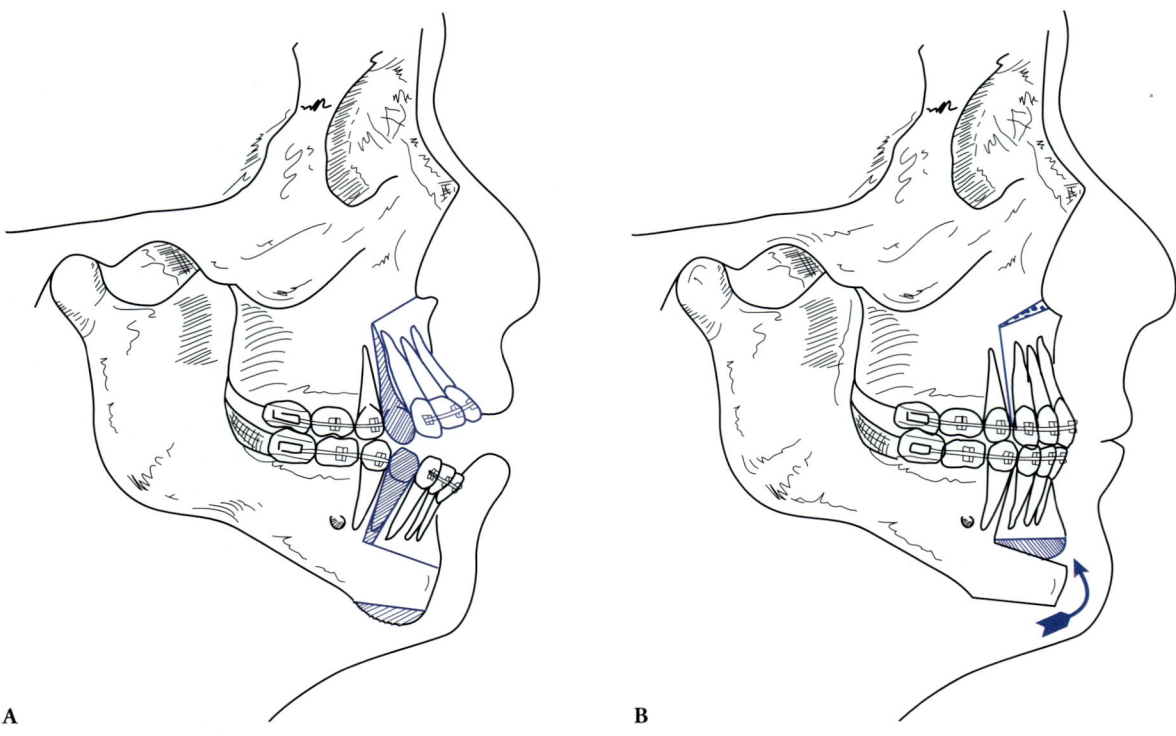

Figure 26–8A and B: Correction of bimaxillary prognathism, excessive facial length, and open bite by alveolar osteotomies and excision of inferior border.

molar. Subperiosteal reflection of the lateral surface of the ramus and very limited posterior border reflection allow for placement of special retractors. A slightly curved oblique osteotomy is performed with oscillating saws from the anterior sigmoid notch to the angle of the mandible, avoiding the lingual area. The mandible is set back by overlapping of the ramus with the condylar segment (Figures 26–9A to C). Direct wire fixation is sometimes used if bone apposition is questionable or condylar sag is apparent. Intermaxillary fixation with wires or elastics is necessary for 6 to 8 weeks. Relapse in the form of a Class III open-bite condition is seen if excessive soft tissue is detached from the condylar segment or if inadequate bone contact occurs between segments. Injury to the inferior alveolar nerve is possible but uncommon. The results are usually quite satisfactory with the VSO, a procedure used for over 45 years extraorally and for over 30 years intraorally.

The inverted "L" osteotomy, a modification of the VSO that maintains the coronoid process, is indicated when the ramus of the mandible is lengthened at surgery to close an anterior open bite with prognathism. Bone blocks are wedged along the horizontal cut to maintain the normal condylar–fossa relation. The sagittal split osteotomy, also used for correction of prognathism with or without an open bite, is more frequently used for mandibular deficiency, and the technique is described in that section.

The body ostectomy is indicated in unusual and very specific cases of prognathism sometimes seen with open bite that is not attributable to excessive maxillary growth or deep bites. If orthodontics and ramus surgery cannot produce an acceptable Class I occlusion and correct a posterior molar crossbite, a body ostectomy may be indicated. The anterior segment is repositioned according to the ostectomy cut, which may be triangular, rectangular, or stepped. The inferior alveolar nerve may require repositioning to perform the ostectomy. Injury to the nerve during this procedure is possible. Fixation of the segments is with wires or bone plates along the inferior border (Figures 26–10A and B).

Surgical Orthodontic Correction of Dentofacial Deformity

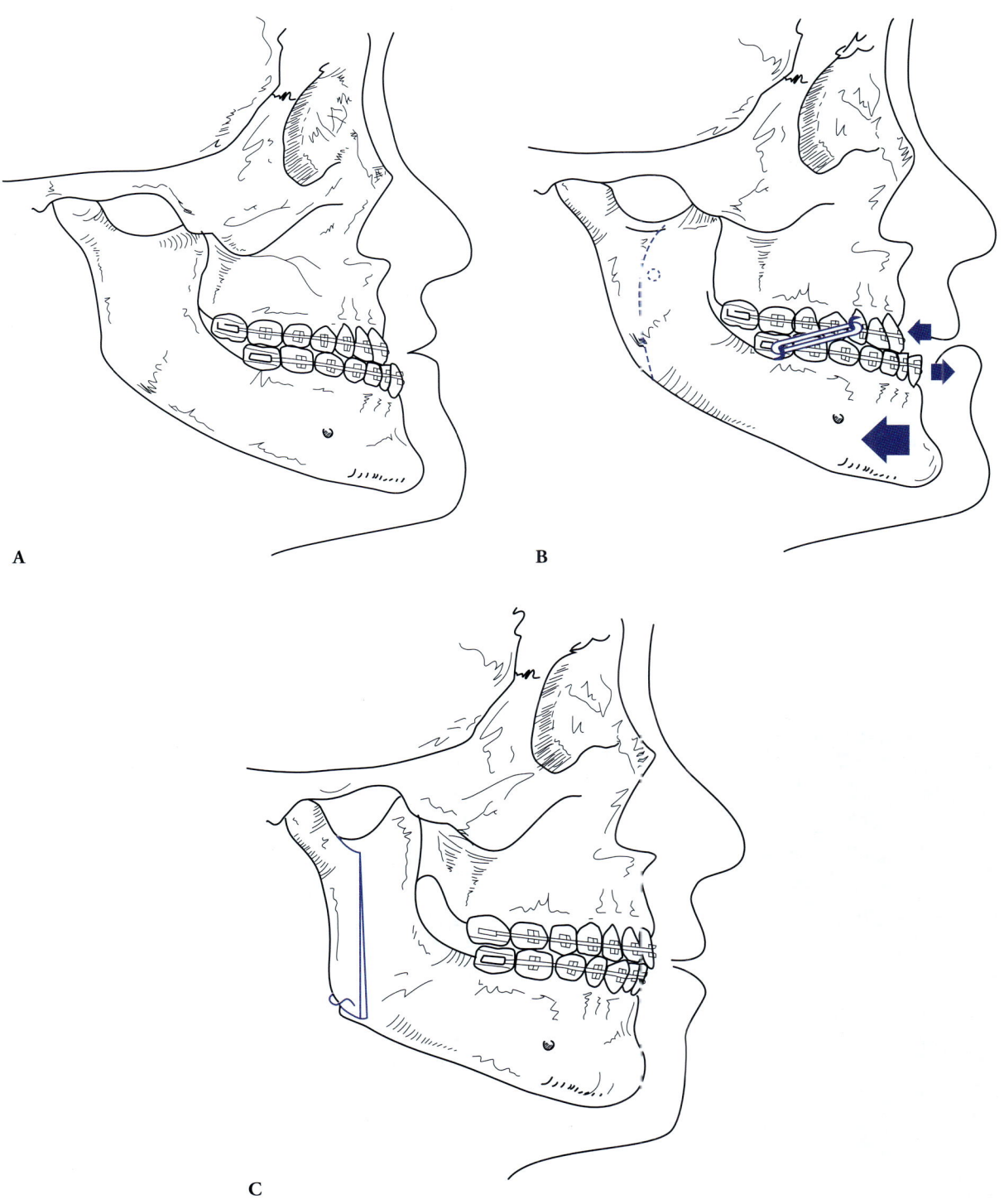

Figure 26–9A to C: *(A)* Profile of hard and soft tissues in classic mandibular prognathism with Class III malocclusion. *(B)* Preoperative orthodontic tooth movement reverses dental compensations, produces correct inclination of incisors, and worsens facial appearance so that mandibular setback maximizes esthetic results. Note the outline of the proposed vertical subcondylar osteotomy. *(C)* Postoperative position of mandible and Class I occlusion following vertical subcondylar osteotomy.

Mandibular prognathism combined with maxillary deformities such as VME or others may result in extreme deformities requiring surgical correction in both jaws (Figures 26–10C and D).

Mandibular Deficiency

In mandibular deficiency, or retrognathism, the soft-tissue characteristics are manifested primarily in the profile view (Figures 26–11 A and B and

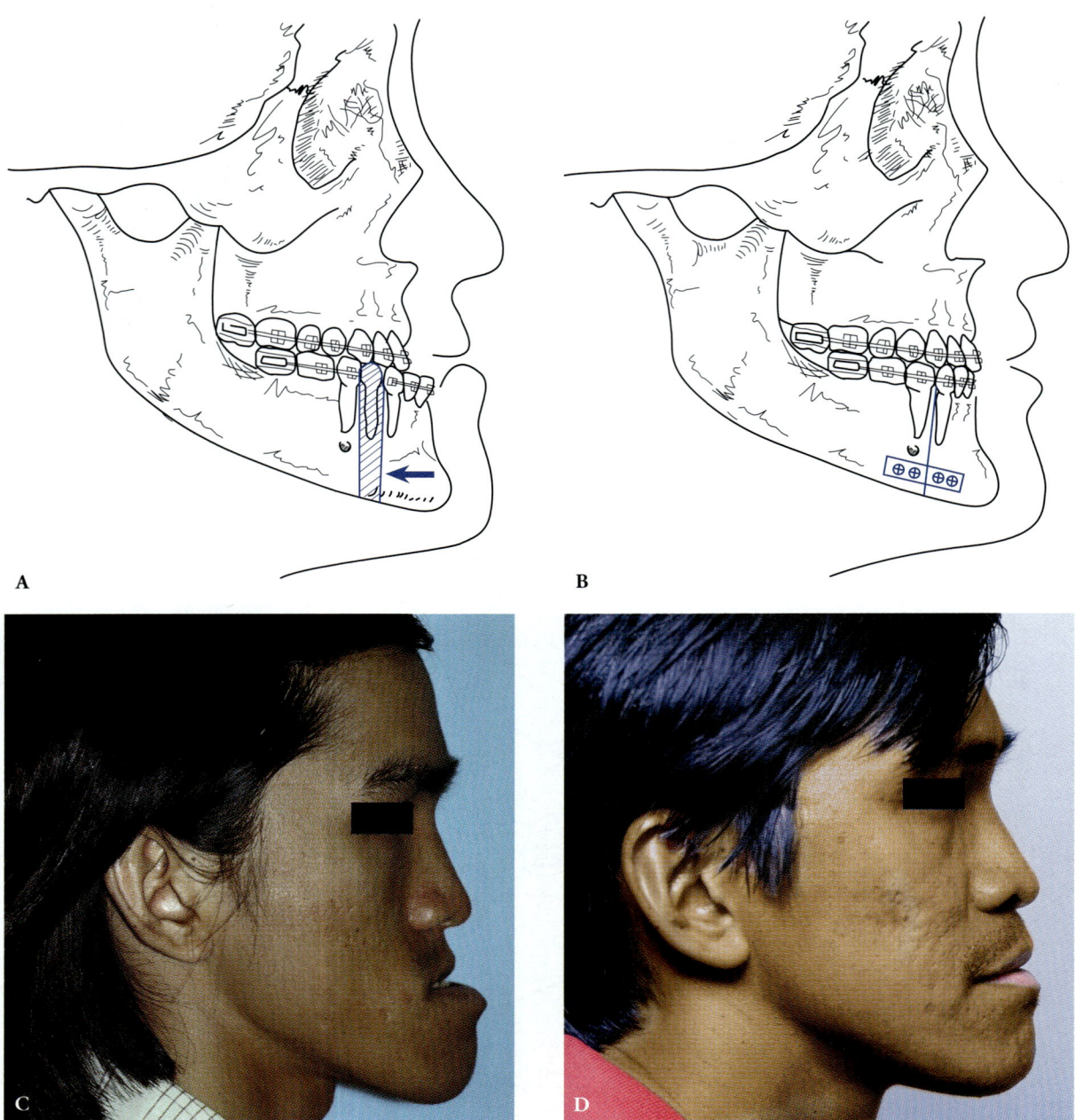

Figure 26–10A to D: *(A)* Correction of mandibular prognathism by body ostectomy through the first premolar site. *(B)* Postoperative stabilization of the mandible with bone plates. *(C)* and *(D)* Presurgical and 5-year postsurgical correction of severe mandibular prognathism and maxillary deficiency by body ostectomy of the mandible (setback) and Le Fort I osteotomy of the maxilla (advancement). Postoperative stabilization of the mandible with bone plates.

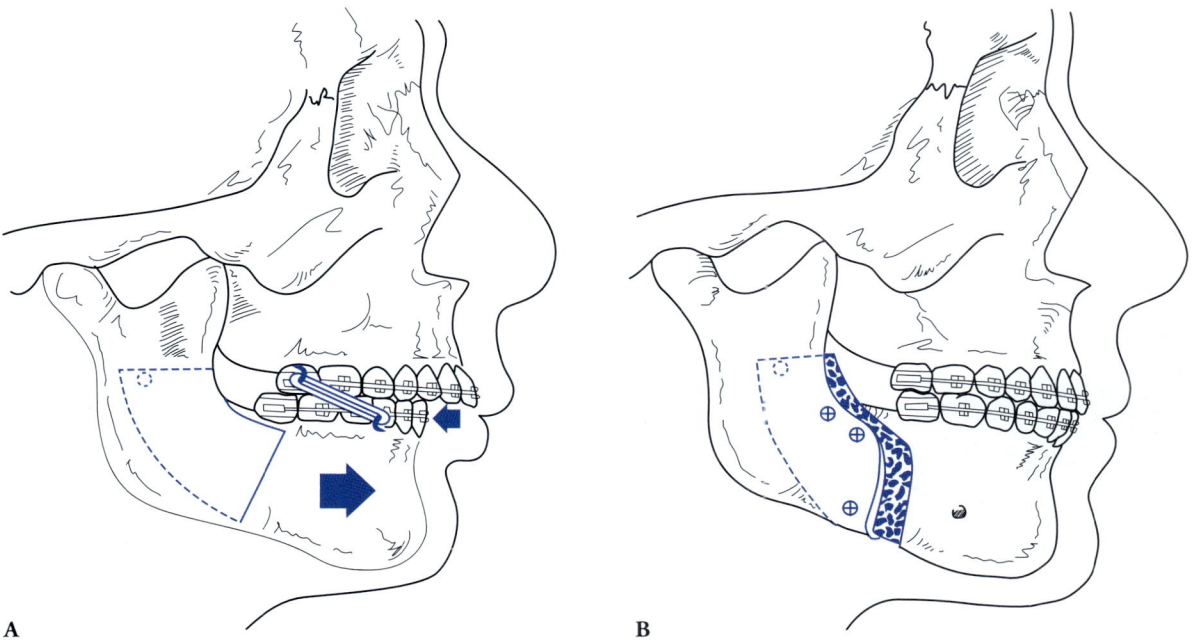

Figure 26–11A and B: *(A)* Profile of hard and soft tissues typical of mandibular deficiency or retrognathism and Class II malocclusion. Preoperative orthodontic treatment reverses dental compensation by uprighting the lower incisors. This permits maximum advancement of the mandible by surgery. Note the outline of the proposed sagittal split osteotomy. *(B)* Mandible advanced by sagittal split osteotomy and stabilized by rigid fixation bone screw technique. Intermaxillary fixation is not required.

26–12 A to D). There will be a short or normal facial height, a deep or normal labiomental sulcus, horizontal deficiency of the lower lip and chin, but a sometimes adequate chin contour. The maxilla may be normal or slightly protrusive, depressing the lower lip. When the patient protrudes the mandible to a Class I posture, the relative protrusion of the maxillary teeth disappears, and the profile view improves. From the frontal view, only the deep mentolabial fold may be apparent (see Figure 26–12A), although often there is evidence of mentalis strain. Cephalometrically, the ANB angle will be increased, the SNB and facial angles will be decreased, and the lower incisors will be protrusive. In Class II, Division 2 types, the maxillary incisors will be retrusive. Dentally, there is an increased overjet, a deep impinging overbite, Class II cuspid and molar relationships bilaterally, and a narrow maxillary arch with transverse discrepancy when the mandible is moved forward.

Orthodontic reversal of dental compensations is necessary to position the teeth over basal bone. The severely flared lower incisors often seen in these cases require lower first premolar bicuspid extractions to achieve significant uprighting. If the horizontal position of the upper incisors is satisfactory, the maxillary second bicuspids may be extracted to exaggerate the Class II molar relationship and minimize the retraction of the maxillary incisors. Seldom are these cases treated with extractions only in the lower arch since Class III molar relationships rarely function well in the occlusal scheme. Class III mechanics are used to retract and upright the lower incisors to the proper axial relationship (see Figure 26–11A). The reciprocal effect of the elastics on the maxillary arch will preclude retraction of the upper incisors, accentuate the overjet, and facilitate maximal surgical advancement of the mandible for improved facial esthetics.

It is preferred to presurgically level the lower arch, although in Class II, Division 2 cases, leveling of the exaggerated curve of Spee, which usually accompanies these types, may be quite difficult. Bite plates are often used to facilitate the leveling. Crowding in the upper arch is usually resolved once the upper incisors have been flared forward to their proper relationship. Class II cases with an acceptable transverse relationship preoperatively may develop posterior crossbites after mandibular advancement. These cases may require significant preoperative maxillary orthodontic expansion or provisions for concomitant surgical expansion of the maxilla.

All surgical procedures for correcting Class II deformities are directed at correcting the majority of horizontal changes with mandibular osteotomies and vertical changes with maxillary osteotomies. Maxillary procedures are described under VME. The sagittal splitting osteotomy (SSO) of Obwegesser is by far

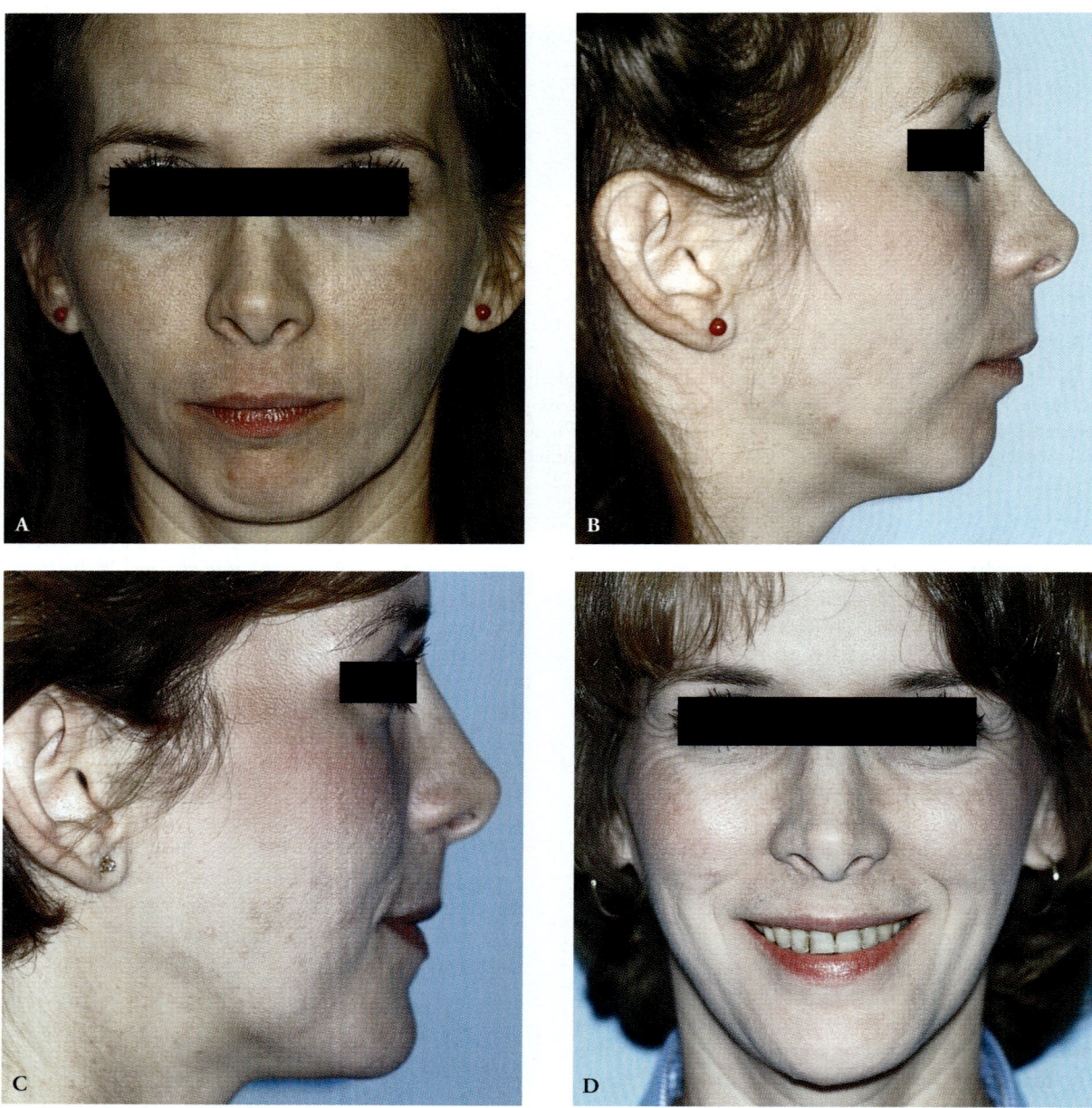

Figure 26–12A to D: Correction of severe mandibular deficiency with microgenia. (A) and (B) Preoperative facial appearance. Note that the chin is retruded and deficient in contour. (C) and (D) Postoperative facial appearance following advancement of the mandible and chin by sagittal split osteotomy and chin implant.

the most frequently used and time-honored procedure for correction of mandibular deficiency with and without open bite and limited facial asymmetry (see Figure 26–11B). The intraoral incision is similar to that used in the VSO procedure. Soft tissue is detached on the medial surface of the ramus and lateral surface of the body but not the lateral ramus surface. Medial ramus and lateral body cortical cuts are joined with an osteotomy cut along the anterior border of the ramus and external oblique ridge. Splitting of the mandible is performed with wide, thin osteotomes and gentle prying. Visualization of the inferior alveolar nerve prior to final separation is key to avoid injury to the nerve. Detachment of the medial pterygoid muscle usually allows full advancement. When anterior border wiring is used to approximate segments, 6 weeks of IMF are usually adequate because of the large area of cancellous bone apposition. More commonly, rigid fixation with bone screws allows for immediate movement of the mandible; however, patients must still be maintained on a liquid diet for several weeks. Temporary anesthesia of the inferior alveolar nerve is frequent, but, fortunately, permanent anesthesia is infrequent. Inappropriate splitting, extensive swelling, and hemorrhage are very infrequent but can occur.

Other procedures such as "C" or "L" osteotomies may be performed either intraorally or extraorally. They are, however, reserved for micrognathia, extreme advancement, or other unusual conditions and may require bone grafting. Additional chin advancement by horizontal osteotomy of the symphysis or chin implant for retrognathia or micrognathia is frequently necessary. These procedures are described below.

Maxillary Excess

Maxillary excess with a normal mandible rarely occurs as a single entity. It is usually accompanied by mandibular deficiency, mandibular excess, or mandibular asymmetry. The facial soft-tissue characteristics of VME are manifested equally in both the frontal and profile views. The facial features are dominated by a long tapering face with a narrow alar base, increased nasolabial angle, lip incompetence, a highly convex profile, a flat mentolabial fold, and usually a deficient chin. Excessive display of maxillary anterior teeth is seen with the lips at rest, and a "gummy smile" is apparent (Figures 26–13A and 3). Cephalometrically, there will be a large increase in the lower anterior facial height and mandibular plane angle and a decrease in posterior

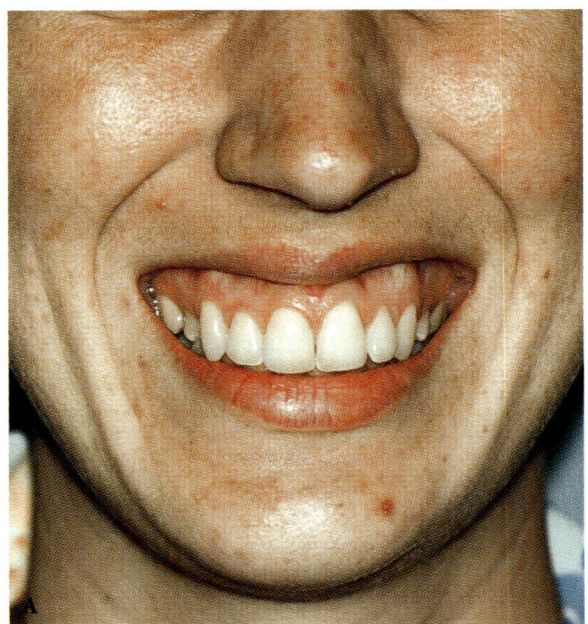
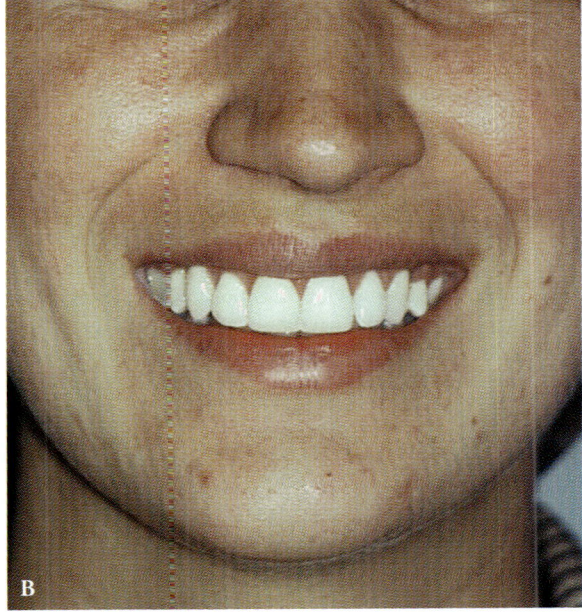

Figure 26–13A and B: Malocclusion and exposed gingiva corrected by superior repositioning of the maxilla with Le Fort I osteotomy.

facial height. Vertical maxillary excess occurs with or without an anterior open bite. Horizontal excess or protrusion of the incisors may be seen, and bilateral posterior crossbites are common.

The mandible may be rotated clockwise (down and back) because of VME (Figure 26–14A).

When a prediction tracing moves the maxilla superiorly to a normal lip–incisor relationship, the mandible will rotate upward and forward toward a more normal position. If this is not the case, surgery to advance the mandible may also be necessary (Figures 26–14B and C). If VME is accompanied by a normal mandible or mandibular excess,

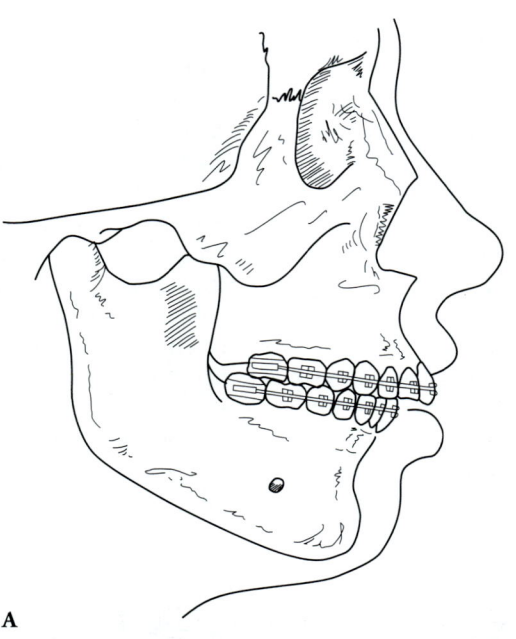

A

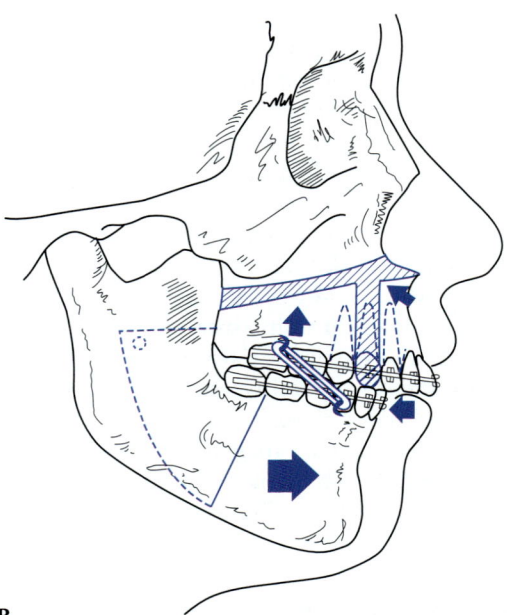

B

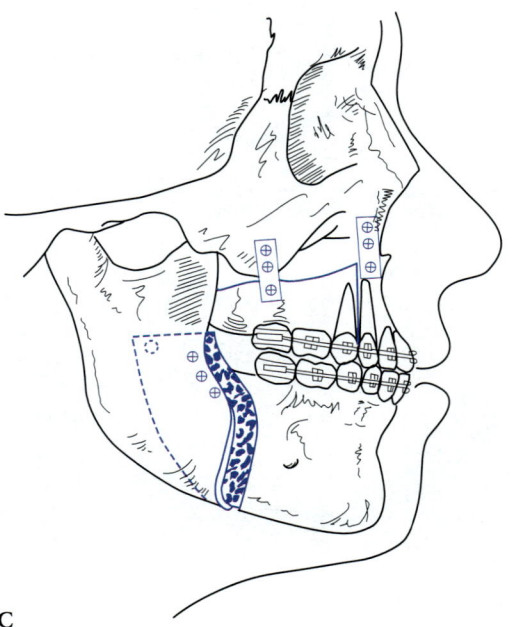

C

Figure 26–14A to C: *(A)* Vertical maxillary excess is characterized by excessive exposure of incisors, lip incompetence, mandibular deficiency, and increased anterior facial height. *(B)* Preoperative tracing shows orthodontic changes that preserve the deformity by uprighting lower incisors and maintaining the maxillary arch position. Treatment is extraction of maxillary premolars, maxillary and mandibular movement through Le Fort I osteotomy of the maxilla with anterior/posterior splitting, and mandibular advancement by sagittal split osteotomy. *(C)* Stabilization of maxilla and mandible by rigid fixation—bone plates and screws.

mandibular setback surgery may be necessary to correct a protruding mandible that is rotated forward secondary to maxillary superior positioning.

Although extractions are frequently required to alleviate crowding, it is often desirable to delay extractions in the upper arch until the time of surgery, using the teeth to be extracted to aid in the leveling and alignment of the posterior segments and to preserve the alveolar bony dimensions. By performing segmental osteotomies with a Le Fort I osteotomy, the surgeon can retract and upright protrusive maxillary incisors and expand or advance posterior segments (see Figure 26–14B). If space is required in the arch, the extraction sites should be closed completely preoperatively. The curve of Spee in the lower arch should be leveled completely.

Presurgical orthodontic treatment of VME cases differs greatly from that of prognathic or retrognathic cases. Since the extrusion of teeth via conventional orthodontic mechanics is potentially unstable, mechanics that would produce this effect are avoided in all instances. Intramaxillary mechanics are used extensively, rather than Class II, Class III, or headgear forces, and deliberate care is taken to ensure the preservation of any open bite. Segmental rather than complete arch leveling is necessary in the maxilla to preserve an exaggerated compensating curve or "stepped" occlusion in the canine region (see Figure 26–14B). In those cases in which the maxilla is to be surgically segmentalized and no extractions are contemplated, it is helpful to diverge the dental roots for passage of the surgical saw. Historically, maxillas were segmentalized between the canines and first premolars. With orthodontic support, more osteotomies are performed between the canines and lateral incisors. Since bilateral crossbites often accompany VME cases, it is often preferable to plan for surgical expansion in the posterior segments at the time the osteotomies are performed.

Vertical changes in the maxilla through Le Fort I osteotomy and concomitant vertical and horizontal changes in the mandible by surgery may produce tremendous functional and esthetic results (Figures 26–15A to C). Le Fort I osteotomy of the maxilla is usually performed through a vestibular incision 5 mm superior to the mucogingival junction from the first molar to the first molar. Tunneling beneath the mucoperiosteum to the pterygoid plates and reflection of the nasal mucosa from the floor of the nose allow for osteotomes and air-driven saws to produce osteotomies for down-fracture of the maxilla from pterygoid plates, nasal septum, lateral maxillary, and nasal walls. The amount of bone to be excised is determined from mock surgery and measurements on models mounted on an anatomic articulator. Division of the maxilla in the canine area or between the central incisors allows for a variety of vertical, horizontal, and transverse movements of all segments. Turbinectomy, nasal septal straightening, palatal repositioning, and buccal lipectomies are frequently done to anatomically correct all aspects of VME. An intermediate splint keyed to the unoperated mandible ensures correct superior positioning of the maxilla. Once the maxilla is stabilized with wires or bone plates, mandibular surgery is performed if necessary. The mandible is stabilized with a final splint to the newly positioned maxilla. Intermaxillary fixation is rarely indicated. Rather, light elastics between the maxilla and mandible will correct any minor occlusal discrepancies into the final occlusal splint.

Maxillary Deficiency

Maxillary deficiency most commonly associated with other deformities can occur in all three planes of space: anteroposterior, vertical, and transverse. Transverse deficiency or posterior crossbite can be bilateral or unilateral and is most commonly associated with other deformities. The apparent transverse deficiency accompanying true mandibular prognathism is usually resolved with the surgical repositioning of the mandible. Class II deformities usually do not have posterior crossbites until the mandible is advanced into the planned Class I position. Concomitant maxillary posterior segmental osteotomies may be required if palatal expansion is not possible. Many VME cases, especially the open-bite types, have transverse deficiency, which is corrected with segmental Le Fort I osteotomies.

Vertical maxillary deficiency usually has the appearance of an edentulous patient not wearing an upper denture (Figures 26–16A and B) The soft tissue will appear squashed, with the teeth in occlusion, and the mandible may appear to be prognathic. With the mandible in the normal rest position, significant freeway space is seen, and a more normal profile is observed. Cephalometrically, the SNA will be normal, the SNB may be increased, the mandibular plane may be decreased, and anterior facial dimensions and the ANB will be decreased. The occlusion will vary from borderline Class I to Class III. It is important to note the lack of display of a normal amount of the maxillary incisor with the upper lip at rest. The rest position must always be used for diagnosis and treatment planning since smile patterns vary too much and have only limited value. We treat to idealize the incisor shown at rest, not at smile.

Anteroposterior or horizontal deficiency will have a soft-tissue appearance similar to that of true mandibular prognathism. A decreased SNA and ANB and an obtuse nasolabial angle are characteristic. The addition of several wide strips of wax or a cotton sponge under the upper lip may improve

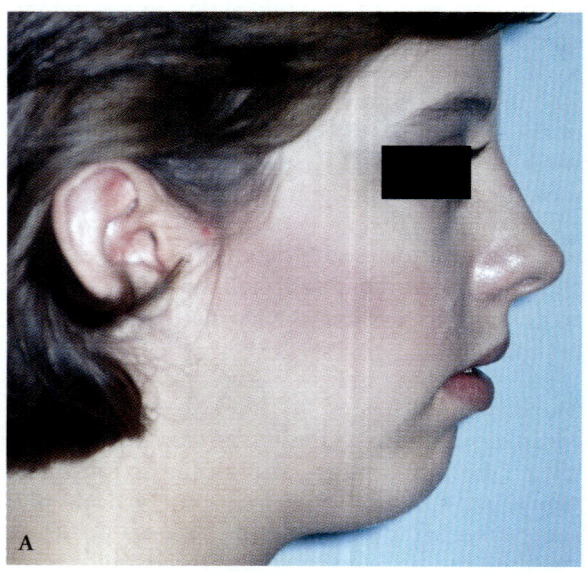

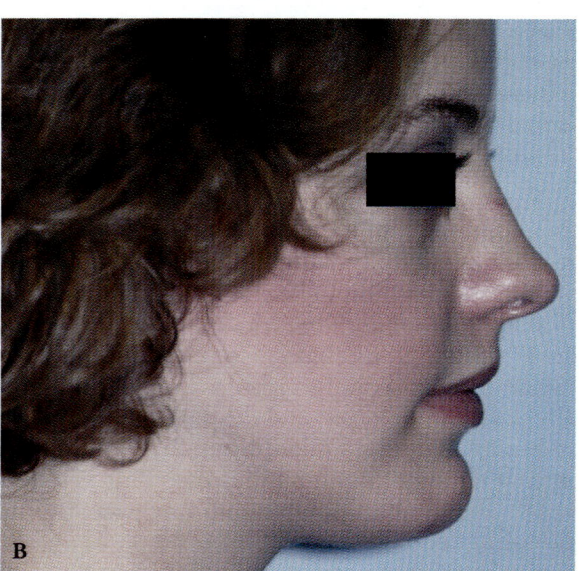

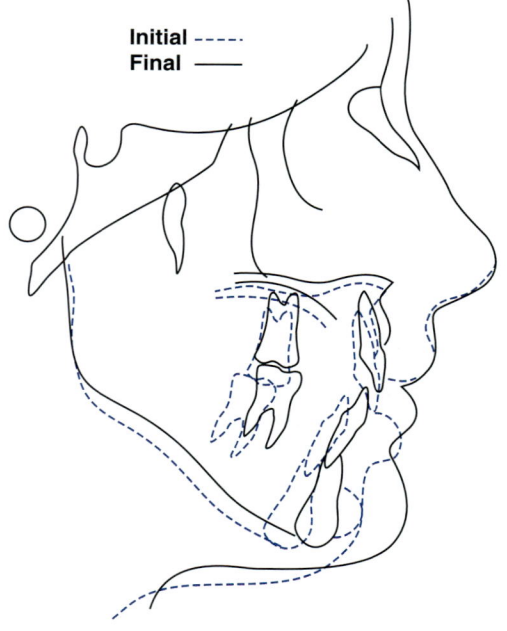

Figure 26–15A to C: Severe convex dentofacial deformity with vertical maxillary excess, mandibular deficiency, and Class II malocclusion. *(A)* Preoperative profile with relaxed lips shows true amount of lip incompetence. *(B)* Three-year postoperative profile following orthodontic treatment, superior repositioning of the maxilla by Le Fort I osteotomy, advancement of the mandible by sagittal split osteotomy, and an alloplastic cheekbone and chin implant. *(C)* Initial pretreatment and 3-year final cephalometric tracing.

the profile. Patients with cleft lip and palate with failure to develop the normal horizontal and vertical positions of the maxilla represent a common type of horizontal maxillary deficiency (Figures 26–17A to D).

Vertical and horizontal maxillary lengthening or advancement through Le Fort I osteotomy can produce dramatic results (see Figures 26–16 and 26–17). Special consideration must be given to methods of stabilization and fixation. In horizontal deficiencies, the bone of the maxilla is characteristically very thin. With advancement, bone contact may be minimal or inadequate. Stable results are obtained with the use of autologous bone from the iliac crest or cortical-cancellous demineralized bone products placed in defects of the lateral maxillary wall and between the posterior maxillary wall and pterygoid plates. Rigid internal fixation with wires or malleable bone plates will produce predictable results without IMF. If simultaneous mandibular surgery is necessary, rigid fixation of the sagittal split osteotomy may also eliminate IMF.

Facial Asymmetry

Diagnosis and surgical orthodontic treatment of facial asymmetry such as condylar hyperplasia or hemifacial microsomia is perhaps more difficult, challenging, and dramatic than any other deformity. Variations of asymmetry are common, corrective procedures are less standardized, and, in many cases, much original thought is required. An elaborate preoperative work-up from multiple radiographic views is required to confirm the diagnosis, eliminate uncommon pathology as an etiology, and arrive at a treatment plan.

There is always a certain amount of asymmetry to the face and to the mandible. In many instances, the face, although slightly asymmetric, is attractive, projects warmth, and is an integral part of an individual's character. Pronounced asymmetry, however, has been detrimental to character development and social and economic progress. Equally important but only recently appreciated are the functional deficits associated with facial or mandibular asymmetry. Fortunately, correction of form almost always improves function.

It is the dentist's responsibility to seek surgical evaluation of patients for whom restorative dentistry is proposed to correct an asymmetric mandible or maxilla. In more recent times, numerous uncomplicated surgical procedures have produced dramatic

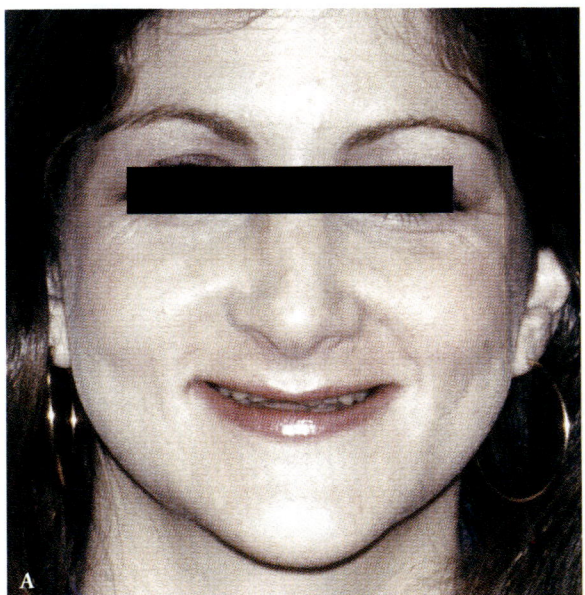
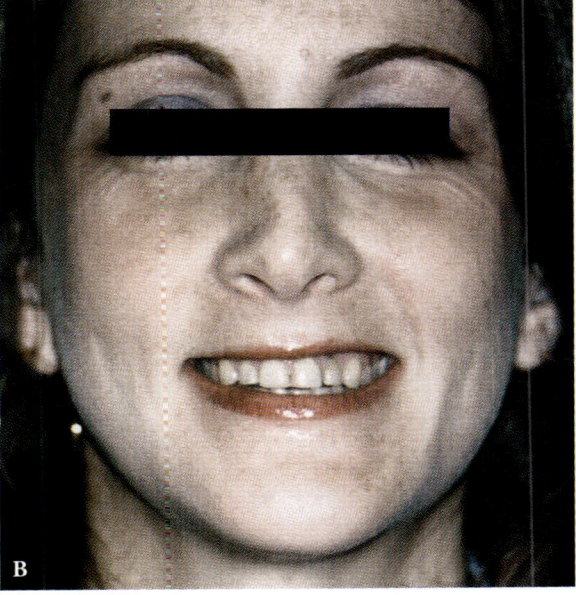

Figure 26–16A and B: Vertical maxillary deficiency corrected by inferior repositioning of the maxilla (downgrafting) with Le Fort I osteotomy and autogenous iliac crest bone graft. (A) Preoperative frontal view demonstrates decreased facial length and hidden maxillary incisors on smiling. (B) Postoperative view demonstrates increased facial length and exposure of maxillary incisors.

796 Esthetics in Dentistry

improvements in appearance and function for patients formerly considered beyond help. Because of the complexity of the deformity, treatment is individualized and may involve osteotomies, recontouring, and associated soft-tissue surgery.

A classification of asymmetry is necessary for proper diagnosis and treatment (Table 26–1).

Condylar hyperplasia is the most common cause of asymmetry, resulting from overproduction or

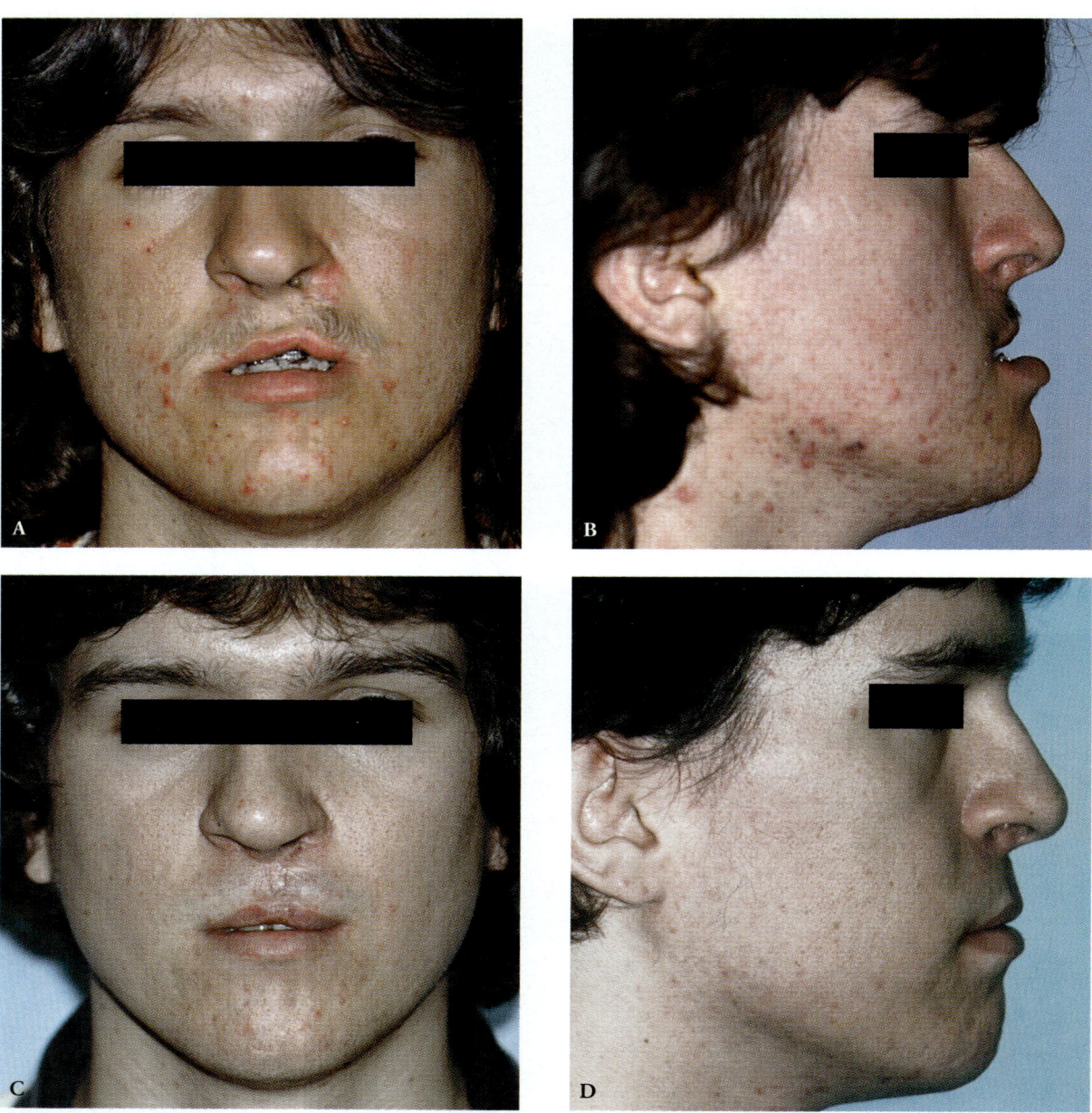

Figure 26–17A to D: Vertical, horizontal, and transverse maxillary deficiencies in a patient with cleft lip and palate and severe Class III malocclusion. (A) Preoperative facial appearance. (B) Profile before surgery following orthodontic treatment to correct dental compensations. (C) Postoperative frontal view at 3 years. (D) Profile 3 years following orthodontics, advancement, and expansion of the maxilla by Le Fort I osteotomy with autogenous iliac crest bone graft, closure of oronasal fistula, and secondary repair of the lip.

prolonged production of cartilage in the condyle. The usual deformity is an enlarged condyle and elongated condylar neck. The result is an outward bowing of the ramus and the body and a downward growth of the mandible that may produce an open bite on the involved side and a crossbite on the opposite side. If the onset is before puberty, the maxilla grows downward and maintains some degree of occlusion with the mandible. If the onset were late, one would not expect to find a downgrowth of the maxilla but instead a developing open bite.

Treatment planning for facial asymmetry involves careful notation of all facial and dental relationships. The facial, chin, and dental midlines are marked (Figure 26–18A). The vertical differences in right to left mandibular inferior borders are noted, including the degree of occlusal plane cant (Figure 26–18B). Bone scans and serial radiographs are helpful to determine remaining condylar growth potential. Photographs, cephalometric analysis, and models mounted on an anatomic articulator aid in treatment planning. Model surgery determines the exact bony movements to be carried out during surgery (Figures 26–18C to F).

As in the case presented, a Le Fort I osteotomy is performed first to achieve normal tooth lip esthetics and a level maxilla with correct positioning in all directions. Ramus osteotomies and possible condylectomy follow maxillary surgery. A condylectomy may be indicated in cases of hyperplasia and hypertrophy where additional growth is anticipated and pain and dysfunction are noted. Otherwise, a subcondylar osteotomy is used on the side being shortened, and a sagittal split, or "L" osteotomy with graft, is used on the side being lengthened (Figures 26–18A to H). Inferior border leveling by ostectomy and genioplasty by sliding horizontal osteotomy may be necessary in severe cases. Facial onlay procedures with alloplasts or tissue transfer are also used to refine symmetry. Space limitation does not permit a discussion of hemifacial microsomia and other facial asymmetries.

Adjunctive Hard-Tissue and Soft-Tissue Procedures

The most common adjunctive procedure performed at the time of orthognathic surgery is the genioplasty (chin reshaping). Other procedures commonly performed simultaneously include rhinoplasty, septoplasty, onlay augmentation, submental lipectomy/liposculpture, buccal lipectomy, platysmaplasty, lip augmentation, reduction cheiloplasty, V-Y lip advancement (to lengthen the upper lip), and alar cinch (to narrow the alar base).

Osteotomies and alloplastic implant augmentation are commonly employed when facial contour deficit exists in the presence of a normal occlusion or when maxillary or mandibular surgery to correct malocclusion fails to satisfy esthetic requirements. When properly performed, both the osteotomy and alloplastic augmentation are quite stable. Chin contour correction by an osteotomy is usually performed through an intraoral vestibular incision. Horizontal augmentation or advancement of a deficient chin occurs with a sliding horizontal osteotomy of the symphysis (Figure 26–19), a chin implant, or a combination thereof for extreme deformity. The chin is pedicled to the genioglossus and geniohyoid muscles to maintain blood supply, and direct wiring or plating stabilizes the segment. The soft-tissue augmentation change is at least 70% of the amount of bone advancement (Figures 26–20A to D).

If excessive vertical dimension exists, a wedge of bone may be removed. Likewise, a short chin may be lengthened by interposing bone or hydroxylapatite

Table 26–1. Classification of Asymmetry

1. Overdevelopment
    Hemihypertrophy (facial)
    Condylar hyperplasia
    Mandibular hypertrophy (macrognathia)
    Deviation prognathism (laterognathia)
    Unilateral masseteric hypertrophy
    Alveolar (maxillary or mandibular)

2. Underdevelopment
    Hemifacial microsomia
    Condylar hypoplasia
    Mandibular hypoplasia
    Alveolar (maxillary or mandibular)
    Treacher Collins syndrome
        (mandibulofacial dysostosis)

3. Acquired states of asymmetry
    TMJ ankylosis from trauma
    Tumors
    Infections
    Inflammation

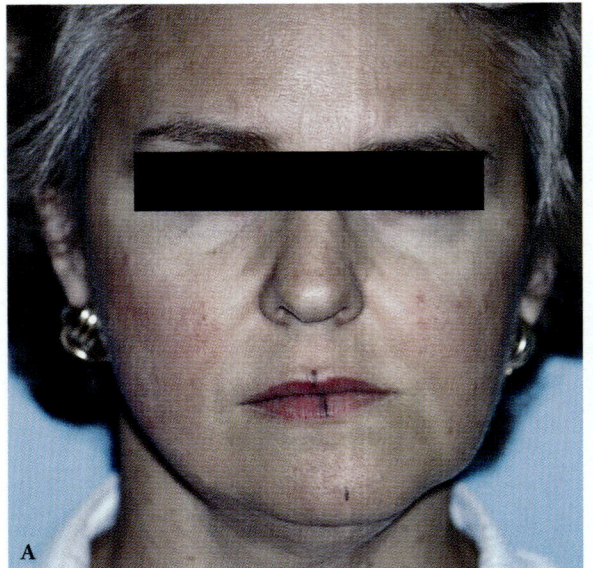
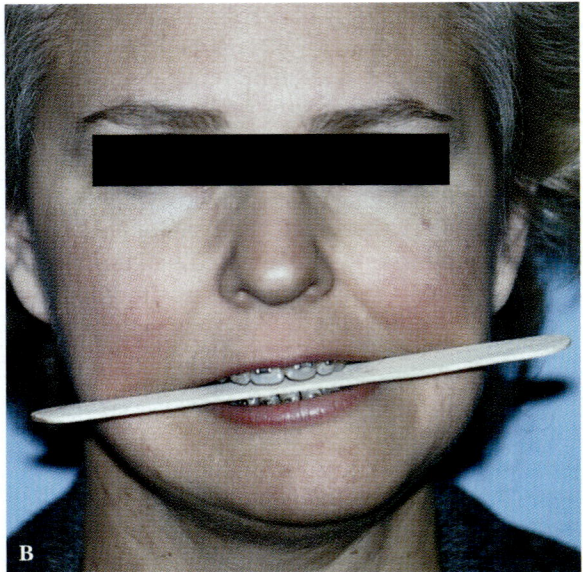
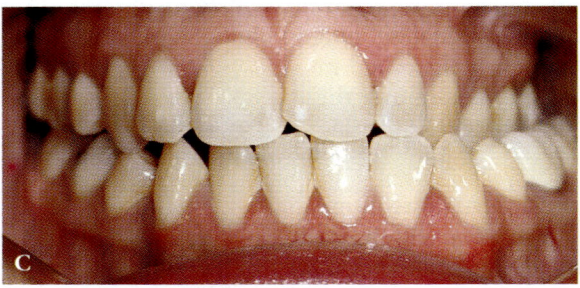
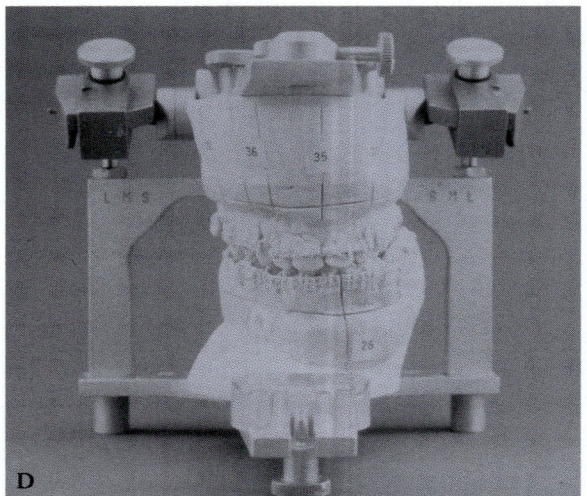
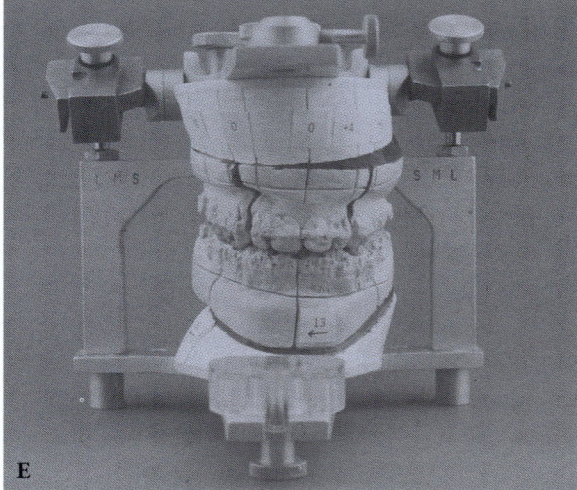

Figure 26–18A to E: *(A)* Maxillary and mandibular dental midlines and chin midline are marked on a patient with facial asymmetry secondary to right condylar hypoplasia. *(B)* Occlusal plane cant. *(C)* Pretreatment occlusion. *(D)* Study models mounted on an anatomic articulator properly scored prior to model surgery. *(E)* After "mock" surgery employing maxillary and mandibular osteotomies with measured movements.

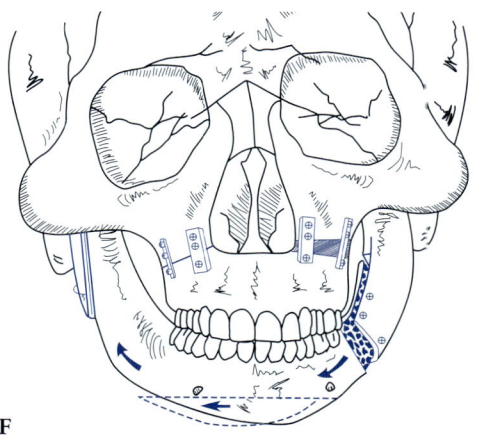

F

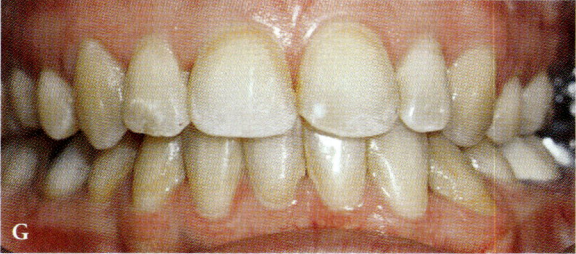

G

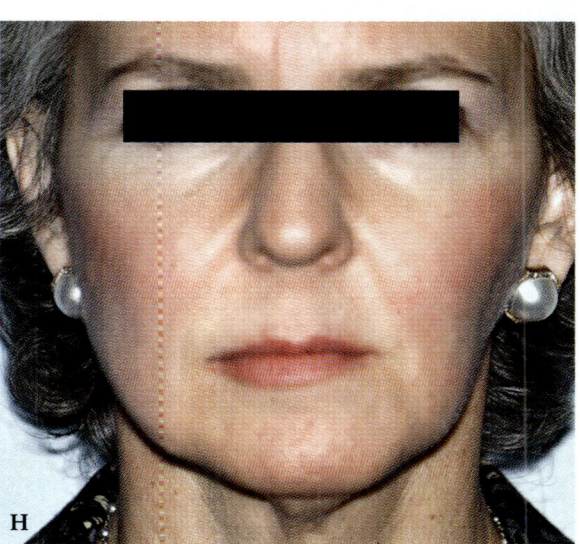

H

Figure 26–18F to H: *(F)* Facial asymmetry secondary to right condylar hypoplasia corrected by Le Fort I osteotomy of the maxilla downgrafting the left side, left sagittal split osteotomy advancement and rotation, and right vertical subcondylar osteotomy setback of the mandible. If required, horizontal osteotomy of the mandible permits additional lateral movement of the chin. *(G)* Two-year postoperative occlusion. *(H)* Two-year postoperative frontal appearance of the patient with correction of right condylar hyperplasia and facial asymmetry.

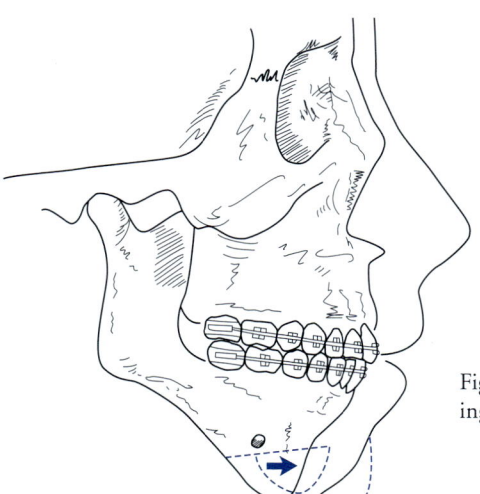

Figure 26–19: Advancement genioplasty by intraoral sliding horizontal osteotomy of the symphysis.

blocks. Prominent and excessively long chins may be reduced by chin shaves but are more accurately corrected by reverse sliding of the symphysis with a horizontal osteotomy and/or ostectomy of excess bone.

Alloplastic implants used for mandibular, facial, and cranial augmentation most commonly employed today include silicone rubber (ie, Implantech, Ventura, CA), porous polyethylene (ie, Medpore, Porex Surgical, Newnan, GA), and expanded polytetrafluoroethylene (ie, Gore-Tex, W.L. Gore and Associates, Flagstaff, AZ). These materials are preformed to fit particular anatomic areas and can be trimmed and or recontoured. They are placed sub-

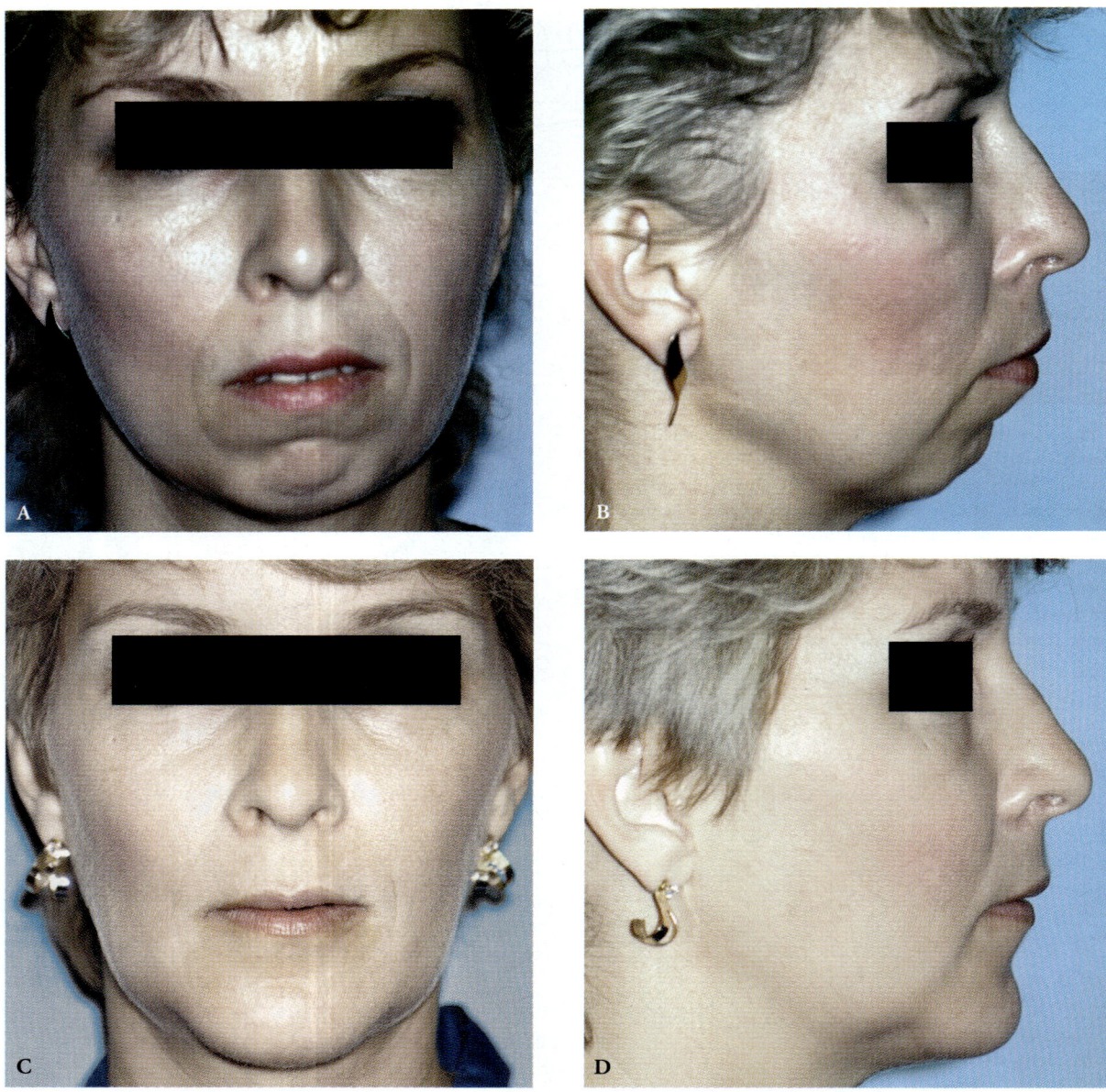

Figure 26–20A to D: *(A)* Preoperative frontal view of patient with chin deficiency. *(B)* Preoperative profile appearance. *(C)* Postoperative appearance following advancement of the chin with sliding horizontal osteotomy and chin implant placed over advanced chin. *(D)* Postoperative profile appearance.

periostally through intraoral incisions and secured with sutures, wires, or bone screws. Chin and cheekbone augmentations with alloplast are very commonly used to enhance the surgical treatment of dentofacial deformities (see Figures 26–7C, 26–15B, and 26–20D).

Additional Resources

Bell WH, ed. Modern practice in orthognathic and reconstructive surgery. Philadelphia: WB Saunders, 1992.

Bell WH, Jacobs JD, Quejada JG. Simultaneous repositioning of the maxilla, mandible, and chin. Treatment planning and analysis of soft tissues. Am J Orthod 1986;89:28–50.

Carlotti AE Jr, Aschaffenburg PH, Schendel SA. Facial changes associated with surgical advancement of the lip and maxilla. J Oral Maxillofac Surg 1986;44:593–6.

Carlotti AE Jr, Schendel SA. An analysis of factors influencing stability of surgical advancement of the maxilla by the Le Fort I osteotomy. J Oral Maxillofac Surg 1987;45:924–8.

Crawford SD. Class II division 1 history of TMJ trauma—maxilla and mandible orthognathic surgery. Orthod Rev 1988;2:18–25.

Ellis E III. Bimaxillary surgery using an intermediate splint to position the maxilla. J Oral Maxillofac Surg 1999;57:53–6.

Epker BN. Esthetic maxillofacial surgery. Philadelphia: Lea & Febiger, 1994.

Epker BN, Stella JP, Fish LC, eds. Dentofacial deformities: integrated orthodontic and surgical correction. St. Louis: CV Mosby, 1995.

Fonseca RJ, ed. Oral and maxillofacial surgery. In: Betts NJ, Turvey TA, eds. Orthognathic surgery. Vol 2. Philadelphia: WB Saunders, 2000.

Gallagher DM, Bell WH, Storum KA. Soft tissue changes associated with advancement genioplasty performed concomitantly with superior repositioning of the maxilla. J Oral Maxillofac Surg 1984;42:238–42.

Gao YM, Qiu WL, Tang YS, et al. Evaluation of the treatment for micromandibular deformity by distraction osteogenesis with submerged intraoral device. Chin J Dent Res 1999;2:31–7.

Hiranaka DK, Kelly JP. Stability of simultaneous orthognathic surgery on the maxilla and mandible: a computer-assisted cephalometric study. Int J Adult Orthodon Orthognath Surg 1987;2:193–213.

Lapp TH. Bimaxillary surgery without the use of an intermediate splint to position the maxilla. J Oral Maxillofac Surg 1999;57:57–60.

Major PW, Philippson GE, Glover KE, et al. Stability of maxilla downgrafting after rigid or wire fixation. J Oral Maxillofac Surg 1996;54:1287–91.

Manna LM, Berger JR. Technique for vertical positioning of the maxilla after Le Fort osteotomy. J Oral Maxillofac Surg 1996;54:652.

Masui I, Honda T, Uji T. Two-step repositioning of the maxilla in bimaxillary orthognathic surgery. Br J Oral Maxillofac Surg 1997;35:64–6.

Posnick JC. Craniofacial dysostosis. Staging of reconstruction and management of the midface deformity. Neurosurg Clin N Am 1991;2:683–702.

Posnick JC, Tompson B. Modification of the maxillary Le Fort I osteotomy in cleft-orthognathic surgery: the unilateral cleft lip and palate deformity. J Oral Maxillofac Surg 1992;50:666–75.

Posnick JC, Tompson B. Modification of the maxillary Le Fort I osteotomy in cleft-orthognathic surgery: the bilateral cleft lip and palate deformity. J Oral Maxillofac Surg 1993;51:2–11.

Rosen HM. Segmental osteotomies of the maxilla. Clin Plast Surg 1989;16:785–94.

Schendel SA, Williamson LW. Muscle reorientation following superior repositioning of the maxilla. J Oral Maxillofac Surg 1983;41:235–40.

Schwestka R, Engelke D, Kubein-Meesenburg D, et al. Control of vertical position of the maxilla in orthognathic surgery: clinical application of the sandwich splint. Int J Adult Orthodon Orthognath Surg 1990;5:133–6.

Shetty V, Caridad JM, Caputo AA, et al. Biomechanical rationale for surgical-orthodontic expansion of the adult maxilla. J Oral Maxillofac Surg 1994;52:742–9.

Song HC, Throckmorton GS, Ellis E III, et al. Functional and morphologic alterations after anterior or inferior repositioning of the maxilla. J Oral Maxillofac Surg 1997;55:41–9.

Sperber GH. Craniofacial development. Hamilton, ON: BC Decker, 2001.

Stanchina R, Ellis E III, Gallo WJ, et al. A comparison of two measures for repositioning the maxilla during orthognathic surgery. Int J Adult Orthodon Orthognath Surg 1988;3:149–54.

Sullivan SM. Isolated inferior repositioning of the maxilla, with or without bone grafting, is a very unstable orthognathic procedure which is confirmed by these surgeons' results. Aesthetic Plast Surg 2000;24:72–5.

Turvey TA. Simultaneous mobilization of the maxilla and mandible: surgical technique and results. J Oral Maxillofac Surg 1982;40:96–9.

Vu HL, Panchal J, Levine N. Combined simultaneous distraction osteogenesis of the maxilla and mandible using a single distraction device in hemifacial microsomia. J Craniofac Surg 2001;12:253–8.

Wessberg GA, O'Ryan FS, Washburn MC, et al. Neuromuscular adaptation to surgical superior repositioning of the maxilla. J Maxillofac Surg 1981;9:117–22.

Wilmot JJ, Barber HD, Chou DG, et al. Associations between severity of dentofacial deformity and motivation for orthodontic-orthognathic surgery treatment. Angle Orthod 1993;63:283–8.

Zarrinkelk HM, Throckmorton GS, Ellis E III, et al. Functional and morphologic alterations secondary to superior repositioning of the maxilla. J Oral Maxillofac Surg 1995;53:1258–67.

Part 6

Esthetic Problems of Special Populations

Chapter 27

Esthetics in Pediatric Dentistry

Claudia Caprioglio, DDS, MS, Alberto Caprioglio, DDS, MS, Damaso Caprioglio, MD, MS

In the period ranging from the end of the primary dentition to the first phases of the early mixed one, the esthetics and harmony of dental arches are determined by the physiologic change of dental elements, the presence of diastemas, the correct canine relationship, and the correct occlusive plane. The occlusion of the primary dentition should be considered as a biological unit, having special esthetic, functional, and skeletal characteristics. In fact, the main duty of the pediatric dentist is the monitoring of growth through adolescence.

The dual duty of the pediatric dentist is expressed not only by the application of preventive and/or conservative dentistry but also by the space management required to produce a morphic-functional recovery.

MATERIALS AND TECHNIQUES

In the primary dentition, it is necessary to consider a therapeutic strategy evaluating the physiologic state of the deciduous element and the efficacy of the treatment. A careful diagnosis must be carried out to define the relevant prognosis. Insignificant therapeutic improvements can result from a poor awareness of pulpal treatment options and lead to unnecessary treatment procedures and materials. The introduction of light-cured composite resins has changed clinical pediatric dentistry. In fact, these materials are welcome treatment options that address both esthetic and functional issues. Their advantages are represented by considerable hardness, high rigidity, and a high level of resistance to compression. However, these materials are very sensitive to technique and can show marginal infiltrations, a reduced resistance to wear, polymerization contractions, surface roughness, and discoloration.

Composite resins are the material of choice to restore anterior teeth. The composite resins recommended are microfilled hybrid composite resins. More research into these materials has led to considerable improvements, particularly in traumatology, thus making possible the tooth fragment reattachment. This, in turn, has allowed dentists to proceed to a true biological restoration to achieve a good anterior guide, improved resistance to wear, and higher color stability in the follow-up years.[2]

Composite resins for posterior teeth can be used for Class I and II restorations, where etching time is extremely important. Some authors emphasized that few statistical differences were found for surface roughness in the primary dentition.[15,16] Further, the use of a glass ionomer cement as a cavity base and the reconstruction of the tooth by applying the incremental technique and using a rubber dam have reduced the wear index and improved cavity adhesion. The kind of (direct or incremental) polymerization influences the marginal adaptation.

Glass Ionomers and Modified Ionomer Cements

These materials appeared for the first time in the early 1970s.[20] They are composed of a powder, a calcium-fluoride-aluminium silicate glass, and a liquid, generally a polyacrylic or polymaleic acid. Considering their link with dentin, fluoride-leaching properties, and high resilience range, the use of these materials has been advantageous in the treatment of caries lesions in primary molar teeth.

Although the percentage of failure is higher in comparison with the amalgam (33% versus 20% for amalgam), and although they lack resilience to abrasion and have a low brightness, they have a great advantage: they result in minimal destruction of sound tooth tissue and a reduced use of local anesthetic.

Berg described the resin-modified glass ionomer cements as materials that can be polymerized and whose resin compound improves the resistance to fractures.[6] They are suggested for Class I and II restorations in primary teeth, which typically do not last beyond 3 years.

Compomers

These materials were introduced in the early 1990s. They are composed of a mixed composite resin with an acid modification, which makes them more similar to composite resins than to glass ionomers. They do not have the improved characteristics of resins but are easy to handle, which reduces operative time and makes them a good restorative solution.

A recent study by El-Kalla and Garcia-Godoy evaluated and measured the resistance to compression, resistance to flexing, microhardness, and roughness of the surface of three different compomers (Compoglass [Ivoclar Vivadent, Amherst, NY], Dyract [DENTSPLY/Caulk, Milford, DE], and Hytac [3M ESPE, St. Paul, MN]).[12] Subsequently, these values have been compared to those of a composite resin (Z 100 [3M ESPE]) and to a modified glass-ionomer (Vitremer [3M ESPE]). The results demonstrated that the tested compomers had flexing, compression, and microhardness qualities that were higher than cement but lower than composite resin, whereas no significant differences in surface roughness were reported.

The properties of compomers consist of

- A good adhesion to dental tissues (a dentinal adhesive is used instead of acid etching);
- Easy handling, enhanced by the possibility of incremental polymerization;
- A reduced marginal fissure due to their property of absorbing water during hardening;
- A good fluoride adsorption-release system; and
- An acceptable range of colors and brightness that produces good esthetics, although not quite comparable to that of composite resin.

Because of the availability of these restorative materials, the pediatric dentist can apply preventive measures and perform early conservative therapy or, in the most severe cases, restore function and improve esthetics.

The increased predictive capabilities of the outcome of treatment along with improvement in materials enable compliance with the relevant postulates for successful pediatric dentistry:

- improvement of esthetic restoration
- elimination of infection, inflammation, and pain
- maintenance of the arch perimeter length
- stimulation of the alveolar growth

See Table 27–1 for a selection of materials for clinical use.

The improved treatment techniques, better materials, and heightened awareness of the benefits of preventive dentistry have led to better management and predictable results. There are also additional means of cavity excavation, representing alternative therapeutic solutions: Carisolv and air abrasion.

Carisolv

Carisolv (Mediteam Dental, Sävedalen, Sweden) is a chemical mechanical system that is used to remove the decayed dentin already deeply modified in its collagen component by the same carious process. The system is composed of a jelly that removes the decayed dentin and a series of metal, spoon-shaped excavators to remove dentinal residues. Carisolv jelly acts only on the dentin involved in the carious process and is totally inactive on healthy dentin and on both healthy and decayed enamel. The jelly contains three amino acids: glutamine, leucine, and lysine, as well as a low concentration of sodium hypochlorite, erythrosin, carboxymethylcellulose, sodium chloride, and sodium hydroxide.

Obviously, to intervene on a closed cavity or one with a small opening in the enamel, it will be necessary to use rotating instruments or excavators to reach the dentin affected by the carious process.

The softening mechanism induced by Carisolv on the decayed dentin develops mainly through the destruction of collagen fibrils already denatured by the carious process. This is a very complex process called chloramination, involving interaction between chlorine ions freed from hypochlorite and amine

TABLE 27–1. Selection of Materials for Clinical Use

INTERVENTIONS	GLASS IONOMER CEMENT	MODIFIED GLASS IONOMER CEMENT	COMPOMERS	COMPOSITE RESINS
Class I or preventive restoration	Primary teeth, permanent teeth (small cavities)	Primary teeth, permanent teeth (small cavities)	Primary teeth, permanent teeth (small cavities)	Whenever good esthetics is needed
Class II	Primary teeth (small cavities)—good for the high fluoride release	Primary teeth (small cavities)—good for the high fluoride release	Primary teeth, permanent teeth (small cavities or temporary treatments = intermediate therapy)	Whenever good isolation is needed
Class III	Primary teeth (temporary treatments) whenever high fluoride release is needed	Primary teeth (small cavities), permanent teeth (temporary treatments)	Primary teeth, permanent teeth (case to be selected)	Whenever good isolation can be applied and good esthetics is required
Class IV	Primary teeth (intermediate therapy)	Primary teeth (intermediate therapy)	Primary teeth (small cavities), permanent teeth (intermediate therapy)	Required for esthetic reasons (anterior areas)
Class V	Primary and permanent teeth where fluoride release is more important than esthetics	Primary teeth, permanent teeth	Whenever good isolation and good esthetics are required	Whenever good isolation can be applied and good esthetics is required

groups of the three amino acids in a highly basic environment.

The Carisolv system can be used without anesthesia because it is not invasive and is without the troublesome vibration and thermal dentinal stimulations produced by rotating instruments. Therefore, it is suitable for phobic or anxious persons and for young patients whenever there are contraindications to conventional anesthesia and in all cases in which there is a risk of accidentally reaching the pulp chamber. This last possibility is considerably frequent in very deep cavities in very close proximity to the pulp. For all of these reasons, Carisolv is a useful operative means. In fact, due to the system selectivity (as already mentioned, this jelly acts exclusively on the decayed dentin), it is able to detect even the thinnest amounts of healthy dentin as opposed to the more aggressive rotating systems that easily reach into the pulp after passing the thin dentin barrier.

Statistical surveys have shown that this system results in a high level of satisfaction and compliance. It seldom requires anesthesia, and the remaining dentinal substratum is receptive to current adhesives. Therefore, Carisolv represents a valid alternative to conventional methods for removing decayed dentin.

Air Abrasion

Air abrasion is a caries excavation system that, as opposed to other conventional or unconventional means, bombards the dental surface with small particles of aluminium oxide projected by a high-pressure air jet. This method was invented in 1954 by Robert Black. It was re-introduced about 20 years ago and in the recent past has enjoyed wider acceptance by dentists and patients alike.

At present, several air-abrasive instruments are available at a reasonable cost for the cavity preparation. Although these systems provide valid assistance to the daily practice of the pedodontist, they are still not positioned to replace conventional instruments for cavity preparation. In fact, they are suitable for the treatment of small carious processes in fissure sealing, amelogenes imperfecta, and whenever an adhesive restoration technique is performed. The various systems are all able to achieve rapid, effective removal of enamel and of healthy dentin (the action on the decayed dentin is less invasive). Various particle sizes may be used (those approved by the U.S. Food and Drug Administration measure 27.5 microns); however, the abrasive effect is conditioned by the particles' kinetic energy, particles' outlet nozzle size, and the distance between the powder outlet hole and the surface to be treated. The advantages of this technique are the absence of vibration, reduced or elimination of anesthetics for small cavities, no need to change rotating instruments as excavation continues, and absence of pulpal exposure. The disadvantages are a lack of tactile sensitivity (which is present with usual rotating instruments), reduced control in depth of dentinal tissue removal, possible toxicity of aluminium oxide particles if inhaled (hence the need for a rubber dam), the need for protection of the dentist and his or her assistants, and the need for a very efficient air-aspiration system to avoid the dispersion of particles into the environment. The system may be improved by using particles of a different nature, transported not only by air but also by water, thus inducing the particles to fall and be more easily removed by aspiration.

RESTORATION OF PRIMARY ANTERIOR TEETH

In the last 15 years, a great evolution has taken place in composite resins. Their adhesion, polish, and esthetics have improved so much that they are now the best restorative material for anterior teeth damaged by caries or by either direct or indirect traumas. Among the undeniable merits of this kind of restoration is the fact that this is a "reversible" treatment; therefore, it can be redone when necessary.

Procedure

Step 1. Carefully evaluate the tooth shape and the place of the contralateral tooth, thus predicting the reconstruction.

Step 2. Choose the restoration color, as the subsequent isolation with a rubber dam prevents an accurate survey.

Step 3. Isolate the area and remove the carious lesion while aiming to maintain as much sound tooth tissue as possible.

Step 4. Treat the dentin and enamel to obtain good adhesion (compliance with instructions described for the selected material).

Step 5. Reconstruction. Ensure modeling is as precise as possible to reduce chair time and improve the esthetic final result.

Step 6. Finishing. Use a flame-shaped diamond bur to reproduce microanatomy of the rather irregular enamel surface. The finishing phase is completed by using a needle-shaped bur.

Step 7. Remove the rubber dam and evaluate the results. Next, polish the interproximal areas with pop-on disks and abrasive strips, taking care not to remove the contact point. Then, polish the other areas of the buccal face using rubber cups and polishing pastes with decreasing particle size.

Step 8. Color check. After initial dehydration, the tooth regains its original color. Note that chromatic considerations should be postponed to the subsequent visit.

CASE STUDIES

Caries Lesions in Anterior Teeth

A male patient, 2 years and 8 months old, with interproximal caries of D, E, F, and G (Figures 27–1A and B).

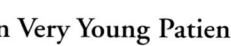

PROBLEM: The patient was not compliant, but an initial radiographic examination was accomplished.

TREATMENT: Under conscious sedation, in only one visit, caries lesions are removed, and the morphic-functional restoration with composite resin is placed.

RESULT: The restoration achieved the esthetic goal and restored function and anatomy. Furthermore, in a situation of tooth crowding, the arch length was preserved. Both the patient and his parents were pleased.

Rampant Caries in Very Young Patients: Conservative Approach

A male patient, 36 months old.

PROBLEM: He presented with rampant caries involving four maxillary anterior teeth and caries in the lower arch. The parents hoped that the teeth could be saved. Initial radiographs were taken (Figures 27–2A and B).

Figure 27–1A and B: Interproximal caries of frontal anterior teeth are removed, and a morphic-functional composite restoration is performed.

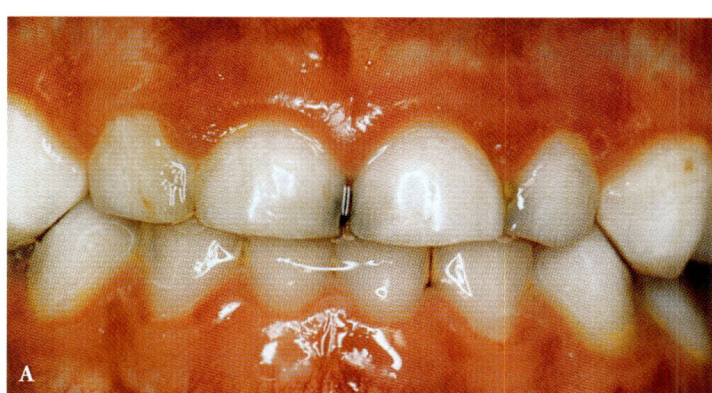
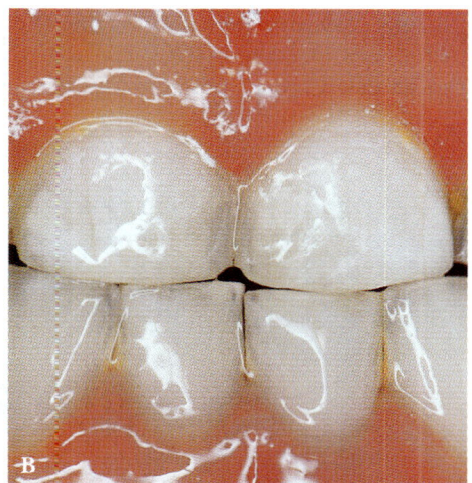

TREATMENT: Caries were removed, and endodontic treatment was performed. Aluminum oxide posts were used. A rubber-base impression was made for laboratory-processed full acrylic crowns (Figure 27–2C).

RESULT: Crowns were seated with an acceptable result. Figures 27–2A and D show the sharp contrast between before and after treatment. The child was able to resume his usual activities without discomfort or fear of future embarrassment.

Nursing Bottle Syndrome and/or Tooth Loss due to Caries of the Anterior Teeth: The Pedodontic Prosthesis

The consequences of this pathology are serious because of the possible loss of one or more anterior teeth due to serious caries lesions. The most critical teeth are the maxillary incisors and, in relation to their eruptive succession, the first primary molars.

When children present with chronic and recurrent fistulas and abscesses (Figures 27–3A and B), tooth function becomes limited. Radiographic investigation and clinical evidence frequently show an infectious necrosis of the pulp in an advanced phase, and the involved teeth (if an endodontic restorative therapy is not possible) are extracted and a pediatric prosthetic appliance is constructed. The correct space management and maintenance allow for the normal physiologic evolution and eruption of the permanent teeth and improved esthetics and speech.[9,14,18]

Pedodontic prostheses (also used in cases of trauma and/or tooth agenesis) are removable appliances that can offer a simple, safe, and efficient therapeutic solution because they can lead to reduction of the orthodontic treatment time. The decision to use these prostheses is guided by the child's and parents' cooperation and by precise clinical conditions (tooth class, available space, both general and oral health conditions).

Removable space maintenance appliances present considerable advantages: they can determine orthodontic movements and can help prevent orofacial muscle imbalance and/or harmful sucking habits, such as finger or thumb sucking or lip sucking. Furthermore, they can be modified during the patient's growth, improve esthetics, and reduce psychological problems. On the contrary, they can be uncomfortable to the young patient because of their volume; they need periodic checks and high patient and parental cooperation and can be more prone to breakage than fixed appliances.

A male patient, 3 years, 9 months old.

PROBLEM: The patient presented with rampant caries, loss of the anterior teeth, and advanced caries in the posterior teeth (Figure 27–4A).

TREATMENT: The root of G is extracted, and the posterior teeth are restored with composite resins. An attempt to maintain pulp vitality is made by

810   Esthetics in Dentistry

placing calcium hydroxide on the pulp. A pedodontic prosthesis has been used to maintain the anterior space, preserve the vertical dimension, improve alveolar growth, and avoid supereruption of the lower anterior teeth (Figures 27–4B to D).

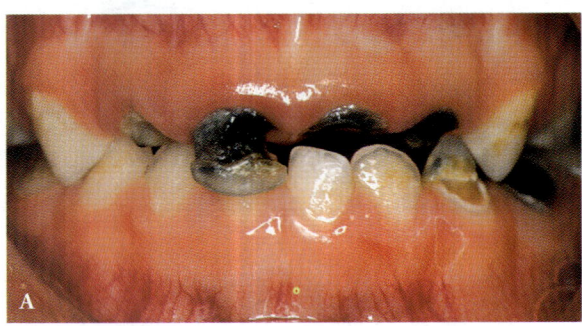
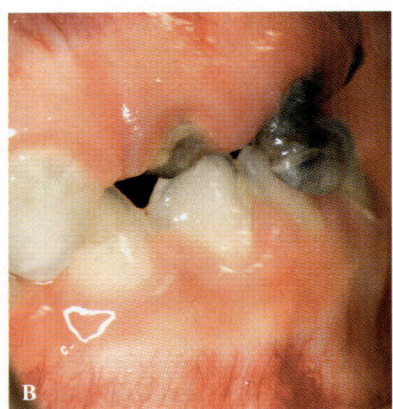

Figure 27–2A and B: Rampant caries involving the anterior teeth and the lower arch.

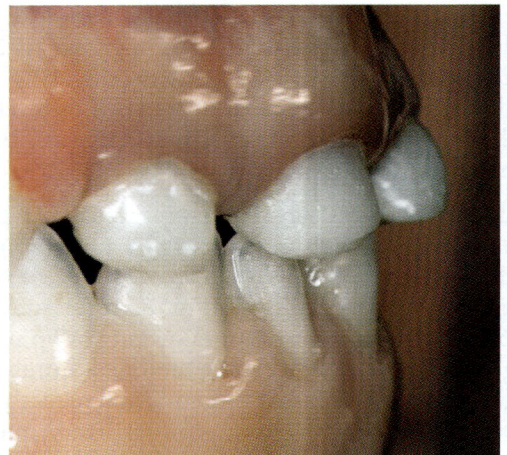

Figure 27–2C: Crowns are seated with an acceptable result.

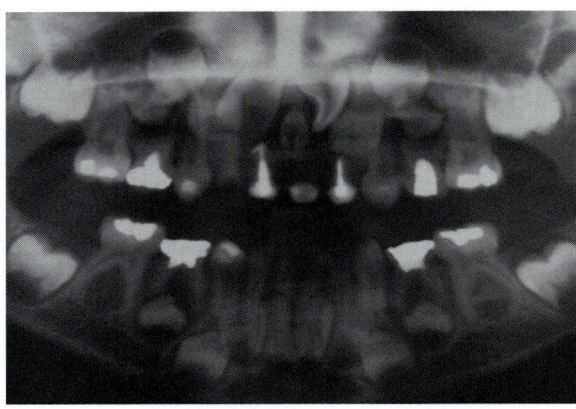

Figure 27–2D: The radiograph shows the endodontic treatment performed and the restoration of the lower caries.

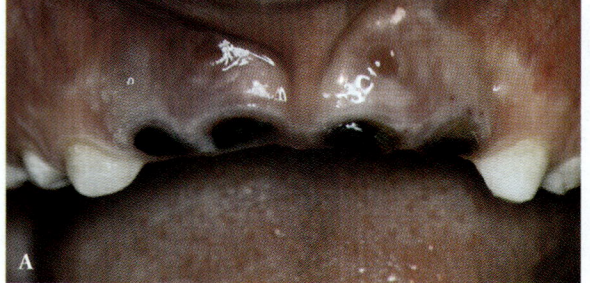
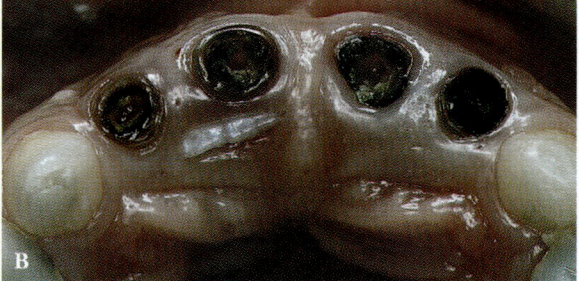

Figure 27–3A and B: When chronic and recurrent fistulas and abscesses are present and a conservative therapy cannot be performed, teeth are extracted.

RESULT: Good function is restored, and the desired psychological result has been achieved, with lasting benefits. The patient has undergone periodic yearly visits: teeth #3 and #14 have erupted (Figures 27–4E and F).

TRAUMA MANAGEMENT IN PRIMARY DENTITION AND IN THE FIRST PHASE OF MIXED DENTITION

In pediatric dentistry, trauma is a very frequent event. Often it is very difficult to make an accurate diagnosis as to the extent and severity of the traumatic injury, manage the initial treatment of the acute aspect of the injury, and determine the long-term follow-up. Dental traumas (as well as dental caries) represent a true emergency and need an accurate diagnosis to provide guidance in saving teeth, restoring the function of the dental arches, improving esthetics, and avoiding complications.

As this is a high-incidence pathology, effective preventive measures need to be taken to reduce the effects of trauma and ensuing complications that can occur in young patients. It is extremely important to develop an effective prevention and information plan for the public. The goal of this plan should be the reduction of the functional and esthetic damage, the reduction of the biological damage involving the orofacial area, and the awareness and sensibility of both patients and practitioners to reduce sequelae, avoid unnecessary treatment procedures, and provide the biological basis for healing after injury.

Among the most effective preventive measures, we specify a timely orthodontic correction to reduce the increased overjet; early correction of habits such as finger sucking, thumb sucking, lip sucking, and abnormal swallowing; use of a mouthguard to protect permanent teeth during sport activities; and correct initial diagnosis and timely treatment, which are essential to produce a correct initial treatment, avoid overtreatment, and avoid sequelae in the long-term follow-up.

Trauma to the Primary Dentition

Andreasen and Andreasen's epidemiologic studies reported that one child in three undergoes dental trauma. In fact, primary teeth, mainly because of their anatomic characteristics, report more luxations than fractures, and 25% of them suffer avulsions.[1]

Regarding trauma to hard tissues, young patients often present with crown fractures (with or without pulp exposure). Therefore, the treatment plan depends on the extent of the pulp exposure, the patient's and the family's cooperation, the skill of the dentist, and the time interval between the trauma and emergency care. If the pulp exposure is very small, the exposed area should be cleaned and a pulp capping applied to the exposed pulp. For a larger pulp exposure, pulp extirpation and root canal treatment should be performed. Examining and diagnosing children's teeth can be especially challenging because accurate radiographs may be difficult to obtain.

The treatment plan for primary teeth is usually different from one for permanent teeth. There are several different reasons to be considered: the healing mechanism of pulp and periodontal tissues in the primary dentition is different than in permanent dentition. The healing mechanism characteristic in permanent teeth may not occur in primary teeth, and sometimes extraction is necessary to limit damage to permanent successors. Often treatment cannot be performed because of the uncooperative behavior of children.

Reimplants of Primary Teeth

Traumatic avulsion is a frequent event in the primary dentition. It is essential to conduct a differential diagnosis in the presence of a total intrusive luxation, and in case of a multiple loss, it is necessary to verify that the teeth have been neither swallowed nor inhaled. Actually, the debate is open as to whether to reimplant only one tooth or even multiple primary teeth.

Avulsed primary teeth in which the roots have begun normal resorption are not indicated for reimplantation. There is little value in reimplantation because of the possibility of rapid root resorption or infection.

However, in young patients, the absence of teeth until the eruption of permanent ones may cause esthetic and functional problems, as well as psychological complications (such as anxiety), not only for the patients but also for their parents. Therefore, attempting reimplantation is sometimes worthwhile. Reimplantation cannot be performed when the tooth is not far from normal resorption, radicular pathologic processes are present, or there is a risk of infection and damage to the permanent tooth bud.

812 Esthetics in Dentistry

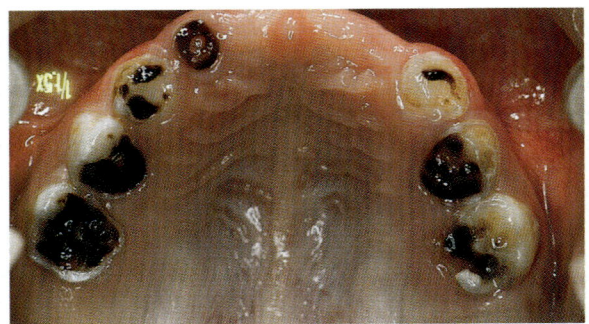

Figure 27–4A: A patient of 3 years, 9 months, with rampant caries and loss of an anterior tooth.

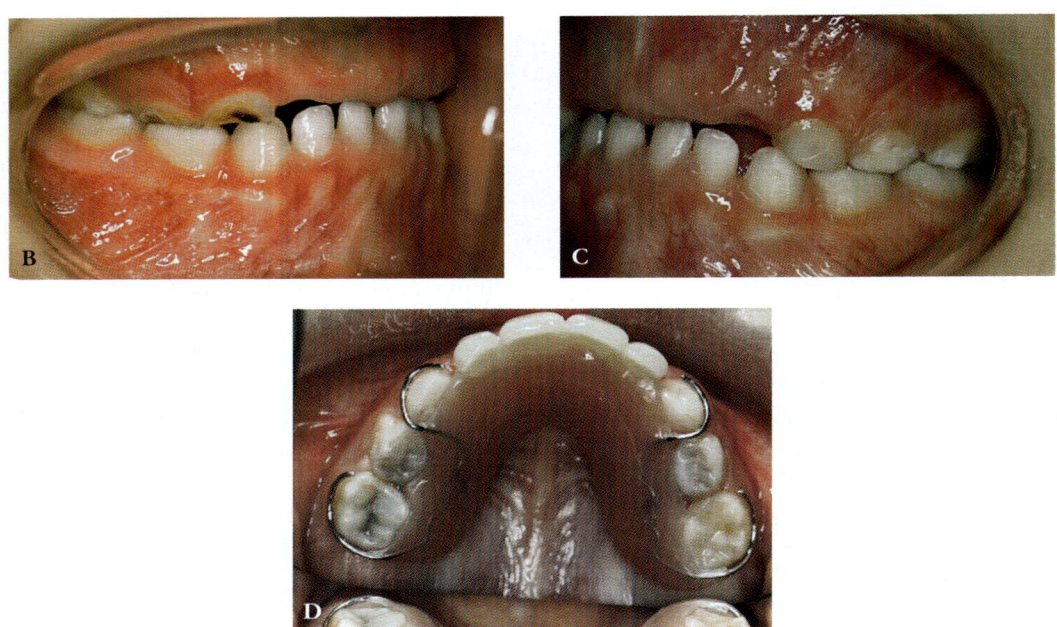

Figure 27–4B to D: The posterior teeth are restored with composite resin, and a pedodontic prosthesis is placed.

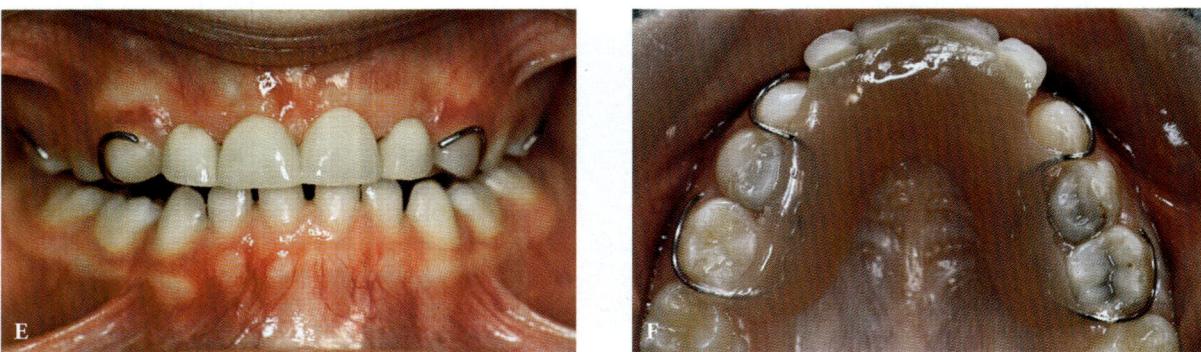

Figure 27–4E and F: Proper function is reached and the desired psychological result has been achieved in the long-term follow-up. Note that teeth #3 and #14 have erupted.

Recent clinical investigations carried out by Caprioglio et al.[10] and Tsukiboshi[19] have begun to define specific guidelines and protocols. The tooth can be reimplanted only if these clinical situations are present: (1) the child has acceptable occlusion, has no harmful habits, and is in good health and (2) the avulsed tooth is far from root resorption, has been avulsed not more than an hour, and has been stored hydrated. In the most successful cases, the tooth will remain vital; otherwise, the root canal will be treated with calcium hydroxide (for necrosis of the pulp). Unlike permanent teeth, with reimplantation of primary teeth, healing of the pulp and periodontal membrane should not be expected.

Sequelae after Trauma to Primary Teeth

One of the problems of trauma to the primary dentition is the possibility of damaging the permanent successor tooth buds. The patient's age and the degree and direction of the malposition of the primary teeth, as well as the type of trauma, are some of the most important factors to be considered. The effect may be either direct or indirect. An accurate diagnosis at the time of injury ensures that appropriate care is prescribed. Combined with careful follow-up, this care will, in many cases, prevent hypoplasia and hypomineralization affecting the permanent successors.

The most serious deciduous tooth injuries in terms of damage to permanent successors are intrusive luxation, avulsion, extrusive luxation, and subluxation. The permanent teeth that are most often affected are the central incisors. The effects on the successional tooth may be discoloration and hypoplasia of the enamel, bending and malformation of the anatomic crown and root, hypoplasia of the root, and retarded eruption. These problems may occur regardless of the treatment of the traumatized primary teeth. It is very important to inform parents about these possibilities; therefore, regular reviews are clearly important to try to avoid or resolve the problems.

A male patient, 5 years, 8 months old.

PROBLEM: Occasionally, parents complain about discoloration of their children's primary teeth, or the discoloration may go unnoticed. Discoloration of primary teeth, as in this case, may be due to slight damage, such as concussion or subluxation. If discoloration continues without pulp obliteration, there is a possibility of pulp necrosis. Because of the original trauma, a malformation of the anatomic crown of teeth #8 and #9 is observed.

TREATMENT: After the complete eruption of the two upper central incisors, the pigmentation (hypoplasia) of the teeth is restored with composite resins.

RESULT: Because enamel hypoplasia is superficial damage, it can be easily and esthetically resolved (Figures 27–5A and B).

Traumas in the Early Mixed Dentition

Although we acknowledge the importance of providing guidelines and promoting informative and preventive protocols, for the purpose of brevity, we are not addressing any reference to classifications, clinical examinations, medical history, or special investigation, which are absolutely essential for comprehensive treatment planning. We simply describe some clinical trauma cases in which the cooperation between the pedodontist and the orthodontist has led to a good esthetic and functional result.

Reattachment of the Tooth Fragment in the Fracture of Anterior Teeth

As far back as 1961, Chosak and Aidelman proposed a technique to manage the reattachment of the tooth fragment after trauma.[11] Therefore, if the fragment is available, this treatment procedure achieves excellent esthetic results, particularly if the fragment is complete.

Another advantage is the ability to reconstruct the palatal face, which will benefit the occlusal stability.

The fragment must be kept hydrated (water, milk, physiologic saline solution, or other special storage media). Alternatively, dehydration will distort the tooth color. The tooth must not have additional fractures, and the soft tissues must not have lacerations, contusions, or bleeding.

Before reattachment, the fit of the tooth fragment to the remaining tooth should be confirmed and checked for enamel defects. A fragment that is highly damaged may be unsuitable for reattachment.

After the pretreatment preparation, local anesthesia is administered, and the tooth is isolated with a rubber dam, the tooth fragment is cleaned and prepared, and the pulp is dressed, if necessary.

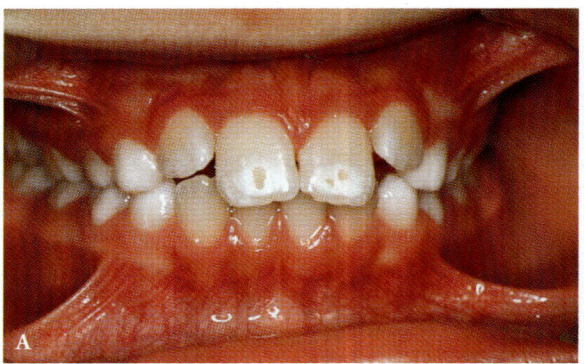 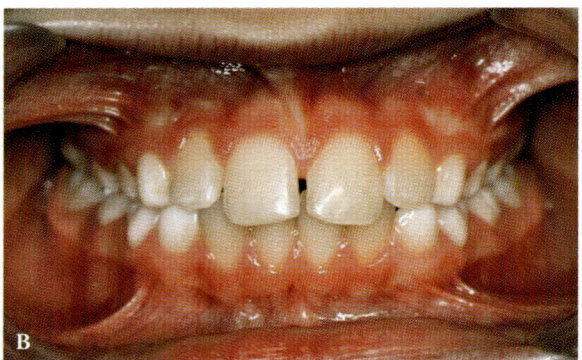

Figure 27–5A and B: Due to a trauma to primary teeth, a malformation of the anatomic crown of teeth #8 and #9 is observed (hypoplasia). Teeth are restored with composite resin.

The remaining tooth is beveled, the tooth fragment is tried in, the tooth is etched, and the fragment is bonded with composite resin. Next, the tooth fragment is attached to the remaining tooth, and the resin is reshaped and polished. The patient should be examined after 1 week, 1 month, and 3 months and then checked annually for discomfort and possible pulp necrosis and to evaluate esthetics.

A female patient, 9 years, 2 months old.

PROBLEM: This patient presented with an extended, noncomplicated enamel and dentin fracture of teeth #8 and #9. Four days had passed since the trauma occurred, and the fragments had not been hydrated (Figures 27–6A and B).

TREATMENT: After performing routine clinical, instrumental, and radiographic examinations, it was decided to try to rehydrate the tooth fragments by putting them in a physiologic saline solution for 1 day. In the meantime, the fit of the tooth fragments was confirmed (Figures 27–6C and D). The following day, the two rehydrated tooth fragments had reached their normal color, and the reattachment of the two fragments proceeded as described above.

RESULT: The result obtained was much better functionally and esthetically than it would have been using only composite resin. This one-appointment procedure (due to a perfect fitting of the fragments) has restored the anterior guide and has reached a correct reproduction of the biting edge (Figures 27–6E and F).

When physiologic effects are more important than cosmetic ones; this technique allows a "true biological restoration" with a true "restitutio ad integrum" of the tooth crown. No additional treatment has been required on the teeth other than periodic examinations.

A male patient, 8 years, 3 months old.

PROBLEM: The patient presented with a complicated enamel–dentin fracture of the left central incisor with an immature apex. The patient had poor oral hygiene and a class II molar relationship. The tooth fragment was available, although it was not complete (Figures 27–7A and B).

TREATMENT: After cleansing and stopping the flow of blood, the restoration was done in accordance with standard procedures. After pulp capping with calcium hydroxide, the tooth fragment was reattached. However, because the fragment was not complete, the missing parts were reconstructed with composite resin, and the entire periphery of the fractured surface of the remaining tooth was beveled to improve esthetics (Figure 27–7C).

RESULT: Immediately after restorative treatment, the patient expressed his satisfaction. After 18 months, the patient returned, reporting an extrusive luxation of tooth 9 following a school incident. The tooth was immediately repositioned and splinted orthodontically (Figure 27–7D). A .018 nytinol wire was used for 15 days. It was subse-

Esthetics in Pediatric Dentistry

Figure 27–6A and B: An extended but not complicated enamel and dentin fracture of teeth #8 and #9.

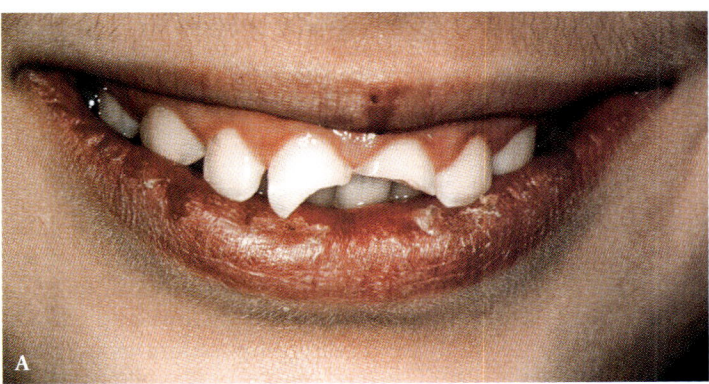
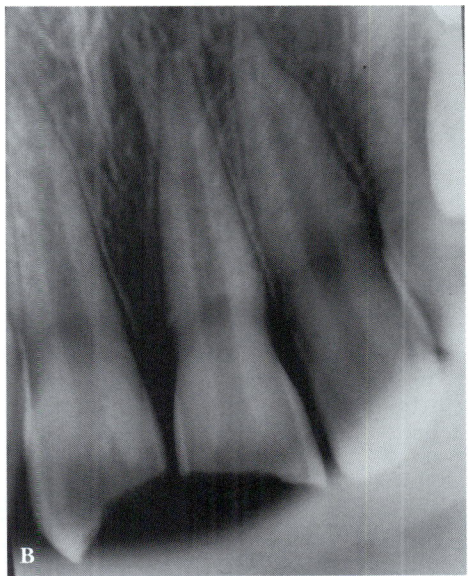

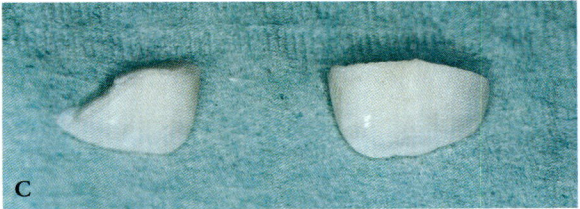
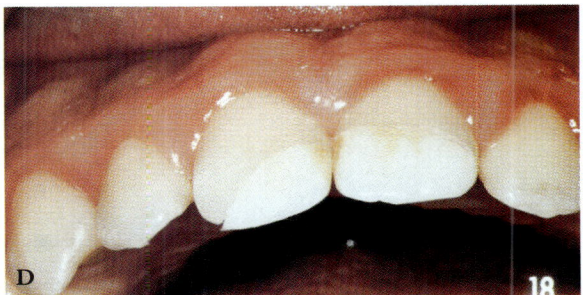

Figure 27–6C and D: The tooth fragments have not been hydrated for 4 days. They fit perfectly but are discolored.

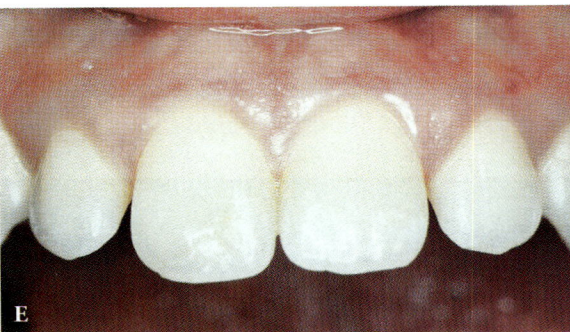
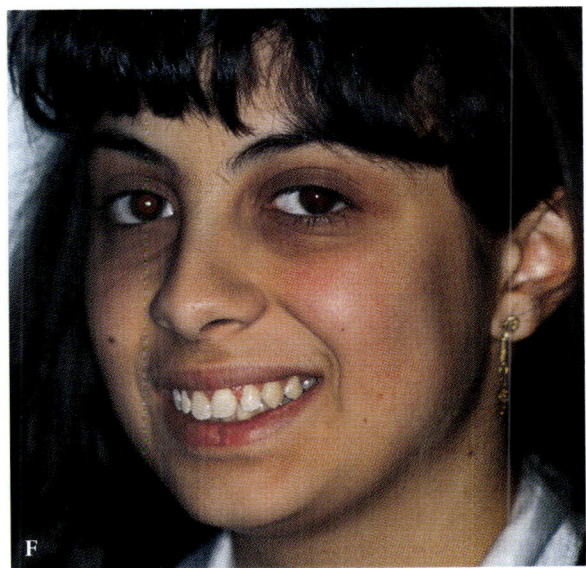

Figure 27–6E and F: The fragments have been rehydrated for 1 day and then reattached. The final result and the patient's smile are satisfying.

quently removed after clinical and radiographic confirmation of results.

~

The patient had periodic radiographic examinations and sensitivity tests to monitor pulp and root healing, as well as tooth vitality (Figure 27–7E).

From an orthodontic perspective, a serious skeletal Class II with deep bite is becoming more and more evident. Therefore, orthodontic treatment has been initiated in both arches to align the dentition over the basal bone in harmony with the surrounding hard and soft tissues, as well as to achieve good esthetics (Figures 27–7F and G).

Traumatic Avulsion

A traumatic avulsion is a serious clinical event. The traumatic loss of one or more teeth, particularly when they are immature, represents a highly dramatic event. Recommended therapy will vary according to the time elapsed from the trauma to the first visit as follows:

- Immediate reimplantation (45 minutes or less) if the tooth is preserved in milk or in a preservative solution and it is reimplanted within 24 hours

- Delayed reimplantation

There are three factors that affect the success of the reimplantation:

1. Time elapsed since the trauma occurred. If the tooth is preserved hydrated or in saliva for a period of 20 to 120 minutes, it can be reimplanted as vital and then followed up periodically to avoid pulp complications or ankylosis.

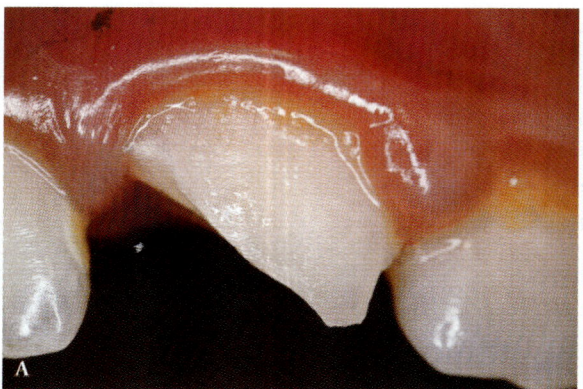
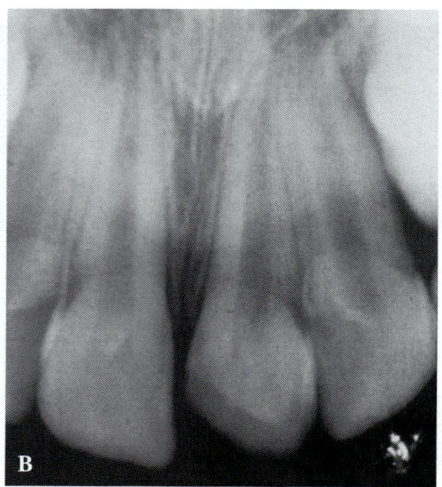

Figure 27–7A and B: A complicated enamel–dentin fracture of tooth 9 and the radiograph.

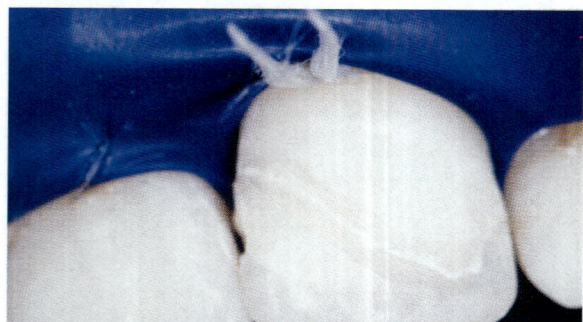

Figure 27–7C: The tooth fragment is reattached with a bevel to improve esthetics.

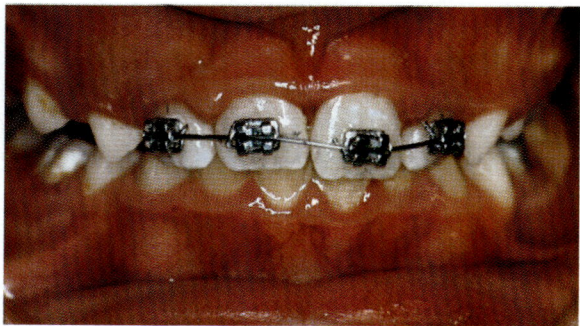

Figure 27–7D: After 18 months, the same tooth has an extrusive luxation and is orthodontically splinted.

Esthetics in Pediatric Dentistry

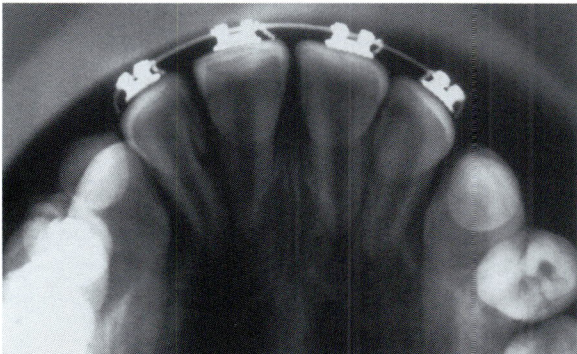

Figure 27–7E: The radiograph after the reposition.

If 2 hours have elapsed since the trauma or after 30 minutes of dryness, the tooth must be treated endodontically with calcium hydroxide and then monitored periodically.

2. Preservation of the avulsed tooth. The tooth must be kept in a liquid in osmotic balance with the tissues. These include saliva, a physiologic saline solution, milk, or special storage medium. It should be noted that teeth kept in water and reimplanted have shown a high percentage of ankylosis.

3. Treatment plan. It is essential for the dentist to have a wide experience in endodontics, pediatric dentistry, orthodontics, and oral surgery to perform the treatment plan correctly to achieve an esthetic result and reduce sequelae.

RESTORATION OF POSTERIOR TEETH

When reference is made to the fundamental concepts governing pediatric dentistry, the importance of the awareness of the correct evolution of arches, as well as treating any irregular condition, must be a primary focus.

The first primary molars are the ones that, during eruption, determine the first proprioceptive reflexes on the transversal plane. Their role, as well as their maintenance, comes second when compared with the second primary molars. The presence of the second primary molar is strategic to guide the eruption and the articulation of the first permanent molars. The restoration and preservation of the posterior primary teeth are vital to maintain the arch length and eliminate mesial drift of the permanent molars.

Arch length and arch anatomy can be modified by

1. Tooth crowding: loss of space (unilateral or bilateral) due to a premature extraction because of caries or loss from a traumatic event or ectopic eruption, impaction, transposition, ankylosis, agenesis, or supernumerary teeth.

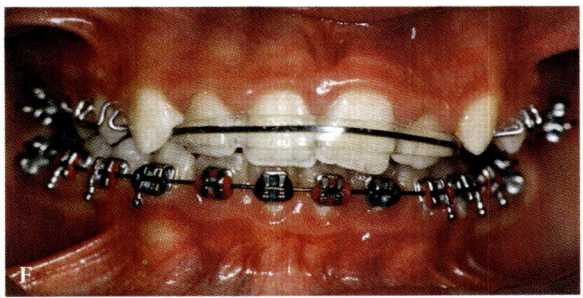
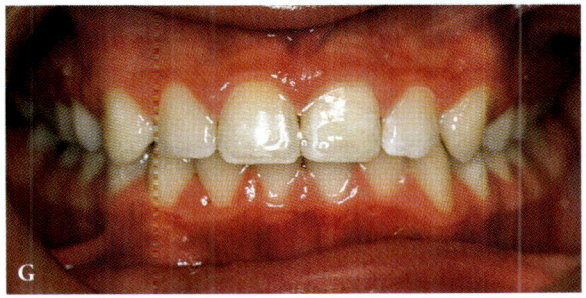

Figure 27–7F and G: The same patient during the orthodontic treatment and after. Good esthetics has been achieved.

2. Presence of habits such as oral breathing, sleep apnea syndromes, and thumb sucking. In the presence of a harmful oral habit, these patients usually present with a reduction of transversal (cross) diameters, as well as the loss of one or more primary molars, which could lead to a further collapse of the arch.

3. Presence of a malocclusion: Class II with an increased overjet and/or overbite or Class III with an anterior crossbite and/or posterior crossbite and/or open bite.

The pedodontist, often working with the orthodontist, must perform a careful analysis of the dentition. The goal is arch harmony and good balance among function, arch form, and oral tissue condition.

Optimum space maintenance therapy is the preservation of the primary molars until natural exfoliation. Dental education and improved prevention have reduced the number of children who develop malocclusion because of premature loss of primary teeth. Therefore, it has become one of the most controllable causes of malocclusion. When posterior teeth are damaged or lost, stainless steel crowns for grossly broken-down teeth, space maintainers (fixed or removable appliances), or esthetic posterior restoration techniques can be used to maintain arch length.

Interproximal caries in primary teeth, due to the different thickness of enamel and dentin, can more easily extend to the pulp, requiring endodontic therapy. This aside, compomers and composite resins are the materials of choice for their easy handling, reduced tooth preparation, reasonable wear properties, good esthetics, and release of fluoride leaching.

Preventive Resin Restoration
Composite resin is the material of choice for the treatment of early occlusal caries in the permanent dentition. The development and use of preventive resin restoration has greatly changed the management of occlusal caries in very young patients. The indications are an enamel-only lesion, incipient lesion just into the dentin, and a small Class I lesion.

A male patient, 7 years, 2 months old.

PROBLEM: The patient was a high-caries–risk subject with poor oral hygiene and an enamel-only lesion of tooth 3.

TREATMENT: Preventive resin restoration. After local anesthesia and rubber dam isolation, a small high-speed diamond burr was applied to the questionable fissure. It was essential to have adequate access to the underlying dentin to be certain of complete caries removal. A glass ionomer liner was placed over the dentin, extended to the amelodentinal junction, and light-cured. An etching gel was placed on the enamel margins and on the occlusal surface, washed, and dried. The bonding resin and the composite resin were placed and polymerized, and, finally, a fissure sealant was placed over the restoration and cured. After the rubber dam was removed, the occlusion was checked (Figures 27–8A and B).

RESULT: The durability of preventive resin restoration has been proved to be as good as amalgam, with less removal of sound tooth tissue and with better esthetics.

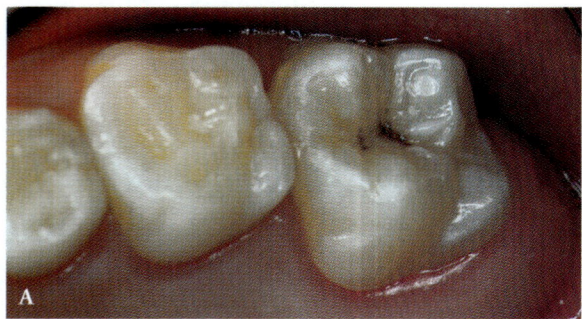
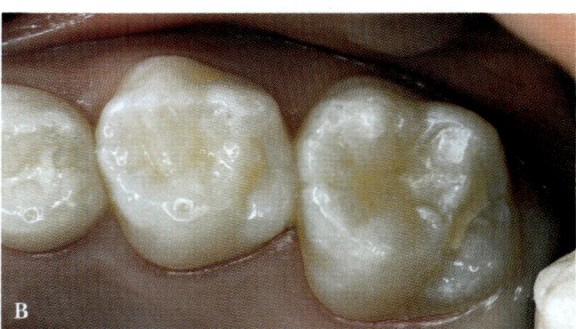

Figure 27–8A and B: An enamel caries is treated with a preventive resin restoration.

ESTHETICS AND HARMONY OF DENTAL ARCHES: SPACE MANAGEMENT IN PEDIATRIC DENTISTRY

Correct space management, starting from the emergence of primary dentition through the late phase of mixed dentition, requires cooperation between the pedodontist and the orthodontist. The preventive strategy not only simplifies the subsequent orthodontic therapy by making it less complex and more reliable, it also helps to improve esthetics and function.

Considering some fundamental concepts and new therapeutic trends focused on the resetting of shape and the esthetics and harmony of the dental arches, it is necessary to balance the arch symmetrically and to check the eruption of the first permanent molar (tipping, uprighting) to prevent mesialization of the first lower molars. Next, a correct dentoskeletal analysis, cephalometric study, and careful evaluation of the means and materials must be done before formulating a diagnosis and logical prognostic evaluation. Last, if orthodontic brackets are applied to primary teeth, the advantages include reduced demineralization risks; the possibility of good anchorage, which decreases the reaction counterforce; and the reduction of acid-etching time and of problems associated with the removal of orthodontic brackets (bonding and debonding).

The dentist can perform several different treatments:

1. Slicing of the primary cuspids and/or primary second molars
2. Lip bumper on the primary second molars
3. Mechanics of symmetrically balancing the arches following a premature loss or extraction of the primary cuspid
4. Uprighting of the first permanent molars

A female patient, 6 years, 7 months old.

PROBLEM: The patient's frontal view showed a serious bimaxillary crowding with deviation of the midline. When teeth #7 and #10 erupted, crowding problems greatly increased. Also, tooth #10 was in crossbite (Figure 27–9A).

TREATMENT: After a short observation period, while the lateral incisors erupted, the pediatric dentist and the orthodontist initiated therapy. M and R were sliced, and a lip bumper was applied to K and T. The occlusal surface rose to resolve the crossbite of the upper left lateral incisor. The maxillary arch was treated orthodontically to correct the alignment (Figure 27–9B).

RESULT: The patient underwent an early orthodontic treatment for 1 year that achieved arch balance, improvement of esthetics, and health of the oral tissues. Furthermore, the improved smile contributed to greater self-confidence and an improved sense of well-being (Figures 27–9C and D).

It is important to emphasize that the correct space management may require, in addition to orthodontic treatment, consultation with and/or treatment by an endodontist, prosthodontist, or oral surgeon. In fact, dental anomalies in number (such as agenesis, supernumerary tooth and/or teeth) or in shape (micro- or macrotooth) may require the cooperation of many different specialists to improve esthetics and/or function.

A female patient, 9 years, 10 months old.

PROBLEM: The initial orthopantography showed agenesis of tooth #10 (with deviation of the middle line), microdontia of tooth #7, and skeletal dental Class III. These are often interrelated (Figure 27–10A).

TREATMENT: After applying a fixed orthodontic appliance, the dental arches were aligned, and a correct transversal relationship was obtained with a reduction in midline deviation. To improve esthetics in the anterior region, tooth #7 was restored with a composite material, and tooth #10 was replaced with a resin-bonded fixed Maryland bridge (Figures 27–10B and C). This bridge has esthetic appeal because it does not require the use of full crowns on either side of the missing tooth, and little or no tooth reduction is involved. The metal framework was bonded to the tooth with resin cement. If the adjacent teeth to a missing tooth are intact and in good condition, a resin-bonded bridge may be the method of choice.

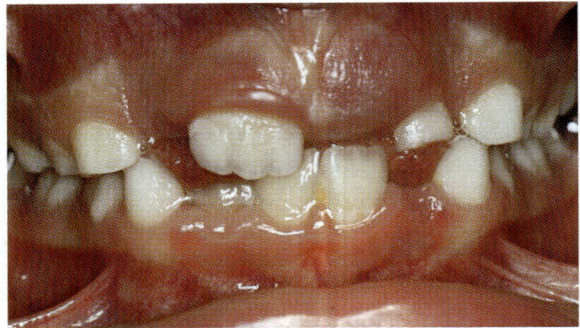

Figure 27–9A: A serious bimaxillary crowding with deviation of the midline in a 6-year, 7-month-old female.

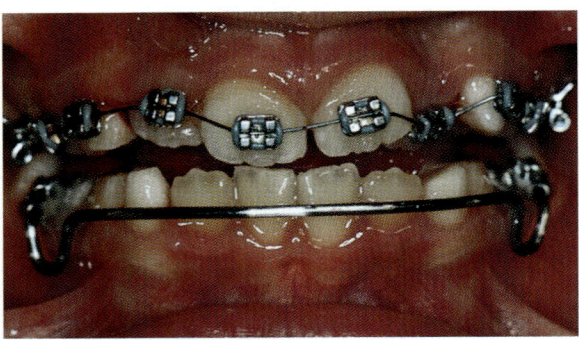

Figure 27–9B: After a short observation period, the early orthodontic therapy is started.

RESULT: This intervention resulted in an acceptable masticatory and esthetic function. Maximum oral hygiene was emphasized to the patient.

A male patient, 8 years, 3 months old.

PROBLEM: The patient presented with a supernumerary incisor and a double tooth in place of the central upper left incisor (tooth #9) (Figures 27–11A and B). This anomaly manifests itself as a structure resembling two teeth that have been joined together. In the anterior region, the anomalous tooth usually has a groove on the buccal surface and a notch in the incisal edge. Radiographs are necessary to determine if there is a (fusion) union of the pulp chambers. Fusion exists when there is a joining of two teeth by pulp and dentin. Two canals are usually present, as in this case.

TREATMENT: Both the supernumerary tooth and fused tooth were extracted (Figure 27–11C); also, the fixed orthodontic appliance was applied to the maxillary arch to close the anterior diastema. Subsequently, the incisal margin and the interproximal area of tooth #9 were restored to improve esthetics (Figure 27–11D).

RESULT: The team work of several specialists created a good morphic-functional recovery (Figures 27–11E and F) and an esthetic result that satisfied the patient (Figures 27–11G and H).

THE FACE IN PEDIATRIC DENTISTRY: ESTHETIC KEYS

The concept of "beauty" has always been subjective. As to the individual esthetic aspect, many attempts have been made during the centuries with

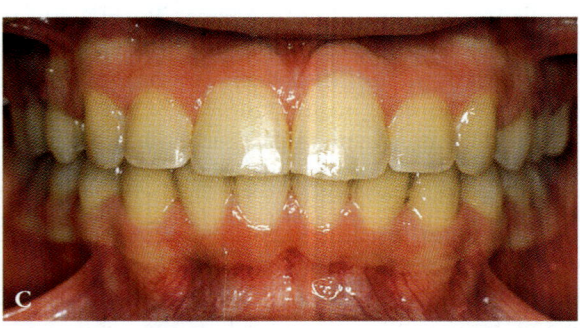

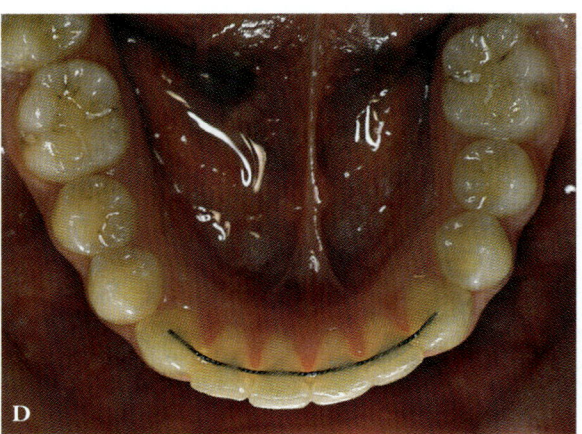

Figure 27–9C and D: The patient's smile and the lower arch after the orthodontic treatment: good balance and esthetics are achieved.

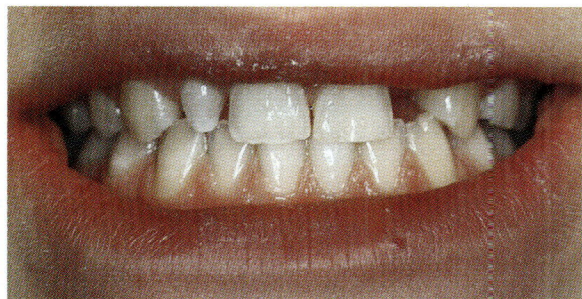

Figure 27–10A: After orthodontic treatment, the patient with microdontia of tooth 7 and agenesis of tooth 10 shows a good alignment.

the purpose of extrapolating the golden cut or divine proportion. In spite of all efforts of standardization, each age and every century has its own esthetic canons, as each individual may have his or her own esthetic ideals. However, our society is continuously creating new ideals of beauty, new trends to which people would like to aspire. During the last few decades in the Western world, an individual's appearance has assumed much more importance and is essential in establishing self-image. Ultimately, it contributes to success in all aspects of professional and social life. For this reason, many branches of medicine that have an esthetic component continue to research and improve their techniques. Among these entities is orthognathodontics, which is enlarging its field of activity from the smile to the entire face of the patient. As Goldstein says, "The way you see yourself and think others see you has a great deal to do with the way you feel about yourself. A charming smile can open doors; our own self-image is the key to our happiness."[17]

Several authors have shown that orthodontic treatment can improve facial harmony, including orthognathic surgery. Traditional cephalometrics, based on angular and linear measurements of the soft and hard tissues of the patient, have proven to be less than reliable for correct diagnosis and a satisfactory esthetic result. It suffices to say that there is no cephalometric analysis that has universal appeal. Most cephalometric analyses use as a reference some intracranial skeletal plans. Diagnosis and treatment planning are based on them because of the assumption that the correction of definite dental and bone parameters achieves facial esthetics, harmony, and facial balance. However, many authors now agree that a careful analysis of the soft tissue is also needed.

For this reason, cephalometrics now includes studies and measurements involving soft tissues by using in general the usual teleradiographies of the skull in norma lateralis or the photographic records of the patient in lateral view or, more rarely, in frontal view.

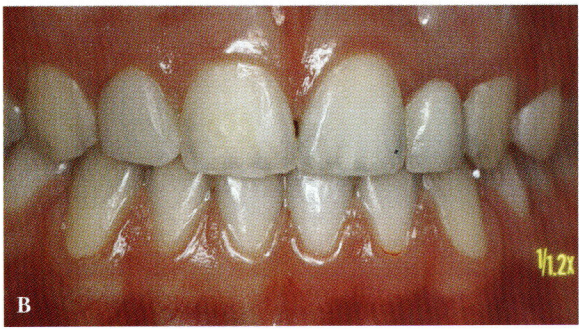
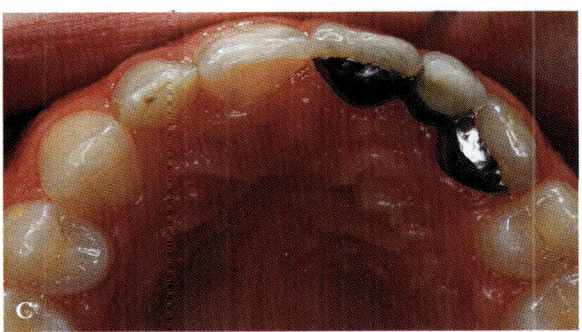

Figure 27–10B and C: A resin-bonded Maryland bridge is placed to improve esthetics in the anterior region.

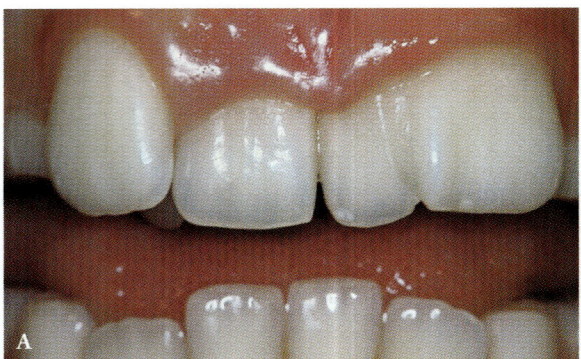
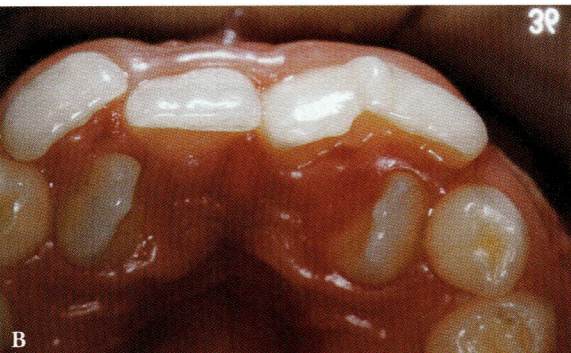

Figure 27–11A and B: A supernumerary incisor and a double tooth in place of the central upper left incisor. Frontal and occlusal views.

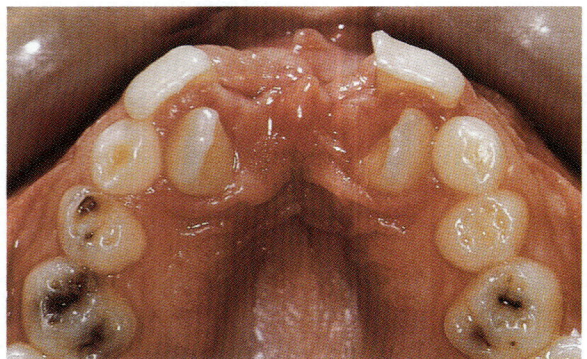

Figure 27–11C: Both the supernumerary tooth and fused tooth are extracted.

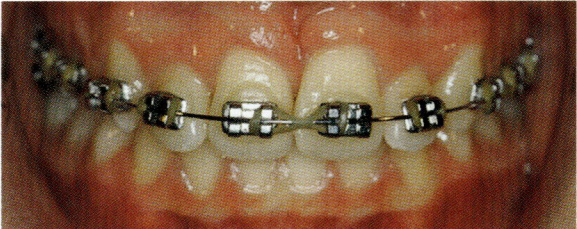

Figure 27–11D: An orthodontic appliance is applied to the maxillary arch to close the anterior diastema.

At issue is the fact that a good functional occlusion with the usual skeletal parameters does not always correspond with an esthetically pleasing facial balance. This phenomenon is mainly due to the thickness of the soft tissues covering the skeleton of the face, which can make the dentoskeletal analysis unreliable in the evaluation of facial harmony. (In other words, if the lips are not well balanced and closed at rest, facial dysmorphosis can be present in the absence of dentoskeletal alterations.)

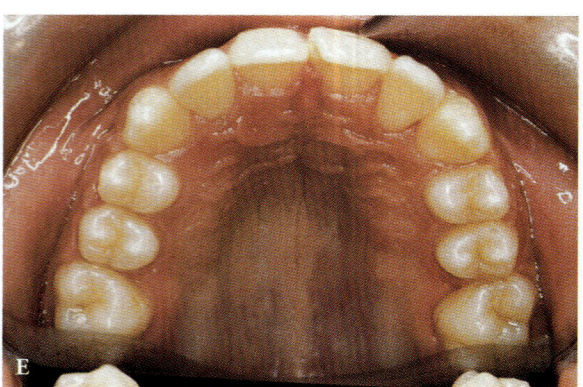
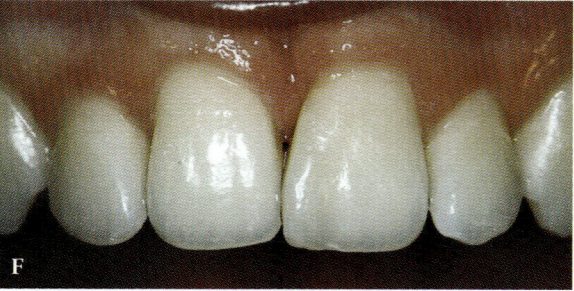

Figure 27–11E and F: The morphic-functional recovery at the end of the orthodontic treatment.

Figure 27–11G and H: The final result showing the patient's smile at the end of the treatment.

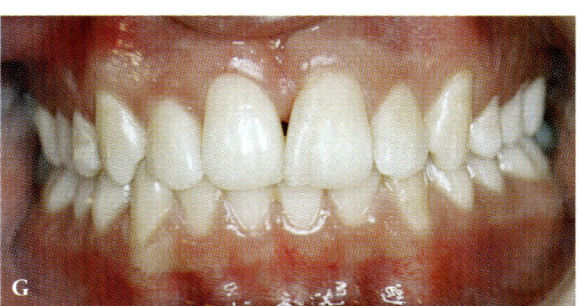

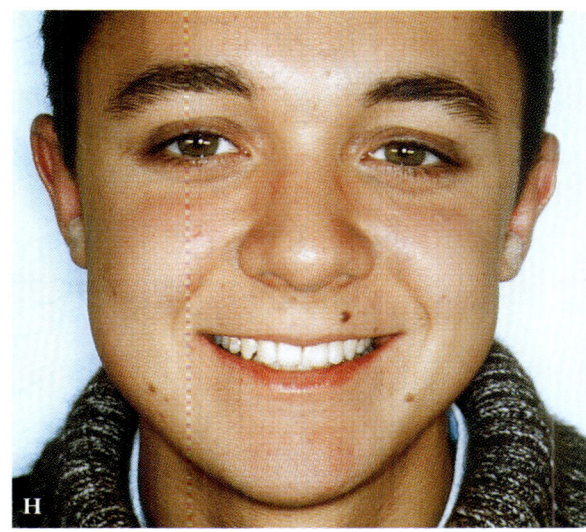

According to Blanchette et al., soft tissues have a tendency to mask discrepancies of the bone base (maxilla and mandible); therefore, we would have thinner soft tissues in low-angle subjects and thicker soft tissues in high-angle ones.[7] Perhaps it was for this reason that Ferrario et al. found significant correlations between the skeletal class and the soft tissues,[13] and that Burnstone et al. argued that any dentoskeletal standard can present unpredictable final esthetics of the face.[8]

At present, the purpose of an orthodontic treatment should be the achievement of a good functional occlusion along with appealing dentofacial esthetics, thus maintaining the integrity of the dentoperiodontal tissues. For these reasons, several practitioners have started to focus their interest mainly on the study of the patient's face rather than the skeleton. Therefore, the transition has been from a diagnostic system, which can be defined as "centrifugal" and which, starting from the skeleton, goes outward, to a "centripetal" system, which begins instead with the analysis of soft tissues to determine the corrections to be effected on hard tissues. Arnett and Bergman's[3,4] and Ayala's[5] cephalometric analyses visually evaluated the facial contour of the patient's soft tissue exclusively in a natural position, both frontal and lateral views, to determine the diagnosis and treatment plan.

Currently, all of the existing diagnostic systems based on the analysis of soft tissues refer to adult subjects, especially those who must undergo orthognathic surgery. The purpose of this chapter is to propose a method of analysis that can determine esthetic reference parameters that are reliable for the child's face (in the different ages of growth) and be useful to create a clinical alternative to cephalometric analysis of the soft tissues. Moreover, this method could help the clinician to integrate and complement the usual cephalometric analysis to achieve not only esthetic facial harmony but also good balance.

By analyzing the different methodologies used by authors to evaluate the harmony of soft tissues in adults, reference parameters and data have been selected that would be useful and reliable when evaluating growing patients. These parameters and data have been subsequently modified after considering craniofacial growth. At birth, in fact, the splanchnocranium is considerably hypodeveloped if compared with the neurocranium (Figure 27–12). Furthermore, the mandible is the least developed of the face's lower third and tends to grow more and for a longer period of time when compared with the rest of the face. Moreover, a sequence exists both in the maxilla and in the mandible. This has been defined as a completion of growth in the three planes of space: first, growth completes in width, then in length, and then in height. The transversal growth of both bones (including width of the dental arches) tends to be complete before the pubertal growth peak and is scarcely influenced by growth variations during adolescence.

824 Esthetics in Dentistry

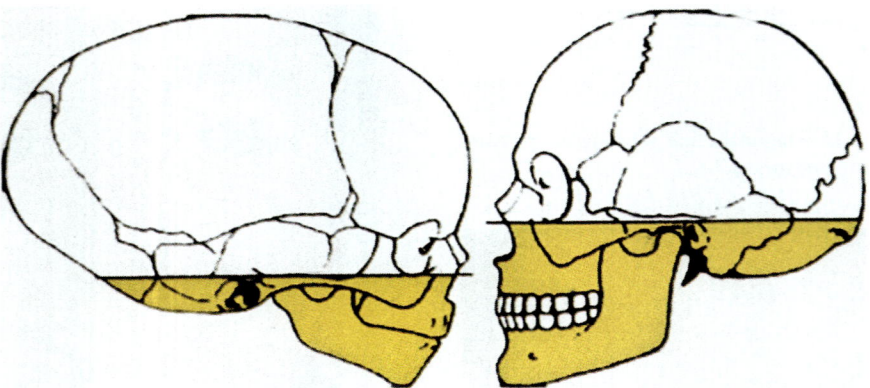

Figure 27–12: At birth, the splanchnocranium is considerably hypodeveloped if compared with the neurocranium.

Sagittal growth of the two maxillaries continues during puberty. In girls, it stops almost immediately, on average between 14 and 15 years of age. In boys, such growth usually does not stop before 18 years of age. The maxillaries' and face's vertical growth continues longer in both sexes when compared with the growth in length.

In light of these considerations, canons of esthetic evaluation have been altered to adapt them to growing patients. The selected reference parameters do not predict deliberate linear measures as the growing patient, unlike adults, cannot have fixed values.

Frontal View Considerations

Symmetry among the Different Parts of the Face. Like in adults, the child's face (Figure 27–13) must show perfect symmetry with the eyes, ears, and mandibular angles placed at the same height.

Correct Distance between the Eyes, Nose, and Lips. The 1:1 ratio between the width of the lips and the distance between the inside margins of the iris (Figure 27–14) remains valid. However, the child's nose base should be smaller than the intercantal distance as it will grow considerably.

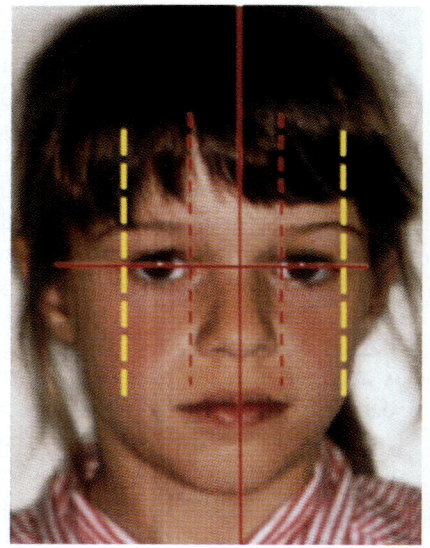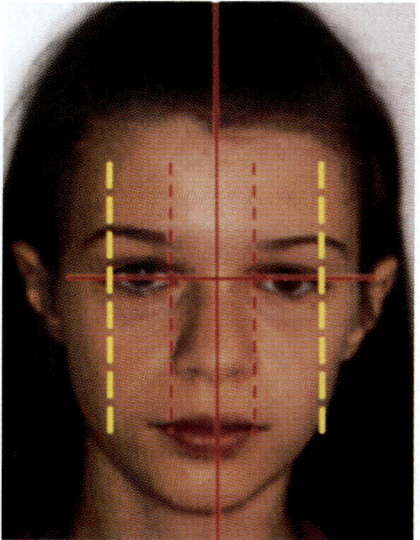

Figure 27–13: These children's faces appear to be in perfect symmetry.

Middle to Lower Facial Third Ratio. The reliable parameters for adults cannot be the same as those for children (Figure 27–15). As previously stated, the neurocranium grows earlier than the splanchnocranium; therefore, the middle third of the face develops before the lower third. In fact, the lower third should be smaller than the middle and upper thirds. Furthermore, when the lower third of the face develops earlier, it is of special concern as it is indicative of excessive growth in a vertical direction. Such considerations are inversely proportional to the patient's age.

Ratio for Esthetic Balance. This is the division of the face by a symmetry line passing through the glabella, nasal tip, midpoint of the upper lip, midpoint of the chin, and the suborbital line. The Tr-Me/ZA-ZA ratio, which in the adult is 1.35 for the male and 1.3 for the female, should have a lower value for the adolescent, who will grow more vertically than in width (Figure 27–16). Therefore, the value shall start from about 1 in younger subjects to increase gradually during growth and ultimately to reach normal (adult) reference values.

Tr = trichion: the point of the hardline in the midline of the forehead. In early childhood, identification of this landmark may be difficult because of an irregular or indistinguishable hairline.

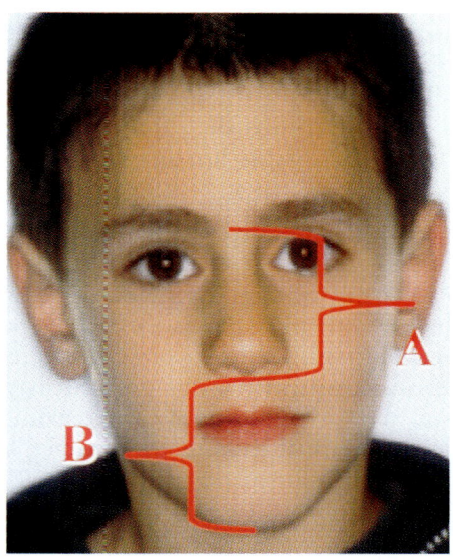

Figure 27–15: The middle third of the face develops before the lower third.

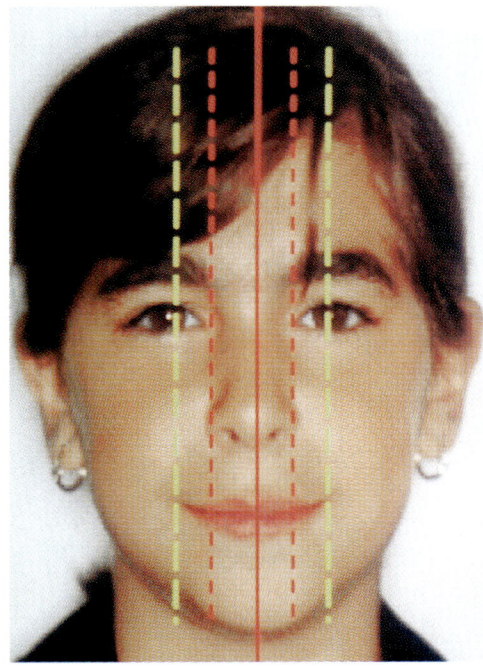

Figure 27–14: Correct distance between the eyes, nose, and lips.

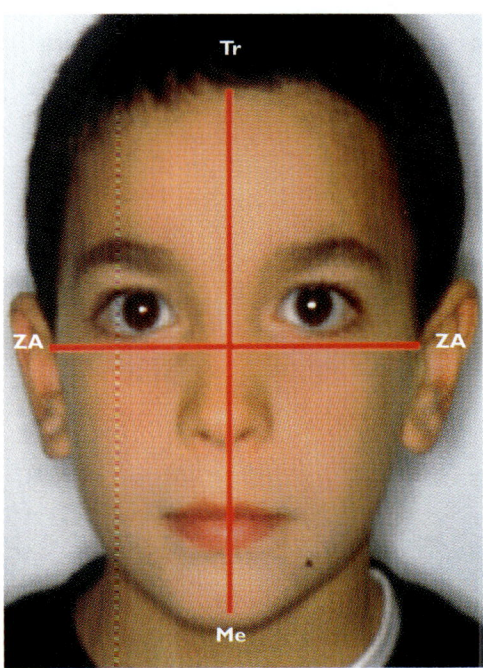

Figure 27–16: The ratio for esthetic balance.

ZA = Zygion angle: the most lateral point of each zygomatic arch. It is identical to the bony zygion of the malar bone.

ME = Menton (chin): the lowest median landmark on the lower border of the mandible.

Sclera Exposure. An excessive exposure of sclera, the firm white fibrous membrane that forms the outer covering of the eyeball, implies a developmental deficit of the middle third of the face. If this is visible and other symptoms are present, such as oral breathing with a narrow pointed nose, reduced transversal diameters of the upper maxillary with crossbite, and, dentally, upper arch crowding with a tendency to cuspal inclusion, a skeletal Class III with maxillary hypoplasia is present.

Incisal Exposure. In children, when teeth can be exfoliating or erupting, there are no reliable reference points. However, if, when smiling, a considerable quantity of marginal gingiva is exposed, an excessive facial anterior vertical growth or a maxillary excessive protrusion could exist.

Lip Closure without Tissue Strain. Over time, all soft tissues have the tendency to relax or strain; therefore, it is acceptable for a young subject to have the upper lip slightly shorter than that of an adult and, hence, moderate lip incompetence. However, this should be present no longer than 7 to 8 years of age.

Profile View Considerations

Skeletal Convexity from the Zygomatic Area to the Interlabial Gap. Considering that, in children, the lower facial third develops ahead of the middle third, it is normal that the cheek's profile is more convex than in adults (Figure 27–17). Also, a curve indicating a trend to high-angle mandibular growth is alarming, even more so if it appears in children rather than adults.

Nose Prominence. This is measured from the subnasal (the point at which the columella merges with the upper lip in the midsagittal plane) to the pronasal (the most prominent anterior point of the nose) parts of the nose. Such distance, which ranges from 16 to 20 mm for normal values in adults, will obviously have a lower value in children (Figure 27–18). It is important to note that a prominent nose is generally a contraindication to an extractive treatment. (See also Chapter 9, *Esthetics in Dentistry*, Volume 1, 2nd edition.)

The shape of the nose must also be considered. In fact, with growth, the point of the nose tends to

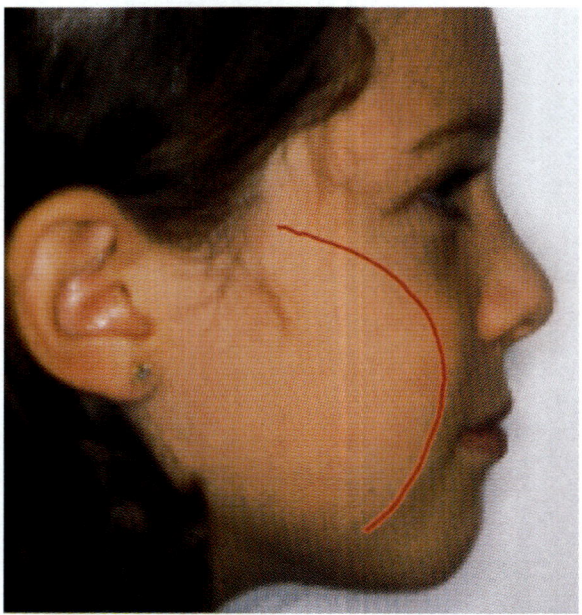

Figure 27–17: In children, the cheek's profile is more convex than in adults.

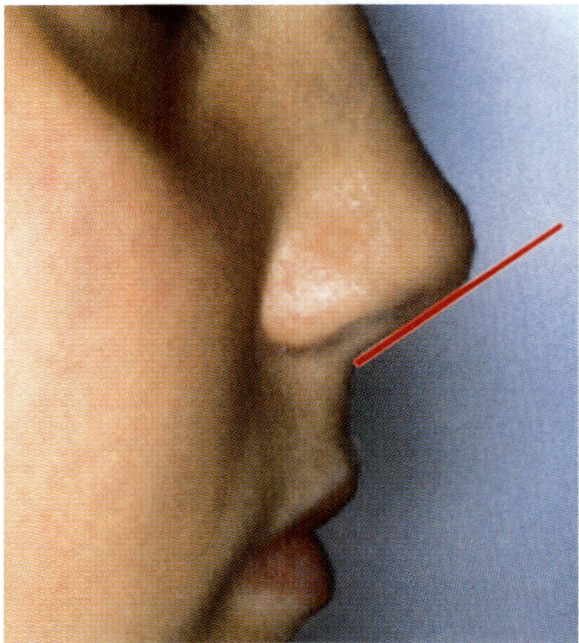

Figure 27–18: The nose prominence (subnasal – pronasal).

move downward and forward. Therefore, it is evident that a convex nose shape in a child worsens considerably with growth. On the contrary, prognosis improves in young subjects with a concave or flat nose shape. In these cases, it is also very useful to observe the child's parents. In fact, the eyes and nose are the somatic features of the face, which present the highest heredity level.

An increased nasolabial angle must not be an absolute contraindication to a protocol of serial extractions but only one of the clinical factors evaluating the case.

Lip Curvature. Both the upper and lower lips must present a slight curvature, with concavity pushing forward.

A very marked labiomental sulcus in a child may indicate a sagittal mandibular and maxillary vertical deficit, thus presupposing a low-angle facial typology (Figure 27–19). Alternatively, the total disappearance of this sulcus can indicate a mandibular sagittal and vertical development involving both planes and therefore a high-angle facial typology. High-angle subjects camouflage the dentoskeletal Class III and the low-angle subjects the Class II, improving the dental compensations that are present in such cases.

Nasolabial Angle. The nasolabial angle can be more open in the child because the nose tip grows lower. Generally, in adults, all soft tissues tend to relax and become less toned. In fact, for this reason, it is acceptable for a young patient to have the upper lip slightly short or strained and a gingival smile not more than 3 to 4 mm.

Correct Ratio between the Submental Area and the Lower Facial Third Inferior: NTP-Gn/Sn-Gn*

This ratio, which in adults has a normal value of about 0.8, will be higher in children even though the mandible will still develop in length, for two reasons: the lower third of the face will continue to develop in height, and the chin-neck contour is modest in children. Therefore, the usual value in the young patient ranges between 1 and 1.2. Lower values indicate a hypomandible; conversely, higher values indicate a hypermandible.

The skeletal type of the patient also has to be considered. For example, a decrease in the normal value of this ratio in an obese child and an increase in an athletic, long-limbed child are expected.

CONCLUSION

The esthetic measurements and treatments considered available and reliable for adults cannot be considered for children. Research must eventually supply reliable data and modify the well-worn cliché of the ideal face and proportion for the Caucasian population during growth. The result should be to alter existing esthetic analyses and adapt them to growing patients by following the predictable craniofacial growth mechanism.

When we are familiar with the growth mechanism and the different factors determining it, it will be possible to reduce the need for orthopedic-orthodontic treatments. True esthetic orthodontics may be a protocol to obtain true facial esthetics and balance when combined with effective pediatric esthetic dentistry.

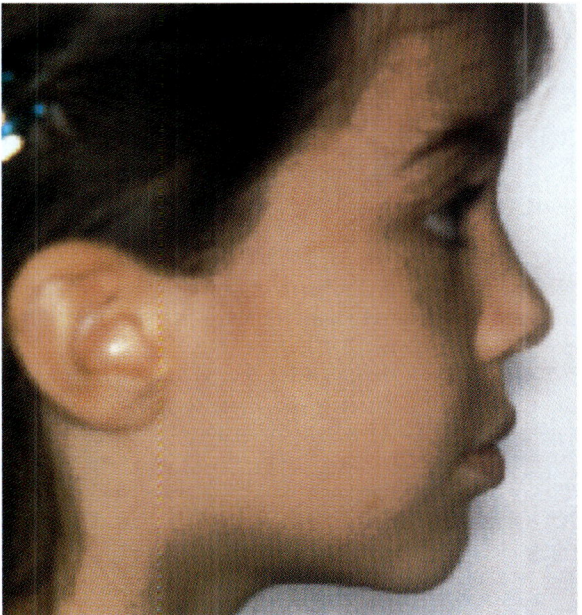

Figure 27–19: In a child, a very marked labiomental sulcus may indicate a sagittal mandibular and maxillary vertical deficit.

---

*NTP = nose tip point
Gn = gnathion: a point located by taking the midpoint between the anterior (pogonion) and inferior (menton) points of the bony chin
Sn = subnasal

As Goldstein has proposed in Volume 1, 2nd Edition of *Esthetics in Dentistry*, esthetics is the fourth dimension in dentistry, in addition to the biological, physiologic, and mechanical dimensions. Esthetic balance is increasing in importance because in the 21st century, our culture is more aware of the essentials of attractiveness in the face and smile and in general physical appeal.

Esthetic harmony is synonymous with skeletal, dental, and neuromuscular harmony and temporal mandibular joint harmony. The concept of note is that esthetics in pediatric dentistry is the basic guideline for esthetics in adults and will become a subject of growing interest in the decades ahead. As a clinical issue, esthetic considerations are increasing in frequency and importance in pediatric dentistry. The pedodontist must work in close cooperation with an orthodontist to apply correct preventive or early interceptive orthodontics and esthetic principles. This close cooperation can reduce treatment times and costs and increase long-term stability because space management will also reduce extraction cases. It is imperative to understand that esthetic harmony can lead to psychological health and higher self-assurance; it improves intrapersonal relationships and strengthens self-confidence.

To quote Jean Cocteau, "A defect of our body, if corrected, can improve our soul," or, to paraphrase an old Jewish saying, "He who gives a smile to a child gives a smile to the world."

References

1. Andreasen JO, Andreasen FM. Traumatic dental injuries—a manual. Copenhagen: Munskgaard, 1999.

2. Andreasen JO, Borum MK, Jacobsen HL, Andreasen FM. Replantation of 400 avulsed permanent incisors: 1–4. Endod Dent Traumatol 1995;11:51–89.

3. Arnett WG, Bergman RT. Facial keys to orthodontic diagnosis and treatment planning. Part I. Am J Orthod Dentofac Orthop 1993;103:299–312.

4. Arnett WG, Bergman RT. Facial keys to orthodontic diagnosis and treatment planning. Part II. Am J Orthod Dentofac Orthop 1993;103:395–410.

5. Ayala M. Estetica facciale. Atti congresso SIDO Roma 2/12/99.

6. Berg JH. The continuum of restorative materials in pediatric dentistry—a review for the clinician. Petriatr Dent 1998;20:93–100.

7. Blanchette ME, Nanda RS, Currier FG, et al. A longitudinal cephalometric study of the soft tissue profile of short- and long-face syndromes from 7 to 17 years. Am J Orthod Dentofac Orthop 1996;109:116–31.

8. Burnstone CJ, James RB, Legan H. Cephalometrics for orthognathic surgery. J Oral Surg 1978;36:269–78.

9. Caprioglio C. Odontoiatria infantile. Cap. 2. In: Paglia L, ed. Progressi in odontoiatria. Milano: Utet, 1999: 33–83.

10. Caprioglio C, Caprioglio D, Garcia-Godoy F. Traumatic dental injuries. In: Garcia-Godoy F, ed. Clinical pediatric dentistry. Heidelberg: Springen (in press).

11. Chosak A, Aidelman E. Rehabilitation of fractured incisor using the patients natural crown-case report. J Dent Child 1961.

12. El-Kalla H, Garcia-Godoy F. Bond strength and interfacial micromorphology of four adhesive systems in primary and permanent molars. J Dent Child 1998;65: 169–76.

13. Ferrario VF, Sforza C, Serrao G, et al. Reliability of soft tissue references for anteroposterior measurement of dental bases. Int J Adult Orthodont Orthognath Surg 1998;13:210–6.

14. Fortier JP, Demars-Freemault CH. Pedodonzia. Milano: Masson, 1988.

15. Garcia-Godoy F, Flaits CM, Hicks MJ. Secondary caries adjacent to amalgam restoration lined with fluoridated dentin desensitizer. Am J Dent 1998;11:254–8.

16. Garcia-Godoy F, Hosoya Y. Bonding mechanism of compo-glass to dentin in primary teeth. J Clin Pediatr Dent 1998;22:217–20.

17. Goldstein RE. Change your smile. 2nd rev. edn. Carol Stream, IL: Quintessence, 1988:22.

18. Pinkam JR, Casamassimo PS, Fields M, et al. Pediatric dentistry: infancy through adolescence. Philadelpha: WB Saunders, 1994.

19. Tsukiboshi M. Treatment planning for traumatized teeth. Tokyo: Quintessence, 2000.

20. Wilson AD, Kent BE. A new translucent cement for dentistry: a glass isonomer cement. Br Dent J 1972; 32:133–5.

Additional Resources

Andreasen JO. Atlas of replantation and transplantation of teeth. Fribourg: Mediglobe, 1992.

Andreasen JO, Andreasen FM. Text book and colour atlas of traumatic injuries to the tooth. 3rd edn. Copenhagen: Munskgaard, 1994.

Bass NM. The esthetic analysis of the face. Eur J Orthod 1991;13:343–50.

Berkman MD, Goldsmith D, Rothschild D. Evaluation-diagnosis-planning. The challenge in the correction of dentofacial deformities. J Clin Orthod 1979;13:526–38.

Black RB. Application and re-evaluation of air abrasive technique. J Am Dent Assoc 1955;50:408–14.

Cameron AC, Widmer RP, et al. Handbook of pediatric dentistry. London: Mosby, Wolfe, 1997.

Caprioglio D, Falconi P. Odontoiatria infantile pratica. Milano: Libraria internazionale, 1992.

Caprioglio D, Manna A, Paglia L, et al. Manuale di traumatologia dento-alveolare. Milano: Ciba, 1996.

Ericson D, et al. Clinical evaluation of efficacy and safety of a new method for chemo-mechanical removal of caries. Caries Res 1999;33:171–7.

Goldstein RE. Esthetics in dentistry. Philadelphia: JB Lippincott, 1976.

Goldstein RE, Parkins FM. Air-abrasive technology: its new role in restorative dentistry. J Am Dent Assoc 1994;125:151.

Holdaway RA. A soft-tissue cephalometric analysis and its use in orthodontic treatment planning. Part I. Am J Orthod 1983;84:279–93.

Jacobson A. Planning for orthognathic surgery—art or science? Int J Adult Orthodont Orthognath Surg 1990;5:217–24.

Loevy HT. Dental management of the child patient. Chicago: Quintessence, 1987.

McDonald RE. Dentistry for the child and adolescent. Mosby, 1982.

Park YC, Burstone CJ. Soft-tissue profile—fallacies of hard-tissue standards in treatment planning. Am J Orthod Dentofac Orthop 1986;90:52–62.

Staele HJ, Koch MJ. Kinder und Jugendzahn heilkunde. Köln: Ärzte-Verlag Grubtl, 1996.

Steiner CC. Cephalometrics in clinical practice. Angle Orthod 1959;29:8–29.

Tweed CH. Indications for extraction of teeth in orthodontic procedure. Am J Orthod Oral Surg 1944;30:405–28.

Worms FW, Spiedel TM, Bevis RR, Waite DE. Post-treatment stability and esthetics of orthognathic surgery. Angle Orthod 1980;50:251–73.

Wylie GA, Fish LC, Epker BN. Cephalometrics: a comparison of five analyses currently used in the diagnosis of dentofacial deformities. Int J Adult Orthodont Orthognath Surg 1987;2:15–36.

Chapter 28

Esthetics: The Complete Denture

Walter F. Turbyfill Jr., DMD

We see all about us the emphasis placed on beauty and health. Dental esthetics and the beauty of the smile are of prime importance in today's society. The edentulous patient is no exception, yet creating a natural-appearing smile for this patient is very difficult to obtain. The edentulous patient will no longer accept the prosaic straight line over the ridge denture esthetics of the past (Figure 28–1A). Dentists, not patients, must be educated that it does not have to be this way. The dentist has an awesome responsibility to the edentulous patient to produce a prosthetic appliance that appears so natural that it defies detection as a prosthetic replacement (Figure 28–1B).[3,7,9]

This chapter is primarily concerned with denture esthetics; however, comfort and function must be addressed. The failure of a complete denture treatment can be traced to three areas: comfort, function, and esthetics. A denture can be functional and comfortable. If, however, it is ugly in the eyes of the patient, it is a total failure. On the other hand, a denture can be esthetically superior, and if it is not functional and comfortable, it is still a failure.

Complete denture prosthetics has been taught in schools the very same way since the turn of the century.[4] Materials are far superior (ie, impression materials, teeth, acrylic, base tints, and precision processing equipment); however, the basic approach to satisfying the patient's needs has remained the same. Impressions are made, and bases and wax rims are constructed. The wax rims are adjusted in the mouth for tooth display, high lip line, and midline, and a jaw relation is determined. The teeth are set on the articulator by the technician or the dentist many times, with few guidelines. Then the wax-up is presented for patient approval. This is frustrating and may result in several resets to achieve patient acceptance. The denture is processed and delivered. In many cases, it is now when the patient begins to speak, eat, and observe the esthetics over a

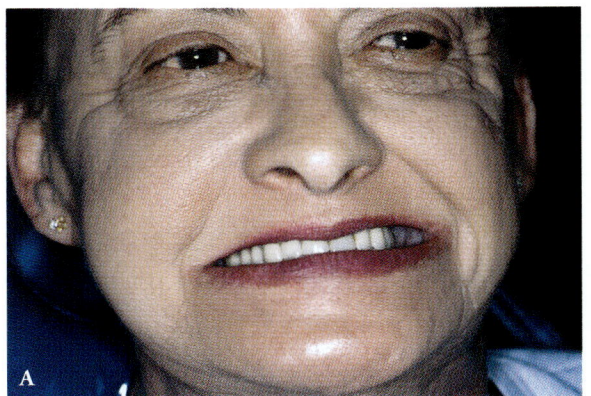 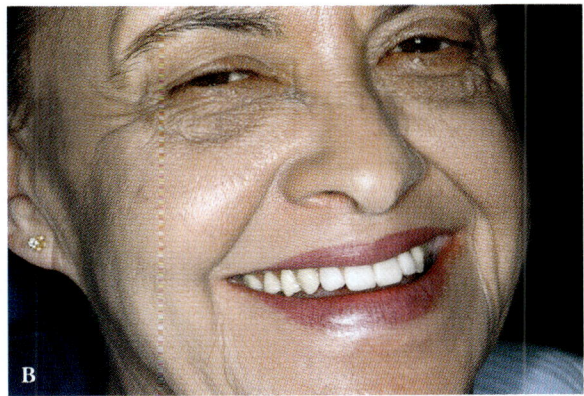

Figure 28–1A and B: *(A)* Unesthetic denture. *(B)* Esthetic denture. Maxillary anterior teeth are in the proper position; therefore, the entire denture is esthetic. The proper positioning of the anterior teeth guide all of the teeth in the denture.

period of several days that the real problems arise. Unfortunately, many patients and dentists are far too familiar with the heart-breaking results using this unpredictable approach.

In the practice of fixed restorative dentistry, comfort, function, and patient acceptance of the esthetics are ensured prior to final prosthesis construction by first providing a provisional prosthesis (Figures 28–2 and 3). In the modern practice of complete denture prosthetics, the edentulous patient is first provided with a provisional denture.[2,10,25,27,28] This provisional denture will allow the dentist to refine all of the functional esthetic aspects of the denture to his or her and the patient's satisfaction (Figures 28–4 and 5). After complete acceptance by the dentist and the patient, the provisional denture is used much like a blueprint to construct the final continuance denture. This approach leads to patient happiness without the frustrating surprises of the past. This technique makes the practice of denture prosthetics very predictable. While the patient wears the treatment denture, an added benefit is the creation of functional impressions (Figures 28–6 and 7). It is the author's experience that after final delivery of the denture, few, if any, postinsertion adjustments are necessary.

OCCLUSION: THE COMPLETE DENTURE

No discussion of complete dentures can be complete without addressing the occlusion. Of all of the causes of denture failure, the lack of a balanced occlusion in centric relation accounts for 90% of all denture failures. The most difficult challenge in denture prosthetics is occlusion. All of the denture teeth must occlude evenly as the mandible opens and closes on the arc of closure. Personal experience tells the dentist that patients with natural teeth many times function for a lifetime in a maximum intercuspal position that is not coincidental with centric relation. This is not true with the edentulous patient. These patients have lost most of the occlusal awareness, and the occlusion must be built to the repeatable position of centric relation.

This is often a difficult task because the precise jaw relation must be registered on two movable bases. In the treatment denture in Figure 28–5, the mandibular posterior teeth are replaced with a noninterfering bite block. This bite or chewing block acts as a superior repositioning splint to help the dentist obtain the optimum position of centric relation.

Registering and confirming the occlusal relation position is done with various waxers and central-bearing recording devices.

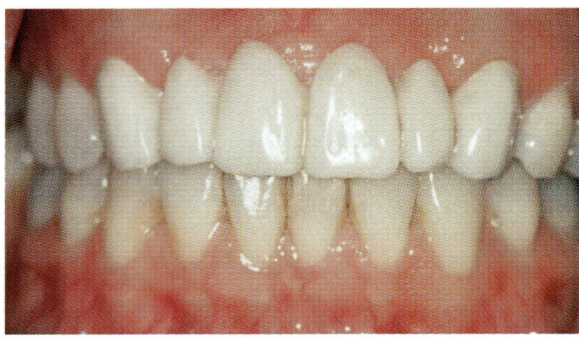

Figure 28–3: Provisional prosthesis placed to gain patient acceptance and to test esthetic and functional values.

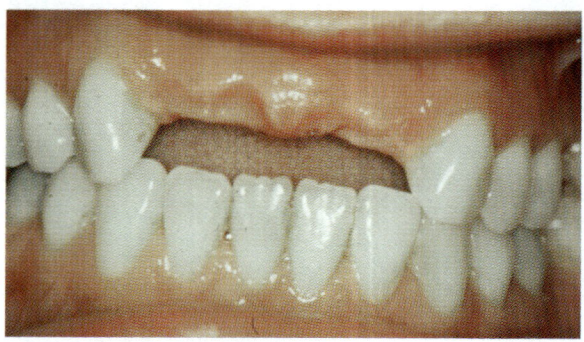

Figure 28–2: Maxillary anterior edentulous area to be treated with a fixed partial denture.

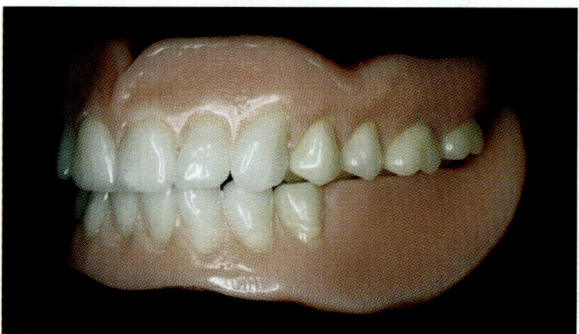

Figure 28–4: Maxillary and mandibular provisional training denture.

Esthetics: The Complete Denture

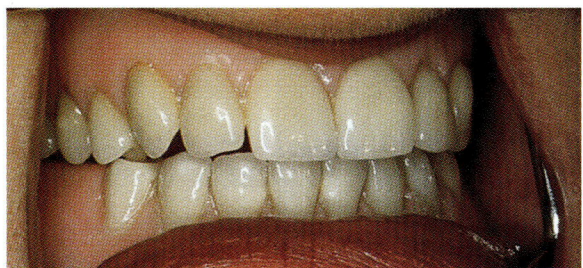

Figure 28–5: Provisional training denture placed to prove all aspects of denture function, esthetics, and comfort and to gain patient acceptance.

The occlusal scheme is referred to as a lingualized occlusion that is characterized with a single maxillary lingual cusp that functions into a mandibular fossa. This occlusion seems to be very efficient and stable for the denture patient (Figures 28–9 and 10).

Figure 28–9 shows the posterior esthetics of lingualized occlusion with the natural maxillary facial cusp.

THE ART OF CREATING ESTHETIC DENTURES: THE ESTHETIC HARMONIES

There are four esthetic harmonies that must be considered to produce a denture that will satisfy the patient's esthetic demands. These esthetic harmonies are (1) tooth size and form, (2) tooth color, (3) tooth position, and (4) background. The background is the denture base, which should be formed and colored to look like human gingiva and tinted to blend with the patient's overall complexion.

Of the four harmonies, the most important are tooth position and size. If the teeth are placed into the position that the natural teeth once occupied and in a size that is in harmony with the face, most of the esthetic requirements will have been achieved. In the consideration of tooth position and arrangement, it must be understood that everything that is done in this area has an influence on the esthetics. These considerations include the proper midline, incisal plane, posterior occlusal plane, horizontal and vertical positions of the maxillary anterior teeth, and horizontal and vertical positions of the mandibular anterior teeth.

Tooth Selection

Size and Form. Tooth size and form are considered simultaneously. The selection of the maxillary incisors is the starting point in creating esthetic dentures. There are many suggested ways to select teeth, including (1) pre-extraction records, (2) patient photographs, (3) patient desires, and (4) facial measurements.

The four methods of tooth selection are used routinely in complete denture prosthetics. There have been several theories set forth. It must be understood that none of these ways are accurate in all cases.[16–18,33,36] However the selection is made, it is a guide or a starting place.

In 1887, the temperamental theory was proposed.[13] It was one of the earliest to propose that a person's personality might influence the morphology of the teeth. In 1914, Williams[37] rejected the temperamental theory as a fallacy, proposing what is known as the geometric theory, and concluded that the shape of the face and the shape of the cen-

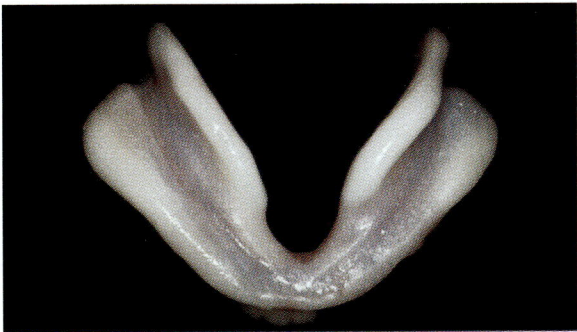

Figure 28–6: Mandibular functional impression is created as the patient wears the provisional denture.

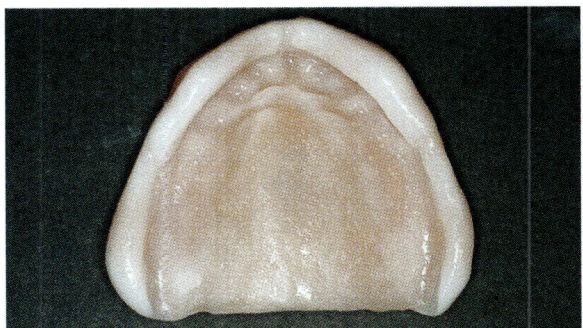

Figure 28–7: Maxillary functional impression is created as the patient wears the provisional denture.

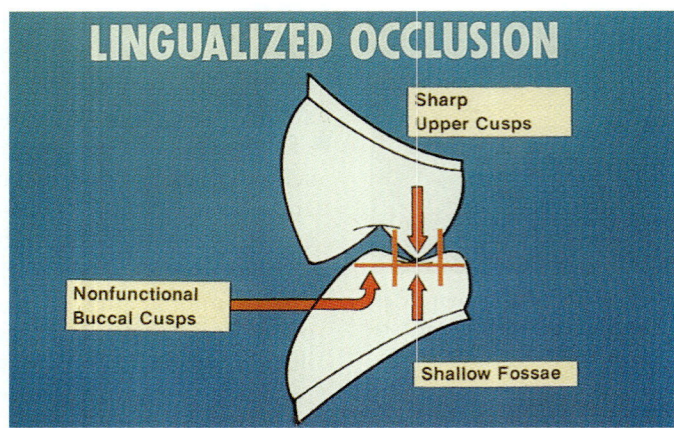

Figure 28–8: Schematic of lingual contact occlusion. Maxillary lingual cusp will function in a mandibular central fossa with no contact of the mandibular buccal cusp and the occlusal incline of the maxillary buccal cusp. (Reproduced with permission from Turbyfill WF. Regaining pleasure and success with complete denture services. Int J Prosthet 1989;2:472–82.)

tral incisor are related. This approach is still being used by many dentists. In 1939, House and Loop[12] expanded on Williams's works to include not only pure typal forms (square, tapered, and ovoid) but also combinations of typal forms and the discovery of the relationship of the width of the face and the width of the central incisor. In a study of 555 subjects, House and Loop found that the majority of central incisors were not only in harmony with facial outlines, they were also one-sixteenth of the size of the face. A study by LaVere and colleagues has confirmed their findings.[15] The author still uses this method as a basic starting place for tooth selection when other data are not available.

In 1955, Frush and Fisher[8] brought forth the sex, personality, and age (SPA) theory of tooth selection. By 1959, five additional articles followed describing the methods of applying the SPA factors. They concluded that tooth size is related to the width of the nose. With the use of the Alameter (Productivity Training Corporation, Morgan Hill, CA), it is determined whether the patient needs a small, medium, or large central incisor. Although the esthetics achieved using the SPA method is very good, one study shows that it may not be anatomically accurate.[1]

At the annual session of the American Academy of Esthetic Dentistry in 1981 in San Francisco, an interesting study was conducted by Abrams.[1] One hundred slides of human teeth were chosen, and the audience, consisting of several hundred dentists, was asked to choose whether each slide was a male or a female (lips were blocked out so that only the teeth were visible). After the results were tabulated, it was determined that (1) gender cannot be determined by tooth morphology or arrangement and (2) the older the patient, the more the audience thought that the patient was a male purely because wear denotes vigorousness to most dentists. Nevertheless, using this approach can produce many quite esthetic and pleasing results.[30] Although none of these methods is absolutely accurate,[16–18,33] it must be reiterated that there must be a starting point.

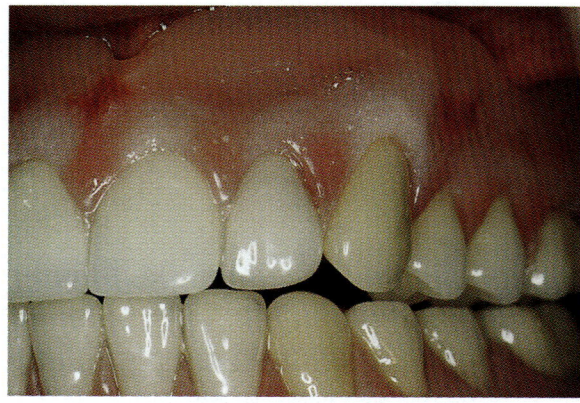

Figure 28–9: Lingualized occlusion in the completed denture.

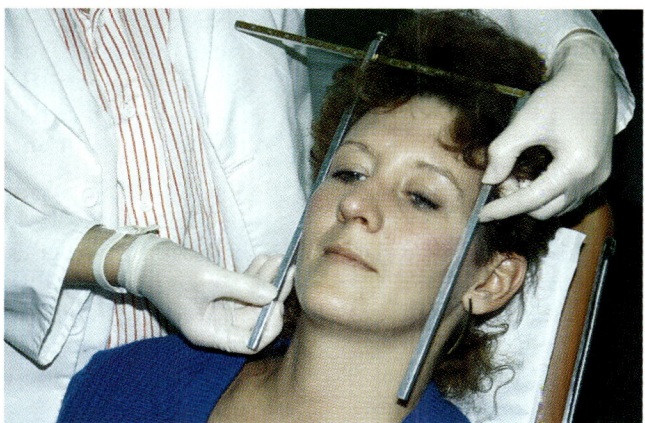

Figure 28–10: The width of the face is measured from 1 inch behind the outer canthus of the eye. (Reproduced with permission from Turbyfill WF. The union of natural contour, color, and shape. Signature 1995; Fall:14–17.)

Clinical Tooth Selection. From a clinical standpoint, measurement of the face is the first step. House and Loop have shown that the width of the central incisor is one-sixteenth of the width of the face as measured from 1 inch behind the outer canthus of the eye (see Figure 28–10). The length of the tooth is determined by measuring from the hairline to the lower border of the chin. If there is hair loss, then the top furor of the forehead is used. The measurement is made by using a device first described by House and Loop (Figure 28–11). The measurements have been interpolated to read in millimeters one-sixteenth of the width of the face.

Tooth Form and Mold. Most instruction on tooth selection suggests that tooth form be matched to the patient's facial form, that is, square, tapered, ovoid, or, in some manufacturers' teeth, combination form types. These combinations include square/tapered, square/ovoid, tapered/ovoid, etc. Some tooth manufacturers make only the basic square, tapered, and ovoid but do not make the combination forms. Other manufacturers make only different size teeth and no teeth designated for the different facial forms. These manufacturers do, however, make molds that exhibit different amounts of incisal wear.

The author rarely considers tooth mold in terms of square, tapered, or ovoid. Once the proper tooth size is selected, the mold is selected to fit the patient's maturity. Younger patients get more rounded molds with unworn tips on the cuspids. More mature patients will get teeth that show more incisal wear and cuspids where the incisal tip is worn flatter. The author puts tapered teeth in ovoid faces or square teeth in tapered faces and does not like ovoid teeth in most cases (see Tip 2 below).

After the upper anterior teeth are selected, the lower anterior teeth are selected as recommended by the manufacturer. For example, the 44E (DENTSPLY/Trubyte, York, PA) maxillary anterior mold is opposed by mandibular mold F (DENTSPLY/Trubyte), and the Universal Lactona maxillary anterior mold M45 (Universal Lactona Dental, Montgomeryville, PA) is opposed by mandibular mold M45 (Universal Lactona Den-

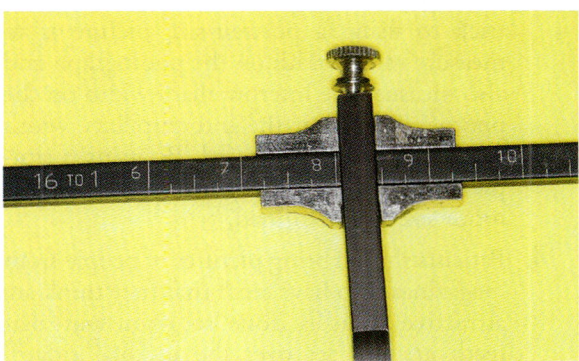

Figure 28–11: The measuring device reads the facial width in millimeters at a ratio of 1 to 16.

tal). The combined width of the recommended six lower anterior teeth is generally 10 mm less than the combined width of the upper six anterior teeth (see Tip 6 below).

Tips on Tooth Selection.

1. Facial width of one-sixteenth is determined to give the width of the central incisors. The laterals and cuspids in any mold are sized to be in harmony with this measurement. The facial length is never used because the length of the teeth is more determined by lip height and the size of the residual ridge. This maxillary central size is always in harmony with the size of the patient's face. Next, the shape or mold of the teeth must be selected. The author uses another method that is called "heart and imagination." This is hard to explain. Credit is to be given to Fillastre (Fillastre, Lakeland, FL, personal communication, 1980). After the appropriate size is selected, the dentist will picture the patient in his mind's eye with the mold chart in front of him and picture what mold would look good for the patient.

2. Facial types—square, tapered, or ovoid—have little to do with mold selection. The amount of incisal wear is a more appropriate guideline. The older the patient, the flatter the incisal edges. The younger patient will require more rounded edges that show less wear. Older patients tend to have flatter, more worn cuspids. There is basically no difference in molds for male or female.

3. Patients should be asked to bring pictures of themselves before they lost their natural teeth. This can show anterior tooth arrangement and situations such as diastemas. A trick to using a portrait-size picture is to measure tooth width on the photograph and also measure the interpupillary width on the photograph. Then the interpupillary width on the patient is measured. By using a simple mathematical proportion, the actual tooth size is determined.

4. Patients should bring pictures of people from magazines who have teeth that they think are attractive. This is done to point out that teeth are not set over the residual ridge[27] with small teeth hidden back in the mouth. Pretty teeth are prominent and support the lip. Most pretty people show all of their teeth when they smile, and many show some or all of their gingiva. This exercise allows the teeth to be placed more in the position that the natural teeth once occupied.

5. The molds are mixed. For example, the central and cuspids from one mold and the laterals from another are used. Also, the use of laterals from two different molds can create a nice effect. The patient must be educated to the fact that bilateral symmetry does not occur in nature and that this is not esthetic.

6. Manufacturers' suggestions for a mandibular anterior mold to use with a specific maxillary anterior mold are dictated by a combined upper and lower width that will allow the first bicuspids, maxillary and mandibular, to blend in harmony with the maxillary and mandibular cuspids and with the cuspids in a Class I relationship. To be esthetic, a denture must be in harmony with nature. It is good to remember that in establishing natural denture esthetics, the teeth are to be set in harmony with original jaw relations, whether it is Class I, II, or III. In these cases, the mandibular anterior mold may have to be varied in size to produce a nice harmonic transition from the cuspids to the first bicuspids during set-up.

7. In selecting posterior teeth, the author's preference is to use an anatomic maxillary posterior tooth (33-degree cuspid tooth) that occludes in a lingualized fashion into the central fossae of the lower.[5,27] The esthetics is far superior to flat plane and other lesser degree teeth. The beautiful maxillary buccal cusps look natural (see Figure 28–9). The purpose of the maxillary buccal cusp is esthetics, food manipulation, and overjet to prevent jaw biting.

8. Facial profiles can be important in denture tooth selection. For example, an individual with a flat profile might look better with a flat mold tooth, and the patient with a curved profile might look better with a more curved or rounded facial contour.

9. A choice is made between porcelain or acrylic teeth. Porcelain teeth keep their luster. They will not wear excessively, causing loss of vertical dimension, which leads to serious esthetic

problems. There are times when, because of interarch space, acrylic teeth must be used. In these cases, metal occlusal surfaces should be used to prevent further loss of vertical dimension. The use of acrylic teeth does not reduce the pressure on the underlying bone. Rapid bone loss is caused by malocclusion. With plastic teeth, the malocclusion is soon worn in; with porcelain teeth, the malocclusion is there forever.

10. The newer composite resin teeth have certain advantages. Ro Youdalis pointed out that the hardness of these teeth will make many metal occlusal surfaces unnecessary because of their wear resistance (personal communication, 1985).

Tooth Color. The hues found in most natural teeth fall into the ranges of yellow, brown, and orange. The lightness and darkness of teeth are controlled by the value (degree of gray or white). Chroma (the saturation of hue) increases with advanced age, whereas the value decreases.

Tooth color and gingival tissue seem to be related to tissue tones and the general overall complexion of the individual. The light-complexion, blue-eyed blond will usually display very light teeth, with little or no yellow. Contrasting this is the dark-complexion brunette and redhead whose teeth generally show more yellow, brown, and orange.

As these individuals grow older, the yellow-brown of the brunette is intensified by a deeper color and lower value. As the blue-eyed blond advances in age, the greatest change is lower value. The teeth become more gray but still exhibit very little yellow-brown.

There are always exceptions. It is not unusual at all to see a dark-complexion brunette with very white teeth with no yellow. There are exceptions to all of these rules.

Tips on Tooth Color.
1. Consultation with the patient is the best way to establish rapport in the matter of tooth color.[11] No attempt should be made to convince a patient to accept any other shade than what he or she wants.[35] All patients want nice white teeth, and the older denture patient is no exception. (A personal note on this subject is in order. In the early days, the author tried to select teeth as his mentor did to be in harmony with the patient's age and complexion. It seemed that he was always at odds with patients who wanted white teeth.) Seminars are conducted during which dentures are provided for patients. Since all of the shades cannot be available during the seminars, only light shades are stocked. There is never a discussion about shades at the seminars. The fact that every patient gets young bright teeth is a key to success.

2. Every female patient is asked when looking at their old denture, "Wouldn't you like a brighter, more youthful tooth on your new denture?" The response is interesting: it is always yes.

3. Many patients love to see the artist in their dentist emerge. The dentist could try using central incisors of one shade and then change the shades of the laterals. The patient with the love of naturalness will respond.

4. Lower anteriors one shade darker than the upper incisors should be used.

Tooth Arrangement

Once a proper tooth has been selected for the patient, the maxillary anterior teeth will be positioned on the base. *The most important consideration in creating an esthetic denture is the position of the maxillary anterior teeth.* This position will directly influence the position of every other tooth in the denture.

Frank Lloyd Wright said, "Form and function are one." So it is with dentures: the closer the artificial teeth are placed to the position once occupied by the natural teeth, the better the function will be. Another advantage of natural tooth placement is that they will fall within the neutral zone, which is the neutral point of muscle balance between the lips and cheeks and the tongue.

E. Pound (personal communication, 1975) said that, in the early days, when motion pictures became talking pictures, many actors lost their jobs because of poor dentistry and poor phonetics. He said that the sound people at the studios knew as little about speech as he did. Pound said that he strove to make dentures exquisitely esthetic and that the better they looked, the better they spoke. This is how his lifetime study of phonetics began.

In the practice of complete denture prosthetics, if the dentist can position the artificial teeth in the position the natural teeth occupied, the better the esthetics and function will be.

Key to Superior Denture Esthetics

The single most important thing that must be done to create an esthetic denture is proper placement of the maxillary anterior teeth. The key is the placement of the maxillary central incisors. If these two teeth are correct, they will directly influence the position of every other tooth in the denture. Correctly placed, the maxillary six incisors should be as close as possible to the exact position once occupied by the natural teeth. The notion that teeth should be set over the ridge to gain a mechanical advantage is simply outdated and untrue. If the teeth are set to anatomic harmony, then they will be in the neutral zone and vice versa.

Setting the Maxillary Anterior Teeth in Anatomic Harmony

Over the years, the author has measured casts of natural maxillary anterior teeth to find a common position. A common average position of the maxillary anterior teeth to constant landmarks has been found by measuring hundreds of casts of natural healthy teeth. These measurements are (1) the distance of the incisal labial one-third of the maxillary central incisors from the center of the incisive papilla (Figure 28–12) and (2) the distance down the incisal edge from the general height of the maxillary anterior labial vestibule (Figure 28–13).

This position will not be appropriate for every patient. It will put the teeth in a reasonable position all of the time. Variations from this position require a judgment on the dentist's part. The author has observed that when positioned in this manner, about 4 in 10 patients are close to ideal. The other 60% will need slight changes.

In Figure 28–14A, the patient has very unesthetic dentures. The ridges are healthy and well formed (Figure 28–14B). A stabilized base is constructed onto the cast of the maxillary edentulous ridge. A wax rim is placed onto the stabilized base. The wax rim is built 10 mm out from the center of the incisal papilla and 20 mm down from the general height of the labial vestibule. In addition, the wax rim is built level to the interpupillary line and parallel to Camper's line. Camper's line runs from the middle of the tragis of the ear to the base of the ala of the nose. The wax rim is tried into the edentulous mouth. The level of the incisal plane and Camper's line is verified. The facial midline is marked (Figures 28–14C to E).

The maxillary central incisors are set onto the wax rim (Figure 28–14F) and confirmed in the mouth (Figures 28–14G and H).[14,21,23] Once the proper position of the central incisors is verified, then the remainder of the maxillary incisors is set (Figure 28–14I). At this point, the basic tooth position has been determined. Detailed esthetics, such as lapping of the lateral incisors and tipping of the cuspids, is done in the laboratory.

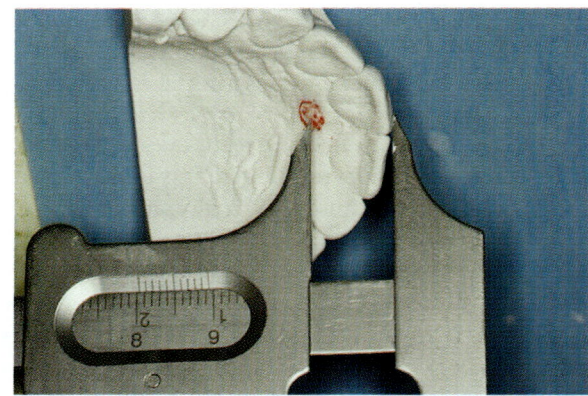

Figure 28–12: Average horizontal position of the maxillary central incisors is determined by measuring the distance from the center of the incisive papilla and the labial incisal one-third of the central incisors.

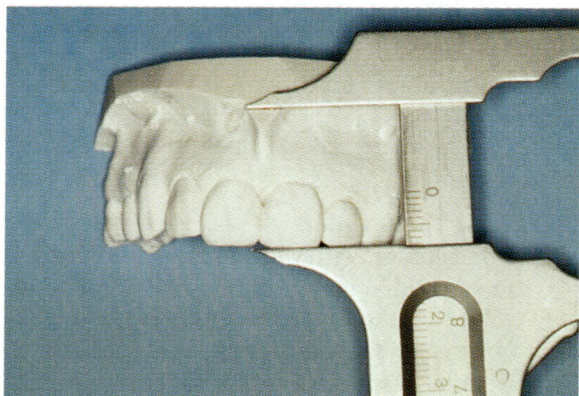

Figure 28–13: Average vertical position of the maxillary central incisors is measured from the general height of the anterior labial vestibule down to the incisal edge of the central incisors.

Esthetics: The Complete Denture 839

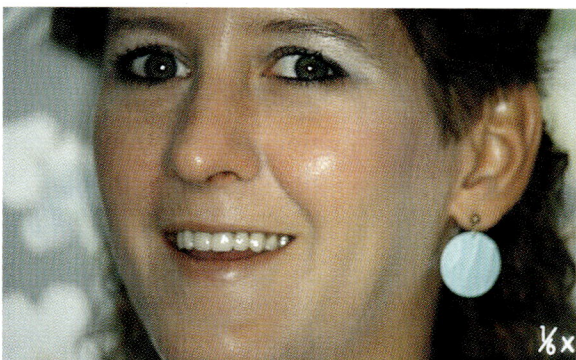

Figure 28–14A: A 32-year-old edentulous patient with teeth set over the ridge with a straight line set-up resulting in the typical denture look.

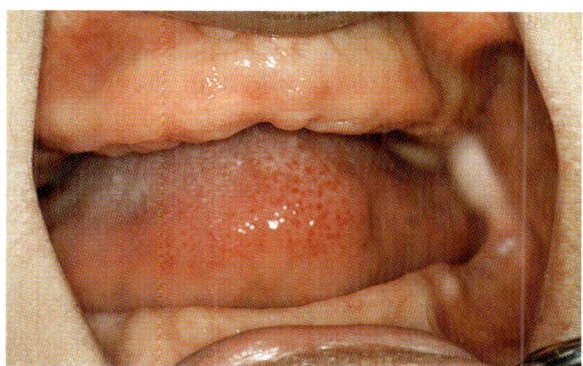

Figure 28–14B: The edentulous ridges appear adequate and healthy.

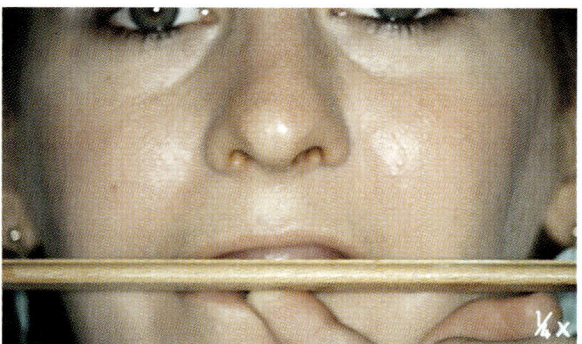

Figure 28–14C: The maxillary bite rim is built 10 mm anterior from the center of the incisive papilla horizontally and vertically 20 mm down from the general height of the labial vestibule. It is built level so that it is parallel to the interpupillary line. (Reproduced with permission from Turbyfill WF. Union of natural contour, color, and shape. Signature 1995; Fall:14–17.)

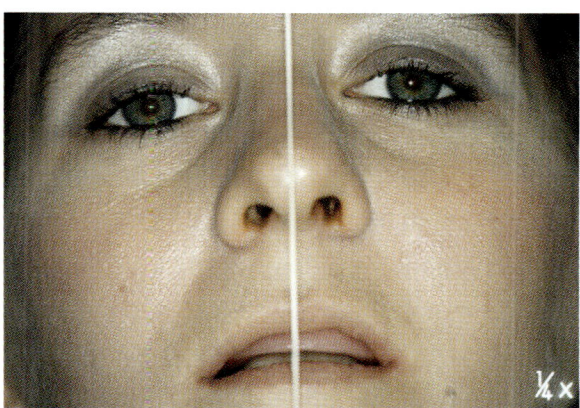

Figure 28–14D: The midline is marked.

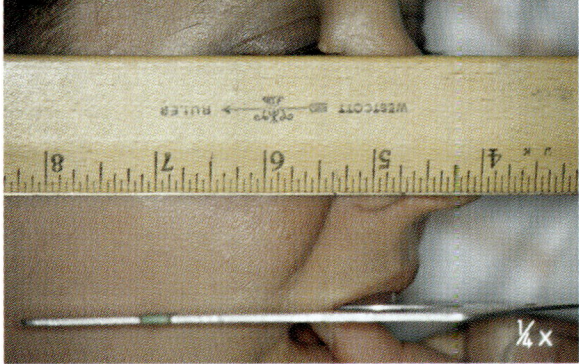

Figure 28–14E: The maxillary bite rim is built parallel to Camper's line.

Once the maxillary anterior basic tooth position has been verified, as a demonstration, a silicone matrix has been made onto the set-up. In this case, the central incisors ended up 9 mm anterior to the center of the incisive papilla. The teeth follow the curvature of the edentulous ridge (Figure 28–14J). If the ridge should be more square or more "V" shaped, this would have been reflected in the arrangement. The cuspid begins to be tucked closer to the ridge as the corner is turned from the anterior ridge to the posterior area of the ridge.

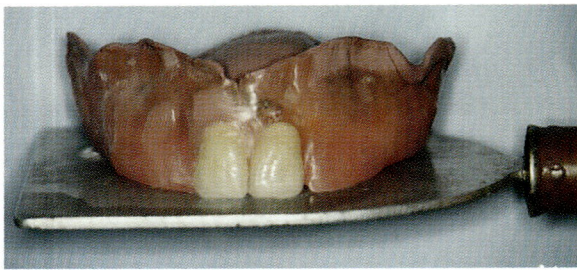

Figure 28–14F: The maxillary central incisors are set to the previously determined midline and the horizontal and vertical determinants. (Reproduced with permission from Turbyfill WF. Union of natural contour, color, and shape. Signature 1995; Fall:14–17.)

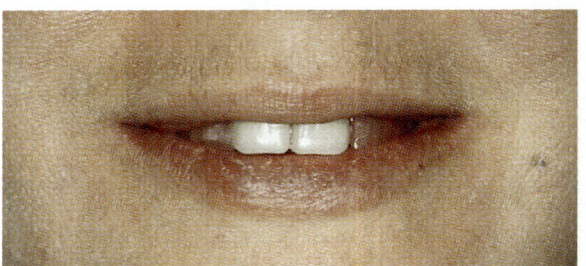

Figure 28–14G: The central incisor position is verified in the patient's mouth as to tooth display and midline.

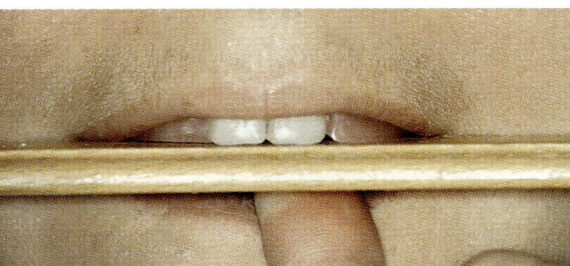

Figure 28–14H: The level of the central incisors is verified. (Reproduced with permission from Turbyfill WF. Union of natural contour, color, and shape. Signature 1995; Fall:14–17.)

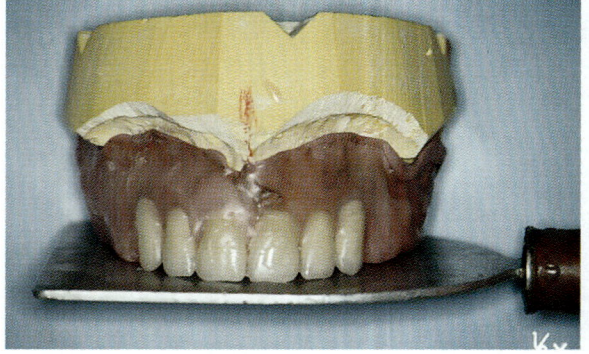

Figure 28–14I: The maxillary anterior tooth position is completed.

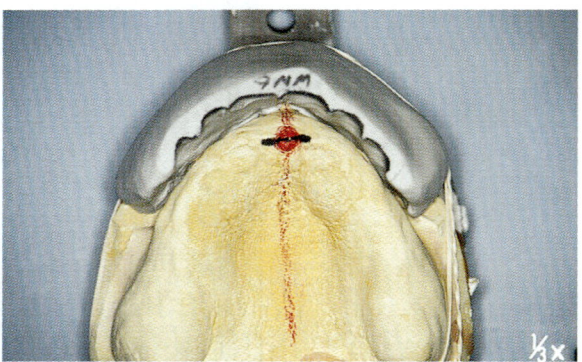

Figure 28–14J: The natural position of the maxillary teeth to the edentulous ridge.

Esthetics: The Complete Denture

The much improved esthetics of the finished denture is shown. Figure 28–14K shows the superior esthetics that has been achieved using this approach.

Once the maxillary teeth are set to anatomic harmony and the dentist is satisfied with this position, the mandibular anterior teeth are set so that they exhibit one half to 1 mm of clearance as the sibilant sounds are being enunciated (Figure 28–14L). The vertical dimension of occlusion is recorded by arcing the mandible in the arc of closure in centric relation and closing the vertical down until the anterior stop comes into contact (Figure 28–14M).

A denture may appear to be reasonably esthetic at first glance, as is the maxillary denture shown in Figures 28–15A to C. The denture was remade because of poor function and comfort. The teeth are now set to a position more in keeping with anatomic harmony. This position is 20 mm down from the height of the maxillary vestibule and 10 mm out from the center of the incisive papilla. Figures 28–15D to F show the subtle but exquisite improvement in esthetics and maxillary lip support.

Placement of the Mandibular Anterior Teeth

The mandibular anterior teeth are set using phonetics. Dawson[6] noted that the vertical dimension of occlusion that has been lost can be regained by noting the closest speaking level and then establishing the vertical dimension of occlusion slightly more closed from that closest speaking position. Pound[24] referred to this as the vertical dimension of speech, and since the teeth are not to touch while a person is speaking, then the vertical dimension of

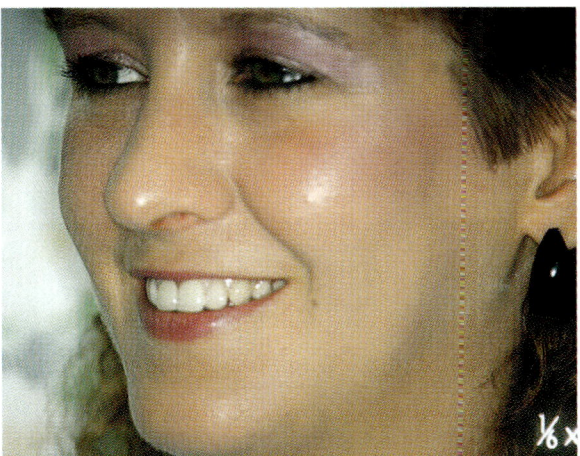

Figure 28–14K: The superior esthetic results achieved by placing the maxillary anterior teeth to anatomic harmony.

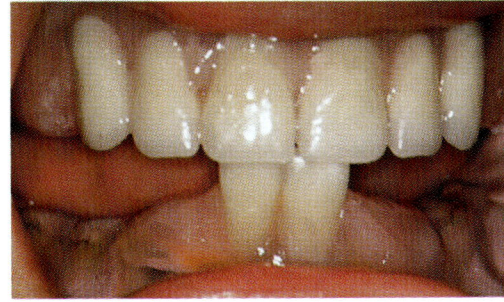

Figure 28–14L: The mandibular anterior teeth are positioned to exhibit a 1- to ½-mm clearance with the maxillary anterior teeth as the patient enunciates "S" sounds.

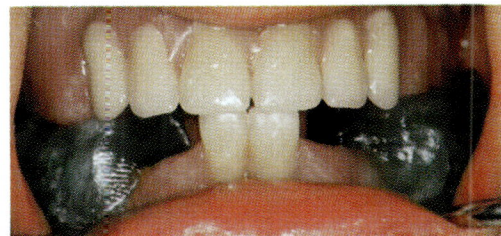

Figure 28–14M: The mandibular position of centric relation is determined by a simple wax recording. This is considered a treatment position, and final centric relation determination is achieved by using a central bearing point and Gathic arch tracing.

842 Esthetics in Dentistry

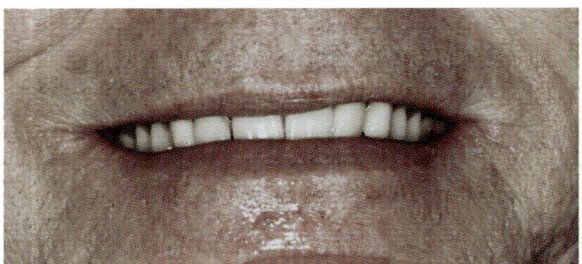

Figure 28–15A: A denture with a poor maxillary anterior tooth position.

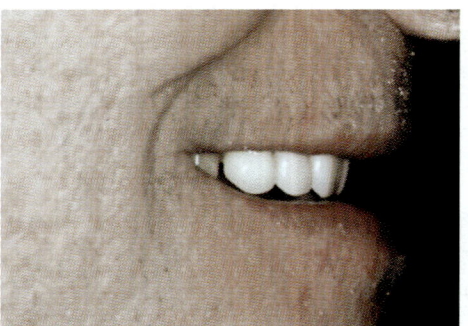

Figure 28–15B: Note the depressed position of the incisors.

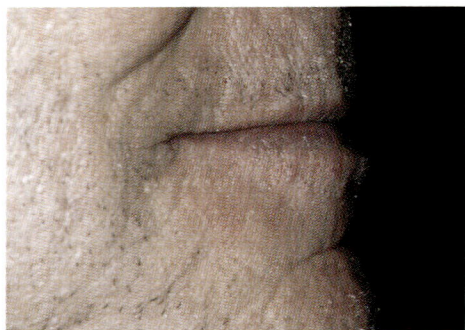

Figure 28–15C: Note the look of the maxillary lip support.

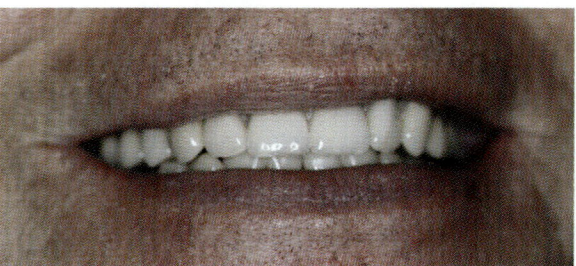

Figure 28–15D: An esthetic denture with the maxillary central incisors set to the 10 × 20 rule.

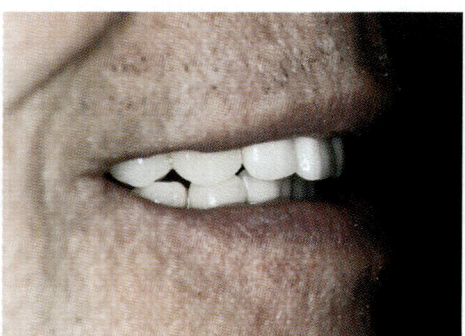

Figure 28–15E: Note the more natural tooth position.

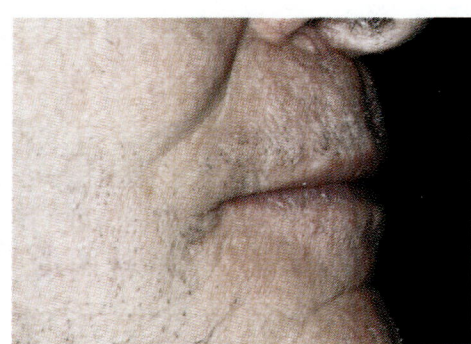

Figure 28–15F: Note the improved lip support.

occlusion should be slightly more closed than the "S" position. Further, the "S" position is the most forward, most closed position the mandible ever assumes during speech.

Two mandibular incisors are set to the "S" position. Pound defined the "S" position as the most intimate relationship of the teeth during speech.[24] There are intimate relationships that occur between the incisal edges of the mandibular teeth and the incisal edges and lingual surfaces of the maxillary anterior teeth. This allows the dentist to verify the accuracy of the maxillary tooth arrangement and place the mandibular incisors in an anatomically natural position that produces an articulate speech pattern.

After this position is verified, the anterior stop has been re-established (see Figure 28–14L).

Anterior Denture Occlusion

No anterior teeth should be in contact when the posterior teeth are in maximum occlusion. This anterior pressure will cause destruction of the bone of the premaxilla. It also causes instability of the dentures. Once the anterior teeth are set to exhibit a phonetic clearance when the "S" sounds are enunciated, the centric relation registration is then taken with the anterior stop in contact. In Class I and II jaw relationships, the mandible leaves the centric relation posture position and moves forward to the phonetic "S" position. Therefore, the articulator pins are opened slightly on Class I and II occlusions so that the anterior teeth will not contact in the centric relation. Since the mandible always moves forward in phonetics, the condylar guidance will keep the posterior teeth from contacting in speech.

In Class III occlusion, there is no forward movement of the mandible during speech. Slight anterior contact in the Class III jaw relationship is inevitable. The occlusal contact should be heavier in the posterior than in the anterior.

Vertical Dimension

The author uses phonetics and the closest speaking position to develop the incisal edge position of the mandibular anterior teeth, and the vertical dimension of occlusion is determined from this. It must be understood that this method is not always accurate. Some patients exhibit an adapted position that is obviously overclosed. In cases like this, the vertical is opened on the trial bases until the facial profile looks more normal. In other words, the patient should not look older below the nose than above the nose. Since all patients are treated with a provisional treatment denture, this "arbitrary" vertical dimension is tested before denture finalization. Even though phonetics is not accurate in every case, it is still the preferred way because the different movements of the mandible for the different classes of occlusion help to position the incisal edges in a more natural position.

There are many ways to establish the vertical dimension of occlusion on dentures, such as phonetics, relaxation of the mandible to establish the resting level of the mandibular free way space, having the patient wet the lips and breathe out, and measuring dots on the nose and chin and other facial dimensions. Volumes have been written about vertical dimension. The subject of vertical dimension is a very emotional one, and some heated arguments can erupt over it.

The most important thing that the dentist must remember about vertical dimension is that if the vertical is opened too far so as to cause the posterior teeth to hit as the patient speaks, a failure will always result. Another important observation is that the dentist should give each denture patient the greatest vertical dimension possible. The patient will look, chew, and feel better.

Improper vertical dimension can have a profound effect on esthetics. In Figure 28–16A, the patient looks prognathic and old below the nose with a vertical dimension that is overclosed. Figure 28–16B shows excellent esthetics when the vertical dimension is properly restored. Figure 28–16C demonstrates the poor esthetics created by improper vertical and horizontal positioning of the maxillary anterior teeth and the denture look. Figure 28–16D shows the improved esthetics with proper maxillary anterior tooth positioning.

Consideration of the vertical dimension of the occlusion for the edentulous patient as it differs from the patient with natural teeth needs to be addressed. Patients with natural teeth are very adaptive to changes in the vertical dimension of the occlusion because of the exquisite proprioception of natural teeth. Many times, a slight opening of the vertical dimension is needed to facilitate restorative procedures. Edentulous patients do not adapt near-

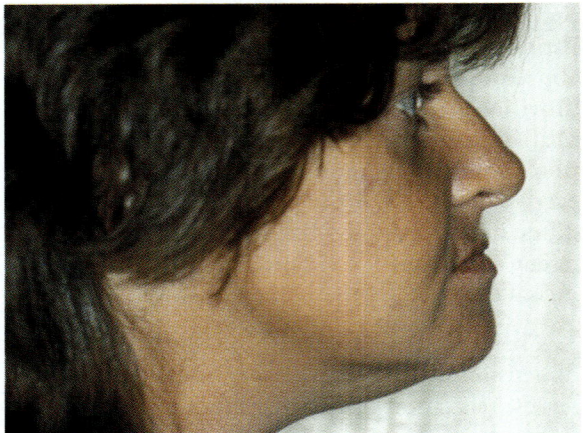

Figure 28–16A: Overclosure of the vertical dimension of the occlusion. Note the prognathic appearance and decreased lower facial length.

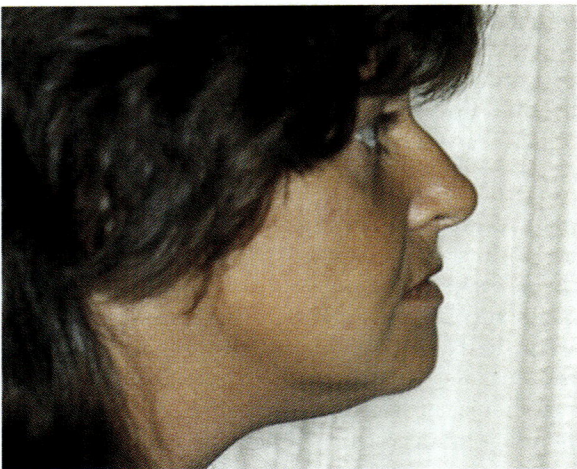

Figure 28–16B: Proper vertical dimension of occlusion. Note how much younger the patient appears.

ly as well. Generally, when the closest speaking position is determined, any opening from that position should be done while the patient is wearing the provisional training denture. An excessive vertical dimension of the occlusion in complete dentures results in a restriction of normal muscle activity, and the posterior and anterior teeth will hit during speech. When opened experimentally using the training denture, if the teeth continue to hit during speech for 1 week, then adaptation is not possible, and the teeth will hit during speech forever.

Posterior Occlusion As It Relates to Denture Esthetics

One area often overlooked or misunderstood is the effect of the posterior tooth position on esthetics. An extremely poor esthetic denture can result by establishing the posterior plane of occlusion too high or too low. This is demonstrated by the patient who smiles, and the maxillary posterior teeth can be seen hanging down below the plane of the maxillary incisors. Camper's line will position the posterior occlusal plane on a line beamed from

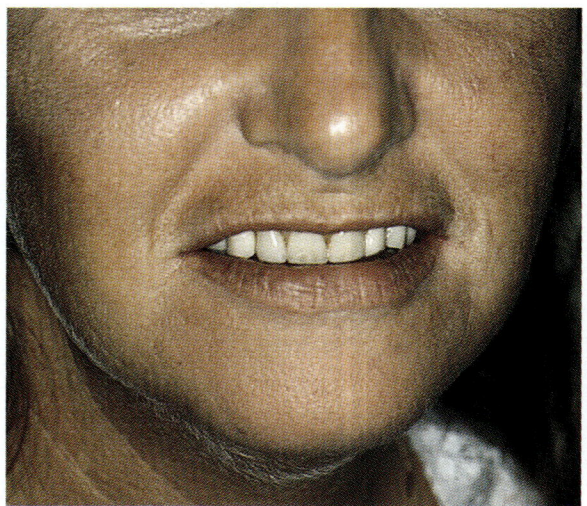

Figure 28–16C: Everything looks bad: the denture look.

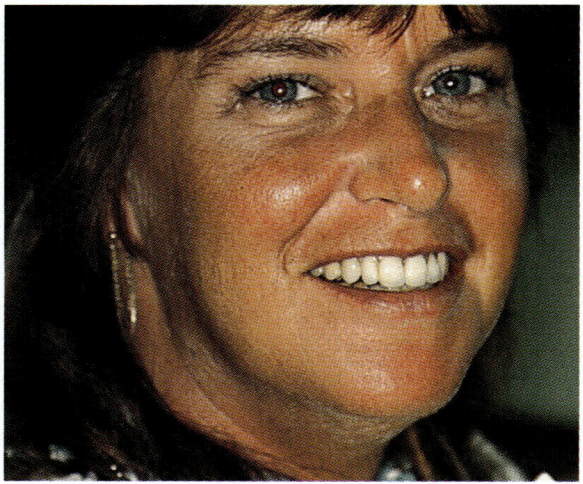

Figure 28–16D: The natural look: correct maxillary anterior tooth placement and correct vertical dimension of occlusion.

the maxillary anterior incisal edge posterior to the middle of the retromolar pad (Figure 28–17).

The buccolingual placement of the posterior teeth can also affect esthetics. If the maxillary teeth are placed too far to the buccal aspect, then the buccal corridor between the maxillary posterior teeth and the corner of the mouth is lost. If the maxillary teeth are placed too far lingually or palatally, then they appear not to exist. Either extreme produces unacceptable esthetics. The guideline for the maxillary posterior tooth position is found in the mandibular arch. The lingual central line is from the mesial contact of the cuspid to the lingual aspect of the retromolar pad. The lingual surface of the mandibular posterior teeth should fall on this line. The mandibular posterior teeth are positioned closer to the tongue than this line (Figure 28–18).

Tips for Tooth Arrangement

1. The position of the maxillary central incisors is the key to denture esthetics. Once they are placed and accepted, all other tooth positions are a product of these two teeth.

2. Placement of the anterior teeth *must* be done at chairside in the presence of the patient. The author never lets the patient see the results of this initial placement because the setting is a very straight-line prosaic set-up and represents basic tooth position. Detailed esthetics is done at the laboratory bench.

3. The appointment for this initial setting is from 1 to 1 1/2 hours. The rapport that is built with

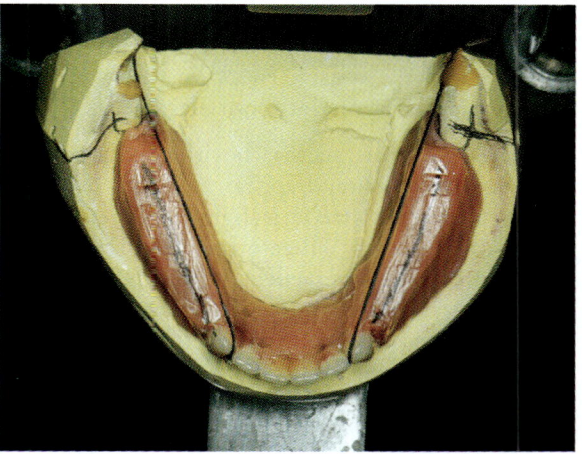

Figure 28–18: Buccolingual placement of the posterior occlusal plane. The lingual control line runs from the mesial contact of the cuspid to the lingual aspect of the retromolar pad.

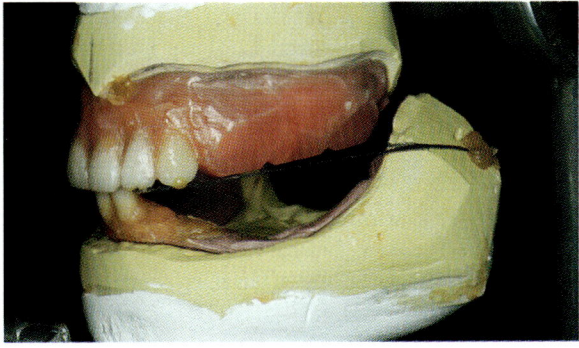

Figure 28–17: Posterior occlusal plane lines up from the maxillary incisal edges to a point halfway up the retromolar pad (Camper's line).

the patient at this time is unbelievable. The patient will always say, "I've never had a dentist spend so much time with me."

4. The "S" position is the most intimate relationship of any teeth during speech.[22,26] As the "S" sounds are formed, the anterior teeth will exhibit a space of 1 to 1 1/2 mm. The "S" sounds are produced by forcing air between the incisal edges of the maxillary incisors and the mandibular incisors. The "S" sounds can also be produced by forcing air between the incisal edges of the mandibular incisors and the lingual surfaces of the maxillary incisors, as will be found in many Class II occlusal relationships. It should be remembered that the teeth do not touch when the "S" sounds are being enunciated.

5. The vertical dimension of occlusion is very easy to determine since it is always less than the vertical dimension of speech.[19,20,32] Therefore, when the anterior teeth are set to the "S" position, the mandible is retruded and closed down 2 mm to tooth contact or, if no teeth touch, merely closes in a centric relation 2 mm less than the vertical dimension of speech.

6. The "F" and "V" sounds are produced when the incisal edges of all six maxillary anterior teeth make a fleeting seal at the vermilion border or the wet dry line of the lower lip. If the maxillary

teeth are placed in anatomic harmony, the "F" and "V" position will always be correct. This is an extremely valuable check on the accuracy of the maxillary anterior tooth placement.

7. The anterior teeth, both maxillary and mandibular, should appear as if they are coming from the bone at a slightly different angle. Sharry[31] wrote, "There is one prominent guide for providing an excellent arrangement of anterior teeth; they must be separate." Bilateral symmetry is not found in nature. The laterals can be mesially lapped or winged out distally. Laterals can be set to be shorter than the centrals or cuspids; however, the older the patient, the more even the incisal edges should be. If photographs are available and show diastemas, they can be placed subject to patient approval. It should be remembered that the younger the patient, the more open the incisal embrasures.

8. Always keep the incisal plane level and slightly curved to follow the smile line of the lower lip. There is nothing more unesthetic than a slanted occlusal or incisal plane.

9. In a few patients, flaring of the cuspid can be esthetic, but, in most cases, it is best to set the cuspid so that only the mesial surface can be seen.

10. It should be remembered that the first introduction to dental esthetics to dental students and dental technology students was a Columbia Dentiform.

11. Pictures of "pretty" people should be used to show how beautiful smiles are made in nature. Dentists should point out the asymmetry and how prominent the teeth appear in a full smile.

12. There are some interesting studies being done concerning the arrangement of teeth for the edentulous patient by the use of cephalometric radiographs.[29] Orthodontists use the method of fixed bony landmarks to determine the ideal placement of natural teeth. It seems that this would be a valuable aid for tooth placement in complete denture prosthetics, particularly in the advanced resorbed dental arch.

13. The author uses "heart and imagination" in selecting and arranging teeth. In the laboratory, there should be a large selection of teeth, and as the dentist looks at the basic tooth position set at chairside, he or she must picture the patient in his or her mind's eye and set and select teeth to what he or she feels will be pleasing.

BACKGROUND

The denture base is important in esthetics.[34,38] Its normal contour aids in support of the soft tissues of the lips and face. If the patient has a short upper lip and would normally show gingival tissues in a broad smile, an unesthetic denture base can destroy an otherwise esthetically successful denture.

An anatomically accurate denture base is important to function since "form and function are one." The food tables that we find facially at the tooth neck in normal healthy tissue help the buccinator muscles keep food out of the vestibule and up onto the occlusal surfaces. The form of the lingual surfaces is important in that it departs a feeling of naturalness to the tongue. It is also paramount that the neutral zone of the tongue not be violated by an overcontoured mandibular lingual flange.

The denture base that copies nature is also self-cleaning. The interdental papilla are full and rounded, and there are no "festoons." These only create food traps and prevent a sweeping of the tongue from its cleaning action.

Tinting of the denture base is important in several respects (Figure 28–19). A natural-looking base is desirable on the facial aspect and on the palatal as well. Nothing gives away a denture faster than an individual laughing with head held back as the slick mono color of the palate is viewed by others (Figure 28–20).

Tips on Creating a Natural-Looking Denture Base

1. Casts of human tissue should be studied, noting stippling, gingival collars, and the interdental papilla. There should be no slick, flat, and shiny surfaces in human gingival tissues.

2. Whatever is wanted in the finished base should be carved in wax. No carving with rotary acrylic finishers can be done after it is processed (Figures 28–21 to 23).

3. The denture should be invested with the same degree of care as was used in investing an inlay (Figure 28–24).

Esthetics: The Complete Denture   847

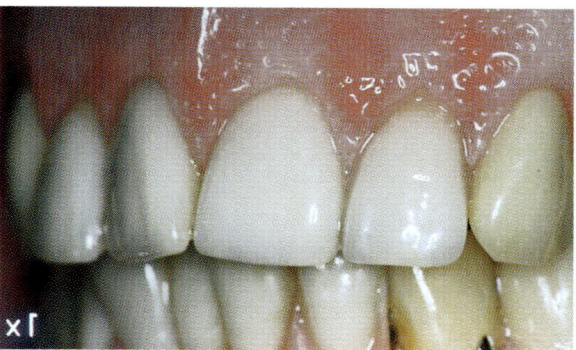

Figure 28–19: Denture base carved and tinted to appear natural. (Reproduced with permission from Turbyfill WF. Regaining pleasure and success with complete denture services. Int J Prosthet 1989;2:474–82.)

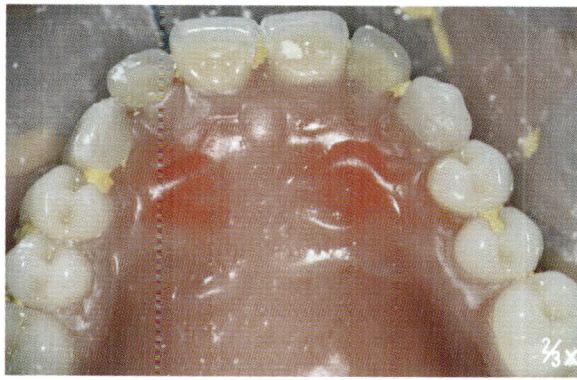

Figure 28–20: Correct anatomy of the palate with singulum carved on anterior teeth and lingual surfaces carved on the posterior teeth. The palate is also tinted.

4. A denture base tinting acrylic (Kay-See Dental Manufacturing, Kansas City, MO) should be used (Figure 28–25).

5. Tints should be placed in eye dropper bottles with the glass droppers turned upside down to control the placement of the tints.

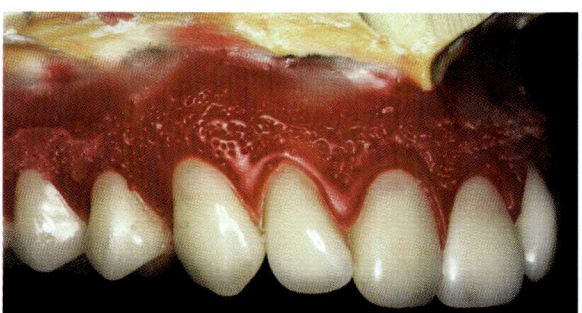

Figure 28–21: Anatomic wax-up.

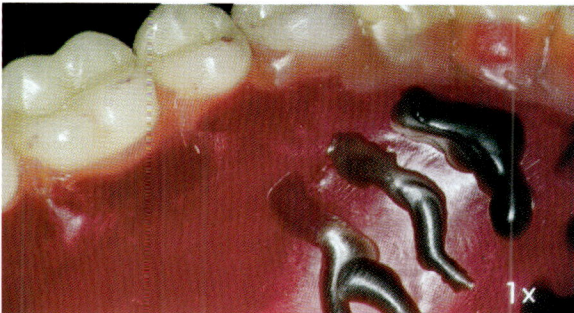

Figure 28–22: Anatomic wax-up.

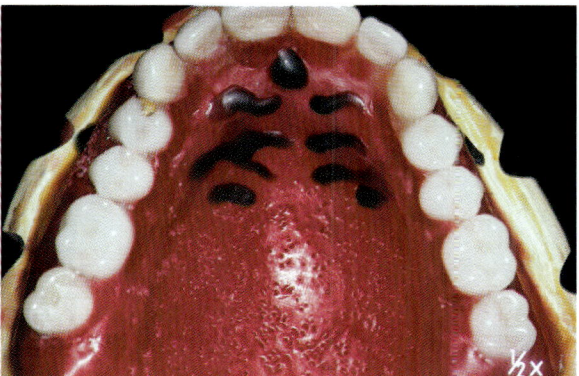

Figure 28–23: Anatomic wax-up. Note that the palate is lightly stippled so as not to appear shiny.

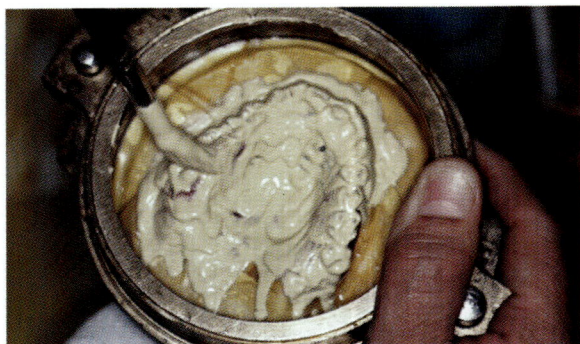

Figure 28–24: Investment is poured using a sable brush to capture the full anatomic wax-up.

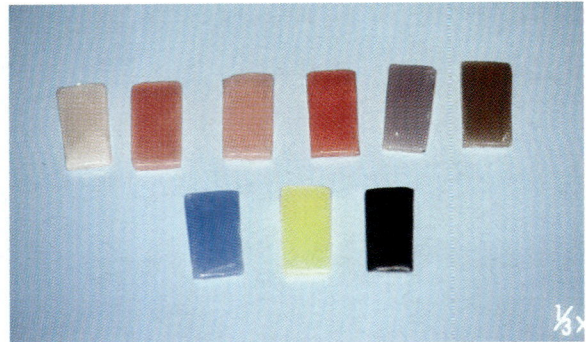

Figure 28–25: Shades of tints available for the wax-up. There is no carving of the base with rotary instruments.

6. The tints are sifted into the boiled out flasks and then are wet with monomer as the technician goes around the arch three or four teeth at a time (Figures 28–26 to 28).

7. Cases are tinted in four basic shades: (1) light-complexion blue-eyed blonds, (2) medium-complexion brunettes, (3) dark-complexion brunettes, and (4) non-Caucasians.

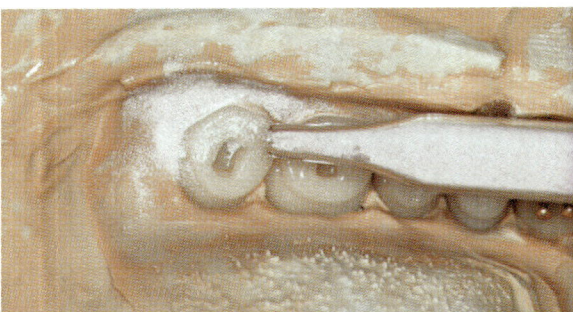

Figure 28–26: Tints are sifted around teeth.

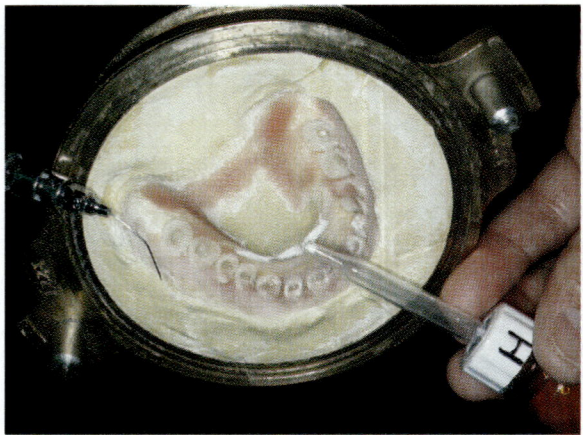

Figure 28–27: The palate is tinted.

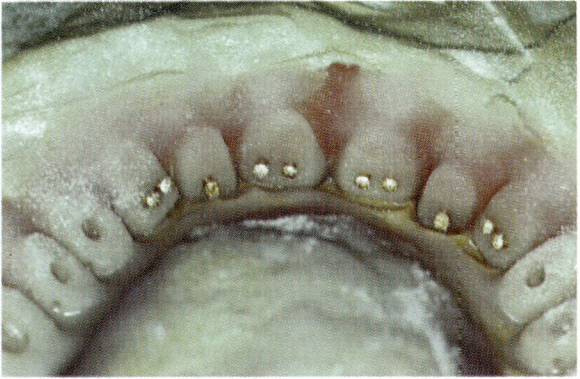

Figure 28–28: The maxillary case tinted. Dentures are then processed with acrylic of a color to complement the overall complexion of the patient.

EXAMPLES OF ESTHETIC DENTURES

Figures 28–29A to F are examples of esthetic dentures.

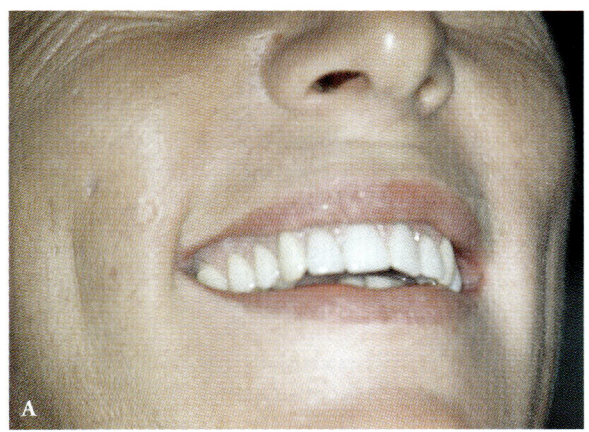

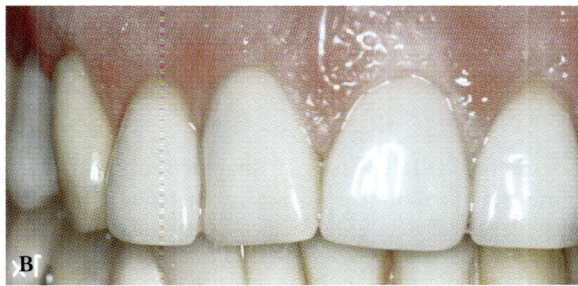

Figure 28–29A and B: *(A)* Full smile view of esthetic dentures. *(B)* Close-up of esthetic dentures. (Reproduced with permission from Turbyfill WFJ. The provisional denture: key to denture success. Aurum Ceramic Classic News 1995;8(2):1–4.)

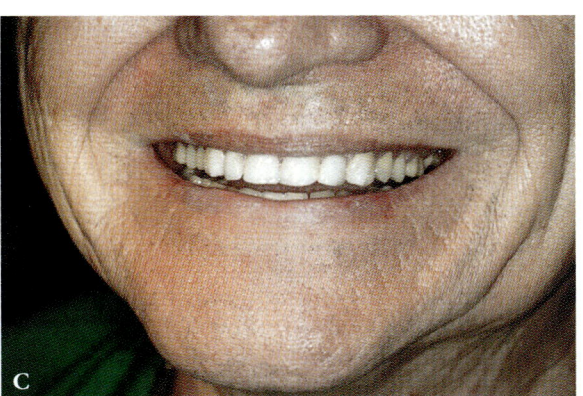

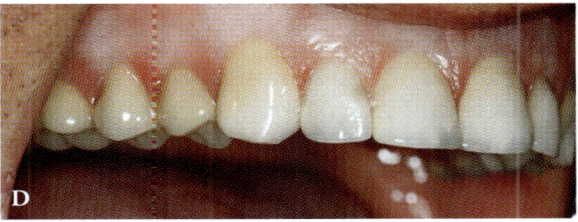

Figure 28–29C and D: *(C)* Full smile view of esthetic dentures. *(D)* Close-up of esthetic dentures.

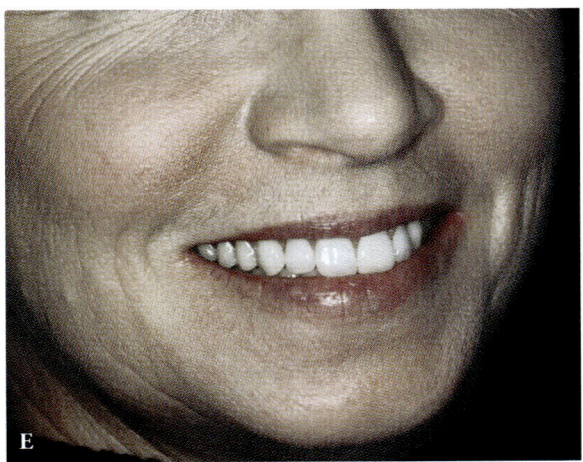

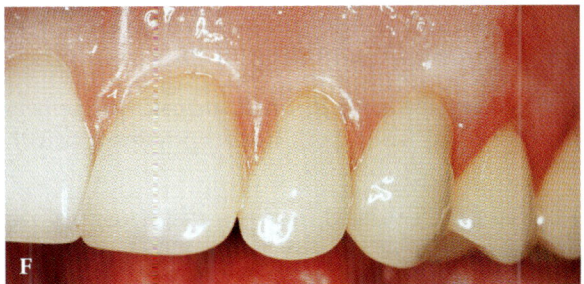

Figure 28–29E and F: *(E)* Full smile view of esthetic dentures. *(F)* Close-up of esthetic dentures.

References

1. Abrams L. Male or female—can you tell by the teeth? Report of sexual dimorphism study. San Francisco: American Academy of Esthetic Dentistry, 1981.

2. Appelbaum MB. The practical dynamics of the interim denture concept: a comparison with the conventional immediate denture technique. J Am Dent Assoc 1983;106:826–30.

3. Berg E, Johnson TB, Ingebretsen R. Patient motives and fulfillment of motives in renewal of complete dentures. Acta Odontol Scand 1984;42:235–40.

4. Boucher CO. Complete denture prosthodontics—the state of the art. J Prosthet Dent 1975;34:372–83.

5. Clough HE, Knodle JM, Leeper SH, et al. A comparison of lingualized occlusion and monoplane occlusion in complete dentures. J Prosthet Dent 1983;50:176–9.

6. Dawson P. Evaluation, diagnosis, and treatment of occlusal problems. St. Louis: CV Mosby, 1989.

7. Fisher RD. Personalized restorations vs. plates. J Prosthet Dent 1973;30:513–4.

8. Frush JP, Fisher RD. Introduction to dentogenic restorations. J Prosthet Dent 1955;5:586.

9. Goldstein RE. Study of need for esthetics in dentistry. J Prosthet Dentist 1969;6:589–98

10. Hansen CA. Diagnostically restoring a reduced occlusal vertical dimension without permanently altering the existing dentures. J Prosthet Dent 1985;54:671–3.

11. Hirsch B, Levin B, Tiber N. Effects of patient involvement and esthetics preference on denture acceptance. J Prosthet Dent 1972;28:127–32.

12. House MM, Loop JL. Form and color harmony in the dental art. USA: MM House (privately printed), 1939.

13. Ivy RS. Dental and facial types. In: Litch WF, ed. American system of dentistry. Vol. 2. Philadelphia: Leaman Brothers, 1887.

14. Krajicek D. Guides for natural facial appearance as related to complete denture construction. J Prosthet Dent 1969;21:654–62.

15. LaVere AM, Marcroft KR, Smith RC, Sarka RJ. Denture tooth selection: an analysis of the natural maxillary central incisor compared to the length and width of the face. Part 1. J Prosthet Dent 1992;67:661–3.

16. Lieb ND, Silverman SI, Garfinkel L. An analysis of soft tissue contours of the lips in relation to the maxillary cuspids. J Prosthet Dent 1967;18:292–303.

17. Marunick MT, Chamberlain BB, Robinson CA. Denture aesthetics: an evaluation of laymen's preferences. J Oral Rehabil 1983;10:399–406.

18. Mavroskoufis F, Ritchie GM. The face-form as a guide for the selection of maxillary central incisors. J Prosthet Dent 1980;43:501–5.

19. Murray CG. Re-establishing natural tooth position in the edentulous environment. Aust Dent J 1978;23:415–21.

20. Murrell GA. Phonetics, function, and anterior occlusion. J Prosthet Dent 1974;32:23–31.

21. Pound E. Apply harmony in selecting and arranging teeth. Dent Clin North Am 1962;Mar:241–58.

22. Pound E. Controlling anomalies of vertical dimension and speech. J Prosthet Dent 1976;36:124–35.

23. Pound E. Fine arts in the fallacy of the ridge. J Prosthet Dent 1954;4(1).

24. Pound E. Mandibular movements of speech and their seven related values. J Prosthet Dent 1966;16:835.

25. Pound E. Preparatory dentures: a protective philosophy. J Prosthet Dent 1965;15:5–18.

26. Pound E. Utilizing speech to simplify personalized denture service. J Prosthet Dent 1970;24:586–600.

27. Pound E, Murrell GA. An introduction to denture simplification. J Prosthet Dent 1971;26:570–80.

28. Pound E, Murrell GA. An introduction to denture simplification. Phase II. J Prosthet Dent 1973;29:598–607.

29. Rayson JH, Rahn AO, Wesley RC, et al. Placement of teeth in a complete denture: a cephalometric study. J Am Dent Assoc 1970;81:420–4.

30. Ruffino AR. Personality projection in complete dentures: traits transmissible to the viewer through vari-

ations in maxillary anterior tooth arrangement. J Prosthet Dent 1984;50:661–2, 664.

31. Sharry J. Essential concepts in denture esthetics. In: Esthetics in dentistry. Philadelphia: JB Lippincott, 1976.

32. Sherman H. Phonetic capability as a function of vertical dimension in complete denture wearers—a preliminary report. J Prosthet Dent 1970;23:621–32.

33. Smith BJ. The value of the nose width as an esthetic guide in prosthodontics. J Prosthet Dent 1975;34:562–73.

34. Starcke EN Jr. The contours of polished surfaces of complete dentures: a review of the literature. J Am Dent Assoc 1970;81:155–60.

35. Tau S, Lowenthal U. Some personality determinants of denture preference. J Prosthet Dent 1980;44:10–2.

36. Turner LC. The profile tracer: method for obtaining accurate pre-extraction records. J San Antonio Dent Soc 1970;25:13.

37. Williams JL. The temperamental selection of artificial teeth. A fallacy. Dent Dig 1914;20:63.

38. Zimmerman DE, Cotmore JM. Denture esthetics (I). Denture base contour. Quintessence Int 1982;13:543–9.

CHAPTER 29

GERESTHETICS: ESTHETIC DENTISTRY FOR OLDER ADULTS

Linda C. Niessen, DMD, MPH, MPP, Ronald E. Goldstein, DDS

Of all human beings who have ever lived to be sixty-five years or older, half are currently alive.

John W. Rowe and Robert Kahn, *Successful Aging*

In 1900, the average life expectancy in the United States was 47 years. By the year 2000, the average life expectancy had increased to 74 years. As adults live longer, they want to make the most of their years. This chapter explores esthetic dentistry for older adults. It reviews the demographics of these aging populations and the market for esthetic services and discusses the clinical issues associated with providing esthetic dental services.

DEMOGRAPHICS

Aging is a worldwide phenomenon. Developed countries have higher percentages of their populations over age 65 years. Table 29–1 lists a sample of countries and the percentage of their populations over age 65.[3] Japan and Sweden lead the world, with about 17% of the population over age 65 years compared with 13% in the United States. Developing countries have a far lower percentage of older adults, primarily because of lower life expectancies in general and higher birth rates, both of which increase the proportion of their younger population.

In addition to an increasing number of people over age 65, those reaching age 65 can expect to benefit from increasing life expectancies as a result of improved medical care and healthier lifestyles. Table 29–2 lists the remaining life expectancies for

TABLE 29–1. Aging Throughout the World

COUNTRY	ESTIMATED PERCENT OF POPULATION OVER AGE 65 YEARS
Australia	13
Canada	12
Japan	17
Mexico	4
Russia	13
Sweden	17
United States	12

Adapted from CIA World Factbook.[3]

TABLE 29–2. Remaining Life Expectancies: U.S. Adults, Age 50 and Over

		CAUCASIAN		AFRICAN AMERICAN	
AGE IN 1990 (YR)	TOTAL	MALE	FEMALE	MALE	FEMALE
50	29.2	27.0	31.7	22.8	28.3
55	24.9	22.8	27.2	19.3	24.3
60	20.9	18.9	23.0	16.2	20.6
65	17.3	15.4	19.0	13.4	17.1
70	14.0	12.3	15.3	10.8	13.9
75	10.9	9.5	12.0	8.7	11.1
80	8.3	7.1	8.9	6.7	8.5
85+	6.0	5.2	6.4	5.0	6.3

Reproduced from U.S. Bureau of the Census.[17]

adults aged 50 and older. At each age, women outlive men, and Caucasian Americans outlive African Americans. Half of all of the women who reached age 50 in 2000 will live to be 80.[16] At age 65, American adults can expect to live another 17 years, or about 20% of their lives, in the retirement years. These adults expect to make the most of these years.

Goldstein cited the revolutionary concept that esthetic dentistry is, in fact, a health service.[6] During the last decade, older adults who elected to have treatments that involved all esthetic disciplines embraced this concept of oral health. A good example of an older adult undergoing extensive esthetic dental treatment appears in Figures 29–1A to O.

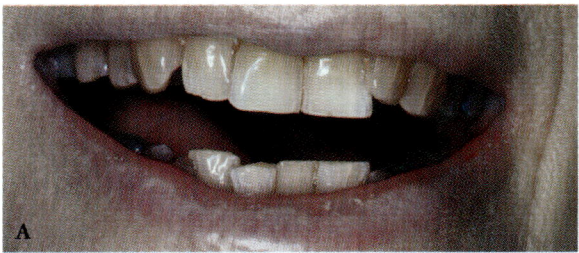
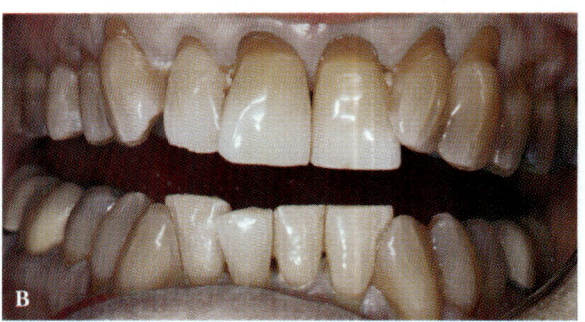
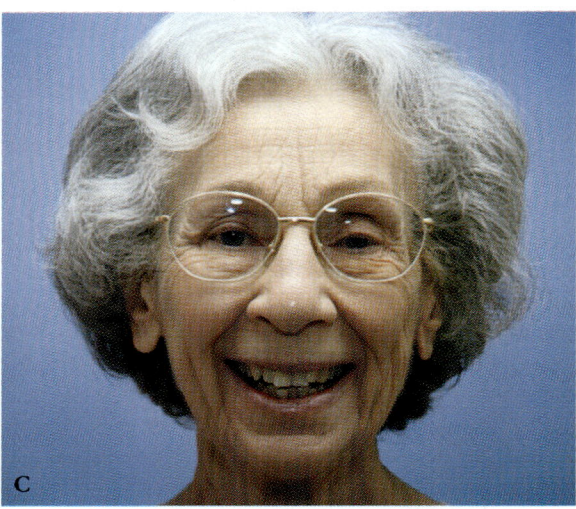

Figure 29–1A to C: This 76-year-old lady presented for treatment after a lifetime of dissatisfaction with her crowded teeth.

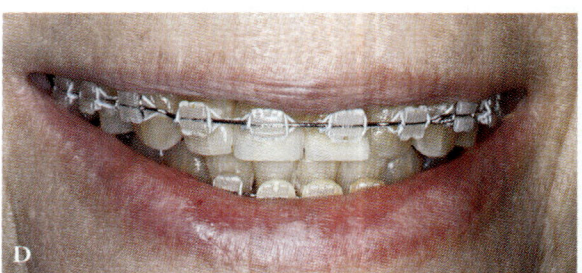
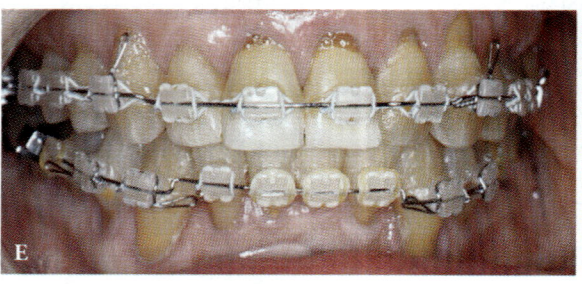
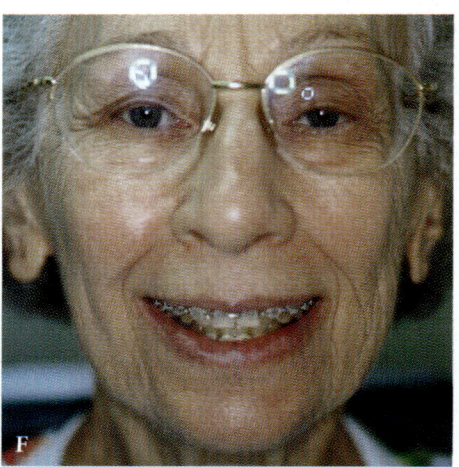

Figure 29–1D to F: Tooth-colored brackets were applied because their esthetic appearance gave the patient the confidence to smile during treatment.

Individuals born between 1946 and 1964 (known as the baby boomers in the United States) are fueling concern about aging in the United States. In the United States, a baby boomer turns 50 every 7 seconds.[15] This group, comprised of 76 million people in the United States, represents almost 30% of the U.S. population. Perhaps more significant than its size is its educational attainment. Twenty-five percent of this group has a college education.

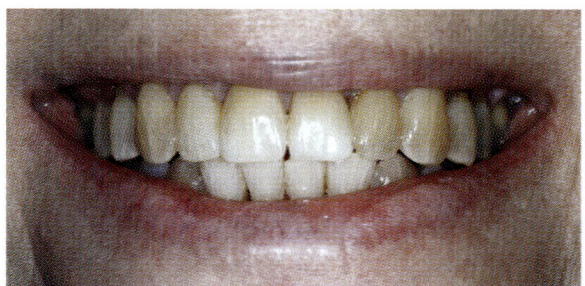

Figure 29–1G: After the removal of the orthodontic appliances, the teeth are much straighter but still discolored.

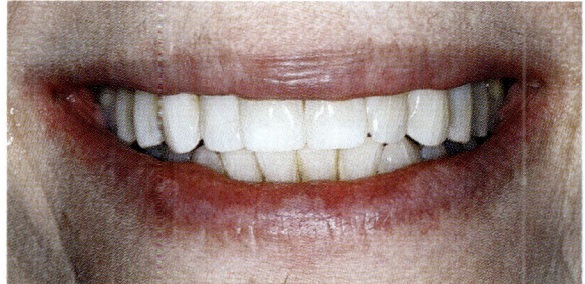

Figure 29–1H: After restorative treatment featuring tooth-colored restorations and bleaching, the patient has the smile she has always wanted.

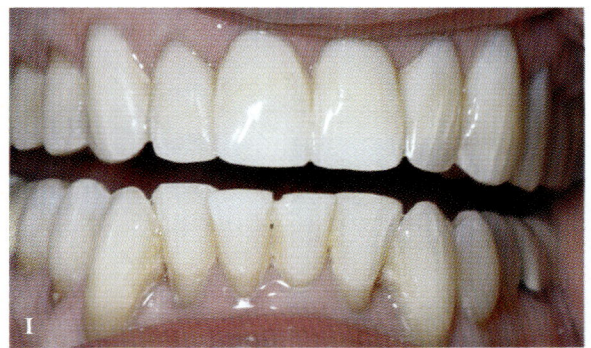
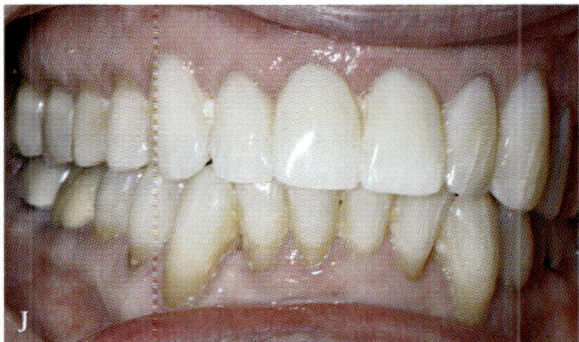

Figure 29–1I and J: Note that the formally eroded cervical areas have better contour and will deflect food particles better.

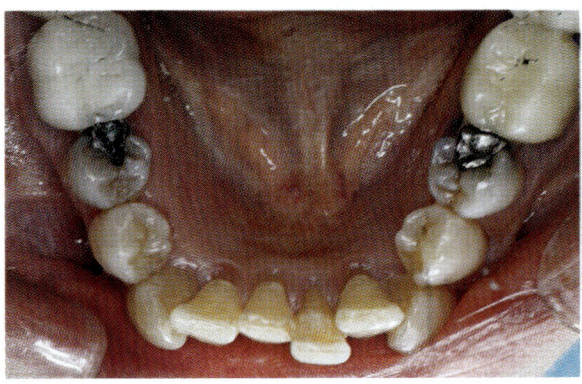

Figure 29–1K: Note the crowding of the mandibular anterior teeth.

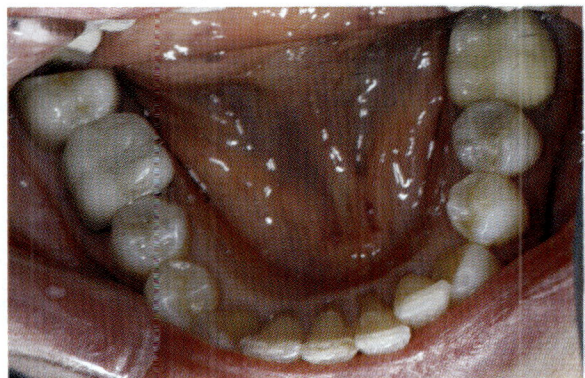

Figure 29–1L: The teeth are less crowded, and the new tooth-colored restorations have been placed.

As the baby boomers age and their World War II generation parents die, Americans will witness one of the greatest transfers of wealth from one generation to the next. Table 29–3 lists the estimated wealth transfer to be between 12 and 18 trillion dollars based on various economic assumptions.

From a dental perspective, the baby boom generation represents the first to have benefited from widespread community water fluoridation and preventive dentistry programs. As a result, they will be the first generation to reach 65 with virtually an intact natural dentition.[7]

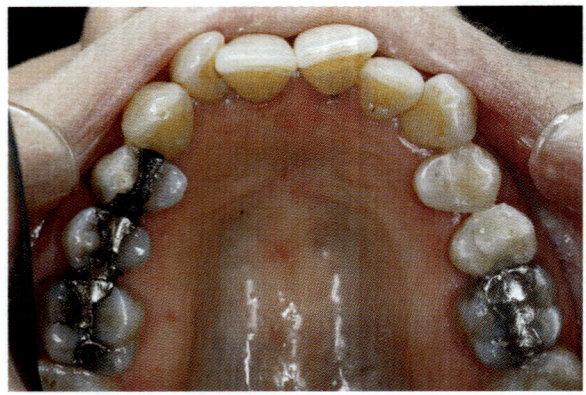

Figure 29–1M: The maxillary arch shows anterior crowding and defective amalgam restorations.

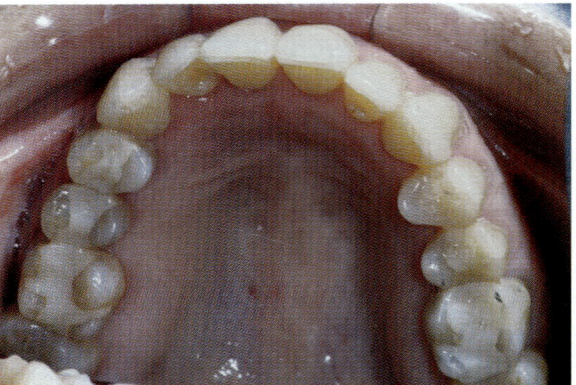

Figure 29–1N: Following 12 months of orthodontic treatment, the patient's amalgam restorations were replaced with posterior composite resin.

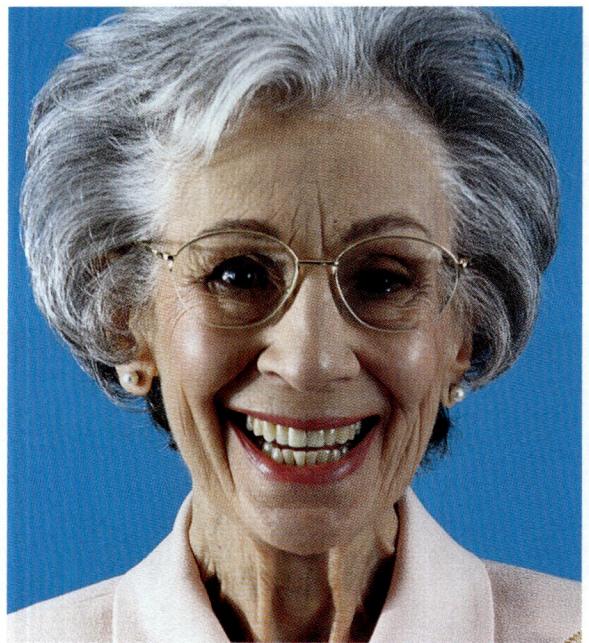

Figure 29–1O: Interdisciplinary therapy including orthodontics, periodontics, and restorative dentistry combined to produce this attractive result 2 years following the initiation of treatment in this now younger-looking 78-year-old lady.

TABLE 29–3. Wealth and Asset Transfer in the United States (1998–2017)

ASSET APPRECIATION	WEALTH TRANSFER	NUMBER OF ESTATES OVER $1 MILLION
Low growth (2%/yr)	$12 trillion	1.8 million
Mid growth (3%/yr)	$14 trillion	2.2 million
High growth (4%/yr)	$18 trillion	2.8 million

Data from Havens and Schervish.[8]

THE MATURE ESTHETIC DENTAL CONSUMER

Today's older adults and tomorrow's baby boomers will be far more willing to invest in themselves. Their oral health goals will include keeping their teeth, keeping their teeth healthy, and keeping their teeth attractive. They will want to erase the effect of years on their dentitions and improve their appearance. Figures 29–2A to H show an attractive woman approaching 60 with an unwanted aging smile. Full mouth reconstruction comprised of posterior maxillary and mandibular crowns plus anterior composite resin bonding lasted 24 years until she died at 80.

Our colleagues in the marketing arena have described baby boomers as "the new health care consumers." These new health care consumers are characterized as more aggressive, demanding, and self-directed in their health care. In fact, a study in the United States on sources of consumer health information has found that slightly more consumers (40%) received their health care information from television than from health care professionals (39%).[18] In addition, the Internet and the World Wide Web are leveling the playing field, so to speak, between health professionals and consumers. With virtually all professional journals now online, health professionals and consumers can be informed about new scientific advances simultaneously. In addition to online health journals, new

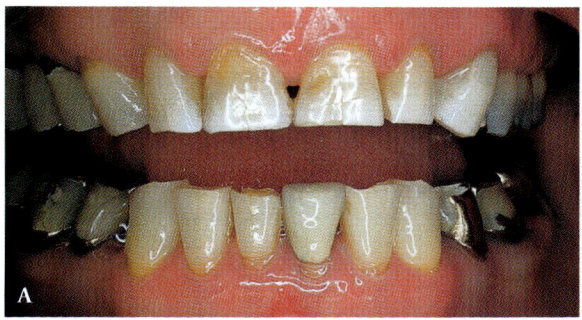
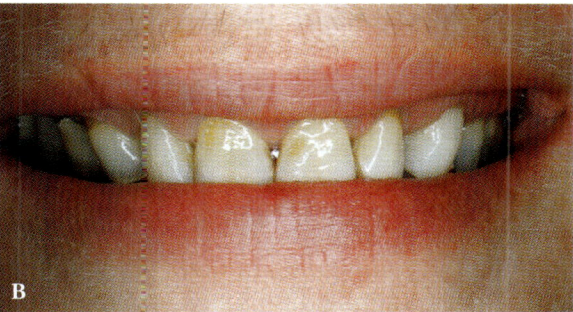

Figure 29–2A and B: This 57-year-old woman had worn down her posterior teeth so much that she was traumatizing the anterior teeth, which had also worn considerably.

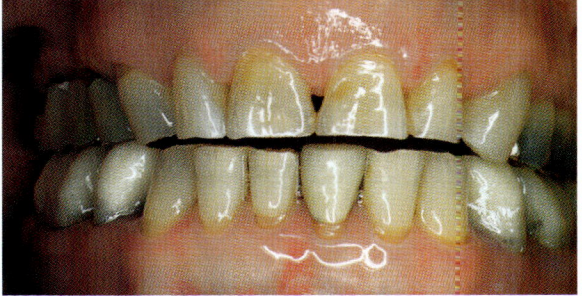

Figure 29–2C: Treatment crowns to restore vertical dimension were constructed for the patient to wear to determine if she would tolerate the new occlusal position.

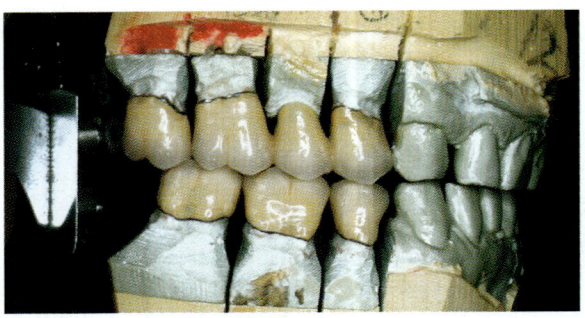

Figure 29–2D: After 3 comfortable months of wearing temporary crowns with an increased vertical dimension, final metal-ceramic crowns were constructed for the posterior teeth.

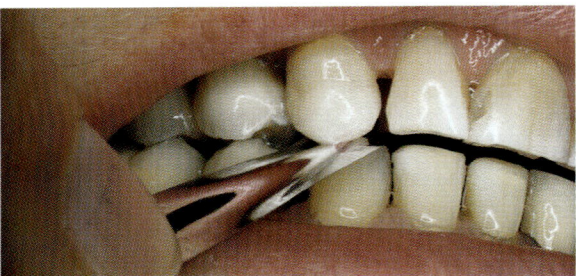

Figure 29–2E: Artus strips (5/10,000 inch thick) were used to make sure the occlusion was perfect. Note sufficient open space for composite resin bonding to be able to lengthen the maxillary anterior teeth.

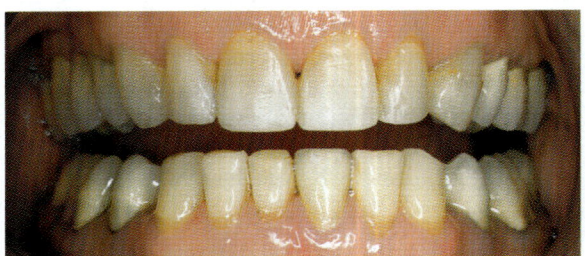

Figure 29–2F: The maxillary anterior teeth were next bonded with a hybrid composite resin. Note the increased length.

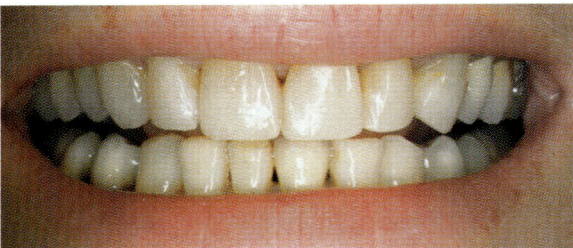

Figure 29–2G: The final smile helped to create a younger-looking smile line, which lasted for 24 years due in part to the exceptional home care performed by the patient.

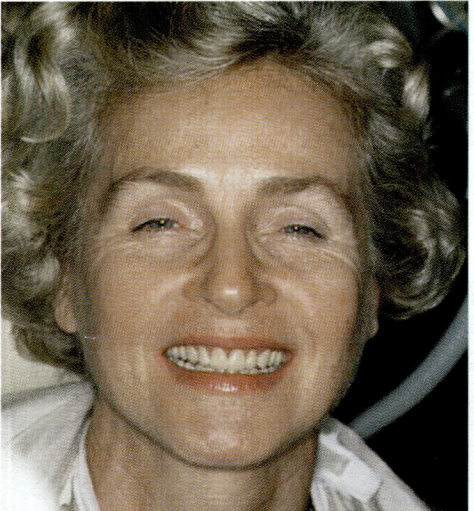

Figure 29–2H: The combined approach of posterior crowns and anterior bonding greatly improved this patient's smile, her appearance, and self-confidence. (Reproduced with permission from Goldstein RE. Change your smile. 3rd edn. Carol Stream, IL: Quintessence 1997:176.)

Internet health sites are being added every day. Chat rooms with consumers having various health conditions have also developed and serve as a source of health information, new treatment options, clinical trial sites, and general support. Consumers will continue to seek health information, including oral health and esthetic dentistry information, via the World Wide Web.

The health and wellness movement, coupled with new oral health research linking periodontal disease with systemic illnesses such as cardiovascular disease and stroke,[2,19] is broadening the interest in and understanding of dental health by consumers. The recently released Surgeon General's Report on Oral Health, *Oral Health in America*, reinforces the message that general health and oral health are related.[11]

Older adults understand better than younger adults that dental health is more than just healthy teeth. It is also the ability to speak, smile, chew, and swallow comfortably. Dental health has become oral health. Patients who receive esthetic dental services readily appreciate this concept of oral health. The ability to smile confidently and improved self-esteem will continue to drive the demand for esthetic dental services by older adults.

Data in the United States show an increased use of esthetic services by older adults.[9] Individuals who may be contemplating plastic surgery such as facelifts, liposuction, or laser skin resurfacing are also contemplating a smile makeover (tooth whitening to eliminate darkened teeth, crowns or veneers to correct shortened clinical crowns, and/or orthodontics to correct malpositioned teeth) as part of their plastic surgery options. This smile makeover, or "instant facelift" as it is being called by some women, may last 20 to 25 years, unlike the plastic surgery changes that may last for only 5 to 10 years.

CHRONIC ILLNESS AND ESTHETIC DENTAL CARE

Baby boomers will soon find themselves caring for their aging parents, who, as they reach the eighth and ninth decades of life, may face issues of how to maintain oral health in the face of declining health. One can anticipate that baby boomers will hold high expectations for their parents' oral health just as they do for their own.

TABLE 29–4. Most Common Chronic Conditions

ALL AGES	AGE 75+
Sinusitis	Arthritis
Arthritis	Hypertension
Orthopedic impairments	Hearing impairments
Hypertension	Heart disease
Hay fever	Cataracts

Adapted from Sumner[14] (based on National Academy on an Aging Society analysis of 1994 National Health Interview Survey data).

Table 29–4 lists the common chronic conditions for individuals of all ages and for those age 75 and over. Whereas arthritis affects 28% of 45 to 74 year olds, it affects over 50% of adults over age 75.[13] Although these chronic conditions may occur in middle age, they may not cause disability or limitation of activities until over age 65. Data from the National Health Interview Survey in the United States found that 34% of 65 to 74 year olds and 45% of those 75 and over reported some limitation in activities because of chronic conditions.[15]

Older adults who visit their dentist may be taking a variety of medications for these various chronic conditions. Thus, the recording and interpreting of the medical history and medication history will often require more time in older adults. These chronic illnesses may also necessitate more frequent consultations with the patient's physicians. Patients with cardiac conditions or orthopedic problems or those on anticoagulation therapy are just a few of the examples of systemic illness for which a physician consultation may be warranted. These systemic conditions may make maintaining any esthetic dentistry more difficult. Patients should be advised that their systemic conditions could affect their oral health.

Even the best dentistry can break down quickly in the absence of oral hygiene self-care and the presence of multiple risk factors such as dry mouth (xerostomia) and a highly refined carbohydrate diet. Patients undergoing esthetic dental services who are about to enter a nursing home or assisted living facility should be assessed for factors that will increase their risk of oral diseases such as dementia, stroke (which may cause the loss of ability to use the dominant hand), or medications that cause dry mouth. Once these risk factors are identified, aggressive preventive therapies must be initiated to avoid dental diseases and breakdown of previous dental work.

MEDICAL/DENTAL HISTORY AND ORAL EXAMINATION

The history and physical examination for older adults will clearly require more time and result in more positive findings than for younger adults. In addition to the routine esthetic questions, it is important to ask each patient what his or her personal goals are for oral health. Does the patient expect to lose any teeth to caries or periodontal disease? Is the patient willing to implement preventive measures to avoid tooth loss? These questions will assist the dental team in understanding the patient's plans and expectations for oral health and whether such plans and expectations are realistic. Clearly, the patient with 7 to 8 mm of probing depths on posterior teeth that are mobile and who would be devastated to lose any teeth may not have realistic expectations given the current level of oral disease present. The sooner this situation is identified, the sooner the dental team can assist the patient in understanding and accepting what goals are realistic.

Questions about the importance of esthetics and the patient's smile will help the patient and dental team understand the patient's self-concept and how esthetic services may affect it. This line of questioning, although not traditional, can result in greater patient understanding and, ultimately, in obtaining the patient's consent for an esthetic procedure. The medical history plays an increasing role in the treatment planning of older adults. The most common chronic diseases seen in older adults include heart disease, arthritis, diabetes, osteoporosis, and senile dementia. Medical conditions must be identified and the stability of the patient's health status assessed. A patient who last took a nitroglycerine tablet 2 weeks previously to control his angina attack would be considered more stable and able to receive dental treatment than the patient who took four tablets for his angina the day before. The latter patient would be better referred to his physician for consultation prior to receiving dental care. Medical history forms should provide an area for comments on the stability of a patient's medical condition. A medical history form that asks "Do you have heart disease?" with a yes or no answer will not provide the dental team with sufficient information to gauge the status of the patient's health. The medical history must include an assessment of both the patient's prescription and over-the-counter medications. Studies have shown that salivary flow does not decrease naturally with age; however, the absence of saliva does put a patient at great risk for root caries.[4]

Salivary flow is much more likely to decrease as a result of multiple medication use. Over 400 medications are estimated to decrease salivary flow. Other medications have been shown to affect oral tissues; for example, nonsteroidal anti-inflammatory medications can cause oral ulcerations, and antihypertensive and antiseizure medications can induce gingival overgrowth.

Esthetic oral health services are not contraindicated for patients with chronic diseases. However, both the dentist and patient must fully understand the effects that one's systemic diseases and medication use will have on dental care and subsequent home care. A patient taking nifedipine for his hypertension is still a candidate for porcelain veneers but must understand that his medication will increase his susceptibility to plaque-induced marginal gingivitis.

Providing esthetic dental services for healthy 65 year olds should not prove difficult for dental practitioners. Rather, the challenge will come when that 65 year old becomes an 85 year old with heart disease, stroke, arthritis, chronic obstructive pulmonary disease, and/or Alzheimer's disease. The patient who has invested significant time and money in one's oral health will find the maintenance of the esthetic dentistry investment more difficult if he or she becomes frail and medically, mentally, or physically compromised. This scenario represents an opportunity for dental professionals to take a leadership role in both patient education and the education of nursing home staff, families, caregivers, and other health care professionals about oral health for compromised patients. Health professionals need to understand that oral health does not have to decline simultaneously with a decline in physical or mental functioning.

TREATMENT PLANNING THE OLDER PATIENT

Options for esthetic dental care are as readily available for 70, 80, and 90 year olds as they are for 20,

30, and 40 year olds. However, with increasing life expectancies, treatment planning the 40-year-old esthetic dental patient requires a life cycle approach. Patients of all ages need to be informed that esthetic dentistry does not last forever and may need to be redone at 60, 70, or 80 years as the dental materials age and wear or the oral tissues change in relation to the face.

In treatment planning older adults, they should be given the opportunity to "say yes." They have seen their children and grandchildren benefit from modern dental materials and techniques, and they are interested in those same procedures. It should not be assumed that the 78-year-old woman is not interested in whitening her teeth, replacing her worn amalgam restorations with new tooth-colored filling materials, or investing in her smile. Older adults in the United States are seeking orthodontic treatment in record numbers to correct long-standing malocclusions and improve their oral function.

Sequencing esthetic dental treatment for older adults will be similar to that for younger and middle-aged adults. Caries control and periodontal therapy may be necessary prior to definitive esthetic treatment. Also, consultations with dental specialists may be required depending on the nature of the patient's oral diagnoses; consultations with the patient's physicians may be required depending on the patient's medical diagnoses.

Because older adults do manage chronic diseases, esthetic treatment may be delayed due to an acute exacerbation of a chronic illness. The patient with hypertension may suffer a stroke and require rehabilitation for 3 to 6 months prior to resuming dental treatment. When dental treatment resumes, the patient may be on anticoagulant therapy and require monitoring of the International Normalized Ratio to ensure that bleeding is not a problem during dental treatment. Similarly, a patient with degenerative joint disease may undergo hip replacement surgery, which may delay dental treatment for a period of time. Once the patient returns for care, he or she will need antibiotic prophylaxis for the first 2 years following the hip replacement (unless the patient has other risk factors) to prevent the possibility of late hematogenous joint infection.[1]

Financing esthetic dental services will most frequently be out of pocket. Although some patients over age 65 may still have dental insurance as part of their employment retirement package, most dental insurance does not reimburse for elective esthetic services. Dental care provided for the treatment of the teeth and/or supporting tissue is generally not reimbursed under Medicare. In some cases, adult children may be willing to incur the cost for esthetic dental services when their parents may not be comfortable spending money on themselves for such care.

Patient attitudes may also affect how individuals make decisions to accept esthetic dental treatment. For some individuals, function and health may be far more important than the esthetic nature of the treatment. Removing oral infection may be the driving force behind dental treatment, and since a restoration has to be placed once the infection is eliminated, it may as well be an esthetic restoration. Others may feel that looking good is important to overall quality of life and have no problem with expending resources for improving their smile. Often during the interview, patients will provide clues behind their motivation for seeking esthetic dental services.

Older adults presenting for esthetic dental care may often arrive at the dental office with an adult "child" as a caregiver. It should not be assumed that the adult child is the decision maker. The treatment plan should be addressed to the older adult. If the older adult needs assistance with the decision making, he or she will seek assistance from the adult child. For the patient who may be medically or physically compromised, the individual's ability to cooperate with the dental treatment should be assessed. The appointments must be timed for the patient's comfort.

Identifying the chief complaint is important when caring for any patient. For older adults seeking esthetic dentistry, it is important to understand precisely what they like and dislike about their appearance. They have lived with their smile a number of years. Often, they know exactly what they would like to achieve. It is critical for the dentist to assist the patient in articulating his or her goals clearly.

Imaging can assist both the patient and dentist in understanding what can be accomplished with esthetic dentistry. Dentists should be wary of the patient who says "I've hated this dental work all my life. I'll be pleased with whatever you do, Doctor." Understanding what the patient does not like should not be assumed. The patient should articulate what he or she likes and does not like. On careful questioning and the use of an intraoral camera and/or imaging, the dental team can usually identify the cause(s) of concern.

For individuals unsure about the decision to pursue esthetic dental treatment, imaging can play an important role in assisting the patient to understand how his or her smile can be altered. By demonstrating the changes overall and changes to be made on each tooth, the patient understands the goal of each dental procedure and how it contributes to the overall result. For patients who are having difficulty making a decision to pursue esthetic dentistry, imaging allows them to share a photograph of the planned results with friends and family. They may be better able to assist the patient in the decision-making process.

Informed consent requires that the patient be presented with treatment options. Imaging can assist the patient in understanding the problems and the potential options for treatment.

As with any dental treatment, maintenance of the oral cavity with appropriate home care is critical to the success and longevity of the dental treatment. Preventive therapies must be an integral part of the treatment planning for esthetic dental care. Professional and home-use neutral sodium fluoride gels or rinses to prevent root caries or recurrent caries should be prescribed for patients who are considered at high risk, such as patients with decreased salivary flow or impaired dexterity. Salivary substitutes may also assist patients with oral dryness to provide comfort and improve oral tissue cleansing by the tongue. Antimicrobial rinses should be used for individuals at risk of gingivitis. Bacterial monitoring may be necessary for individuals particularly at high risk for caries or periodontal disease. Smoking cessation counseling should be provided for patients who use tobacco.

By including a comprehensive preventive plan as part of the overall esthetic treatment plan, the unspoken message the dental team conveys to patients is that the team believes in the patient's future. That future is one of oral health, not oral disease.

ESTHETIC DENTAL CONSULTATION AND ESTHETIC FACIAL SURGERY

Esthetic dentistry can be part of an overall appearance makeover. When a younger appearance is desired through plastic surgery, esthetic dental services should be considered prior to the esthetic facial surgery. The reasons for this include the following: (1) creating a younger-looking smile may be sufficient to please the patient so that plastic facial surgery may not be necessary or less surgery may be sufficient and (2) oral pathology such as caries or severe periodontal disease subsequent to facial surgery will compromise the esthetic surgical result. Patients should be educated as to the benefits of consulting with a dentist prior to undergoing any esthetic surgery procedures.

Another issue that may occur when esthetic dental services are provided after facial surgery involves the use of retractors. When dentists provide esthetic dental services, they may use retractors during the course of treatment. If esthetic dental services are provided after facial surgery, patients may perceive the use of retractors as contributing to "new" wrinkle development that the plastic surgery had removed. In truth, these wrinkles were present prior to the dental treatment, but the patients did not notice them until after the dental procedures. When treating a patient who has had plastic facial surgery, the patient should be photographed in repose and smiling close up and full face without make-up to record any existing facial wrinkling prior to dental treatment.

For a patient considering facial surgery, the consultation with the dentist regarding smile enhancement should occur prior to the facial surgery to maximize the final facial esthetics. In some cases, interdisciplinary dental care such as orthodontics, periodontics, and prosthodontics may be required to achieve the best result and will take several months to accomplish.

ESTHETIC DENTAL PROCEDURES FOR OLDER ADULTS

Vital Tooth Bleaching

Teeth darken and become more yellow as they age. Teeth also tend to take on stain throughout the enamel and cementum surfaces (characterization, as it is euphemistically called). With the trend toward whiter teeth, it is not at all surprising to find patients of all ages requesting tooth-lightening procedures.

Vital tooth bleaching performed either in office or at home has been demonstrated to be effective in older adults. In older adults, sensitivity does not appear to occur as frequently as in younger patients. This is thought to be due to the gradual receding of the pulpal tissue with age. Because aging effects darken teeth in the yellow color range, this color range has been shown to achieve the best results with vital tooth-whitening procedures.

In-office and at-home whitening with trays work equally well. Products containing 10 to 35% peroxide have been shown to work in mature adults. The main determinant is whether the patient desires the whitening results immediately or can wait longer for the at-home whitening agents to begin to work. If a patient has anterior teeth with prominent microcracks, he or she should be advised of these cracks and monitored carefully to ensure that there is no streaking in the whitened teeth.

Figure 29–3A shows a 72-year-old woman who felt that her smile made her look older than she felt. Her teeth were whitened using an in-office 35% hydrogen peroxide solution. Figure 29–3B shows the result of whitening on her maxillary teeth. The in-office whitening procedures provide an instant result when patients do not have the time to wait for the results, do not want to take the time to use at-home whitening agents, or have tried home whitening but had difficulty complying with the daily regimen. Patients will require touch-up treatments after the initial whitening procedures and should be advised accordingly.

Cosmetic Contouring and Bonding

The teeth of 60-, 70-, and 80-year-old people often exhibit the wearing away of hard tissue by erosion, abrasion, or parafunctional habits such as bruxism. Shortened anterior teeth, particularly in the maxilla, result in less of the teeth being seen when one talks or smiles. This shortening of teeth in the maxilla contributes significantly to an older appearance. As hard tissues wear away, patients will lose vertical dimension, resulting in the mandible becoming more anteriorly positioned. The reverse, the so-called "long-in-tooth" phrase that Shakespeare used to describe the aging process, results from periodontal disease.

With age, one shows less of the maxillary teeth and more of the mandibular teeth. The patient at age 50 who wishes to change only the color or shape of the maxillary teeth by age 60 may be requesting similar changes in the mandibular teeth. Both of these age-related changes can add years to an individual's appearance and inhibit oral function. However, esthetic dental treatment can easily transform the patient's appearance, in effect turning back the clock on the aging process.

Cosmetic contouring provides an excellent introduction to esthetic dentistry for patients who are unsure about making significant changes in their smile. It also provides a lower cost option for those patients with limited financial resources.

Figure 29–4A shows a 74-year-old woman who was dissatisfied with her smile but was not sure if she wanted considerable changes made. Her chief concern was that she did not like her malpositioned lower incisors. Orthodontics was not an option owing to the cost and length of treatment time. Cosmetic contouring of the mandibular teeth was

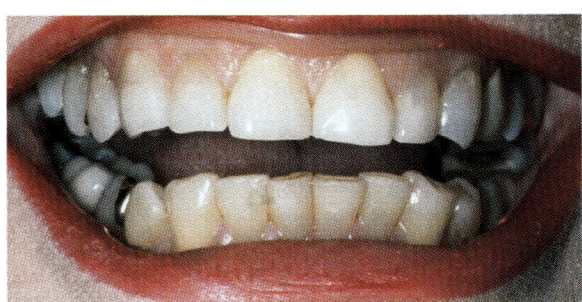

Figure 29–3A: This 72-year-old woman felt that the color of her teeth aged her smile.

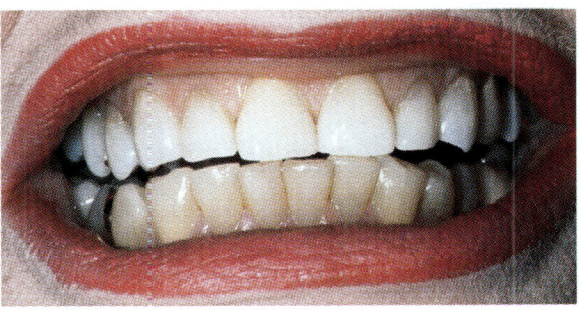

Figure 29–3B: After an in-office bleaching procedure on her maxillary teeth, the patient was pleased with her lightened color.

selected as a compromise treatment because of its conservative approach (Figure 29–4B). The patient liked the changes in the lower teeth and subsequently asked about options for improving the maxillary teeth. Finances remained an issue, so cosmetic bonding was selected as the treatment plan of choice. Figures 29–4C and D show the patient's maxillary teeth before and after cosmetic bonding.

Bonding with composite resin is a particularly useful esthetic technique for the mature adult. With minimal preparation, the tooth or teeth can be altered to achieve an esthetic result. Bonding also enables the dentist to easily repair chipping and fractures that occur in the teeth of older adults.

Although manufacturers have made cosmetic shades lighter to reflect the increasing range of whiter shades of bleached teeth, older patients may require darker composite shades to restore erosion or root caries. Currently, when a patient needs a restoration on a tooth darker than existing composite shades, the dentist may need to use modifiers to make the restoration more natural in appearance and blend with the surrounding teeth. An overlay technique or partial veneer can be used when a spot match is not possible.

Figures 29–5A and B show a patient who did not like the appearance of her front teeth. She felt that her maxillary central incisors were too dark and too short. Cosmetic resin bonding was chosen as the treatment of choice because of the immediacy of the result. Figures 29–5C and D show how the teeth were both lightened and lengthened to provide a younger-looking smile line.

Figures 29–6A to E illustrate a patient who did not care much about his smile. The motivation for pursuing esthetic dentistry was his wife. She thought that his smile made him look much older than his years. She encouraged him to have esthet-

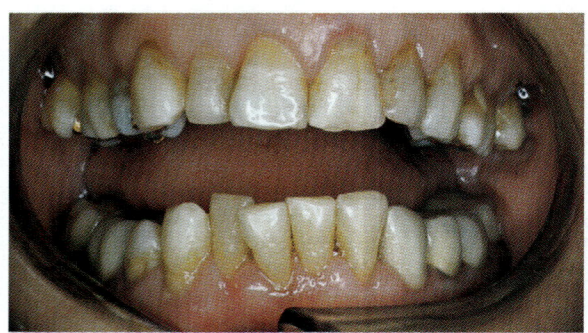

Figure 29–4A: This 74-year-old woman was dissatisfied with the appearance of her teeth.

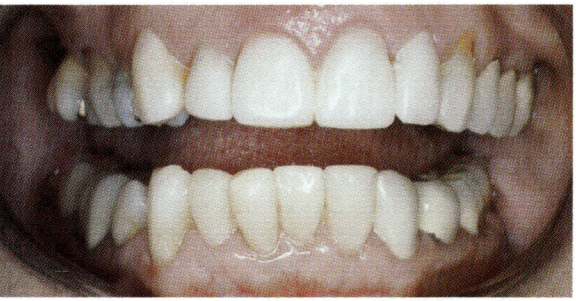

Figure 29–4B: Cosmetic contouring was done to make the mandibular teeth appear straighter; the maxillary incisors were direct bonded with composite resin.

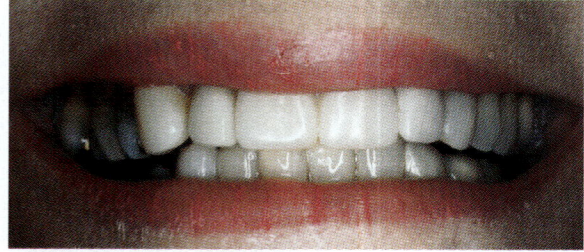

Figure 29–4C: Although a compromise to full restorative esthetics, just treating a limited amount of anterior teeth can satisfy the older patient.

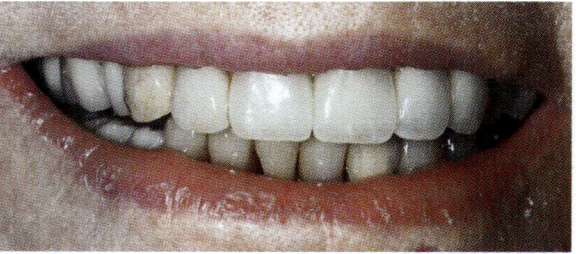

Figure 29–4D: At 90 years of age, this patient is still motivated to improve her smile—now with porcelain laminates. Although the treatment is still a compromise because of her inability to sit through many long appointments, she is slowly involving more teeth in the restorative process.

Geresthetics: Esthetic Dentistry for Older Adults

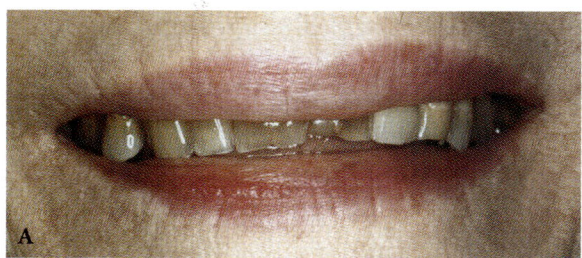

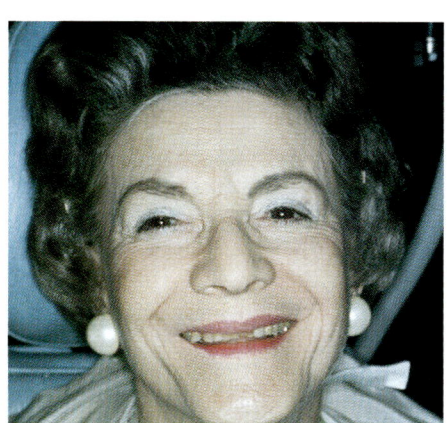

Figure 29–5A and B: This 78-year-old lady had shortened and darkened maxillary central incisors. (Reproduced with permission from Goldstein RE. Change your smile. 3rd edn. Carol Stream, IL: Quintessence, 1997:242.)

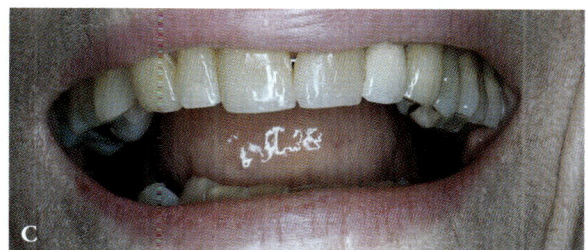

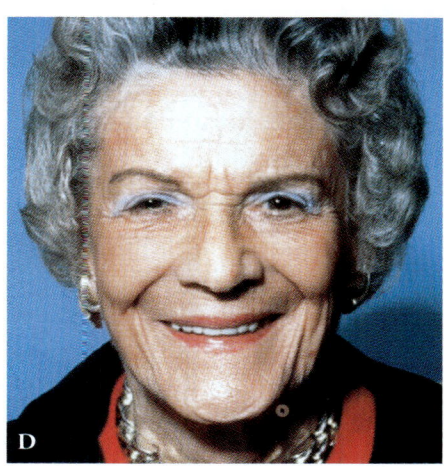

Figure 29–5C and D: Composite resin bonding was done to lengthen and lighten the central incisors. (Reproduced with permission from Goldstein RE. Change your smile. 3rd edn. Carol Stream, IL: Quintessence, 1997:242.)

ic dentistry by telling him that she would not kiss him until he had his smile improved. Figures 29–6A and D show the worn and discolored central incisors and the crowded lower anterior incisors. Figure 29–6B shows cosmetic contouring of the lower incisors. Figures 29–6C and E illustrate the completed esthetic improvement following composite resin bonding of the central incisors.

Esthetic dentistry requires excellent listening skills to identify what patients like and dislike about their appearance. Figures 29–7A and B show an older man who had worn his lower incisors. He also had diastemas between his maxillary teeth. Although he requested bonding to improve the appearance of his lower teeth, he did not want the diastemas closed since he felt that they were an important part of his personality. Therefore, Figure 29–7C shows the result of the esthetic procedure the patient wanted, which was composite resin bonding of the mandibular incisors.

ORTHODONTICS

Research has shown that teeth can be repositioned successfully at any age. Orthodontics should always be considered as an option in the cases of facial-dental arch discrepancies. Often, orthodontics is the most conservative treatment option to improve malocclusion. It is a mistake to assume that the older adult would not be willing to invest the time or money in orthodontics as a treatment option.

For adult orthodontic patients with missing teeth or insufficient numbers of teeth for orthodontic anchorage, palatal implants are being used to assist with the necessary support.

Orthodontically repositioning teeth may prevent the need for more aggressive crown and bridge coverage. In baby boomers who may not have as many restored teeth as the previous generation, preserving the natural enamel through orthodontics may be preferable to removing enamel and

866 Esthetics in Dentistry

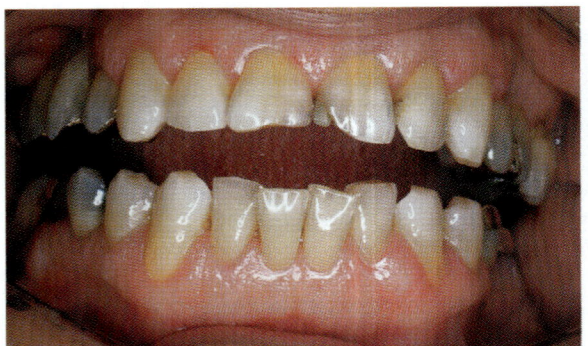

Figure 29–6A: This 65-year-old man displayed worn, discolored maxillary central incisors with a fractured anterior composite restoration on tooth #9.

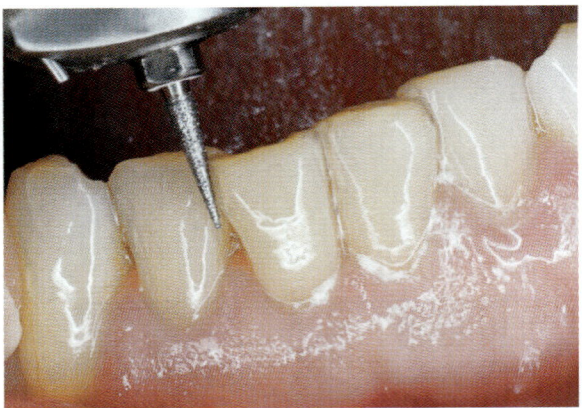

Figure 29–6B: Cosmetic contouring of mandibular incisors.

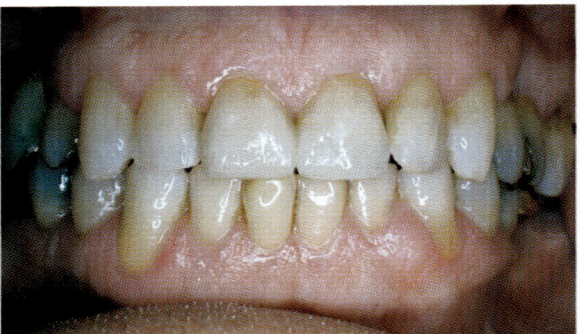

Figure 29–6C: The view after composite resin bonding of his central maxillary incisors.

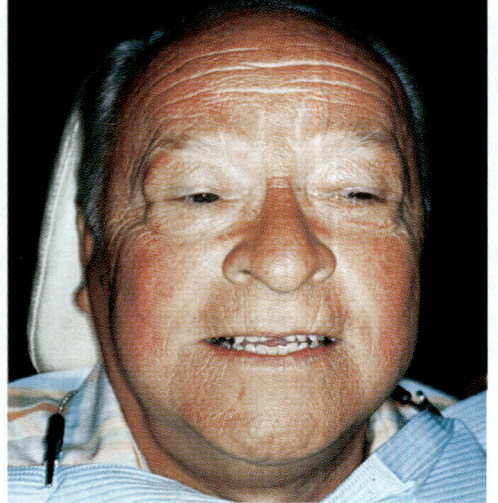

Figure 29–6D: This man avoided smiling to hide his worn, discolored, and fractured central incisors.

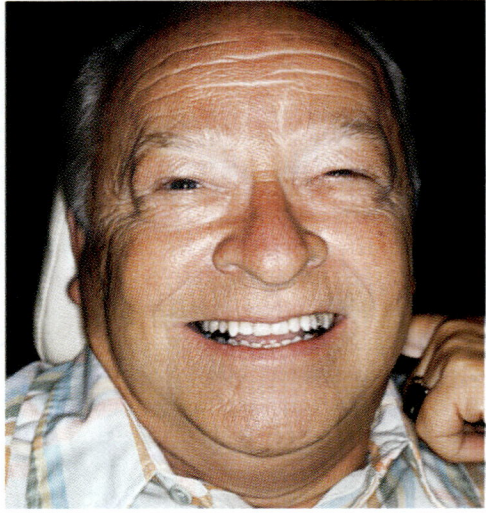

Figure 29–6E: Note how much younger and happier the patient is following his esthetic dental treatment.

Geresthetics: Esthetic Dentistry for Older Adults 867

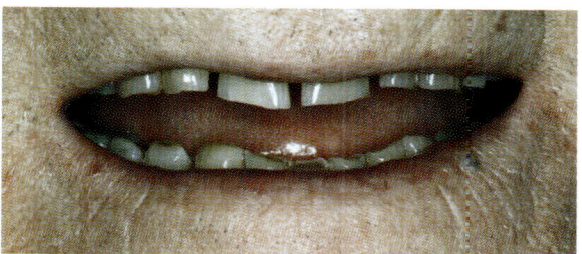

Figure 29–7A. This 70-year-old man was unhappy with the look of the worn enamel on his mandibular incisors but felt that his maxillary diastemas were an integral part of his personality.

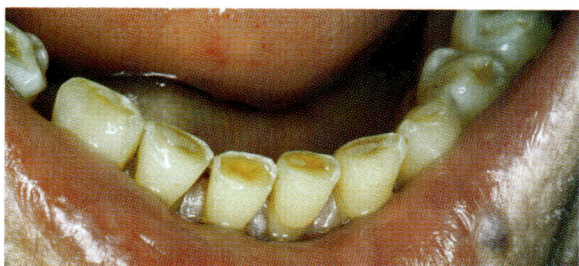

Figure 29–7B: The extent of tooth loss due to bruxism.

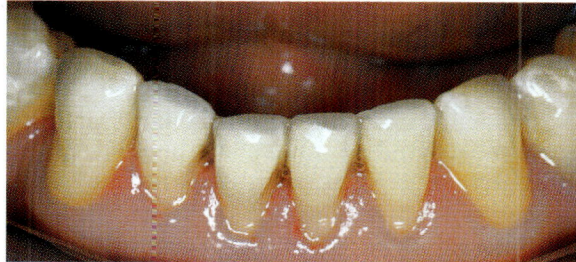

Figure 29–7C: Composite resin bonding and cosmetic contouring helped to improve the appearance of the mandibular anterior incisors.

dentin for crowns or veneers. The orthodontics may also be less costly in the long run than the prosthodontic procedures.

Figure 29–8A shows a 56-year-old woman who was unhappy with her smile and sufficiently health conscious to want to correct her malocclusion. She was also conscious of her appearance and opted for tooth-colored brackets (Figure 29–8B). The teeth were repositioned in 18 months. The patient maintained her newly esthetic dentition very well. Figure 29–8C shows this woman 24 years after initial orthodontics and cosmetic resin bonding. She demonstrates the effectiveness of long-term orthodontic results, particularly when retainers are used regularly.

PERIODONTAL THERAPY

Esthetic dentistry procedures require a foundation of good periodontal support. Periodontal tissues frame the teeth and need to be healthy and in harmony with the teeth. Age is not a contraindication for periodontal plastic surgery or periodontal surgery of any type. New periodontal regeneration procedures are providing older adults who have lost periodontal bone support with new options for retaining teeth.

Esthetic surgery, whether periodontal or oral surgical, should be offered to the older adult if surgery provides the best option for an esthetic result. Frequently, interdisciplinary therapy is necessary to achieve the most esthetic result.

Figure 29–9A shows an older man with discolored and worn teeth and irregular gingival margins. This combination contributed to his unattractive smile. He requested a younger-looking smile. His treatment plan consisted of periodontal surgery to improve the gingival contours and five porcelain veneers plus posterior crowns and inlays. Figures 29–9B and C show the final result with lighter teeth and improved tooth shape and arch alignment.

PROSTHODONTIC AND ENDODONTIC PROCEDURES

Prosthodontic procedures can restore function and an esthetic appearance to a worn dentition.

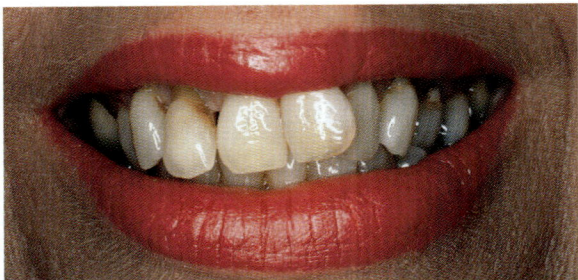

Figure 29–8A: This 56-year-old woman was unhappy with her malpositioned teeth and was willing to undergo orthodontic treatment. (Reproduced with permission from Goldstein RE. Change your smile. 3rd edn. Carol Stream, IL: Quintessence, 1997:247.)

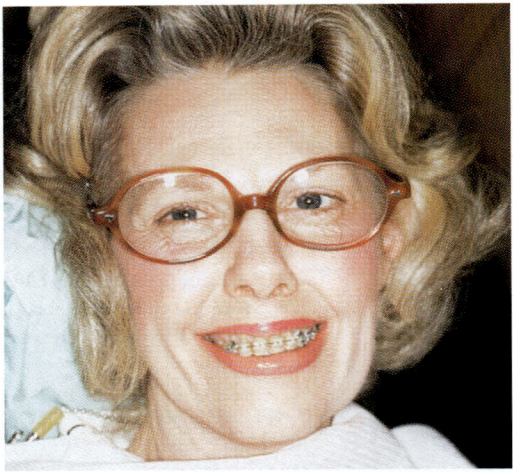

Figure 29–8B: Tooth-colored brackets were applied because of her concerns about her appearance during treatment. (Reproduced with permission from Goldstein RE. Change your smile. 3rd edn. Carol Stream, IL: Quintessence, 1997:247.)

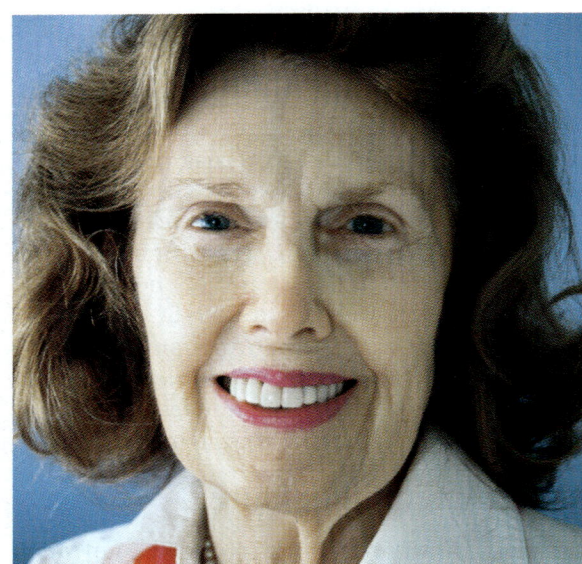

Figure 29–8C: Twenty-four years after treatment with orthodontics and composite resin bonding, as well as regular use of retainers, shows effective esthetic treatment. (Reproduced with permission from Goldstein RE. Change your smile. 3rd edn. Carol Stream, IL: Quintessence, 1997:247.)

Prosthodontic treatment may last longer than composite resin bonding. Often, the bonding procedures serve to introduce the patient to how esthetic dentistry can improve his or her smile. Later, when it needs to be redone, the patient may opt for the longer-lasting prosthodontic procedures.

Endodontic procedures are also not contraindicated in older adults. However, since dental pulps decrease in size with age, endodontics can be more difficult in older adults than in younger adults with larger pulp chambers. Consultation with an endodontist can assist the dentist in performing these procedures successfully.

Porcelain veneers are by far one of the most effective and yet conservative methods to achieve an esthetic result, especially when 8 or more teeth are involved. If the patient's goal is to improve his or her smile, the dentist should first note how many teeth are involved in this smile improvement. Generally, the patient should smile to his or her fullest, and then which of the posterior teeth shows at the corner of the mouth can be noted. Sometimes, it may be a second molar. If so, the esthetic result the patient desires will not be achieved if only 8 teeth are included in the treatment plan. Since the upper lip line varies considerably in older adults, this assessment will be critical to achieving an esthetic result pleasing to the patient. The most artificial result occurs when only the 6 anterior teeth are restored in a lighter shade, with 8 or 10 teeth showing when the patient smiles. The unrestored posterior teeth now appear even darker than previously and detract from the anterior teeth. The result is a false-looking smile on the older adult. If the patient cannot afford to include 10 or 12 teeth in the treatment plan, consider bleaching the posterior teeth first to see if you can avoid laminating all of the

Geresthetics: Esthetic Dentistry for Older Adults

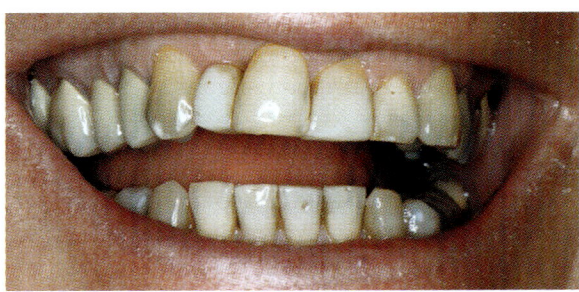

Figure 29–9A: This chief executive officer had discolored and worn teeth and irregular-looking gum tissue, resulting in an aged smile. (Reproduced with permission from Goldstein RE. Change your smile. 3rd edn. Carol Stream, IL: Quintessence, 1997:243.)

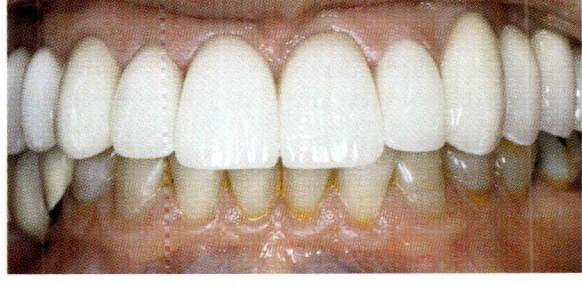

Figure 29–9B: After cosmetic periodontal surgery, during which the gingiva was cosmetically and functionally improved, five porcelain laminates were placed, as well as posterior crowns and inlays.

teeth. The opposite arch should be whitened so that the entire smile will look as natural as possible.

Porcelain restorations of all types offer the ability to retain their color over the years and not darken with age as the natural dentition does. Porcelain veneers can also be used to reshape teeth that show loss of interdental spaces. Newer low-fusing porcelains are showing considerably less wear to opposing teeth than the high-fusing porcelains. This is particularly important for middle-aged patients (eg, age 50) undergoing esthetic dental treatment with a 30-year remaining life expectancy.

When the patient requires complete oral rehabilitation, the full crown is still the restoration of choice. It can be expected to provide a greater functional life than bonding. It can be combined with porcelain veneers to accomplish an esthetic result. In many cases of bite problems that require an esthetic solution, the full crown, rather than porcelain onlays, will offer the most occlusal support against fracture.

Age and dysfunctional habits can contribute to severe wear over the years. Figures 29–10A and B demonstrate evidence of bruxism in an 86-year-old woman who had been advised to wear a bite guard when she was in her mid 50s. She disappeared from the practice and returned 30 years later demonstrating severe wear, loss of vertical dimension, loss of masticatory function, and temporomandibular pain. More importantly, she was embarrassed by her smile. Her treatment plan consisted of a temporary crown and bridge to restore vertical dimension and comfort. She was subsequently treated months later with fixed prosthodontics using metal-ceramic restorations (Figure 29–10C). She regained much of her self-confidence, as well as masticatory function, following the esthetic reconstruction of the maxillary arch (Figure 29–10D) and planned to restore the lower arch.

Fixed and removable prosthodontics can be used to improve appearance and function. The 78-year-old patient in Figures 29–11A and B showed severe wear on his upper and lower incisors, which com-

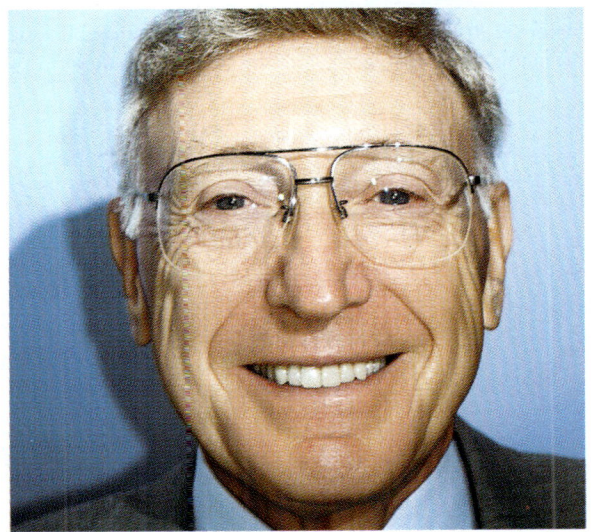

Figure 29–9C: The result was lighter teeth and improved tooth shape and arch alignment to help create a younger-looking smile. (Reproduced with permission from Goldstein RE. Change your smile. 3rd edn. Carol Stream, IL: Quintessence, 1997:243.)

promised his smile line. He also had multiple missing teeth. He was president of a large company and felt that he looked older than his actual years because his smile did not show any teeth. His treatment plan included crowns on his remaining natural teeth and a maxillary precision attachment removable bridge. The final result shows both improved appearance and function (Figure 29–11C).

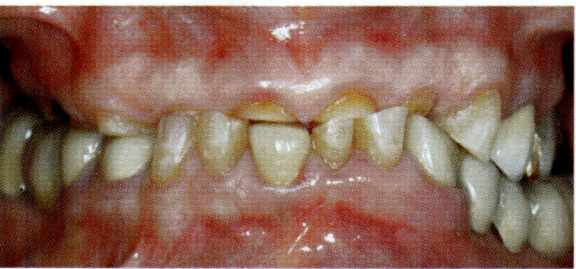

Figure 29–10A: This lady presented with a severe bruxism habit that resulted in virtually all of her maxillary teeth being hidden when she smiled.

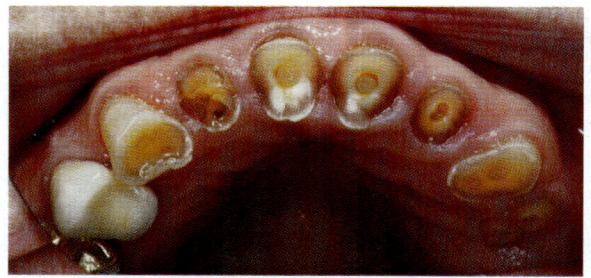

Figure 29–10B: Although she was advised more than 30 years previously to wear a night guard, she chose not to do so.

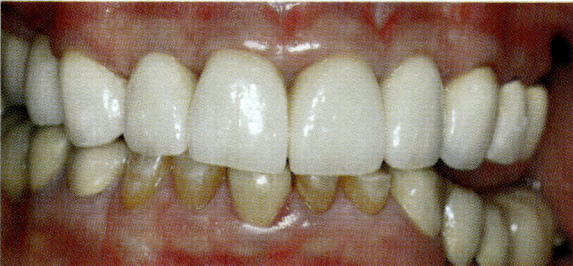

Figure 29–10C: Crown lengthening followed by prosthodontic reconstruction helped to recreate her smile. The next step is for her to rebuild the mandibular arch.

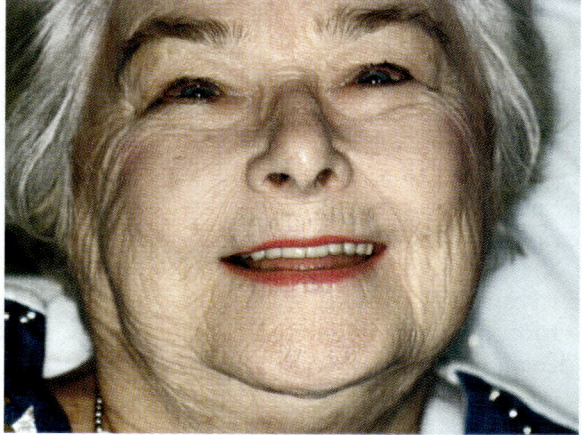

Figure 29–10D: The reconstructed teeth of this 88-year-old lady now enhance her smile

Geresthetics: Esthetic Dentistry for Older Adults

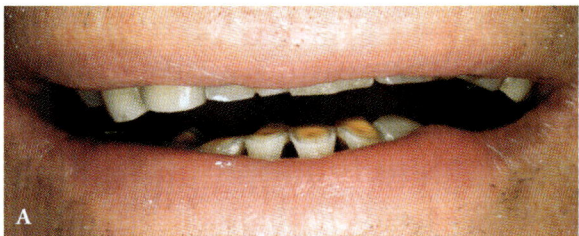
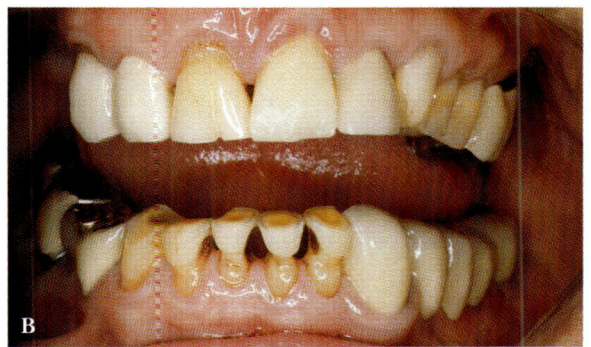

Figure 29–11A and B: This 78-year-old man had worn down his maxillary and mandibular teeth during the course of his life. This negatively affected his smile line.

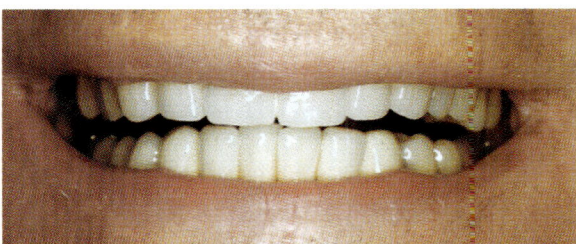

Figure 29–11C: All of the maxillary and mandibular teeth were crowned and a precision attachment partial denture was made to improve both function and esthetics.

Although esthetic dental treatment for older adults may require an interdisciplinary team approach of general dentists and specialists, families may also be involved in helping patients understand the need for dental treatment.

Figures 29–12A to C show a 75-year-old woman who presented with severe root caries and moderate periodontal disease. Her daughter, who disclosed that her mother was difficult to please, referred her. The daughter was very supportive of her mother receiving dental treatment; however, her mother was initially not interested. The mother did not think that the esthetic aspect of dentistry was important. During consultation with the dentist, the mother was informed of the infection in her mouth and the potential effect that this could have on her future health and functionality. The patient consented to have the maxillary arch restored with fixed prosthodontics. She refused to accept treatment for her mandibular teeth, preferring to use her existing partial denture. Figures 29–12D and E show the final result after periodontal and prosthodontic treatment. Although the patient was not particularly grateful to have the dental treatment, her family was thrilled to have the caries infection removed and the esthetic appearance improved. The patient lived with her esthetically improved appearance for an additional 13 years.

There are few things in a dental practice that can be more satisfying than helping a patient to obtain the best esthetic appearance possible; it can be just as important to work toward that goal when the patient is elderly. Although it may be the family and friends who enjoy seeing their loved one look and feel his or her best, ultimately, it is the older individual who has the most to gain with enhanced esthetics and function.

Implant treatment is increasing in older adults. Again, age, in and of itself, is not a contraindication to implant therapy. Many older adults are trading their complete dentures for implant-supported prostheses. Implant therapy is expected to increase as implants become the treatment of choice for replacement of a single missing tooth. Implant therapy often requires a team approach

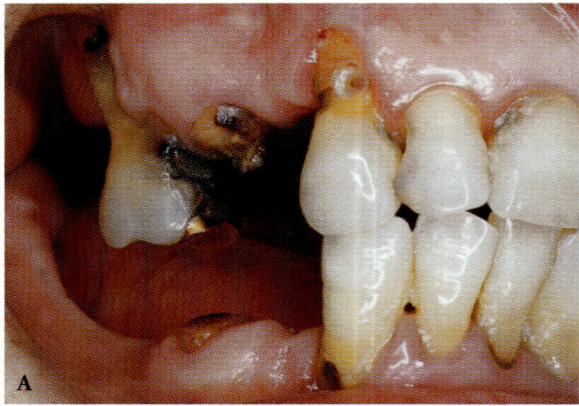

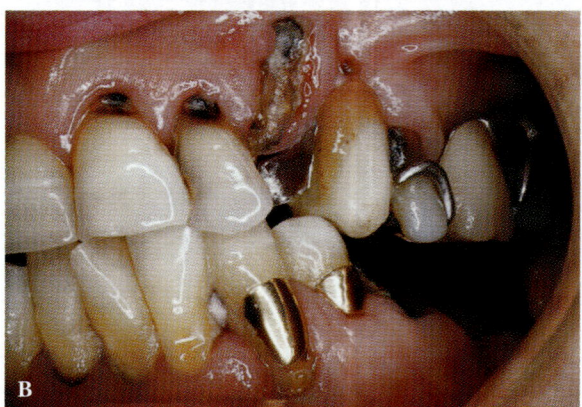

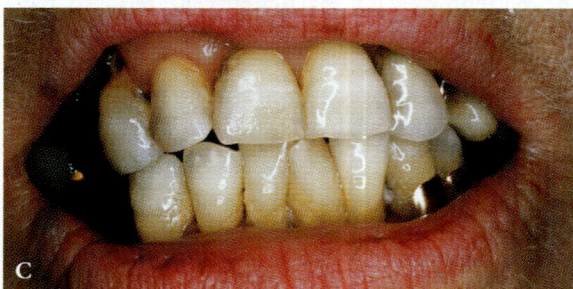

Figure 29–12A to C: This 75-year-old woman had severe root caries and moderate periodontal disease.

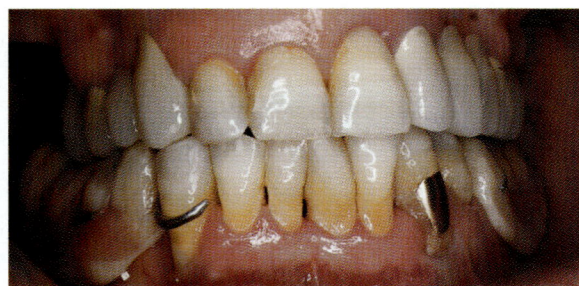

Figure 29–12D: Although this woman stated that she would "just as soon have her teeth extracted," she was motivated to have both periodontal and prosthodontic treatment.

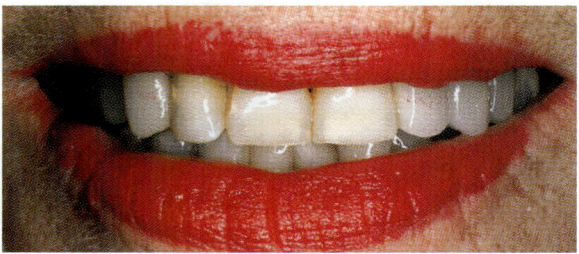

Figure 29–12E: The patient's smile after esthetic dental treatment shows just how much she appreciated her dental treatment.

with excellent communication between the surgical and the prosthodontic teams.

ESTHETIC DENTISTRY AND THE NURSING HOME OR ASSISTED LIVING RESIDENT

The increase in the oldest-old has led gerontologists to define a concept of active life expectancy. Active life expectancy refers to that portion of life in which one can perform the activities of daily living with little or no help. Scientists have estimated that although a 65-year-old man may have an average of 16 years remaining life expectancy, 3 of those years may be periods of dependency, in which the individual requires some type of care.[12]

Dependency results from the disabilities caused by long-standing chronic illnesses. Older adults often require more care from their children, family, or unrelated caregivers. Some may also need nursing home care.

In the United States, only 5% of the population over age 65 resides in a nursing home. However, adults over age 65 have a one in four chance of spending some time in a nursing home. The most frequent scenario is that of the older woman living alone who falls and fractures a hip. She is hospitalized to have the hip surgically repaired and then may enter a nursing home for 3 to 6 months of rehabilitation therapy. More recently, as people age, they consider the concept of assisted living before severe problems arise. Thus, they avoid abrupt change when something adverse does occur. However, good or even adequate home care for them remains a problem.

The risk of residing in a nursing home increases with advancing age and is greatest for those with dementia. In the United States, over 50% of nursing home residents carry a diagnosis of dementia.

Data on the oral health needs of nursing home residents in Ohio found that fulfillment of patients' dental needs was declining.[13] The authors hypothesized that patients and their families are delaying entry into the nursing home, opting instead to care for the family member for as long as possible in their home. During this period of home care, dental appointments are often overlooked as the family struggles to meet the care needs of their family member.

Dental care for residents of nursing homes in the United States remains woefully inadequate.[5] Oral health care in most nursing homes is virtually nonexistent. Studies have shown that education of the nursing staff can help improve the daily oral care and the ability to recognize the oral problems of the residents.[10] As baby boomers care for their aging parents and/or make difficult decisions regarding nursing home placement, they may become aware of the lack of essential health care services in nursing homes and demand improvements for the family members. (One can only hope that they demand improved oral hygiene care.)

Patients who have spent considerable time and money for esthetic dental services should not enter a nursing home only to have the lifetime of restorative and esthetic dentistry become undermined by root caries or periodontal infection. The opportunity for dentistry lies in advocating for a change in the standard of oral health care for nursing home residents. If residents can have their sight and hearing needs met, their oral health needs should be accepted as an important part of their health care needs, particularly given the amount of time that residents spend using their oral cavity to swallow, smile, eat, and, especially, to communicate. These are surely important activities in the life of a nursing home resident.

CONCLUSION

Americans now have the potential to enjoy a lifetime of oral health rather than suffer from a lifetime of oral diseases. The desire to feel good and look healthy is not limited by age. The new procedures, materials, and techniques that have provided an esthetic revolution in dentistry will provide older Americans with improved quality of life, greater self-esteem, and continued oral function.

All patients should be treatment planned based on their needs and wants and not their age. It should not be assumed that patients do not care about their appearance as they age. The relationship between systemic illnesses and oral health must be recognized and understood. A preventive program as part of every treatment plan based on oral and medical conditions, risk factors, and, especially, the physical and mental ability to perform adequate home care should be developed.

Patients should be given the opportunity to learn how esthetic dentistry can improve the quality of their life. Even in the nursing home, life revolves around speaking, smiling, eating and socializing—all functions of the oral cavity. An esthetic smile is an asset in any venue, even the nursing home.

The importance that family and caregivers play in maintaining oral health, particularly in the medically and physically compromised older adult, must be recognized. The dentist should not be shy about inviting family and caregivers to assist in the daily oral care for a patient who has become incapacitated and can no longer perform his or her own oral care.

An accurate diagnosis is the most important first step in providing any esthetic dental service. In the final analysis, *no* treatment is better than the *wrong* treatment. In the words of Hippocrates, "First, do no harm." Esthetic dentistry has the potential to contribute greatly to improving the oral health and quality of life of older adults.

References

1. Antibiotic prophylaxis for dental patients with total joint replacements. J Am Dent Assoc 1997;128:1004–7.

2. Beck JD, Garcia RG, Heiss G, et al. Periodontal disease and cardiovascular disease. J Periodontol 1996; 67(Suppl):1123–37.

3. CIA world factbook, 1999. http://www.odci.gov/cia/publications/factbook/index/html.

4. Fox PC. Differentiation of dry mouth etiology. Adv Dent Res 1996;10:13–6.

5. Gift HC, Cherry-Peppers G, Oldakowski RJ. Oral health care in US nursing homes, 1995. Spec Care Dent 1998;18:226–33.

6. Goldstein RE. Esthetic dentistry: a health service. J Dent Res 1993;72:641–2.

7. Goldstein RE, Niessen LC. Issues in esthetic dentistry for older adults. J Esthet Dent 1998;10:235–42.

8. Havens JJ, Schervish PG. Millionaires and the millennium. Boston: Social Welfare Research Institute, October 1999.

9. Johannes L. Looking good. Wall Street Journal Oct. 18, 1999.

10. Lin CY, Jones DB, Godwin K, et al. Oral health assessment by nursing staff of Alzheimer's patients in a long term care facility. Spec Care Dent 1999;19:64–71.

11. National Institutes of Health. Oral health in America: a report of the Surgeon General. Washington, DC: Government Printing Office, May 25, 2000.

12. Rowe JW, Kahn RI. Successful aging. New York: Pantheon, 1998.

13. Strayer M. "Catching up" with the problem of homebound care. Spec Care Dent 1998;18:52–7.

14. Summer L. Chronic conditions: a challenge for the 21st century. No. 1. Washington, DC: National Academy on an Aging Society. November 1999.

15. Trupin L, Rice D. Health status, medical care use, and number of disabling conditions in the United States. Disability Statistics, Abstr. No. 9, June 1995.

16. U.S. Bureau of the Census. Current population reports. Washington, DC: Government Printing Office, 1998.

17. U.S. Bureau of the Census. Statistical abstract of the United States, 1998. 118th edn. Washington, DC: Government Printing Office, 1998.

18. U.S. Department of Health and Human Services. Wired for health and well-being: the emergence of interactive health communication. Washington, DC: Government Printing Office, 1999.

19. Wu T, Trevisan M, Genco R, et al. Periodontal disease and risk of cerebrovascular disease. Arch Intern Med 2000;160:2749–55.

Additional Resources

Goldstein RE. Diagnostic dilemma: to bond, laminate, or crown. Int J Periodont Restor Dent 1987;87:(5):9–30.

Goldstein RE. Esthetic principles for ceramo-metal restorations. Dent Clin North Am 1988;21:803–22.

Goldstein RE. Finishing of composites and laminates. Dent Clin North Am 1989;33:305–18.

Goldstein RE, Garber DA, Schwartz CG, Goldstein CE. Patient maintenance of esthetic restorations. J Am Dent Assoc 1992;123:61–6.

Goldstein RE. Change your smile. 3rd edn. Carol Stream, IL: Quintessence, 1997.

Goldstein RE, Adar P. Special effects and internal characterization. J Dent Technol 1989;17(11).

Goldstein RE, Feinman RA, Garber DA. Esthetic considerations in the selection and use of restorative materials. Dent Clin North Am 1983;27:723–31.

Goldstein RE, Garber DA. Goldstein CE, et al. The changing esthetic dental practice. J Am Dent Assoc 1994;125:1447–57.

Appendix E

Manufacturer Index

Align Technology
851 Martin Ave.
Santa Clara, CA 95050
1-408-470-1000

Artus
P.O. Box 511
Englewood, NJ 07631
1-201-568-1000

Attachments International
600 S. Amphlett Blvd.
San Mateo, CA 94402
1-800-999-3003

Austenal, Inc.
3206 N. Kilpatrick Ave.
Chicago, IL 60641
1-773-205-6600

Bay Technical Products
1895 Mowry Ave., Suite 110
Freemont, CA 94538
1-510-797-8606

Bisco Inc.
1100 W. Irving Pk. Rd.
Schaumburg, IL 60193
1-800-247-3368

Brasseler USA
One Brasseler Blvd.
Savannah, GA 31419
1-800-841-4522

Cendres & Métaux SA
Route de Boujean 122
CH-2501
Biel-Bienne
Switzerland
41 32 344 2211

COSMEDENT Inc.
401 North Michigan Ave.
Suite 2500
Chicago, IL 60611
1-800-621-6729

DEN-MAT Corporation
2727 Skyway Drive
Santa Monica, CA 93455
1-800-433-6628

DENTSPLY/Caulk
]38 West Clark Ave.
Milford, DE 19963-0359
1-800-532-2855

DENTSPLY/Maillefer
5001E 68th St., Suite 500
Tulsa, OK 74136-3332
1-800-924-7393

DENTSPLY Professional
1301 Smile Way
York, PA 17404
1-800-989-8826

DENTSPLY/Rinn
1212 Abbott Drive
Elgin, IL 60123
1-800-323-0970

DENTSPLY/Trubyte
570 West College Ave.
P.O. Box 872
York, PA 17405-0872
1-800-877-0020

DENTSPLY/Tulsa
5001 East 68th St., Suite 500
Tulsa, OK 74136
1-800-379-3432

Discus Dental
8550 Higuera St.
Culver City, CA 90232
1-800-348-8806

E.C. Moore Co. Inc.
13325 Leonard
Dearborn, MI 48126
1-800-331-3548

Gnathos Dental Prod. Inc.
56 Colpitts Road
P.O. Box 655
Weston, MA 02193
1-800-325-0285

Harry J. Bosworth Co.
7227 North Hamlin Ave.
Skokie, IL 60076
1-800-323-4352

Hu-Friedy Manufacturing Co. Inc.
3232 North Rockwell
Chicago, IL 60618-5982
1-800-483-7433

Hygenic Corp.
1245 Home Ave.
Akron, OH 44310
1-800-321-2135

Implantech
2064 Eastman Ave., Unit 101
Ventura, CA 93003
1-800-733-0833

Ivoclar Vivadent, Inc.
175 Pineview Drive
Amherst, NY 14228
1-800-533-6825

J. Morita USA
9 Mason
Irvine, CA 92618
1-800-752-9720

Jeneric/Pentron Inc.
53 North Plains Industrial Road
Wallingford, CT 06492
1-800-243-3100

Kay-See Dental Manufacturing Co.
124 East Missouri Ave.
Kansas City, MO 64106-1294
1-800-842-8844

KerrDental
1717 West Collins Avenue
Orange, CA 92667
1-800-537-7123

KerrDental
28200 Wick Rd.
Romulus, MI 48174
1-800-537-7123

Masel
2701 Bartram Road
Bristol, PA 19007
1-800-423-8227

Mediteam Dental AB
Göteborgsvägen 74
SE-433 63
Sävedalen, Sweden
46 31 336 91 00

Miltex Dental Technology
589 Davies Drive
York, PA 17402
1-800-221-1344

Pfingst & Co. Inc.
105 Synder Road South
South Plainfield, NJ 07080
1-908-561-6400

Porex Surgical Inc.
15 Dart Road
Newnan, GA 30265-1017
1-800-521-7321

Practicon Inc.
1112 Shugg Pkwy.
Greenville, NC 27834
1-800-959-9505

Premier Dental Products
3600 Horizon Drive
King of Prussia, PA 19406
1-610-239-6000

Productivity Training Corporation
360-A Cochrane Circle
Morgan Hill, CA 95037
1-800-448-8855

Professional Results Inc.
29 Merano
Laguna Niguel, CA 92677
1-800-350-3705

R. Chige Inc.
4531 North Dixie Hwy
Boca Raton, FL 33431
1-800-645-2628

Roth International
669 West Ohio
Chicago, IL 60610-3958
1-800-4450572

Shofu Dental Corp.
4025 Bohannon Drive
Menlo Park, CA 94025
1-415-324-0085

Sterngold
23 Frank Mossberg Drive
Attleboro, MA 02703
1-800-243-9942

Sullivan-Schein Dental
135 Duryea Rd.
Melville, NY 11747
1-800-372-4346

Sultan Chemists Inc.
85 W. Forest Ave.
Englewood, NJ 07631
1-800-637-8582

3M ESPE
3M Center Bldg. 275-2E-03
St. Paul, MN 55144-1000
1-800-634-2249

Ultradent Products Inc.
505 West 10200 South
South Jordan, UT 84095
1-801-553-4200

Universal Lactona Dental Corp.
108 Park Drive
Montgomeryville, PA 18936-0447
1-800-523-2559

Vident
3150 East Birch Street
Brea, CA 92621
1-714-961-6224

W.L. Gore & Associates Inc.
1505 North 4th Street
Flagstaff, AZ 86004
1-800-645-4337

Appendix F

Product Index

Alameter — Productivity Training Corp.
ASC 52 attachment — Attachments International
Beyeler — Attachments International
Biloc and Plasta attachment — Attachments International
Brasseler 801-016 — Brasseler
Carisolv — Mediteam Dental AB
Cavit — 3M ESPE
Cerestore crowns — 3M ESPE
Compo-Disc — Premier
Compoglass — Ivoclar Vivadent, Inc.
Composite — COSMEDENT, Ultradent
Compo-Strip — Premier
Cosmetic Contouring Kit — Shofu
Crismani attachment — Sterngold
Cushee rubber dam clamp cushions — Practicon
Dalbo attachment — Cendres & Metaux SA
Dental Dial Calipers — Masel
Denture base tinting acrylic — Kay-See Manufacturing Co.
Desentize — DEN-MAT
DET-GF diamond stone — Brasseler
Dycal (acid resistant) — DENTSPLY/Caulk
Dycal Caulk — DENTSPLY/Caulk
Dyract — DENTSPLY/Caulk
Endo-Z — DENTSPLY/Maillefer
Endo-Ice — Hygenic
ET diamond burs — Brasseler
ET6, ET9, ETUF4, ETUF6, ETUF, OS1 — Brasseler
44E maxillary anterior mold — DENTSPLY/Trubyte
Fortify — Bisco
Gates Glidden — Miltex
Geristore — DEN-MAT
Gnathos 801-016 — Gnathos Dental Products
Goldstein #3 composite instrument — Hu-Friedy
Gore-Tex — W.L. Gore & Associates
Hader Vertical — Attachments International
Hannes anchor — Attachments International
Horico 139x012 — Pfingst & Co. Inc.
Hytac — 3M ESPE
IC attachment — Attachments International
Inceram — Vident
Invisalign — Align Technology
IRM — DENTSPLY/Caulk
Jacoby plastic clamps — Bay Technical Products
Kerr Vitality Scanner 2006 — KerrDental
Lentulo spiral drill — DENTSPLY/Caulk
Life — KerrDental
LVS System, LVS diamond bur — Brasseler
Nonlatex rubber dam — Hygenic
M45 mandibular mold — Universal Lactona Dental Corp.
M45 maxillary anterior mold — Universal Lactona Dental Corp.
Medpore — Porex Surgical
Novatek 12 — HU-Friedy
Octolink System — Attachments International
Odontotest Thermal Pulp Tester — Miltex
Omega-M — Attachments International
Opalescence with Fluoride — Ultradent
Optiguard — KerrDental
Oraseal Putty — Ultradent
ORS-DE attachment — Attachments
Panavia cement — J. Morita
PDC — Attachments
Peeso reamer — Miltex International
Premier 120F, Premier 365.4F, 982.8 — Premier
ProRoot MTA — DENTSPLY/Tulsa
Prophy-jet air polisher — DENTSPLY Professional
Provit — E.C Moore
Quick Dam — Ivoclar Vivadent
Regisil 2x — DENTSPLY/Caulk
Relief — Discus Dental
Rexillium III — Jeneric/Pentron Inc.
Roth 801 — Roth International
SA SwissAnchor attachment — Attachments International
Schatzmann attachment — Attachments International
Score-BR, Score-PD, and Score-UP attachments — Attachments International
Seek Caries Indicator — Ultradent
Shim-type articulating ribbon — Artus
Silicone rubber — Implantech
SoFlex discs — 3M ESPE
Stern ERA and Stern-RV extracoronal attachments — Sterngold
Stern intracoronal attachments — Sterngold
Super EBA — Harry J. Bosworth
Superoxol — Sultan Chemists Inc.
Swiss McCollum attachments — Sterngold
Swiss Tac/Tach E-Z — Attachments International
TGE diamond — Premier
TPE diamond — Shofu
Thermaseal Plus — DENTSPLY/Tulsa
Tooth Slooth — Professional Results
UltraEZ — Ultradent
UltraSeal — Ultradent
U/P Root Canal Sealer — Sultan
Vita shade guide — Vident
Vitallium — Austenal
Vitrebond — 3M ESPE
Vitremer — 3M ESPE
Wedjets — Hygenic
XCP — DENTSPLY/Rinn
Z 100 — 3M ESPE

Index

Page numbers in italics indicate figures.

Abfraction, 502–505
  bruxism and, 508
  case studies of, 503–505, *503–505*
  defined, 502
  differential diagnosis, 515–516
  stress etiology of, 502, *503*
Abrasion
  case studies of, 505, *505–507*, 507
  defined, 505
  differential diagnosis, 515–516
  due to improper brushing, 507, *508*
  etiology of, 505
Aging, *see* Older adults
Air abrasion, 807–808
Alcohol abuse, oral damage due to, 615, *615*
Amalgams, using composites to mask, 491–492, *492*
Analytical Technology Vitality Scanner, 559–560, *560*
Ankylosis, in avulsion injuries, 593
Anorexia nervosa
  oral damage due to, 612, *613, 614*
  symptoms of, 612
Appliance(s)
  for bruxism, 603, *604*
  Crozat, 754–755, *756–758, 757, 760–761*
  for diastema, 708–709
  for frenum involvement, 705, *705*
  Hawley, 764, *764,* 772, 773
  lingual, 770, *771*
  for lip or cheek biting, 608, *609, 610*
  for lip or cheek sucking, *610,* 611
  removable, 770, *772, 773*
  see also Retainers for missing teeth
Arch, evolution of, in pediatric dentistry, 817–818
Arch space, in treatment of crowded teeth, 733, *734*
Attachments for dentures
  adjunctive procedures with, 682
  biomechanics in, 683
  classification of, 680
  contraindications for use, 682
  defined, 680
  diagnosis and treatment planning, 679–680
  extracoronal, 685, 690–698
    advantages, 690
    ASC 52 ball, 693–694
    Dalbo, 690, *691–692*
    disadvantages, 690
    Dolder bar, 694, *697,* 698
    Hader vertical, 693
    Octolink, 690–691, *693–694*

ORS-DE, 694, *696*
  plunger, 694, *696*
  SA SwissAnchor, 692
  splint bar designs, 694, *697,* 698
  Stern ERA, 692, *695, 696*
  Stern-RV, 692, *695, 696*
general considerations, 681–683
indications for use, 681–682
indirect retention, 684
intracoronal, 685–690
  advantages, 686–687
  Biloc and Plasta, 689, *689*
  Crismani, 688–689
  disadvantages, 687
  Patrix, 689–690, *690*
  Schatzmann, 689
  Score system, 689
  Stern G/A, 687, *687*
  Stern G/L, 687–688, *688*
  Stern G/L ESI, 688, *688*
  Stern McCollum, 688–689, *689*
  Stern Type 7, 687
  Swiss McCollum, 688, *688*
milled lingual bracing arm, 685, *685*
milled lingual ledges, 698
overdenture abutments, 698
path of insertion, 684
precision, 686
selection considerations, 684–686
  cost, 682–683, 686
  dexterity of patient, 682
  function, 686
  location, 685
  oral hygiene maintenance of patient, 683
  retention, 686
  space, 686
semiprecision, 681
tooth preparation, 684
Attrition, 507–514
  bruxism and, 508, *508,* 510–514
  in children, 507, *508*
  defined, 507
  etiology of, 507
Avulsion injuries
  ankylosis in, 593
  in pediatric dentistry, 816–817
  root reabsorption in, 593, *594*

Baby boomers
  aging parents of, 859
  as dental consumers, 857, 859
Bite test, 564
  in endodontic evaluations, 564, *564, 565*
  plastic saliva ejector, 564, *565*

tooth slooth, 564, *564, 565*
Bleaching, 480–491, *482–483, 483*
  at-home, tray design for, *480,* 480–481
  of endodontically treated teeth, 484, 585, *586*
  walking bleach technique, 585–587, *586*
  inside-outside, 482–483, *483*
  closure of internal, 483–484
  in older adults, 862–863, *863*
  porcelain veneers and, 489–490, *490*
  restorations and, 490, *491*
  single dark tooth, *481,* 481–482
  tetracycline staining, *488,* 488–489, *489*
  tooth sensivity during, 484–485, *485*
  vs. microabrasion, 485–488
Bonding, *see* Composite resin bonding
Bruxism, 602–603, *602–603*
  abfraction in, 503, *503,* 508
  case studies of, *513,* 513–514
  damage due to, 508, *508,* 602, 603, 604
  differential diagnosis, 515–516
  as learned behavior, 603
  in older adults, 865, *867,* 869, *870*
  with temporomandibular joint pain, 603
  treatment options
    crowns, 508, *509*
    orthodontic therapy, 510, 637, *638*
    overlay denture, 512, *512*
    prosthodontics, 510, *510–511*
Bulimia
  differential diagnosis, 515–516
  loss of tooth structure and, 502, 516
  oral damage due to, 610, 612, *612*
Burs, in cavity preparation for endodontic procedures, 581–582
  for acrylic veneer and full metallic crowns, 581
  for all-ceramic crowns, 581–582
  for aluminous porcelain, 581
  for porcelain fused-to-metal crown, 581, *582*
  for porcelain inlays and onlays, 582
  for restored teeth, 581

Camper's line, 838, *839,* 844
Cantilever fixed partial denture, 651, *652*
Caries
  materials and techniques for, 805–808
    air abrasion, 807–808
    Carisolv, 806–807, *807*
    compomers, 806, *807*
    composite resin bonding, 805, 808
    glass ionomers, 805–806, *807*

modified ionomer cements, 805–806, *807*
in pediatric dentistry, 808–811
caries in anterior teeth, 808, *809*
composite resin bonding for permanent caries, 818, *818*
nursing bottle syndrome, 809–811, *810, 812*
rampant caries in very young, 808–809, *810*
Carisolv system, 806–807, *807*
Casts, diagnostic, 636
for crowded teeth, 736
Cavity preparation for endodontic procedures, 578–580, *579, 580*
burs for, 581–582
for acrylic veneer and full metallic crowns, 581
for all-ceramic crowns, 581–582
for aluminous porcelain, 581
for porcelain fused-to-metal crown, 581, *582*
for porcelain inlays and onlays, 582
for restored teeth, 581
etched cast bridges, 582, *583*
procedure, *579–580*, 581
radiography use in, *566*, 578–579, *579*
retentive value after, 582–583, *584*
Cavity tests, in endodontic evaluations, 561, *562*
Cement-enamel junction (CEJ), bleaching and, 482
Cephalometric analysis
in pediatric dentistry, 821
in surgical orthodontics, 780, *782, 784*
Cheek biting, oral damage due to, 606, 608
Chewing habits, oral damage due to, 603, 605, *605*
Children
attrition in, 507, *508*
damaging oral habits in, 599–601
thumb sucking in, 600–601
treatment options, 620–621
see also Pediatric dentistry
Chipped teeth, 525–549
see also Fractured teeth
Chromagenic foods, tooth discoloration and, 479, *479*, 491, *492*
Clasp types, in removable partial dentures, 672–676
circumferential, 672
combination, 676, *677*
embrasure, 675–676, *676*
I-bar, 672–673, *673*
mesial groove reciprocation (MGR), 674–675, *675, 676*
modified T-bar, 673–674, *674*
reciprocal arm, 672, *673*
rest-proximal plate-I-bar, 674, *674*
retentive arm, 672, *673*
ring, 675
T- or Y-bar, 673, *674*

Cocaine, oral damage due to, 615
Color of teeth
selection of, in complete dentures, 837
see also Bleaching; Discoloration of teeth
Color of tissue
in denture esthetics, 837
discoloration of, 596
use of tissue-colored material, in pontics, 660, *660, 661*
Compomers, 806, *807*
Composite resin bonding, 805
for anterior teeth, 808
for crowded teeth, *737,* 738
and cosmetic contouring, 738–739, *739, 740*
for diastema, 711, *712*, 717, 717–721, *718*
adjacent teeth, *710,* 710–711, *711*
due to small teeth, *714,* 714–716, *715*
full labial veneer *vs.* partial, 720
microfilled, 720, *721*
posterior, 712–714, *713, 714*
proportionality in, 714, 716
small teeth, 718–719, *719*
discoloration of, 490–491, *492*
in older adults, 864–865, *864–867*
in pediatric dentistry, 805, 808
for permanent caries, 818, *818*
for posterior teeth, 805
use of to mask amalgams, 491–492, *492*
Computer-assisted treatment trays, 769–770, *771*
Condylar hyperplasia
case study, 797, *798–799*
surgical treatment of, 795–797
Contouring, cosmetic
for crowded teeth, *737*
composite resin bonding with, 738–739, *739, 740*
porcelain laminates with, *744–745,* 744–746
for diastema, 711, *712*
of fractured teeth, 525–526, *526,* 530 *531*
in older adults, 863–865, *864, 866*
Corrosion, defined, 501
Cracked tooth syndrome, 525
treatment options, *526*
Crossbite, orthodontic therapy for, 764–766
anterior, 765, *767*
posterior, 765, *766*
severe, 766, *768, 769*
short lower jaw, 765–766, *767*
Crowded teeth, 733–751
composite resin bonding, *737,* 738–739, *739, 740*
cosmetic contouring, *737*
composite resin bonding with, 738–739, *739, 740*
porcelain laminates with, *744–745,* 744–746
diagnostic casts, 736

diagnostic wax-up, 736, 740–744, *741–743*
discing, *737,* 738
matrices for, 736, 740–744, *741–743*
orthodontic therapy for, 574–755, *737,* 738, 757–759
class I crowding with extractions, 758–759, *761, 762*
expansion therapy, 754–755, *756–758*
lower crowding with slight overbite, 755, 757–758, *759*
porcelain laminates, *737,* 739–746
cosmetic contouring with, *744–745,* 744–746
diagnostic wax-up for, 740–744, *741–743*
treatment considerations, *733,* 733–735
arch space, 733, *734*
emergence profile and oral hygiene, 735
gingival architecture, 733–734, *735*
influence of root proximity, 734–735
smile line, 735
treatment options, *737,* 738–749
treatment selection considerations, 750–751
treatment strategy, 735–737
degree of correction, 736
type of restoration, 736–737
unusual clinical presentations, 749–750
lingually locked tooth, 750
malposed or misaligned teeth, 749
protruding tooth, 749–750, *750*
retruded tooth, 750
Crowns
for crowded teeth, *737, 746,* 746–748, *748*
for diastema, 723–729
four crowns, *725,* 725–727, *726*
one crown, *724,* 724–725, *725*
principles in shaping, *726,* 726–727, *727*
six crowns, 272–729, *727, 728*
discoloration of, 587
for endodontically treated fractured teeth, 537–539, *537–539*
fracture of, *587,* 587–588, *588*
lengthening procedures, in conjunction with dentures, 682
in older adults, 869–871, *870–871*
telescoping, 653, *654,* 655, *655, 656*
three-quarter, retainers for missing teeth, 639–640, *640*
for treatment of bruxism, 508, *509*
Crozat appliance, 754–755, *756–758, 757, 760–751*
Cushee rubber dam clamp cushions, *577,* 577–578

Dam, rubber, *see* Rubber dam
Dental floss, improper use of, 617–618, *621*

Dental history, *see* Medical history
Dental surveyor, use in removable partial dentures, 670–671
Dentin
  reparative, *569*, 570
  secondary, *569*, 570
Dentition, wear of, 501–516
  see also Tooth structure, loss of
Dentofacial deformity, surgery for, *see* Surgical orthodontics
Dentures, complete, 831–849
  denture base, 846–848
    fit of, 846
    tips on creating natural looking, 846–849, *847*, *848*
  esthetics in, 831–832
    examples of, *849*
  mandibular anterior tooth placement, 841, *841*, 843, 845
  maxillary anterior teeth placement, 838, *838–842*, 840–841, 845
  occlusion in, 832–833, *833–835*
    anterior, 843
    posterior, 844–845, *845*
  provisional dentures, 832, *832*, 833
  tooth arrangement, 837–838
    tips for, 845–846
  tooth selection, 833–837
    clinical, 835, *835*
    sex, personality, and age theory of, 834
    temperamental theory of, 833–834
    tips on, 836–837
    tooth color, 837
    tooth form and mold, 835–836
  vertical dimension, 843–844, *844*
Dentures, removable partial, 669–698
  attachments, *see also* Attachments for dentures
    adjunctive procedures with, 682
    biomechanics in, 683
    classification of, 680
    defined, 680
    diagnosis and treatment planning, 679–680
    general considerations, 681–683
    indirect retention, 684
    path of insertion, 684
    precision, 680
    selection considerations, 684–686
    semiprecision, 681
    tooth preparation, 684
  biomechanics in, 671–672, 683
    lever system, 671
    occlusion, 672
    residual ridge, 671–672
    tooth, 671
    tooth morphology, 672
  clasp types, 672–676
    circumferential, 672
    combination, 676, *677*
    embrasure, 675–676, *676*
    I-bar, 672–673, *673*
    mesial groove reciprocation (MGR), 674–675, *675*, *676*
    modified T-bar, 673–674, *674*
    reciprocal arm, 672, *673*
    rest-proximal plate-I-bar, 674, *674*
    retentive arm, 672, *673*
    ring, 675
    T- or Y-bar, 673, *674*
  esthetic considerations, 677–679
    adjunctive mechanisms to minimize metal display, 678
    rotational path removable partial dentures, 678–679, *678–681*
  flange design, 676–677
  Kennedy classification of, 669, *669*
  principles of design, 669–670
  problem situations, 672
  radiographic evaluation, 670
  replacement teeth, 677
  rest seats, 676, *677*
  retention enhancement, 676
  use of dental surveyor, 670–671
Diagnostic casts, 636
  for crowded teeth, 736
Diagnostic evaluation
  for endodontic procedures, 553–567
    bite test, 564, *564*, *565*
    cavity tests, 561, *562*
    communication in, 554
    diagnosis, 567
    fiber-optic light assessment, 554–555
    medical history, 554
    palpation, 563–564, *564*
    percussion, 561, 563, *563*
    periodontal probing, 555
    precementation radiographs, 565, *566*, 578–579, *579*
    pretreatment radiographs, 564–565, *566*
    thermal pulp testing, 555, 557–559
    visual examination, 554–555
  for fixed replacement of missing teeth, 635–639
    diagnostic casts, 636
    diagnostic waxing, 636–637
    esthetic considerations, 637
    extraoral examination, 636
    functional considerations, 637
    interdisciplinary consultants, 637, 639
    intraoral examination, 635–636, *636*
    medical and dental history, 635
    radiographs, 636
Diagnostic wax-up, 636–637
  for crowded teeth, 736, 740–744, *741–743*
Diastema, 703–730
  with advance bone loss, 729, *729*, 730
  combined therapy for, 708–710, *709*
  frenum involvement, 704–706, *704–707*
  composite resin bonding for, 711, *712*, *717*, 717–721, *718*
    adjacent teeth, *710*, 710–711, *711*
    due to small teeth, *714*, 714–716, *715*, 718–719, *719*
    full labial veneer *vs.* partial, 720
    microfilled, 720, *721*
    posterior, 712–714, *713*, *714*
    proportionality in, 714, 716
  cosmetic contouring for, 711, *712*
  diagnosis and treatment planning, 707–708
  due to foreign object between teeth, 706
  due to tongue thrust, 706, *707*
  etiology of, 703–704, *704*
  full crowns for, 723–729
    four crowns, *725*, 725–727, *726*
    one crown, *724*, 724–725, *725*
    principles in shaping, *726*, 726–727, *727*
    six crowns, 272–729, *727*, *728*
  immediate temporary closure, 712–714, *713*, *714*
  orthodontic therapy for, 708, 759–760, 764
    correction, 760, *763*
    differential diagnosis, 764, *764*, *765*
    early treatment, 759–760, *763*
    maxillary midline diagnosis chart, *764*
  orthognathic surgery for, 711, *712*
  porcelain laminates for, 720–723, *722–724*
  prosthodontic replacement, 728–729
Digit sucking, *599*, 600–601
  in children, 600–601, 620–621
  damage due to, *600*, 600–601
  intervention, 601
  self-correction, 601
Discing, for crowded teeth, *737*, 738
Discoloration of teeth, 473–495
  amalgams, using composites to mask, 491–492, *492*
  causes of, *474*
    clinical appearance and, *477*
  chromagenic foods and, 479, *479*, 491, *492*
  of class IV restorations, 493–495
  by color
    black, *474*, *475*
    brown, *474*, *475*, *485*, *486*, 555, *558*
    gray, *474*, *475*, 554–555, *557*
    green, *474*
    localized white, *485*, *487*
    orange, *474*, 491, *492*
    pink, 544, *544–556*
    yellow, *474*, *476*, 555, *558*
  of composite resin restorations, 490–491, *492*
  of crowns, 587
  extrinsic stains, 475–477

intrinsic stains, *479, 479*–*480*
in older adults, 479, *479*
of porcelain laminates, 489–490, *490*
around, 493, *494*
of primary teeth, in pediatric dentistry, 813
tetracycline staining, *488,* 488–489, *489*
treatment options, *477, see also* Bleaching
sealants, *477,* 491
toothpastes, 477–478

Eating disorders
damage due to, 608, 610, 612–613, 615
anorexia nervosa, 612, *613, 614*
bulimia, 610, 612, *612*
prevalence of, 610
Ecstasy, oral damage due to, 615
Edentulous ridge, in pontics, 657, 659
classification of, 659
Electric pulp testing, 559–561
Analytical Technology Vitality Scanner, 559–560, *560*
"mini-tip," *560, 560,* 561, *561*
Enamel fluorosis, 475
Endodontically treated fractured teeth, 536–549
anterior teeth, 537, *537*–*539,* 544, *544*
cast post, 537, *538,* 539, *539*
for anterior teeth, *544*
direct *vs.* indirect, 545–546, *547*
post preparation, 545–546, *547*
core restoration
amalgam, *541,* 541–542
composite resin, 541, *541*
material for, 541
crowns for, 537–539, *537*–*539*
preparation, 547–549, *548*–*549*
ferrule design in, *548,* 548–549, *549*
posterior teeth, 537, 539, 541–543, *542*–*543*
post restoration, 537, *539,* 539–541
cementation of post, 547
improper, 545, *545*
material for, 540–541, *541*
mode of attachment, 539
optimum post length, 539, *540*
preparation, 544–547, 549
retention of post, 539, *540*
surface configuration, 539
prefabricated post, 537, *539,* 543, *543, 548*
for anterior teeth, *544*
material for, *540,* 540–541
post preparation, 545, *546*–*547*
premolars, 547, *548*
principles for, 536–539
Endodontically treated teeth, bleaching of, 484, 585, *586*
walking bleach technique, 585–587, *586*

Endodontics and esthetic dentistry, 553–596
clinical evaluation, 553–567
bite test, 564, *564, 565*
cavity tests, 561, *562*
communication in, 554
diagnosis, 567
fiber-optic light assessment, 554–555
medical history, 554
palpation, 563–564, *564*
percussion, 561, 563, *563*
periodontal probing, 555
precementation radiographs, 565, *566,* 578–579, *579*
pretreatment radiographs, 564–565, *566*
thermal pulp testing, 555, 557–559
visual examination, 554–555
in conjunction with dentures, 682
in older adults, 867–872
procedures, 569–587
access cavity preparation, 578–580, *579, 580, see also* Cavity preparation for endodontic procedures
complications from, 573
depth of preparation, 569–571, *570, 571*
instrumentation/debridement, 583–584
pulp capping, 571–572, *572*
rubber dam, 574, 576, 578
sealing the canal system, *584,* 584–585, *585*
stressed pulp, 572–573, *573*–*575*
pulpal response to operative procedures, 567–569
surgery in, 593, *594*–*596,* 596
tissue discoloration, 596
trauma in, 587–593
crown discolorations, 587
crown fractures, *587,* 587–588, *588*
luxation and avulsion, 593, *594*
root fractures, 588–589, *590*–*592, 591, 593*
treatment planning, 553
Endo-Ice refrigerant, 555–556, *560*
Erosion, 514–515
case studies of, 514–515, *514*–*515*
defined, 501–502, 514
etiology of, 514
treatment of, 514
Etched cast bridges, in cavity preparation for endodontic procedures, 582, *583*
Extraoral examination, 636

Face, measurement of, for dentures, *835,* 835–836
Facial asymmetry, classification of, *797*
Facial esthetics, 776–777
age of patient, 776

body type considerations, 776
in pediatric dentistry, 820–827
cephalometric analysis, 821
frontal view considerations, 824–826, *825*
physical development and, 823–824, *824*
profile view considerations, *826,* 826–827, *827*
ratio, 827
soft tissue analysis, 821–823
racial characteristics, 776
symmetry and proportions, 776–777, *776*–*778*
frontal horizontal, 777, *777*
frontal vertical, *776,* 776–777
profile symmetry, 777, *778*
Facial surgery, in older adults, 862
Fiber-optic light, use in endodontic evaluations, 554–555
Flexure of the tooth, 502, *503*
Fluoride ingestion, high, tooth discoloration and, *485, 485*
Foreign objects in mouth
diastema due to, 706
oral damage due from, 615–620
fingernails, 615–616, *616*
ice chewing, 619
nut cracking, 619–620
pen/pencil chewing, 618, *622*
pins or needles, 616–617, *617*
pipe smoking, 618–619, *623*
thread biting, 617, *619*
toothpicks, 617, *619*
Fractured teeth, 525–549, *526*
composite resin bonding for, 526, *527, 528,* 530–531, *531,* 535, *535*
life expectancy of, 535
pros and cons of, 530
cosmetic contouring for, 525–526, *526, 530, 531*
crown restoration for, 526, 536, *536*
pros and cons of, 526, *530*
of crowns, *587,* 587–588, *588*
with pulp involvement, 588, *588*
without pulp involvement, *587,* 587–588
of endodontically treated teeth, 536–549, *see also* Endodontically treated fractured teeth
interdisciplinary consultants for, *532*–*534,* 532–535
porcelain laminates for, 526, *527,* 529, *529*
pros and cons of, 526, *530*
posterior teeth, 535–536, *536*
with pulpal involvement, *525,* 531–535
pulpotomy for, 531–532
reattachment of tooth fragment in, 813–814, *815*–*817,* 816
of the root, 588–589, *591, 593*
in the apical third, 589, *589*

in coronal third, 589, 591, *592*
    extrusion of the root segment, 591, *593*
    in the mid-root, 589, *590*
    Vitallium pin for, 589, *591*
    treatment options, *525*
        considerations in, 525–526, 529
    vertical, assessment of, 555, *559*
    without pulpal involvement, *525*, 530–531, *531*
Frenectomy, 704, *704*
Frenum muscle involvement
    combined therapy for, 704–706, *704–707*
    surgical removal, 704, *704*

Gastroesophageal reflux disease (GERD), loss of tooth structure and, 514, 516
Genioplasty, advanced, 797, *799*
Gingival architecture, in treatment of crowded teeth, 733–734, *735*
Gingival seal, in esthetic considerations for facial composite restorations, 494
Gingivectomy, in conjunction with dentures, 682
Glass ionomer cement, 805–806, *807*
    modified, 805–806, *807*
Gutta-percha, 542
    removal of, 544–545

Hawley appliance, 764, *764, 772, 773*
Hemifacial microsomia, surgical treatment of, 795–797
History, *see* Medical history

Ice pencil, 555, *559*
Implants, 651
    chin, 797, 800, *800*
    material used for, 800–801
    for older adults, 871–872
    as overpartial dentures, 698
    reimplant of primary teeth, in pediatric dentistry, 811, 813
Interdisciplinary consultations
    for fractured teeth, *532–534*, 532–535
    in orthodontic therapy, 769, *770*
    in replacement of missing teeth, 637, 639
    in surgical orthodontics, 775–776
Intermaxillary fixation (IMF) wires, 784
Intraoral examination, 635–636, *636*
Invisalign, computer-assisted treatment trays, 769–770, *771*

Jacoby plastic clamps, 576–577, *577*

Kennedy classification, of removable partial dentures, 669, *669*
Kerr Vitality Scanner 2006, 559–560, *560*

Laminating, *see* Porcelain laminate/veneer
Lingually locked tooth, correcting, 750

Lip biting, oral damage due to, 606, 608
    treatment of, 608
Luxation injuries
    ankylosis in, 593
    root reabsorption in, 593, *594*

Malposed teeth, correcting, 749
Matrices, for crowded teeth, 736, 740–744, *741–743*
Medical history, 635
    in endodontic evaluations, 554
    in older adults, 860
    in replacement of missing teeth, 635
Microabrasion, 485–488, *486*
    defined, 485
Misaligned teeth, correcting, 749
Mouth breathing, oral damage due to, 608

Nursing bottle syndrome, 809–811, *810, 812*
Nursing home, dentistry in the, 872–873

Occlusion
    in complete dentures, 832–833, *833–835*
        anterior, 843
        posterior, 844–845, *845*
        lingual, 833, *834*
    in removable partial dentures, 672
Older adults
    bruxism in, 865, *867*, 869, *870*
    demographics of, 853–856
        by country, 853, *853*
        life expectancy, *853*, 853–854, 872
        in nursing homes, 872
        wealth, 856, *857*
    as dental consumer, 857, 859
        examples, 854, *854–858*, 857
    dental procedures in, 862–865
        chronic illness and, *859*, 859–861
        composite resin bonding, 864–865, *864–867*
        in conjunction with facial surgery, 862
        cosmetic contouring, 863–865, *864, 866*
        medical history, 860
        oral examination, 860
        treatment planning, 860–862
        vital tooth bleaching, 862–863, *863*
    dentistry in the nursing home, 872–873
    endodontic procedures for, 867–872
    esthetic dentistry for, 873
    implants for, 871–872
    orthodontic therapy for, 865, 867, *868*
    periodontal therapy for, 867, *869*
    prosthodontic procedures for, 867–872
        crowns, 869–871, *870–871*
        porcelain laminates, 868–869, *869*
    tooth discoloration in, 479, *479*
Oral examination, in older adults, 860
Oral habits, 599–623
    bruxism, *see* Bruxism

chewing habits, 603, 605, *605*
    in children, 599–601
    concepts, 599
    detection of, 602
    digit sucking, *599*, 600–601
        in children, 600–601, 620–621
        damage due to, *600*, 600–601
        intervention, 601
        self-correction, 601
    eating disorders, 608, 610, 612–613, 615
        anorexia nervosa, 612, *613, 614*
        bulimia, 610, 612, *612*
        prevalence of, 610
    foreign objects in mouth, 615–620
        fingernails, 615–616, *616*
        ice chewing, 619
        nut cracking, 619–620
        pen/pencil chewing, 618, *622*
        pins or needles, 616–617, *617*
        pipe smoking, 618–619, *623*
        thread biting, 617, *619*
        toothpicks, 617, *619*
    habit questionnaire, 616, *618, 623*
    lip or cheek biting, 606, 608
        treatment of, 608
    mouth breathing, 608
    tongue thrusting, 605–606, *605–607*
    treatment options, 620–623
Oral surgery, *see* Surgical orthodontics
Orthodontic therapy, 753–773
    for bruxism, 510, 637, *638*
    in conjunction with dentures, 682
    for crossbite, 764–766
        anterior, 765, *767*
        posterior, 765, *766*
        severe, 766, *768, 769*
        short lower jaw, 765–766, *767*
    for crowded teeth, *737, 738*, 754–755, 757–759
        class I crowding with extractions, 758–759, *761, 762*
        expansion therapy, 754–755, *756–758*
        lower crowding with slight overbite, 755, 757–758, *759*
    for diastema, 708, 759–760, 764
        correction, 760, *763*
        differential diagnosis, 764, *764, 765*
        early treatment, 759–760, *763*
        maxillary midline diagnosis chart, *764*
    esthetic forms of, 769–770, *773*
        computer-assisted treatment trays, 769–770, *771*
        lingual appliance therapy, 770, *771*
        problems and possible solutions, *773*
        removable appliance therapy, 770, *772, 773*
    esthetics in, 753
    interdisciplinary consultation, 769, *770*
    in older adults, 865, 867, *868*
    orthodontic tooth movement, 754, *755*